Textbook of Biochemistry

As per the latest NMC Guidelines | Competency Based Medical Education (CBME) Curriculum under Graduate Medical Education Regulation

Fifth Edition

Textbook of Biochemistry

As per the latest NMC Guidelines | Competency Based Medical Education (CBME) Curriculum under Graduate Medical Education Regulation

Harbans Lal PhD, FACBI

Former Sr. Professor and Head
Department of Biochemistry
Maharaja Agrasen Medical College, Agroha (Hisar)
Former Professor, Department of Biochemistry, PGIMS
Pt. BD Sharma University of Health Sciences, Rohtak
Former Visiting Professor, Department of Biosciences
MD University, Rohtak
Former WHO Fellow and Visiting Assistant Professor
Louisiana State University Medical Centre
New Orleans (USA), and
Visiting Professor, Swami Dayanand Postgraduate Institute of
Pharmaceutical Sciences, Pt. BD Sharma University of Health Sciences, Rohtak

Ashuma Sachdeva MD

Professor
Department of Biochemistry
PGIMS, Pt. BD Sharma University of Health Sciences, Rohtak (Haryana)

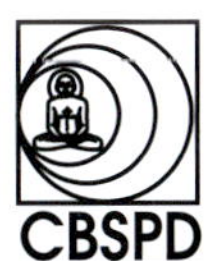

CBS Publishers & Distributors Pvt Ltd

New Delhi • Bengaluru • Chennai • Kochi • Kolkata • Lucknow • Mumbai
Hyderabad • Jharkhand • Nagpur • Patna • Pune • Uttarakhand

Disclaimer

Science and technology are constantly changing fields. New information, research and experience broaden the scope of knowledge. The authors have tried their best in giving information available to them while preparing the material for this book. Although all efforts have been made to ensure optimum accuracy of the material, yet it is quite possible some errors might have been left uncorrected. The authors, the publisher and the printer will not be held responsible for any inadvertent errors or inaccuracies.

Fifth Edition

Textbook of Biochemistry

ISBN: 978-81-979890-5-6

Fifth Edition: 2025

First Edition: 2004
Reprint: 2008, 2010
Second Edition: 2011
Reprint: 2014
Third Edition: 2017
Fourth Edition: 2021

CBS Publishers & Distributors Pvt Ltd
4819/XI Prahlad Street, 24 Ansari Road, Daryaganj, New Delhi 110 002, India.
Ph: 23289259, 23266838 Website: www.cbspd.com
e-mail: delhi@cbspd.com; cbspubs@airtelmail.in
Corporate Office: 204 FIE, Industrial Area, Patparganj, Delhi 110 092
Ph: 011-4934 4934 Fax: 011-4934 4935 e-mail: publishing@cbspd.com; publicity@cbspd.com

Branches

- **Bengaluru:** Seema House 2975, 17th Cross, K.R. Road, Banasankari 2nd Stage, Bengaluru 560 070, Karnataka, India
  Ph: +91-80-26771678/79 Fax: +91-80-26771680 e-mail: bangalore@cbspd.com
- **Chennai:** 18/8B, Subbarayan Street, Shenoy Nagar, Chennai 600 030, Tamil Nadu, India
  Ph: +91-44-42032115, 26681266 e-mail: chennai@cbspd.com
- **Kochi:** 42/1325, 1326, Power House Road, Opp KSEB, Power House, Ernakulam 682 018, Kerala, India
  Ph: +91-484-4059061-65 Fax: +91-484-4059065 e-mail: kochi@cbspd.com
- **Kolkata:** 6/B, Ground Floor, Rameswar Shaw Road, Kolkata-700 014, West Bengal, India
  Ph: +91-33-22891126, 22891127, 22891128 e-mail: kolkata@cbspd.com
- **Lucknow:** Basement, Khushnuma Complex, 7-Meerabai Marg (Behind Jawahar Bhawan), Lucknow-226 001, Uttar Pradesh, India
  Ph: +910522-4000032 e-mail: tiwari.lucknow@cbspd.com
- **Mumbai:** PWD Shed. Gala no. 25/26, Ramchandra Bhatt Marg, Next to JJ Hospital Gate no. 2, Opp. Union Bank of India, Noorbaug, Mumbai-400009, Maharashtra, India
  Ph: 022-66661880/89 e-mail: mumbai@cbspd.com

Representatives

- **Hyderabad** 0-9885175004
- **Patna** 0-9334159340
- **Jharkhand** 0-9811541605
- **Pune** 0-9664372571
- **Nagpur** 0-8692091830
- **Uttarakhand** 0-9716462459

Printed at: Gokul Offset Pvt. Ltd, Okhla Industrial Area, New Delhi

Foreword

It is a pleasure to write a brief introduction to *Textbook of Biochemistry* written by Dr Harbans Lal, Professor, Department of Biochemistry, Pt. BD Sharma Postgraduate Institute of Medical Sciences, Rohtak (Haryana).

Biochemistry deals with the chemistry of life and living processes. The scope of biochemistry is as vast as life itself. It is the most rapidly developing branch of science as it gives an understanding of the functioning of the living body at the cellular and molecular level.

The book written by Dr Harbans Lal will be warmly welcomed both by the students as well as the teachers of various medical institutions in the country, for it is written with clarity and in a simple comprehensive style.

The book is mainly based on the MBBS curriculum; however, recent advances have been covered in almost all the chapters. It gives a thorough understanding of the health and disease status in the human body.

I congratulate Dr Harbans Lal for the enormous efforts he has made in compiling this textbook which will be very useful to the medical students in particular as well as the teaching faculty of various scientific institutions of our country.

Kiranjeet Kaur MD
Professor and Head
Department of Biochemistry
and
Principal
Government Medical College
Patiala

Preface to the Fifth Edition

Welcome to the fifth edition of *Textbook of Biochemistry*. Since its inception, this textbook has aimed to serve as a comprehensive guide for the students and professionals alike in the dynamic field of biochemistry. As we present this updated edition, our goal remains steadfast: To provide a clear and concise exploration of the fundamental principles and latest advancements in biochemistry. The book has focused deeply on competency-based learning of biochemistry for medical students.

Biochemistry continues to evolve rapidly, driven by groundbreaking research and technological innovations. This edition reflects these advances, incorporating new findings and perspectives that shape our understanding of biochemical processes. From molecular interactions to cellular metabolism, from genomics to proteomics, each chapter is meticulously crafted to encompass the breadth and depth of this multifaceted discipline.

In preparing this edition, we have focused on enhancing clarity and accessibility without compromising on scientific rigor. We have updated content to reflect current research findings, expanded sections to cover emerging areas of study, and integrated new illustrations and diagrams to aid comprehension. Recommended Daily Allowances for Indians have been updated as per Indian Council of Medical Research–National Institute of Nutrition Expert Group 2020.

We hope that the textbook continues to serve as a valuable resource for the students embarking on their journey into biochemistry, as well as for professionals seeking to deepen their knowledge. We sincerely hope that it inspires curiosity, sparks inquiry, and fosters a deeper appreciation for the intricate biochemical processes that underpin life itself.

We express our sincere thanks and acknowledgements to the Director, National Institute of Nutrition (ICMR), Hyderabad, for the use of RDAs for Indians, as per recommendations of the ICMR–NIN Expert Group 2020. We are also thankful to Mr Satish Kumar Jain and the entire team from CBS Publishers & Distributors Pvt. Ltd., New Delhi, for bringing out this edition of the book in a very short time.

We would appreciate constructive suggestions for improvement in the book.

Harbans Lal
hl.biopgimsr@gmail.com

Ashuma Sachdeva
ashuma03@gmail.com

Preface to the First Edition

The appreciative response of my fellow teachers and students from various colleges throughout the country, to my previous publication, *Textbook of Biochemistry for Dental Students,* encouraged me to write this book.

Biochemistry is the chemistry of the living matter in its different phases of activity, from the smallest micro-organisms to the most complex and highly evolved human beings. The subject has made a great advances worldwide, backed by intensive research and application.

The purpose of introducing this book *Textbook of Biochemistry* is to convey a knowledge of modern biochemistry to the readers in a simple, precise and lucid manner. The text of the book has been supplemented with the self-explanatory flowcharts, diagrams and tables. Some of the important aspects of clinical relevance/application too have been highlighted in colored boxes for a better understanding of the subject. It is intended that the book will meet the requirement of the students who are to take a basic course in biochemistry, particularly those studying biochemistry in relation to medicine.

This book would never have been accomplished without the encouragement and support of my sincere friends and associates. To each one of them, I extend my most earnest thanks. I am highly indebted to Prof SK Aggarwal, MMES Medical College, Maulana (Haryana), and Dr Vijay Shanker, Associate Professor of Biochemistry, PGIMS, Rohtak, for giving their valuable suggestions. I am also grateful to Dr Rajesh Pandey, Research Associate, Department of Biochemistry, PGI, Chandigarh, for his encouragement and help. I also tender my thanks to Dr Manju Pahwa, Lecturer, and Dr Ashuma Sachdeva; Dr Anjali Singh; Dr Deepa Rao; Dr Richa; Dr Anuj; Dr Munish; Dr Parul and Dr Ekta, Residents, Department of Biochemistry, PGIMS, Rohtak, for their help in completion of the book. My appreciation also extends to Mr SK Jain and his team from CBS Publishers & Distributors, New Delhi, for bringing out this book.

Every care has been taken in preparing the text of this book, however, there could have been a few short-coming oversights. To overcome the same, I welcome comments, criticism along with useful suggestions from the students and faculty for the improvement of this book.

Nov. 2003
Rohtak (Haryana)

Harbans Lal

Contents

CHAPTER

1

Cell and Subcellular Components

Competency Achievement: **The student should be able to:**

BI1.1 Describe the molecular and functional organization of a cell and its subcellular components

PY1.1 Describe the structure and functions of a mammalian cell

MOLECULAR ORGANIZATION OF CELL

Simple precursors, or raw materials, such as CO_2, H_2O, NH_3, N_2 and NO_3^-, and their derivatives like pyruvate, citrate, succinate, 3-phosphoglycerate, etc. (commonly referred to as metabolites) are required to synthesize basic structural molecules known as building blocks. These include:

- Monosaccharides (Chapter 3),
- Fatty acids and glycerol (Chapter 4),
- Amino acids (Chapter 5), and
- Nucleotides (Chapter 7),

These building blocks, either through polymerization or other chemical means, form macromolecules such as polysaccharides, lipids, proteins and nucleic acids. Interaction among various macromolecules results in supramolecular complexes, e.g. multienzyme complexes, cytoskeleton, ribosomes, etc. An orderly assembly of such complexes forms various membrane-bound organelles or nonmembranous entities (subcellular fractions), all of which are defined within a physical boundary, to form a cell (Fig. 1.1).

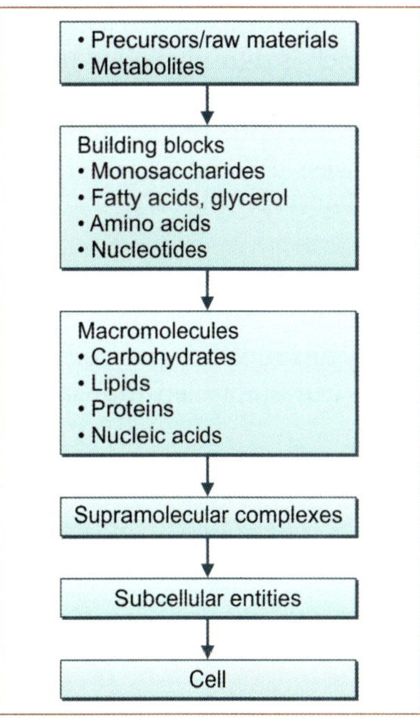

Fig. 1.1: Hierarchy of molecular organization

THE CELL

The cell is a structural and functional unit of life. All animals and plants are made up of a large number of such units, in a manner to the utilization of bricks in the construction of a building. Living cells are divided into two groups, i.e. the prokaryotic cells and the eukaryotic cells. As their name suggests (*pro* = prior to; *karyot* = nucleus; *eu* = true), the fundamental difference between them is the absence or presence of a true nucleus.

Prokaryotic Cells

The simplest form of the cell is a prokaryotic cell. Prokaryotes, e.g. bacteria, are unicellular and have one of the three basic shapes, viz. spheroidal (cocci), rod-like (bacilli) and helically-coiled (spirella).

A prokaryotic cell is small (1 to 10 nm), relatively simple in structure and has only a single membrane called cell membrane which is usually surrounded by

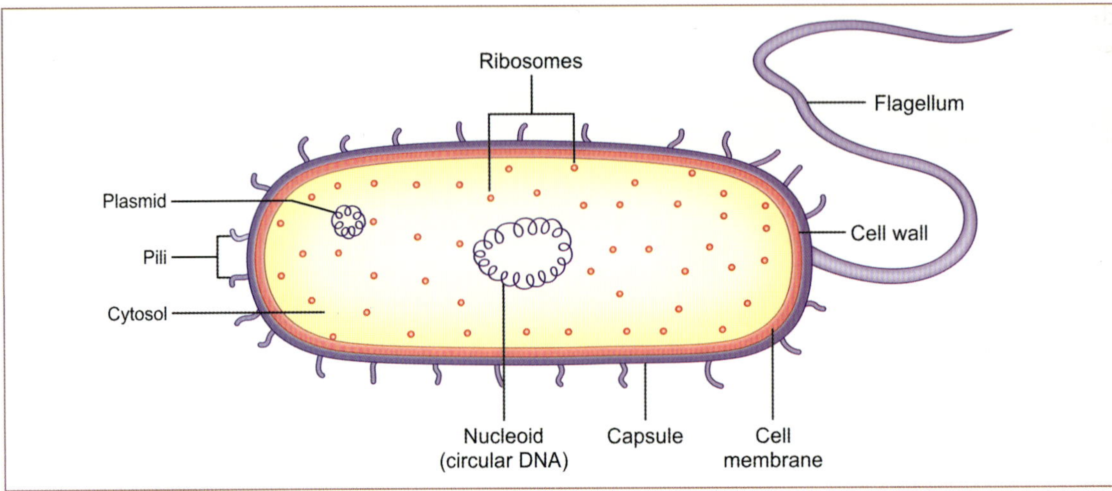

Fig. 1.2: A prokaryotic cell

a rigid cell wall of characteristic structure. There may or may not be a surrounding capsule. Besides, there is a single chromosome comprised of a molecule of double helical DNA which is densely coiled to form a nuclear zone. Reproduction is by asexual division. The best characterized prokaryotic cell is *Escherichia coli*. Some prokaryotes possess pili and flagella for adhesion and movement, respectively (Fig. 1.2).

Eukaryotic Cells

Animals, plant, fungi and protozoa are called eukaryotes which may be unicellular as well as multicellular. Eukaryotic cells are one to ten thousand times larger and are more complex in structure than the prokaryotic cells. They may vary from one tissue to another with respect to its function, e.g. the liver parenchymal cell, adipose cell, nerve cell, renal tubular cell, white blood cell, etc.

Generally, the eukaryotic cell has a well-defined membrane-bound nucleus containing several chromosomes. Their chromosomes undergo replication of DNA during mitosis and get separated into daughter chromosomes, i.e. these cells reproduce by cell division.

A typical eukaryotic cell contains various organelles such as a **nucleus, endoplasmic reticulum, Golgi apparatus, mitochondria,** etc. (Fig. 1.3).

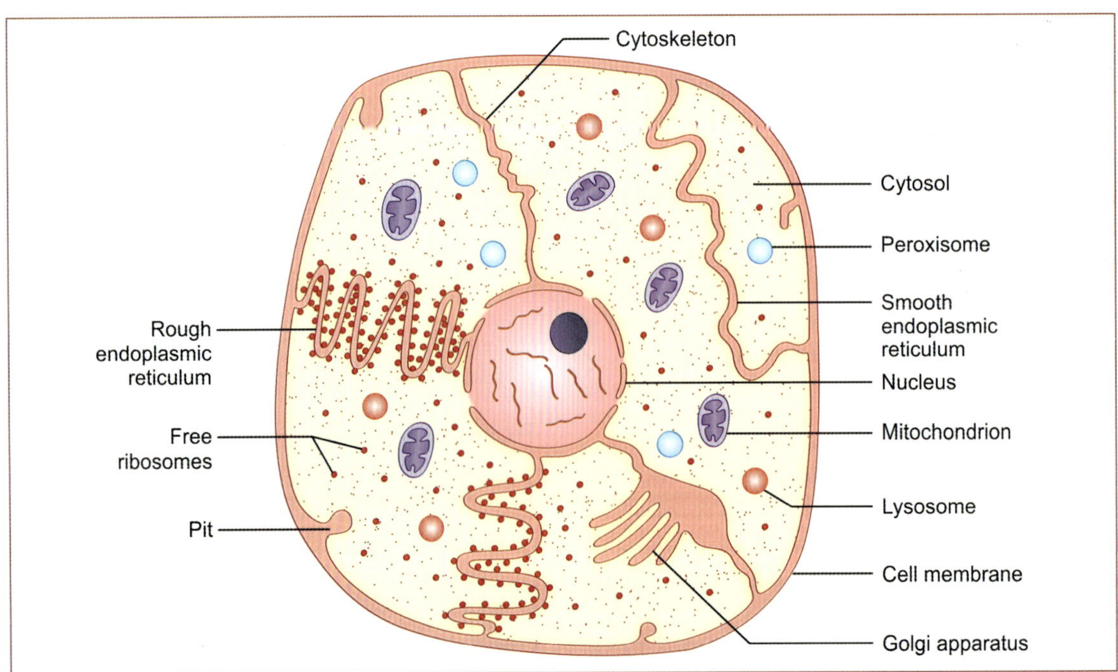

Fig. 1.3: The eukaryotic cell

Major differences between prokaryotic and eukaryotic cell structure are given in Table 1.1.

Table 1.1 Major differences between prokaryotic and eukaryotic cell structure

Parameters	Prokaryotic cells	Eukaryotic cells
Cell size	Small	Large
Overall organization	Simple	Complex
Boundary	Cell membrane and cell wall (sometimes surrounded by a capsule)	Cell membrane
Subcellular entities	Few	Many
Nucleus	Single DNA double helices in a poorly defined region called nucleoid	Well-defined nucleus with a membrane and multiple DNA double helices organized into chromatin
Reproduction	Asexual	Sexual
Examples	Bacteria, blue-green algae	Plant and animal cells

MAMMALIAN CELL AND SUBCELLULAR COMPONENTS

Mammalian cells live and grow, within their normal environment, in the body in contact with other cells and extracellular matrix. They are supplied with energy, in the form of carbohydrates and with nutritional components by the circulating blood. A subcellular component or **organelle** is defined as a subcellular membranous entity, which can be isolated by high speed centrifugation. The nonmembranous entities, such as ribosomes, cytoskeleton and cytosol, are designated as **subcellular fractions**.

Fractionation of Subcellular Components

Functions of different subcellular components can be studied after their fractionation (separation and isolation) from the cell, by various steps. These include:

1. *Preparation of tissue homogenate:* The cells are disrupted under mild conditions, e.g. the tissue may be grinded in a pestle and mortar, or is homogenized by using a **homogenizer.**
   In a homogenizer, a manually operated, or motor driven, pestle is rotated within a glass tube containing a small piece of the tissue in some suitable solution (an isotonic medium such as 0.25 M sucrose solution, adjusted to pH 7.4) between 0 and 4°C to avoid loss of biological activities. Mechanical force disrupts cells and causes liberation of the cellular components into the medium. This is called **tissue homogenate**. Besides homogenization, use of a deter-gent or osmotic shock can also disrupt plasma membrane.
2. *Differential centrifugation:* Due to the differences in their size and density, various cellular components can be separated by centrifugation at variable speeds and timings:
   i. ***Low speed centrifugation:*** The homogenate is first centrifuged at low speed (500 × g for 10 min) to separate nuclear fraction, which contains nuclei and the unruptured cells in the pellet.
   ii. ***Intermediate speed centrifugation:*** The **supernatant** is, thereafter, again centrifuged at an intermediate speed (10,000 × g for 20 min) to get mitochondrial fraction, which contains mitochondria, lysosomes and peroxisomes in the pellet.
   iii. ***High speed centrifugation (ultracentrifugation):*** High speed centrifugation (100,000 × g for 60 min) of the leftover supernatant gives the microsomal fraction. The microsomal fraction contains free ribosomes, fragments of the endoplasmic reticulum and the plasma membrane in the pellet.

   The supernatant, after separation of the microsomal fraction, is a clear solution which corresponds to the cell sap or cytosol and contains free ribosomes and soluble molecules. It is, thus, possible to isolate each subcellular component, from most of the organs and cells, in a relatively pure form, by various modifications of this general procedure, i.e. differential centrifugation (Fig. 1.4).
3. *Identification of subcellular entities:* Each entity can be assessed by the measurement of some suitable marker (an enzyme or chemical constituent of the particular fraction) either by the use of an electron microscope or by biochemical estimation. Various intracellular organelles/subcellular fractions, their functions and markers are given in Table 1.2.

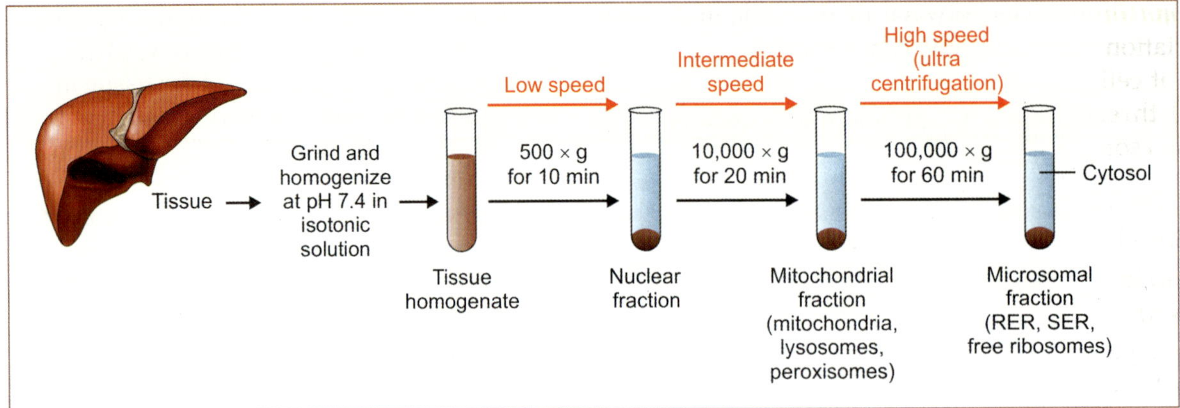

Fig. 1.4: Separation of subcellular fractions by differential centrifugation

Table 1.2: Subcellular entities, their functions and biochemical markers

Subcellular entity	Function	Biochemical marker
Cell membrane	Transport across cell membrane, bears receptor and enzymes, cell-cell recognition	Na^+/K^+-ATPase
Nucleus	DNA replication, cell division, control of RNA and protein synthesis	DNA polymerase
Endoplasmic reticulum	Protein synthesis, lipid metabolism, xenobiotic metabolism	Glucose-6-phosphatase
Golgi apparatus	Post-translational modification of proteins and their sorting	Galactosyltransferase
Mitochondria	ATP synthesis, fatty acid oxidation, Krebs cycle, cytosolic Ca^{2+} regulation	Succinate dehydrogenase, glutamate dehydrogenase
Lysosomes	Intracellular digestion and detoxification	Acid phosphatase
Peroxisomes	Fatty acid oxidation, detoxification of H_2O_2	Catalase, uric acid oxidase
Cytoplasm	Glycolysis, fatty acid synthesis, bears the cytoskeleton	Lactate dehydrogenase

Structure and Functions of Subcellular Components

The Nucleus

The nucleus is the largest component of the cell. It contains DNA, which is organized into separate chromosomes, and is surrounded by a membrane, called nuclear membrane.

Nuclear membrane, or nucleolemma, consists of two layers which are separated by an intermembrane space termed perinuclear space (cisterns). The outer membrane though is continuous with the endoplasmic reticulum but the two layers of the nuclear membrane are fused together at several places producing nuclear pores for the exchange of materials between the nucleus and the cytoplasm. The nucleus is filled with nucleo-
1 plasm which has a discrete body, called nucleolus, and a thread-like structure, called chromatin (Fig. 1.5).

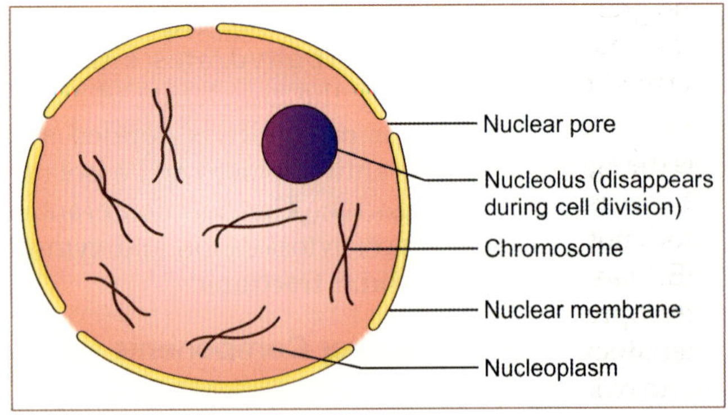

Fig. 1.5: The nucleus

Nucleolus: The number of nucleoli may vary from one cell type to another. The genes for three of the four ribosomal RNA molecules are located in the nucleolus. Nucleoli are rich in RNA and disappear during cell division.

Chromatin: It contains most of the cellular DNA in association with basic proteins termed histones. At the time of cell division, the chromatin is organized into small thread-like structures called **chromosomes**. Human somatic cell contains 23 pairs of chromosomes.

Important functions of nucleus include:

- Control of cell-division (DNA replication).
- Protein synthesis (by controlling the synthesis of RNA).

  The regulation of DNA synthesis and other functions of the nucleus are severely disturbed in some pathological conditions, such as cancer.

  DNA polymerase is a marker of the nucleus.

The Endoplasmic Reticulum

Endoplasmic reticulum is a system of membranes (lipid bilayer structures) with a network of vesicular spaces. This network is present throughout the cytoplasmic matrix and grows by its own synthesis. These membranes run parallel to each other creating channels which are called cisternae. The interior of the endoplasmic reticulum thus is well connected with perinuclear spaces and through pores on the cell surface, with the extracellular space. Cisternae have a role in the exchange of materials between the cell and the extracellular fluid.

The surface of the endoplasmic reticulum may or may not bear ribosomes. Accordingly, endoplasmic reticulum is of two types:

- *Rough endoplasmic reticulum (RER):* It is also called the granular type of endoplasmic reticulum since it has small granules attached to it. These granules are termed ribosomes.
- *Smooth endoplasmic reticulum (SER):* It is also called as the agranular type of endoplasmic reticulum since it consists of the membranous structure only and does not contain ribosomes on its outer surface. The SER has enzymes for the biosynthesis of lipids and glycoproteins. Further, SER are very important in hepatocytes where these are primarily concerned with oxidative metabolism and for the detoxification of many drugs and other toxic organic molecules.

  Glucose-6-phosphatase is a marker enzyme for the endoplasmic reticulum.

The Ribosomes

Ribosomes consist of ribonucleoprotein particles of two sizes, i.e. 50S and 30S in prokaryotes or 60S and 40S in eukaryotes. Because of their high RNA content, ribosomes are the site of protein synthesis. Ribosomes on the RER are associated with the synthesis of proteins for export from the cell. Free ribosomes, on the other hand, are present in the cytoplasm and synthesize proteins for use within the cell.

RNA is used as a marker for the ribosomes.

The Golgi Apparatus

The Golgi apparatus is a smooth membrane system with vacuoles. It is rich in lipids and is considered to be the site where secretions from other organelles are brought and assembled. The newly synthesized proteins are also transferred from RER and stored in the Golgi apparatus temporarily. Some of the synthesized proteins also undergo post-translational modifications within the Golgi apparatus and thereafter are transported to different destinations. The Golgi apparatus is thus especially active in cells which produce proteins for export. They form secretory granules for the proteins after their synthesis on the ribosomes.

Galactosyltransferase is a marker enzyme for the Golgi apparatus.

Endoplasmic reticulum with Golgi apparatus has a role in the formation of other cellular organelles, such as lysosomes and peroxisomes.

The Mitochondria

The mitochondria are the major organelle of eukaryotic cell lacking any direct structural relationship with other organelles and contain their own DNA (Fig. 1.6).

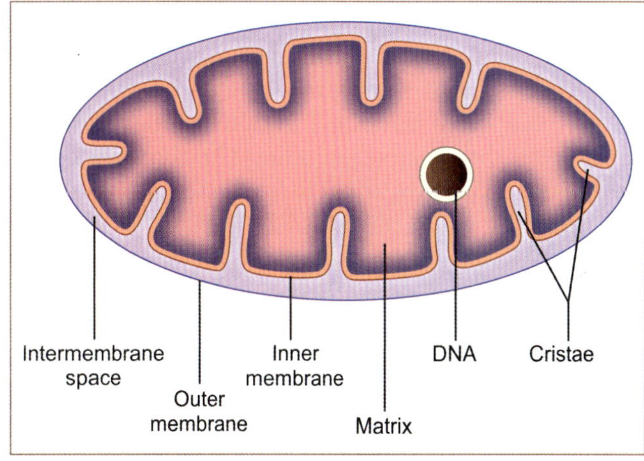

Fig. 1.6: A mitochondrion

A mitochondrion produces energy in the form of ATP for the cellular functions and is thus called a **power house** of the cell. Thus, depending upon energy requirement of the cell, mitochondria may vary in size, shape and number, from cell to cell. Besides producing energy, mitochondria also help to control the level of

1

calcium in the cytoplasm. Most of the cells contain several hundred mitochondria.

Mitochondrial membrane: It is a double-layered structure where the two layers are separated from each other by 50–100Å intermembrane space. Several enzymes especially those involved in the nucleotide metabolism are located here.

- The **outer membrane** of the mitochondria has a smooth structure. It is composed of both lipids and proteins and is freely permeable to most of the small molecules. Several enzymes involved in lipid metabolism such as the enzymes for fatty acid elongation, glycerol phosphate acyltransferase and phospholipase A are associated with the outer membrane of the mitochondria.
- The **inner membrane** of the mitochondria has a denser structure. It has more proteins than lipids. The inner membrane has extensive irregular folding called cristae. Cytochromes, the enzymes of electron transport chain and flavoproteins are localized within the inner membrane of the mitochondria.

Matrix: The intra-mitochondrial space (enclosed within the inner membrane) is called the mitochondrial matrix. This chamber contains enzymes for β-oxidation of fatty acids, for citric acid cycle and glutamate dehydrogenase. In addition, mitochondria also have DNA, referred to as mtDNA.

Succinate dehydrogenase and **glutamate dehydrogenase** are marker enzymes for mitochondria.

Mitochondrial DNA: Mitochondria are the only cellular organelles that contain their own chromosomal DNA (mtDNA), which is maternally inherited. Human mtDNA is a small double stranded circular molecule (about 16,000 base pairs), encoding 13 polypeptides that are integrated into the inner mitochondrial membrane along with other polypeptides encoded by nuclear genes. In addition, it encodes 2 rRNAs and 22 tRNAs that are used in protein synthesis within the organelle. mtDNA differs from nuclear DNA in several aspects.

Differences between nuclear DNA and mitochondrial DNA

A comparison between nuclear DNA and mtDNA is given in Table 1.3.

In contrast to nuclear DNA, the mtDNA is exposed to high levels of mutagenic free radicals and is not protected by the usual DNA repair mechanisms. This results in mutations in mtDNA that affect mitochondrial structure and function, leading to various muscular and neurological disorders. The mtDNA is more vulnerable to damage because:

- Histones (DNA binding proteins) are absent.
- Being located in the mitochondrial matrix, it is exposed to free radicals generated in the respiratory chain.
- Lack of introns.
- A few DNA repair mechanisms.

Mutations in mtDNA are responsible for several disorders associated with the process of oxidative phosphorylation, aging and degenerative diseases such as:

1. Leber's hereditary optic neuropathy.
2. Mitochondrial encephalopathy.
3. Chronic progressive external ophthalmoplegia.
4. Mitochondrial encephalopathy, lactic acidosis and stroke-like episodes (MELAS).

The Lysosomes

The lysosomes are small sac-like organelles surrounded by a membrane. These are intermediary in size between the mitochondria and the microsomes. Lysosomes are rich in all types of hydrolases, such as for

Table 1.3: Comparison between nuclear DNA and mitochondrial DNA (mtDNA)

Parameters	Nuclear DNA	mtDNA
Location	Nucleoplasm	Mitochondrial matrix
Inheritance	Both paternal and maternal	Maternal
Shape	Linear	Circular
Base pairs	3×10^9	16×10^3
Introns	Present	Absent
Histones	Present	Absent
Encoded proteins	Used within the cell as well as exported	Used within mitochondria
Repair mechanisms	Well developed	Poorly developed
Mutation rate	Low	High

1

carbohydrates, lipids, proteins and nucleic acids since digestion of these macromolecules takes place within the lysosomes. Release of lysosomal enzymes as well as absence of lysosomal enzymes is of clinical importance (Chemistry to Clinics 1.1 and 1.2).

Chemistry to Clinics 1.1: Suicide Bags

Various hydrolases are enclosed in the lysosomal membrane in such a way that they are not able to result in lysis of their own cells. However, a disruption of the lysosomal membrane leads to the release of lysosomal enzymes. This in turn causes digestion of cellular components leading to their release from the cell. This process is called autolysis. Due to this specific role of lysosomes these are also called suicide bags. Lysosomal enzymes play key roles in phagocytosis, acute and chronic inflammation such as arthritis.

Chemistry to Clinics 1.2: Lysosomal Storage Disorders

Absence of the specific lysosomal enzyme is seen in a number of genetic disorders. This in turn results in accumulation of various cellular components which cannot be digested (hydrolysed) due to inherited deficiency of the lysosomal enzyme. Lysosomes of the affected individuals become enlarged with the undigested material and thus interfere in normal cellular processes. Various such lysosomal disorders are known:

- *Lysosomal acid lipase deficiency:* It results in Wolman's disease in infants, and cholesterol ester storage disease in adults. There is accumulation of triacylglycerol and cholesterol esters in tissues, particularly in the liver.
- *Maltase deficiency:* It results in glycogen storage disease type II.
- *Alpha-L-iduronidase deficiency:* It results in Hurler's syndrome with accumulation of glycosaminoglycans.

Acid phosphatase is a marker enzyme of the lysosomes.

Age-related pigments: Any foreign particle which enters the cell is completely destroyed by the lysosomal enzymes. The lysosomes are normally active after their fusion with a vacuole. These vacuoles may contain ingested foreign particles, such as dead bacteria and result in their lysis (the process is called heterophagy). Further, in these vacuoles, the destruction of redundant/damaged cellular components such as mitochondria also occurs (the process is called autophagy). If not destroyed, indigestible material gets accumulated in the vesicles which are referred to as residual bodies that may be removed by exocytosis. The residual bodies containing a high concentration of lipids are designated as lipofuscin. Since these residual bodies accumulate in cells of the older individuals, these are also called age-related pigments.

The Peroxisomes

Certain oxidative enzymes, e.g. uric acid oxidase, D-amino acid oxidase and catalase are associated with special organelles called peroxisomes or microbodies. The major function of the peroxisomes is in hepatocytes where these are involved in the oxidation of fatty acids by a modified α-oxidation pathway. Besides, peroxisomes also represent a very primitive cellular organelle which provides protection to the cell from the toxicity of hydrogen peroxide (H_2O_2).

Catalase and **uric acid oxidase** are marker enzymes of the peroxisomes.

Absence of functional peroxisomes results in **Zellweger syndrome**, a rare autosomal recessive disease characterized by abnormalities of several organs due to the decreased levels of plasmalogens.

The Cytosol

The cytosol or cell sap is a structureless material filling the cell (aqueous matrix) in which all the cellular organelles float. It is a colloidal solution of proteins containing nearly 70% water. Besides proteins, the cytosolic fraction also contains various enzymes for glycolysis, gluconeogenesis and HMP shunt, and a variety of organic as well as inorganic substances such as glucose, potassium and magnesium.

The cytosol is in contact with all the cellular organelles and is an important vehicle for the transport of metabolites from one organelle to the other.

The cytosol of all eukaryotic cells also contains a network of fibers, collectively called the **cytoskeleton**, which includes microtubules, intermediate filaments and microfilaments.

Lactate dehydrogenase is a marker enzyme of the cytosol fraction of the cell.

The Plasma Membrane

Plasma membrane or cell membrane is the outer membrane of the cell. It is in contact with the extracellular matrix. In addition to the cell membrane, eukaryotic cells also contain internal membrane systems (nuclear membrane, mitochondrial membrane, lysosomal membrane, etc.) which form specialized compartments within the cell. Cell membrane and other membranes are collectively referred to as **biological membranes** that determine which substances are to enter or exit from the enclosed region.

Na^+, K^+-ATPase is a marker for plasma membrane.

COMPOSITION OF A BIOLOGICAL MEMBRANE

Biological membranes are composed of lipids, proteins and carbohydrates. Different membranes within the cell and between cells, however, have different composition (Fig. 1.7).

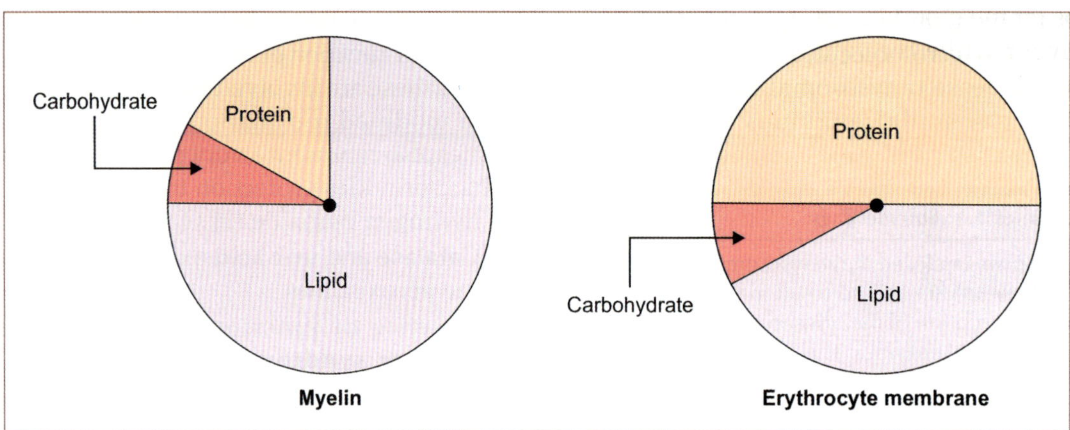

Fig. 1.7: Composition of biological membranes

Lipids

Lipids form >50% of the total membrane constituents. Membrane lipids comprise both hydrophobic as well as hydrophilic regions, and thus are termed **amphipathic** molecules. Fatty acids in lipids have a polar head group and a nonpolar tail (Fig. 1.8).

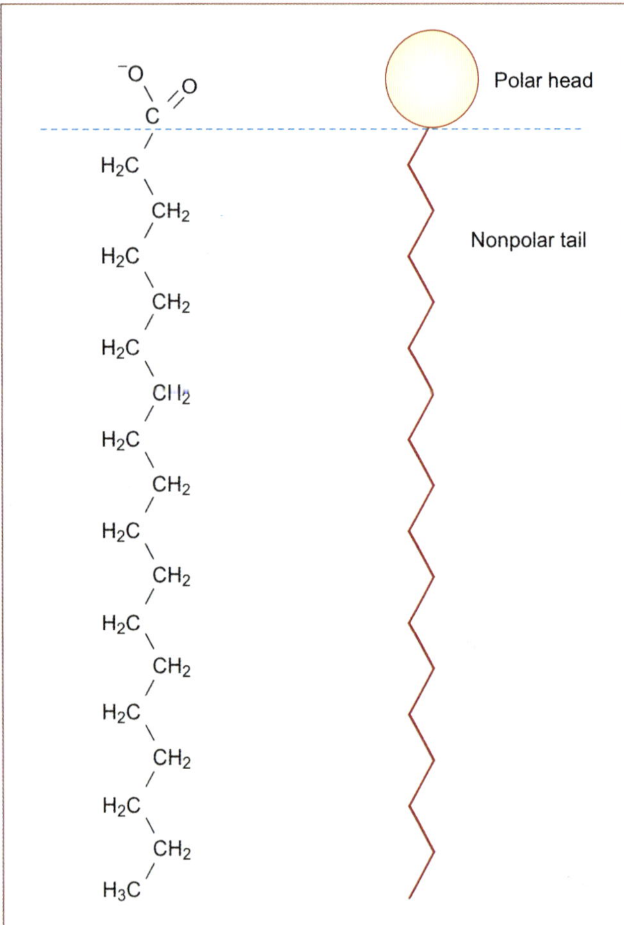

Fig. 1.8: A fatty acid

Fatty acids present in the tail are both saturated as well as unsaturated.

Phospholipids form the major proportion of the lipid component of cell membranes (Fig. 1.9).

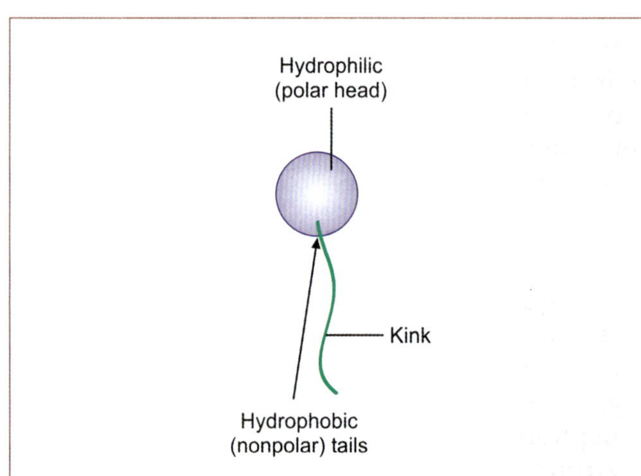

Fig. 1.9: A phospholipid

Besides, **free/unesterified cholesterol** is also present.

There are also qualitative differences between the classes of lipids and the individual lipids in different membranes within the cell as well as between the cells, e.g. plasma membrane has higher concentration of cholesterol and sphingolipids while intracellular membranes primarily contain glycerophospholipids with little sphingolipids or cholesterol.

In an aqueous solution, amphiphilic molecules form structurally ordered aggregates, such as micelles and bilayers, which form the structural basis of biological membranes.

Micelles: A micelle is a spheroidal aggregate where a large number of amphiphilic molecules, e.g. soaps and detergents, are arranged in such a way that their hydrophilic groups (at the globular surface) interact with the aqueous solvent while the hydrophobic groups are associated at the centre, i.e. away from the solvent (Fig. 1.10).

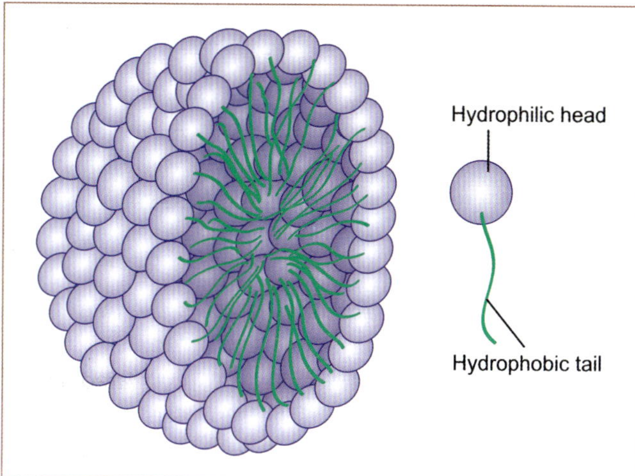

Fig. 1.10: A micelle

Micelles are formed when the cross-section of the hydrophilic head group exceeds that of the hydrophobic tails. This molecular arrangement eliminates unfavourable contact between water and hydrophobic tails of amphiphiles.

Lipid bilayers: Bilayers are formed when the cross-section of the hydrophilic head group of amphiphilic lipids equals that of the hydrophobic tails. Lipid bilayers are the key structures in biological membranes. A lipid bilayer exists as a sheet, i.e. an expanded planer-aggregate, in which hydrophobic regions of phospholipids are protected from the aqueous environment while the hydrophilic regions are immersed in water (Fig. 1.11).

These are extremely stable structures which are held together by noncovalent interactions of the hydrocarbon chains and ionic interactions of the charged head groups with water. Lipophilic molecules such as cholesterol intercalate between fatty acyl residues of phospholipids and have minimal contact with the aqueous phase.

Liposomes are a special type of vesicles surrounded by lipid bilayer and are of clinical significance (Chemistry to Clinics 1.3).

Chemistry to Clinics 1.3: Liposomes

A lipid bilayer when closes on itself and forms a spherical vesicle which separates the external environment from the internal compartment is called a liposome.

Preparation: A variety of techniques have been devised for the synthesis of liposomes in a laboratory. These can be prepared by using synthetic phospholipids or lipids extracted from natural membranes suspended in an aqueous solvent and subjected to very high frequency ultrasonic waves.

Types: Depending on the preparation technique employed, liposomes may either be bound by a single lipid bilayer (**unilamellar liposomes**) or may consist of more than one concentric lipid layers alternating with aqueous layers (**multilamellar liposomes**; Fig. 1.12).

Properties

1. Closed, self-sealing, solvent-filled vesicles formed from a suspension of phospholipids (glycerophospholipids or sphingomyelins) with or without cholesterol.
2. Usually have a diameter of 20–200 nm, and in a given preparation, are uniform in size.
3. Nontoxic.
4. Biodegradable.

Significance

1. The outer structures of liposomes are similar to a biological membrane. Thus, liposomes serve as models of biological membranes.

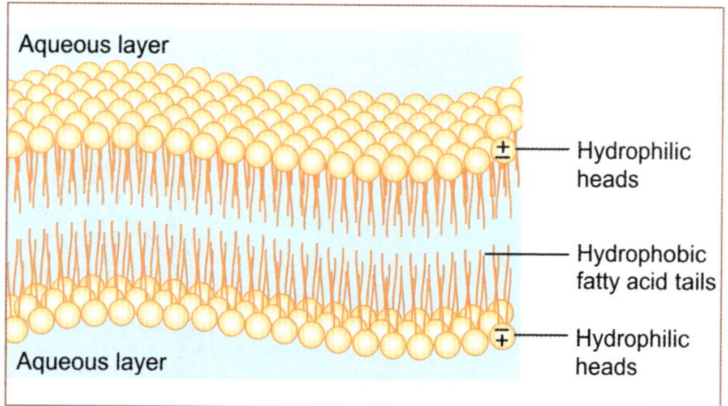

Fig. 1.11: A lipid bilayer

1

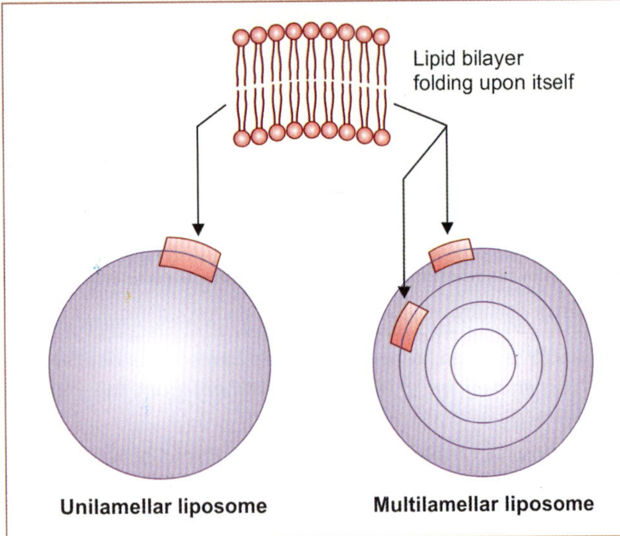

Fig. 1.12: Liposomes

2. When administered intravenously, liposomes are absorbed by many cells through fusion with the plasma membrane. This has a profound clinical application because the technique can be used to deliver those compounds to a patient which cannot be absorbed when administered orally. Thus, they are used as vehicles for drug delivery, e.g. liposomal. Amphotericin B is commercially available for the treatment of systemic fungal infections in immunocompromised patients. Liposomes have also been prepared with enzymes and DNA.
3. A major problem associated with liposomes is their nonspecific uptake by the reticuloendothelial system following intravenous administration. This can be circumvented by a two-fold strategy: Firstly, by coating them with specific ligands so that they are targeted to the tissue bearing the cognate receptors, and secondly, by incorporating polyethylene glycol in the bilayer which avoids uptake by the reticuloendothelial system. Such liposomes act as 'homing devices' for the encapsulated molecules including drug(s). It also minimizes the side effects of the drug(s).

Proteins

Proteins form another major portion of the membrane and play several roles such as the structural components, transport systems, enzymes and recognition sites for hormones. Protein concentration varies from about 20% in the myelin sheath to about 80% in the inner membrane of the mitochondria.

Membrane proteins are classified by their mode of interaction with the membrane, as integral membrane proteins, peripheral membrane proteins and lipid-linked proteins (Fig. 1.13).

Integral membrane proteins: These proteins have the following characteristics:

- Span the cell membrane from one side to the other.
- Also called **transmembrane proteins** or **intrinsic proteins**.

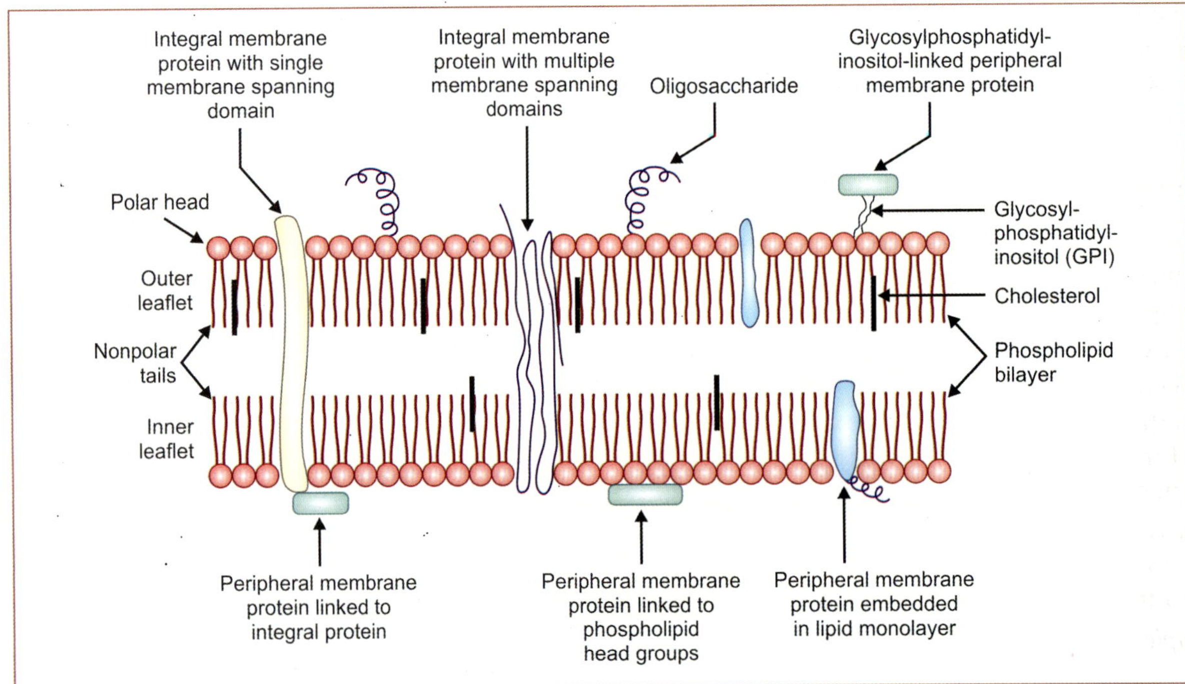

Fig. 1.13: Fluid-mosaic model of biological membrane

- Amphiphilic molecules tightly bound to the membrane by hydrophobic interactions.
- Some proteins contain α-helical structure consisting primarily of hydrophobic amino acids. This, in turn, forms a transmembrane sequence which has three domains, i.e. a sequence exterior to the cell containing the $-NH_2$ terminal end, a transmembrane sequence and a sequence extending into the cell with the –COOH terminal end.
- Can be separated from the membrane only by drastic treatment with certain agents that disrupt membranes, such as organic solvents or detergents.
- *Example:* **Glycophorin A**, which spans the erythrocyte membrane.

Peripheral membrane proteins: These proteins have the following characteristics:

- Proteins which are embedded on any one side of the membrane.
- Also called **extrinsic proteins**.
- Immersed in the membrane only partially and are weakly bound to the hydrophilic region of the specific integral proteins.
- May have various modes of attachment: Some bind to integral proteins, such as an antigen. On the other hand, some peripheral proteins such as cytochrome b5, have sequences of hydrophobic amino acids at one end of the peptide chain which serve as an anchor in the membrane lipid.
- Can be released by relatively mild procedures that leave the membrane intact, such as by treatment with a salt solution of high ionic strength or by extremes of pH.
- *Example:* **Cytochrome** ***c***, in the outer surface of the inner mitochondrial membrane.

Lipid-linked proteins: These proteins have the following characteristics:

- Membrane-associated proteins containing covalently attached lipids.
- Lipids anchor proteins to the membrane and thus mediate protein–protein interaction or modify structure and activity of the protein to which these are attached.
- Removal of the lipid fraction from these proteolipids leads to denaturation of the membrane proteins and loss of their biological functions.
- *Example:* **Lipophilin** presents in the myelin.

Carbohydrates

Some of the membrane proteins and lipids bear short chains of carbohydrates (oligosaccharides), covalently attached either to a protein **(glycoprotein)** or to a lipid **(glycolipid)**. Carbohydrate content of biological membranes varies between 3 and 10%. Oligosaccharide chains are normally located on the outer surface of the membrane or on the terminal side of the endoplasmic reticulum.

STRUCTURE OF A BIOLOGICAL MEMBRANE

As described above, the **lipid bilayer** forms the structural basis of a biological membrane. Some proteins span the lipid bilayer, whereas others are only immersed partially. This is called the **fluid-mosaic model** because the membrane is **fluid** in consistency, consisting of a **mosaic** of proteins and lipids which are **free to drift** about in the plane of the membrane (Fig. 1.13).

The fluid-mosaic model of a biological membrane has following characteristics:

- Sheet-like structure forming a closed boundary; thickness ≈ 7–10 nm.
- Noncovalent, asymmetric assemblies of amphiphilic lipids and proteins.
- Electrically polarized (inside negative with respect to outside).
- Membrane fluidity is regulated by:
    i. The presence of unsaturated fatty acids. Since *cis*-double bonds cause fatty acyl chains to bend (i.e. form kink), the membrane thus becomes less tightly packed and therefore is more fluid in nature (Figs 1.9 and 1.13).
    ii. *The degree of unsaturation of fatty acids:* Higher the unsaturation more is the fluidity.
    iii. Ca^{2+} (increased Ca^{2+} decreases membrane fluidity).
    iv. Cholesterol content of biomembranes.

At high temperature, cholesterol prevents lateral movement of phospholipid hydrocarbon tails thereby preventing an abnormal rise in membrane fluidity. At low temperature, it prevents the close packaging of the same hydrocarbon tails thereby preventing an abnormal fall in membrane fluidity. Hence, it is aptly said that **cholesterol 'modulates' membrane fluidity**. Abnormally high membrane cholesterol is observed in **spur cells** (Fig. 1.14).

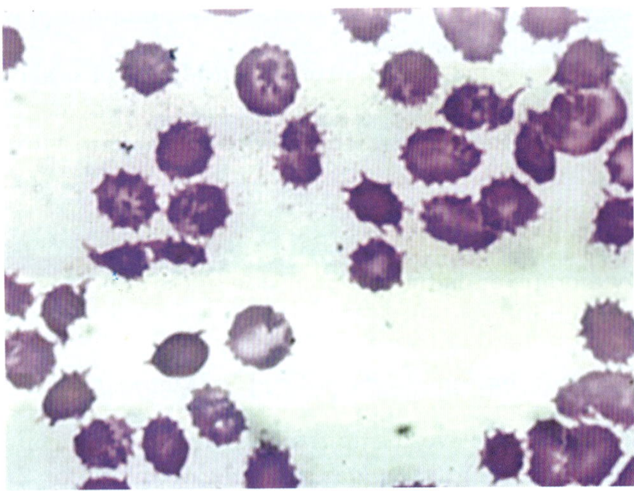

Fig. 1.14: Spur cells or acanthocytes: Red blood cells with multiple irregularly distributed, thorn-like spicules often with drumstick ends, projecting from the cell membrane. These biomembranes have an abnormally high cholesterol content derived from cholesterol-rich plasma lipoproteins

FUNCTIONS OF A BIOLOGICAL MEMBRANE

1. ***Compartmentalization:*** It separates two different microenvironments, e.g. the cell membrane separates the intracellular compartment from the extracellular matrix or extracellular fluid.
2. ***Cell shape:*** Plasma membrane proteins have a structural role, i.e. maintain shape of the cell and define its boundaries.
3. ***Cell movement:*** Specific arrangement of plasma membrane proteins is critical in controlling the movements of some cells, e.g. movement of neutrophils from the intravascular to the extravascular compartment requires a change in cell shape as well as movement, known as diapedesis.
4. ***Enzymes:*** Many of the membrane proteins are enzymes and are located either within or on the cell membrane. The inner mitochondrial membrane is essential for localization and correct orientation of the respiratory enzymes within it for their maximum efficiency. The membrane of the endoplasmic reticulum plays an important role in localizing lipophilic substrates for their oxidation by the enzymes present therein.
5. ***Receptor molecules:*** Membrane proteins act as recognition sites, such as hormone receptors for insulin or glucagon or immunoreceptors present on B lymphocytes for the recognition and response to foreign antigens, etc.
6. ***Signal transduction:*** Various membrane proteins help in the transmission of signals, such as transmission of nerve impulses.
7. ***Translocation of substances:*** Membrane proteins regulate translocation of molecules, such as amino acids, glucose and various ions.

MEMBRANE TRANSLOCATION

'Translocation' versus 'transport': As a general rule, the term 'translocation' should be used to describe any type of transmembrane movement irrespective of the size of the substance to be moved. Further, it may or may not require a 'helper', located in the membrane itself. However, when such a helper or 'transporter' is required, the process should be called 'transport'.

MEMBRANE TRANSLOCATION SYSTEMS

The translocation may or may not require the formation of a membrane-bound vesicle; accordingly, the translocation may be **vesicular or nonvesicular** (Fig. 1.15).

Functional Mechanisms of Translocation

Translocation of a substance across the cell membrane can be described, in a functional sense, according to the number of molecules transported and the direction of their movement (Fig. 1.16):

Uniport: The process which allows the movement of one type of molecules in only one direction, e.g. glucose uptake in erythrocytes.

Cotransport: The process where transfer of one solute depends upon the simultaneous or sequential transfer of the other. It includes:

- ***Symport:*** Two types of molecules when move in the same direction, it is called symport, e.g. the Na^+ glucose transporter 1 (SGLT1) or the Na^+ amino acid transporter in the cells lining the small intestine and proximal renal tubules.
- ***Antiport:*** Two types of molecules when move in the opposite direction, it is called antiport, e.g. the $Na^+ = K^+$ antiport, the $Na^+ = Ca^{2+}$ transporter and the $Cl^- = HCO_3^-$ antiport.

NONVESICULAR TRANSLOCATION SYSTEMS

These are of two types, i.e. the nonmediated translocation system and the mediated translocation system (Fig. 1.15).

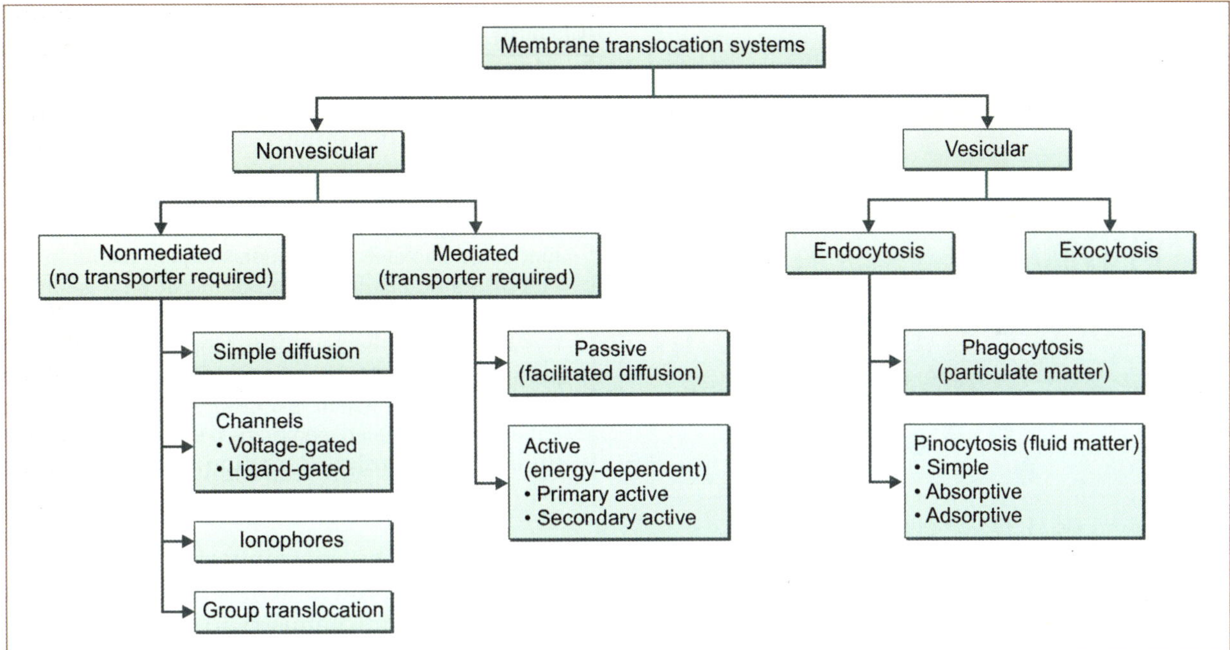

Fig. 1.15: Membrane translocation systems

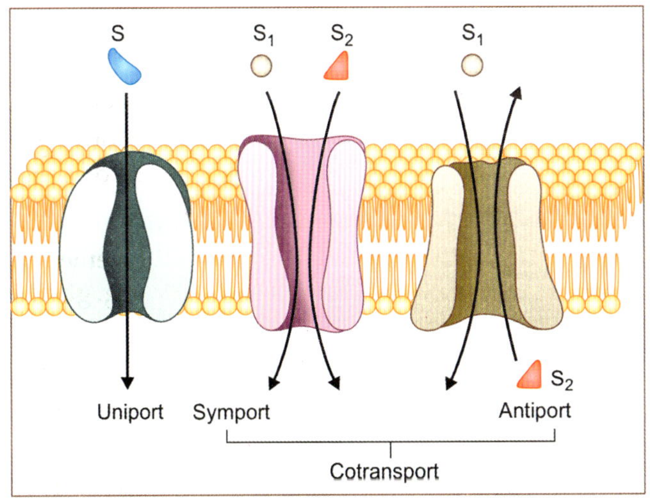

Fig. 1.16: Transport of substances with respect to the number of molecules and the direction of movement

NONMEDIATED TRANSLOCATION

- Some solutes (O_2, N_2, CO_2, NO, urea, etc.) move across the cell membrane by diffusing down an electrochemical gradient and do not require metabolic energy. This, passive nonmediated translocation is called **simple diffusion**.
- It is limited by the thermal agitation of the specific molecule, by the concentration gradient across the membrane, and by its solubility in the hydrophobic core of the membrane bilayer. Electrolytes, since are poorly soluble in lipids, acquire a shell of water by electrostatic interaction. The size of the shell is directly proportional to the charge density of the electrolytes. For example, electrolytes with a large charge density have a larger shell of hydration and thus a slower diffusion rate.
- The direction of flow is always **from a higher to a lower concentration** and the net movement of a molecule from one side to the other continues until concentration on each side is at chemical equilibrium.
- Diffusion of a substance may also occur through membrane channels or pores.

Channels

- Pore-like structures **formed by integral membrane proteins**.
- Permit rapid movement of specific ions or molecules from one side of membrane to the other (Fig. 1.17).
- The permeability of a channel depends upon the size, the extent of hydration, and the charge density on the ion.
- Specific channels exist for Na^+, K^+, Ca^{2+}, Cl^-, etc. These channels are **very selective** and permit the passage of only one type of ions.
- Channels are opened transiently, i.e. they are gated. The channel opening and closing involves a change in the voltage/membrane potential (**voltage-gated channel**) or the binding of a chemical agent (**ligand-gated channel**; Table 1.4).

1

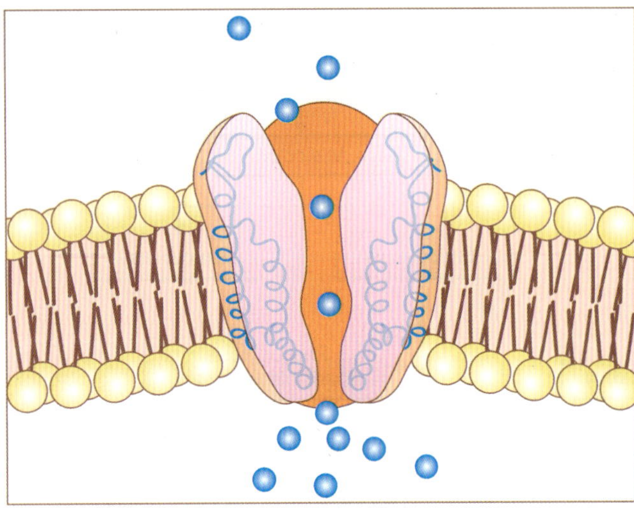

Fig. 1.17: Ion channel

Table 1.4: Types of ion channels

Cannel	Responsive factor
Voltage-gated	Change in membrane potential, e.g. Na^+, K^+ and Ca^{2+} channels in the heart
Ligand-gated	• A specific extracellular molecule, such as acetylcholine.for the acetylcholine receptor channel of the neuromuscular junction. • A specific intracellular molecule, e.g. cAMP for Ca^{2+} channels in myocytes.

- Sometimes, one ion can regulate the activity of the other ion, e.g. a decrease in Ca^{2+} ion concentration in the extracellular fluid increases membrane permeability and diffusion of Na^+. This, in turn, depolarizes the membrane and triggers nerve discharge.
- A number of pharmacologic agents that modulate these channels are used therapeutically.
- Mutations in genes encoding polypeptide constituents of ion channel may lead to certain diseases termed **channelopathies**, e.g. myasthenia gravis and cystic fibrosis (Chemistry to Clinics 1.4).

Movement of water across biological membranes—aquaporins: Water can move rapidly in and out of cells, but the partition coefficient of water into lipids is low; therefore, the permeability of the membrane lipid bilayer for water is also low. Specific membrane proteins that function as water channels explain the rapid movement of water across the plasma membrane. These water channels are small nearly 30 kDa, integral membrane proteins known as **aquaporins** (**AQP**). Many different forms have been discovered so far; at least six forms are expressed in cells in the kidneys and seven forms in the gastrointestinal tract, tissues in which water movement across plasma membranes is particularly rapid (Chemistry to Clinics 1.5).

Chemisty to Clinics 1.4: Channelopathies

1. *Myasthenia gravis:* It is an acquired autoimmune disease characterized by muscle weakness due to decreased neuromuscular signal transmission. Autoantibodies against acetylcholine receptors accelerate their turnover and reduce their number. Acetylcholinesterase inhibitor drugs are given to enhance the stay of acetylcholine at the neuromuscular junction. Ultimately, the patients require the removal of the culprit antibodies from the plasma at regular intervals, a process called 'plasmapheresis'.
2. *Cystic fibrosis:* It though is a multiorgan disease but its gene product is a cystic fibrosis transmembrane conductance regulator (CFTR), which is a cAMP-dependent Cl^- channel. Patients have reduced membrane permeability which impairs fluid and electrolyte secretion and leads to luminal dehydration.

Chemistry to Clinics 1.5: Nephrogenic Diabetes Insipidus

Nephrogenic diabetes insipidus is renamed as arginine vasopressin resistance (AVP-R) and is, primarily, due to pathology of the kidney. This is in contrast to central or neurogenic diabetes insipidus, which is caused by insufficient levels of vasopressin (also called antidiuretic hormone, ADH). Nephrogenic diabetes insipidus caused by an improper response of the kidney to vasopressin, leading to a decrease in the ability of the kidney to concentrate the urine by removing free water. Rarely, a mutation in the "aquaporin 2" gene impede the normal functionality of the kidney water channel, which results in the kidney being unable to reabsorb water. This mutation is often inherited in an autosomal recessive manner.

Ionophores

Besides channels, the other transmembrane route for the nonmediated translocation is through ionophores, whose features include:

- These are small organic molecules such as antibiotics which are synthesized by some bacteria and function as shuttles.
- Ionophores **increase permeability of the membrane to a particular ion** by binding the ion, diffusing it through the membrane and releasing it on the other side. To ensure the net transport, uncomplexed ionophores return to the original side of the membrane and are ready to repeat the process.
- Because of their ability to complex specific ions and facilitate their transport, ionophores contain hydrophilic centres for ion-binding and are surrounded by peripheral hydrophobic regions. This

allows the molecules to dissolve effectively in the membrane and diffuse through it. The net diffusion of a substance thus depends upon:

1. Its concentration gradient across the membrane.
2. The electric potential across the membrane.
3. The permeability coefficient of the substance for the membrane.
4. The hydrostatic pressure gradient across the membrane, and
5. Temperature.

- Each ionophore, e.g. valinomycin or nigericin has definite ion specificity. **Valinomycin** translocates K^+ by an electronegative import mechanism. **Nigericin** is an electrically neutral antiporter which translocates K^+ in exchange for H^+ across the membrane.

Group Translocation

Principle: Group translocation involves chemical modification of the transported substrate. The **γ-glutamyl cycle (Meister cycle)** transports **amino acids** across the plasma membrane. During the translocation, the substrate (amino acid) undergoes alteration and is released into the cell as a different molecule.

Mechanism: The pathway involves the membrane-bound enzyme γ-glutamyl transpeptidase (γ-GT). The amino acid transported is the substrate to which the γ-glutamyl residue of glutathione (GSH), a tripeptide, is transferred. This leads to the formation of a dipeptide containing γ-glutamyl residue of GSH with the transported amino acid. The dipeptide, γ-glutamyl amino acid, is transported into the cell and the complex is then hydrolyzed by a separate cytosolic enzyme to liberate the free amino acid. Glutamate is released as 5-oxoproline while cysteinylglycine is cleaved to its component amino acids (Fig. 1.18).

Salient Features

- Group translocation is especially active in renal epithelial cells, liver and enterocytes.
- All amino acids except proline can be transported by group translocation.
- Rapid process.
- High capacity.
- ***Energetically expensive:*** The energy for the transport comes from the hydrolysis of a peptide bond in GSH. For the system to continue, GSH must be resynthesized which requires 3 molecules of ATP. Hence, for each amino acid translocated across the membrane, 3 ATPs are used.

CARRIER-MEDIATED TRANSPORT

Molecules that cannot freely diffuse through the membrane by themselves, need to be transported in association with specific carrier molecules/transport proteins.

Salient Features of a Transport Protein

- Carrier molecules (variously designated as carriers, permeases, porters, **translocases or transporters**), behave much like enzymes.
- Have a high degree of **structural stereospecificity** for the substances to be transported.
- Demonstrate **saturation kinetics**, i.e. when binding sites on all the transport proteins are occupied, the system is saturated and the rate of transport reaches a plateau.

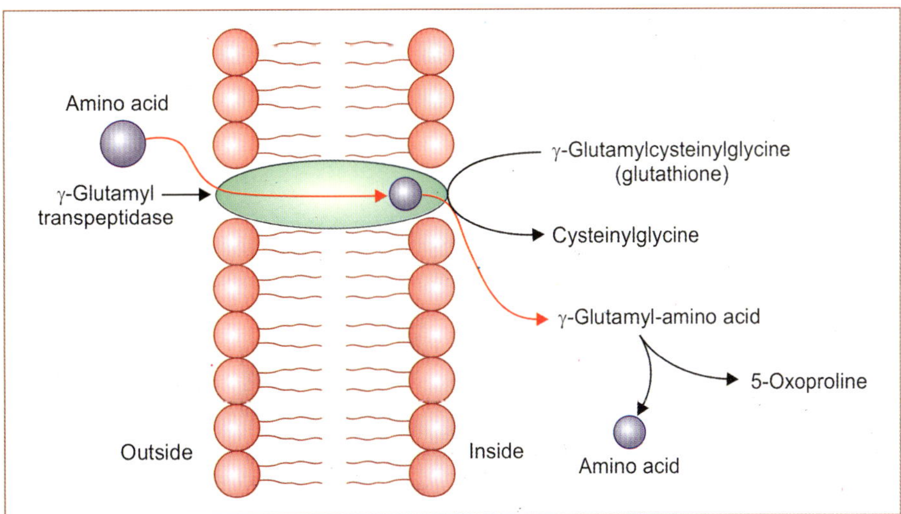

Fig. 1.18: Group translocation (γ-glutamyl cycle)

1

- Can be **inhibited** by both competitive and non-competitive inhibitors. The inhibition can prevent transport by blocking the binding sites or by interacting with the transport protein and altering its conformation so that it becomes non-functional.
- All cell membranes contain highly specific transporters for the movement of ions (Na^+, K^+, Cl^-, HCO_3^-, etc.) as well as organic compounds (such as amino acids and sugars).
- The transport of a solute molecule mediated by a transport protein has four aspects, explained by a **'ping-pong' mechanism** (Fig. 1.19):
  1. ***Recognition:*** Transport proteins have receptor sites to which the solute attaches. The transporter thus recognizes an appropriate solute from the aqueous environment for its translocation across the membrane.
  2. ***Translocation:*** After binding of the solute with the transporter protein, there occurs a conformational change in the transporter protein which translocates (moves) the solute molecule to the opposite side of the membrane.
  3. ***Release:*** A change in the conformation of the transporter protein decreases affinity of the solute and release it to the new environment.
  4. ***Recovery:*** After release of the solute, the transport protein reverts to its original conformation to accept another solute molecule, i.e. the transporter is recovered in its original conformation.
- Carrier-mediated transport includes (Fig. 1.15):
  1. **Passive transport** (passive mediated transport) or **facilitated diffusion**.
  2. **Active transport**.

Polarized epithelial cell: Before discussing the details of carrier-mediated transport, it is useful to understand the concept of polarized epithelial cells lining the **small intestine** and the **renal tubules** (Fig. 1.20).

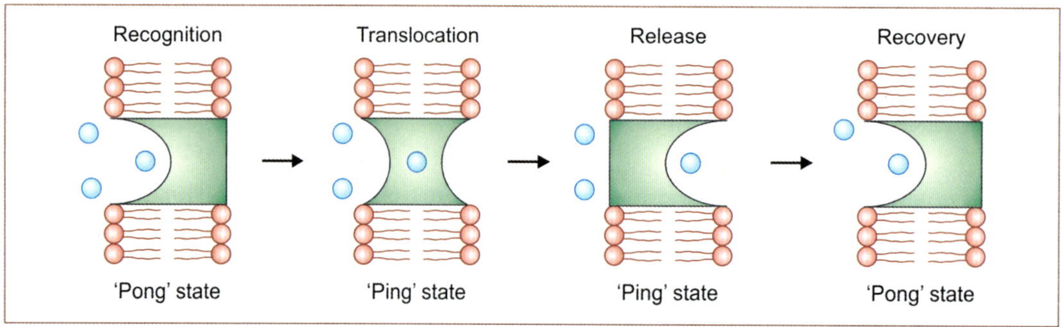

Fig. 1.19: 'Ping-pong' model for mediated membrane translocation

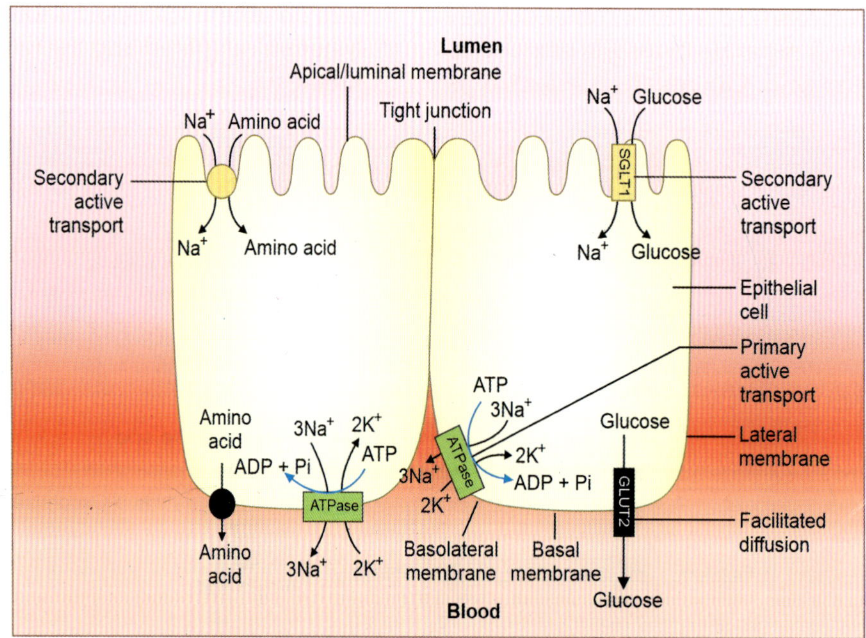

Fig. 1.20: Transport of glucose in epithelial cell

Epithelial cells occur in layers or sheets that allow the directional movement of solutes not only across the plasma membrane but also from one side of the cell layer to the other. Such regulated movement is achieved because the plasma membranes of epithelial cells have **two distinct regions** with different morphologies and different transport systems. These regions are the **apical membrane** facing the lumen, and the **basolateral membrane** facing the blood supply. The polarized organization of the cells is maintained by the presence of **tight junctions** at the areas of contact between adjacent cells. Tight junctions prevent proteins on the apical membrane from migrating to the basolateral membrane and vice versa. Thus, the entry and exit steps for solutes can be localized to opposite sides of the cell. This is the key to transcellular transport across epithelial cells.

PASSIVE MEDIATED TRANSPORT/ FACILITATED DIFFUSION

- Passive mediated transport, also referred to as facilitated diffusion, leads to the translocation of solutes through membrane transport proteins **without the expenditure of metabolic energy**.
- The process can operate either unidirectionally or bidirectionally and the net flux across the membrane occur down a concentration gradient, i.e. the molecules flow from a higher to the lower concentration.
- 'Ping-pong' mechanism explains facilitated diffusion of molecules across the biological membrane with the help of a transport protein which exists in two principal conformations (Fig. 1.19).
- Several hormones (such as insulin, glucocorticoids, growth hormone, etc.) regulate facilitated diffusion by changing the number of transport proteins available.
- Examples of the transport proteins which mediate facilitated diffusion include:
  1. ***Glucose transporters (GLUT):*** A group of transport proteins present in the plasma membrane of mammalian cells for the transport of D-glucose, e.g. GLUT1, GLUT2, etc. These are referred to as glucose permeases. They translocate several D-sugars by a uniport mechanism.
  2. ***Cl^-/HCO_3^- exchanger:*** It is an anion exchanger protein for the antiport movement of Cl^- and HCO^{3-} in RBC membrane.
  3. ***ATP-ADP translocase:*** An antiport for the exchange of anions (ADP^{3-} and ATP^{4-}) between the cytosol and the mitochondrial matrix, located in the inner mitochondrial membrane.

ACTIVE TRANSPORT

In active transport, the transport protein moves a specific molecule against the concentration gradient, i.e. from a lower concentration to the higher concentration. It is a process that requires energy which, in most cases, is coupled to the hydrolysis of ATP (Fig. 1.21).

The active transport can be grouped as:

- **Primary active transport,** and
- **Secondary active transport.**

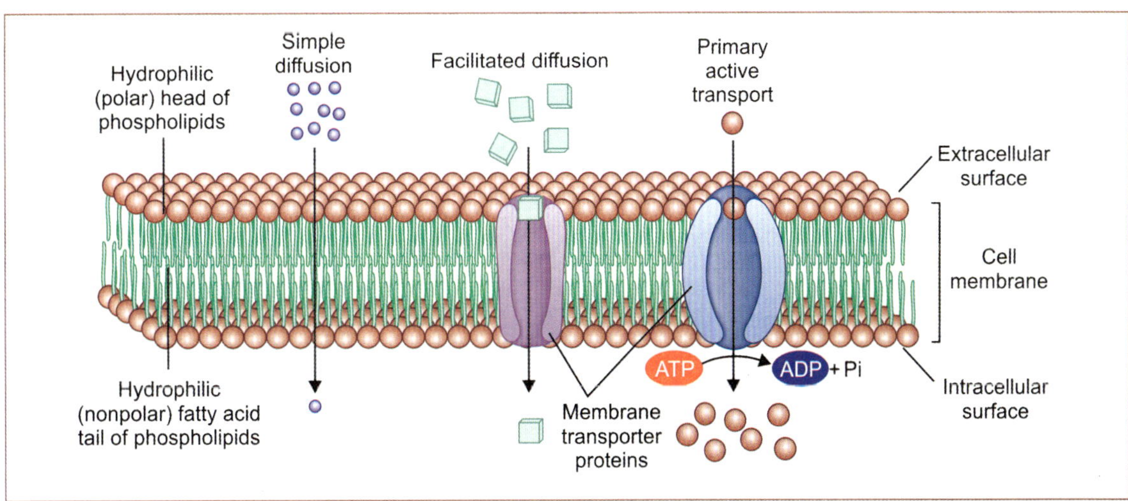

Fig. 1.21: Transport systems

Primary Active Transport

This transport system has the same characteristics as the passive transport system but it is an **endergonic process**. Examples of such transporters include membrane-bound ATPases that translocate cations. They are further classified as:

- ***P type transporters:*** The transporter protein is phosphorylated and dephosphorylated during the transport activity.
- ***V type transporters:*** These are present in the membrane of the lysosomes, the Golgi vesicles and the secretory vesicles. These are responsible for acidification of the interior of these vesicles.
- ***F type transporters:*** These are present in mitochondria and are involved in ATP synthesis.

Some of the Primary Active Transport Systems

Primary active transport systems are important in the maintenance of electrochemical gradient in biological systems and consume nearly one-third of the total energy expenditure of a cell. Examples of primary active transport system include Na^+/K^+-ATPase, Ca^{2+}-ATPase, H^+/K^+-ATPase and neurotransmitter transporters:

1. **Na^+/K^+-ATPase:** The Na^+/K^+-ATPase (Na^+-K^+ pump) is an antiport that moves three Na^+ ions out of the cell in exchange of two K^+ ions into the cell, with the concomitant hydrolysis of intracellular ATP (Fig. 1.22).

   The pump is an integral part of the membrane and has binding sites for both ATP and Na^+ on the cytoplasmic side of the membrane, and K^+ binding site on the extracellular side of the membrane. Drugs that inhibit the Na^+=K^+ pump are of clinical importance (Chemistry to Clinics 1.6).

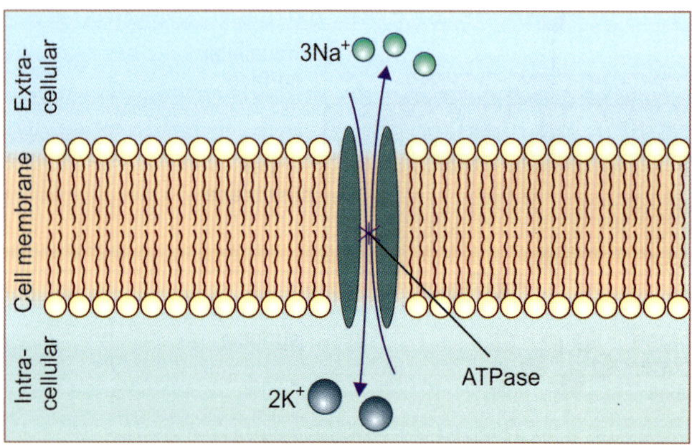

Fig. 1.22: Na^+-K^+ pump

Chemistry to Clinics 1.6: Heart Failure

The cell membrane of cardiomyocytes (cells of the myocardium) contain many transport pumps. Two of them are, Na^+/K^+-ATPase and Na^+/Ca^{2+} exchanger. The Na^+/K^+-ATPase serves its usual function of maintaining low intracellular Na^+ concentrations. The Na^+/Ca^{2+} exchanger relies on this Na^+ gradient to extrude Ca^{2+} out of the cells. Cardiac glycosides (digitalis) such as digoxin and ouabain abolish this gradient by inhibiting the Na^+/K^+-ATPase. High intracellular Na^+ concentration slows the extrusion of Ca^{2+} by the Na^+/Ca^{2+} exchanger. Increased availability of Ca^{2+} results in increased force of contraction that is clinically useful in the management of cardiac failure (Fig. 1.23).

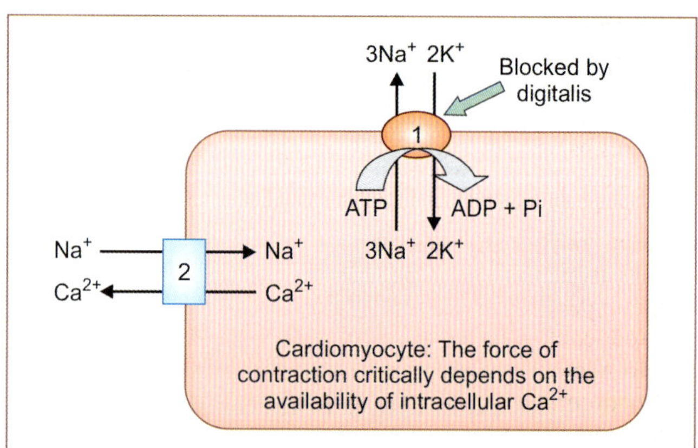

Fig. 1.23: Role of digitalis in heart failure: Normally, the Na^+-K^+-ATPase in the cardiomyocyte membrane moves Na^+ out of the cell in exchange for K^+ (1). The low cytosolic Na^+ maintains the Na^+ gradient for the functioning of the Na^+-Ca^{2+} exchanger so that low cytosolic Ca^{2+} levels are maintained nothing to be done here. In a failing heart, the aim of treatment is to make the myocardium contract with greater force (2). This is achieved with digitalis, which, by inhibiting Na^+, K^+-ATPase, abolishes the Na^+-gradient. Consequently, Ca^{2+} cannot exit the cell and attains sufficiently high intracellular levels to mediate excitation-contraction coupling and generate greater contractile force. As more blood is pumped out, the symptoms of heart failure are alleviated

2. ***Ca^{2+}-ATPase:*** Ca^{2+} is an important intracellular messenger referred to as a second messenger. It regulates various cellular processes such as muscle contraction, release of neurotransmitters and glycogen breakdown. It is also an important activator of oxidative metabolism. In order to maintain low cytosolic Ca^{2+} concentration, it is actively transported out of the cell across the plasma membrane, the endoplasmic reticulum or the sarcoplasmic reticulum. The Ca^{2+}-ATPase (Ca^{2+} pump) actively pumps two Ca^{2+} out of the cytosol at the expense of ATP hydrolysis. The mechanism of Ca^{2+}-ATPase resembles that of the Na^+/K^+-ATPase. In eukaryotes, the Ca^{2+} transporter is regulated by the cytosolic Ca^{2+} level through a calcium binding protein termed calmodulin.

3. ***H^+/K^+-ATPase:*** Parietal cells in the gastric mucosa secrete HCl. Intracellular hydration of CO_2 by carbonic anhydrase forms carbonic acid (H_2CO_3) which splits into H^+ and HCO_3^-. The secretion of H^+ involves the H^+/K^+-ATPase, also called the proton pump, in the luminal membrane. This is an antiport and as H^+ is pumped out, the K^+ which enters the cell is subsequently externalized to the lumen. The chloride channels secrete Cl^- into the lumen so that the overall secreted product is HCl. Inhibition of H^+/K^+-ATPase is of clinical importance (Chemistry to Clinics 1.7).

Chemistry to Clinics 1.7: Peptic Ulcer

Excess production of HCl along with a failure of mucosal defense mechanisms, can damage the gastric mucosa and may lead to peptic ulcer. The H^+/K^+-ATPase of the gastric mucosa is activated by histamine stimulation of the cell surface receptor (type 2 histamine receptors). Compounds, such as cimetidine and its analogs (type 2 antihistamine drugs) block the process by competing with histamine for its binding to the receptor and, in turn, reduce HCl production. These drugs are therefore widely used to alleviate the painful and otherwise fatal symptoms of peptic ulcer. However, proton pump inhibitors such as omeprazole are better because they are selective inhibitors of H^+/K^+-ATPase and are therefore more powerful than the antihistamines. It is now recognized that many ulcers are caused by infection with the bacteria *Helicobacter pylori* and can better be cured by the use of antibiotics besides a reduction in acidity.

4. ***Neurotransmitter transporters:*** Regulating the temporal availability of synaptically released neurotransmitter is critical to normal neuronal function. The removal of neurotransmitter from the synaptic cleft by active transport back into the presynaptic terminal or perisynaptic astrocytes (in the central nervous system) is the major way in which synaptic signaling is terminated at most of the synapses. Many disease processes in the central and peripheral nervous systems are due to disorders of synaptic signaling, and may involve altered function of neurotransmitter transporters (Chemistry to Clinics 1.8).

Secondary Active Transport

Secondary active transport is also called **ion gradient-driven active transport**. In this process, free energy of the electrochemical gradient, generated by an ion-pumping ATPase, drives the transport of another substance, such as a sugar or an amino acid, against its concentration gradient. Na^+ glucose transport system

Chemistry to Clinics 1.8: Neurotransmitter Transport Disorders

Dopamine, serotonin, glutamate, norepinephrine, etc. are some of the well-known neurotransmitters. Each has its own reuptake mechanism mediated by specific membrane transporters which may be affected in several diseases:

- *Defect in the dopamine transporter:* Alzheimer's disease, attention deficit hyperactivity disorder, obesity, Parkinson's disease, schizophrenia and substance abuse.
- *Defect in the serotonin transporter:* Autism, gastric motility disorders, mood disorders and obsessive-compulsive disorder.
- *Defect in the glutamate transporter:* Amyotrophic lateral sclerosis, epilepsy, schizophrenia, and stroke.
- *Defect in the norepinephrine transporter:* Mood disorders, severe orthostatic hypotension and substance abuse.

Knowing the tertiary and quaternary structure of the transporters is important for developing selective drugs to target them.

and the amino acid transport system are the examples of secondary active transport system.

1. ***Na^+ glucose transport system:*** An example is the absorption of glucose in the proximal renal tubules and the small intestine (Fig. 1.20).

   Glucose enters the intestinal epithelial cells by secondary active transport using the electrogenic Na^+ glucose transporter 1 (**SGLT1**) in the apical membrane. This increases the intracellular glucose concentration above the blood glucose concentration, and the glucose molecules move passively out of the cell and into the blood via an equilibrating carrier mechanism (**GLUT2**) in the basolateral membrane. The intestinal GLUT2, like the erythrocyte GLUT1, is a sodium-independent transporter that moves glucose down its concentration gradient. However, unlike GLUT1, the GLUT2 transporter can accept other sugars, such as galactose and fructose for absorption. The **Na^+/K^+-ATPase** that is located in the basolateral membrane pumps out the Na^+ (that enter the cell with glucose via SGLT1). In short, the successful uptake of glucose and sodium (symport) is ***'secondarily'*** dependent on the Na^+ gradient maintained by the primary active transport by Na Na^+/K^+-ATPase (Fig. 1.20). The **polarized** organization of the epithelial cells and the integrated functions of the plasma membrane transporters form the basis by which cells accomplish transcellular movement of both glucose and sodium ions, and is also exploited clinically in oral rehydration therapy (Chemistry to Clinics 1.9).

Chemistry to Clinics 1.9: Oral Rehydration Solution

The administration of oral rehydration solution (ORS) has dramatically reduced the mortality resulting from cholera and other diseases that involve extreme losses of water/solutes from the gastrointestinal tract. The main ingredients of ORS are glucose, NaCl or $NaHCO_3$, KCl and water. The glucose and Na^+ are reabsorbed by the sodium-glucose transporter 1 (SGLT1) in the apical membrane of enterocytes, i.e. epithelial cells lining the lumen of the small intestine. Transfer of solutes on the basolateral aspect of the enterocytes increases the osmolarity compared with the luminal osmolarity thereby favoring the osmotic absorption of water. In this manner, the absorption of glucose accompanied by the obligatory increase in absorption of NaCl and water, help to compensate for the diarrheal losses of water/solutes, and treat dehydration.

A comparison between passive mediated transport (facilitated diffusion) and active transport is shown in Table 1.5.

Table 1.5: Comparison between facilitated diffusion and active transport

Parameter	Facilitated diffusion	Active transport
Specific binding site	Present	Present
Saturation kinetics	Yes	Yes
Inhibition by structural analogs	Yes	Yes
Direction of operation	Uni- or bidirectional	Unidirectional
Mode of operation	Along electrical/ chemical gradient	Against electrical/ chemical gradient
Energy dependent	No	Yes

2. ***Amino acid transport systems:*** Amino acids are transported by luminal epithelial cells of the intestine by the Na-dependent pathway, similar to the Na^+-dependent glucose transport system. At least seven different brush-border specific transport systems have been identified for the uptake of different classes of L-amino acids and the dipeptides in the luminal membrane. These include the amino acid transporter for:
   - Neutral amino acids with short or polar side chain such as serine, threonine and alanine.
   - Neutral amino acids with aromatic or hydrophobic side chain, e.g. phenylalanine, tyrosine, tryptophan, methionine, valine, leucine and isoleucine.
   - Imino acids, e.g. proline and hydroxyproline.
   - β-amino acids, such as β-alanine and taurine.
   - Basic amino acids, e.g. lysine and arginine as well as cystine.
   - Acidic amino acids, such as aspartate and glutamate, and
   - Dipeptides.

   Each one of these transport systems is specific for a group of closely related amino acids and operates as Na^+ symport system. Several pathological conditions due to a defect in the membrane transport system for specific amino acids are known (Chemistry to Clinics 1.10).

Chemistry to Clinics 1.10: Amino Acid Transport Disorders

- *Hartnup's disease* is due to a decrease in the transport of neutral amino acids including tryptophan in the epithelial cells of the intestine and in the renal tubules. It is characterized by pellagra-like features due to niacin deficiency consequent to tryptophan deficiency.
- In *cystinuria* renal reabsorption of cystine and basic amino acids (arginine and lysine) is abnormal. This in turn may result in the formation of cystine stones in the kidney.

VESICULAR TRANSLOCATION

Cells translocate certain macromolecules across the plasma membrane by mechanisms which involve vesicle formation with or from the plasma membrane and are referred to as **endocytosis** and **exocytosis** (Fig. 1.15).

All these processes require energy (ATP), Ca^{2+} and the cytoskeletal system for proper functioning.

Endocytosis

Endocytosis is a mechanism for the uptake of large molecules such as polysaccharides, proteins or polynucleotides into the cytoplasm. In this process, a region of the plasma membrane invaginates, enclosing a small volume of the extracellular fluid and its contents within a bud, and generates endocytotic vesicles. The vesicle then pinches off, as fusion of the plasma membrane seals the neck of the vesicle at the original site of invagination. The resulting small vesicle is called an **endosome**. It moves into the interior of the cell and delivers its contents to some other organelle, bound by a single membrane, e.g. a lysosome, by fusion of the two membranes. This 'hybrid vesicle' is called a **secondary lysosome**. Due to the presence of hydrolytic enzymes, the macromolecular contents are digested to their monomers, such as amino acids, simple sugars or nucleotides, which then diffuse out of the vesicle in the cytoplasm.

There are two general types of processes referred to as endocytosis, i.e. phagocytosis and pinocytosis.

- ***Phagocytosis (or cell eating):*** It occurs only in specialized cells like macrophages and granulocytes for the ingestion of large particles, such as bacteria, viruses, etc.

- ***Pinocytosis:***
  - ***Simple pinocytosis*** (or ***cell drinking***) leads to cellular uptake of fluid and its contents as a result of invagination of the plasma membrane (Fig. 1.24).

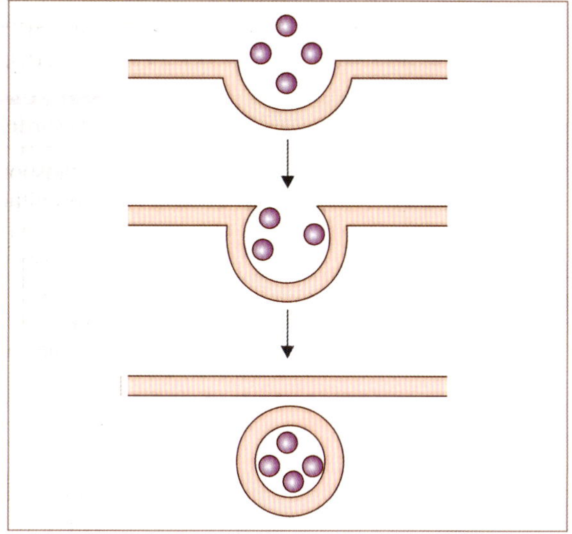

Fig. 1.24: Endocytosis (simple pinocytosis)

  - ***Absorptive pinocytosis*** or ***receptor-mediated pinocytosis*** is a very selective type of pinocytosis that occurs in coated pits, lined with the protein **clathrin**, resulting in the formation of the clathrin-coated vesicles. The high affinity receptors permit selective concentration of the ligand from the medium, e.g. low density lipoproteins (LDL), transferrin, etc. and the receptors are subsequently internalized by means of the coated pits containing the receptors. The coated vesicle may fuse with lysosomes, the contents are digested and clathrin is recycled back to the membrane (Fig. 1.25).
  - Sometimes, in case of some hormones, clathrin is not required for receptor-mediated pinocytosis. The internalized vesicle fuses with another organelle such as Golgi complex, i.e. no secondary lysosomes are formed. The process is known as ***adsorptive pinocytosis***.

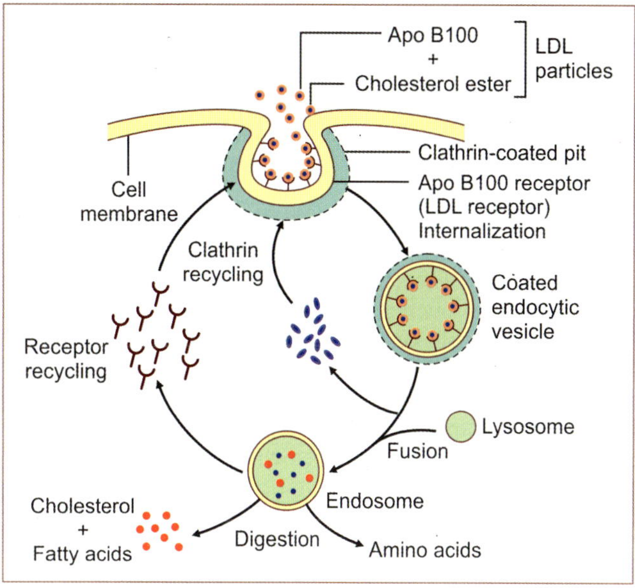

Fig. 1.25: Receptor-mediated pinocytosis

Exocytosis

Exocytosis is the reverse of endocytosis. It involves contact of two inside surface monolayers from the cytosolic side and release of macromolecules to the exterior of a cell. A secretory vesicle in the cytoplasm, originating in the Golgi complex or the endoplasmic reticulum, moves to the inner surface of the plasma membrane and fuses with it, releasing the vesicular contents outside the membrane (Fig. 1.26).

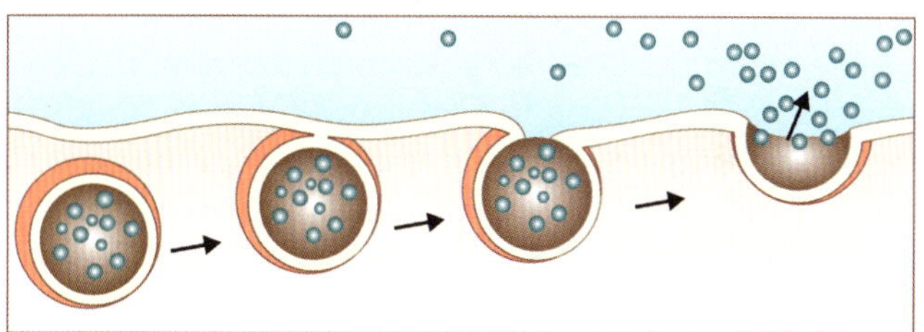

Fig. 1.26: Exocytosis

The secreted/exocytosed molecules may have either of three possible fates:

1. They become a part of the cell membrane surface, e.g. antigens.
2. They become a part of the extracellular matrix, e.g. collagens.
3. They enter the blood and carried to distant sites, e.g. hormones like insulin.

In some diseases characterized by uncontrolled cell division, vesicles may be thrown out to the cell exterior, and contain molecules actually meant for intracellular use only. The process is not a true exocytosis and such vesicles are not true secretory vesicles. They are called **exosomes** (Chemistry to Clinics 1.11).

Chemistry to Clinics 1.11: Exosomes

All cells contain the machinery for the targeted destruction of intracellular macromolecules when they are no longer needed. For example, 'proteasomes' are meant for targeted destruction of proteins and 'exosomes' are meant for targeted degradation of RNA. Exosomes contain RNAse-P activity for RNA cleavage and all the RNA as substrates, marked for degradation. In cells undergoing rapid division, exosomes may be thrown out into the surrounding. Hence, the term 'exosomes' also refers to small microvesicles surrounded by lipid bilayer, shed by tumors into the blood. The exosomes contain the complete set of messenger RNAs (mRNAs) and micro-RNAs (miRNAs), collectively known as the transcriptome. The exosomes can be isolated from the blood and the transcriptome subjected to reverse transcription polymerase chain reaction for detecting DNA mutations. Such blood-based detection of mutations is very valuable in diagnosing tumors where there may be constraints in obtaining a tissue biopsy, as in case of cancers of lungs, pancreas and ovaries.

MEMBRANE ASSOCIATED PHENOMENON: GIBBS-DONNAN EQUILIBRIUM

Consider two solutions separated by a semipermeable membrane as shown in Fig. 1.27.

Both the solutions I and II contain diffusible ions such as Na^+ and Cl^-; in addition, solution I contains impermeable/nondiffusible anions designated as nondiffusible ions (ND^-). According to Gibbs and Donnan, the ND^- create an osmotic gradient and influence the distribution of the permeable ions across the membrane so that **at equilibrium**:

1. The product of diffusible ions in solutions I and II are equal ($36 \times 16 = 24 \times 24 = 576$).
2. Both the solutions remain electrically neutral.
3. The total number of every ion remains the same as that before equilibrium; however, the total ion concentration is higher on the side containing the ND^-.

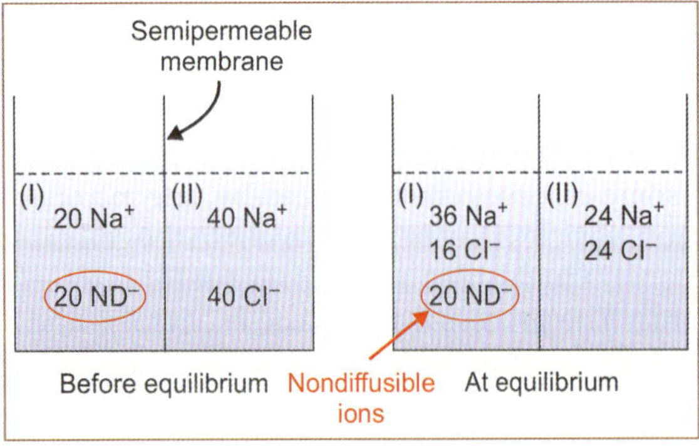

Fig. 1.27: Gibbs-Donnan membrane equilibrium

Gibbs-Donnan equilibrium has **important biological applications:**

- Responsible for the **differential solute** (glucose, urea, electrolytes, etc.) distribution between plasma and other biological fluids such as intracellular fluid, interstitial fluid, gastric juice, cerebrospinal fluid, etc.
- Explains the **osmotic gradient and pH gradient** between plasma and other biological fluids.
- Explains the **'chloride-shift'** in RBC.
- Finds its clinical application in **dialysis** (Chemistry to Clinics 1.12).

Chemistry to Clinics 1.12: Dialysis

Dialysis (Greek *'dialusis'* = 'dissolution'; *'dia'* = 'through'; *'lysis'* = 'loosening'), an artificial means to purify blood, works on the principle of Gibbs-Donnan membrane equilibrium. It is a useful maneuver to partly compensate for the loss of renal function in patients of renal failure. The blood (in case of **hemodialysis**) from a peripheral artery of the patient is allowed to flow on one side of a semipermeable membrane while an artificially prepared fluid of known solute concentration, called the **dialysate**, flows by the other side but in opposite direction (Fig. 1.28).

Proteins present in the blood are the large ND^-. The solute concentration in the dialysate is so designed as to maximize diffusion of water and solutes across the membrane. The net effect is the reduction of toxic molecules to low levels in the blood while improving the levels of the essential ones. The 'purified' blood is returned through a peripheral vein.

The basic procedure is the same in case of **peritoneal dialysis.** Here, the dialysate is run through a tube into the peritoneal cavity and the peritoneal membrane itself serves as the semipermeable membrane. The dialysate is retained for some time and eventually drained out through the tube, removing excess water and waste products.

STEM CELLS

Cell potency: Stem cells are the **master cells** and potential building blocks of the body because they can change into and thus create all other tissues, organs and systems in the body (Fig. 1.29).

This 'changing' is known as differentiation. Thus, 'multipotent' stem cells become 'committed' stem cells once they follow a particular line of differentiation (Table 1.6).

Availability: Stem cells are found in the bone marrow and peripheral blood of adults and the umbilical cord blood of newborn infants. The cord blood cells are preferred because the baby's blood cells have not yet developed their typical set of antigens and because

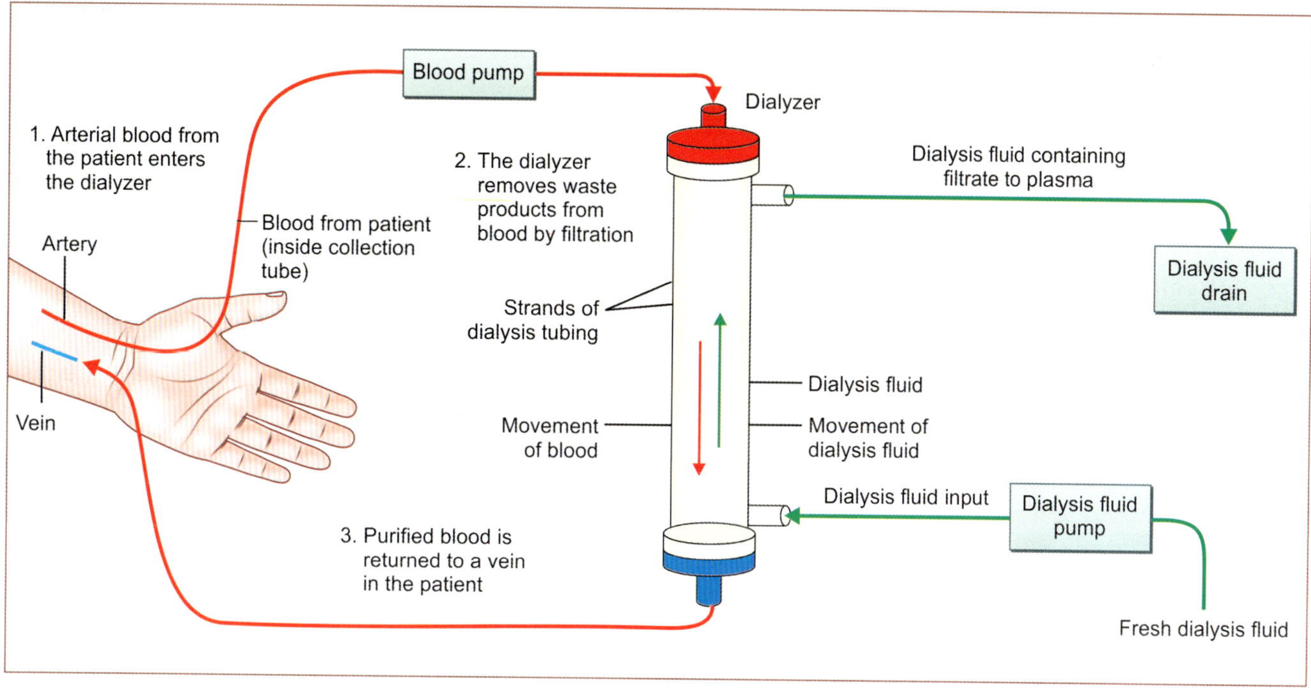

Fig. 1.28: Hemodialysis

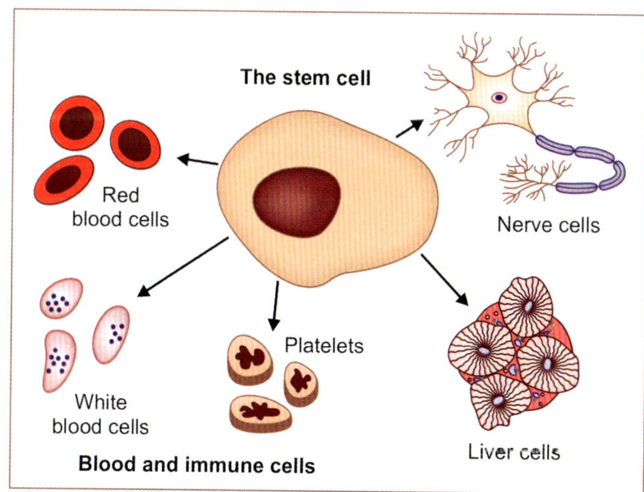

Fig. 1.29: Examples of cells derived from stem cells

umbilical cord blood lacks well-developed immune cells that usually cause graft-versus-host disease.

In addition to cells with blood-forming potential, few mesenchymal stem cells are also found in bone marrow. These cells can give rise to a large number of tissue cells, such as bone, cartilage, fat and connective tissue cells. However, such adult stem cells may be obtained from any tissue, are capable of self-renewal and are multipotent with the potential to form all cell types in the concerned tissue. Thus, **adult stem cells** are 'undifferentiated cells' in a 'differentiated tissue'.

Table 1.6: Stem cell potency

Stem cells	Potency of differentiation
Totipotent stem cells	The zygote and cells derived from it during the first 4 days of conception give rise to all cell types and even whole organism
Pluripotent stem cells	Cells of the inner cell mass after 4 days of conception give rise to all cell types except placenta, but cannot form the whole organism
Multipotent stem cells	Form several cell types restricted to a particular tissue/organ, e.g. hemopoietic stem cells in the bone marrow (forming RBC, WBC and platelets) and neuronal stem cells (forming various cells of the nervous system)
Unipotent/committed stem cells	Form a specific cell type, e.g. erythroid progenitor cells and myeloid progenitor cells

Stem cell therapy: The possibilities for stem cell therapy are unlimited, once we understand how to control their differentiation into all types of tissue cells:

- The major clinical use of stem cells to date has been to restore a patient's hemopoietic system that has been completely disrupted by radiation or chemo-

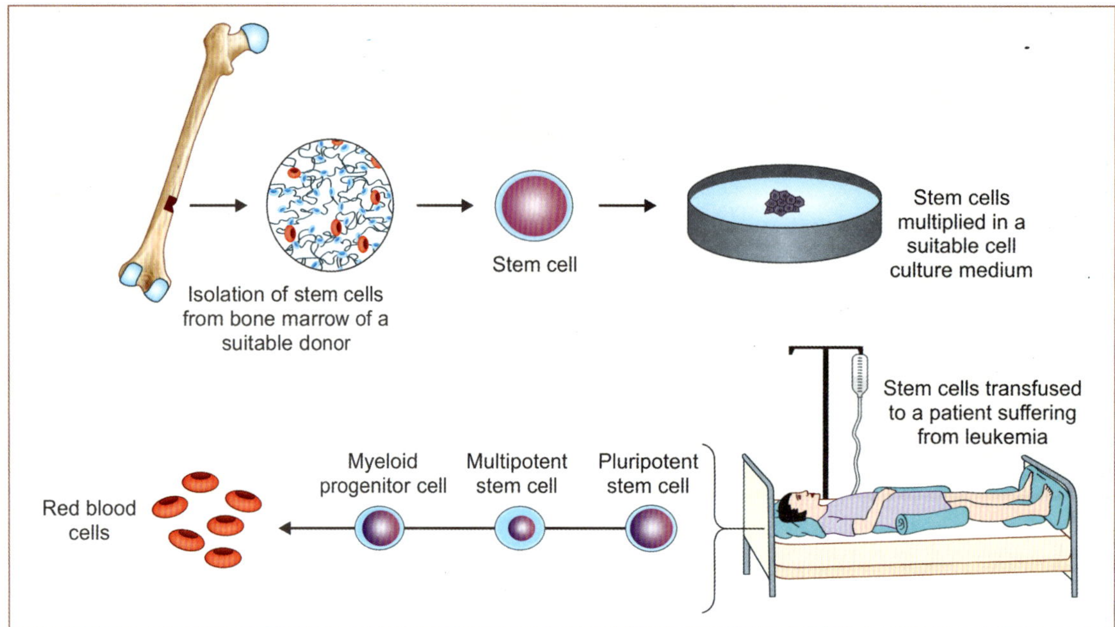

Fig. 1.30: A patient received treatment for leukemia (tumor of white blood cells) due to which his red blood cell count dropped resulting in severe anemia. By selecting a suitable donor and using **stem cell-based hematotherapy,** the red blood cells are restored

therapy for treatment of leukemia and solid tumors (Chemistry to Clinics 1.13).

- Based on the same principle, patients with AIDS could be supported by periodic infusions of T cell precursors.
- Infusions of neutrophil progenitors would help patients with cancer to recover from aggressive cancer therapy.
- Patients with certain anemias would benefit from infusions of red cell progenitors.

Chemistry to Clinics 1.13: Stem Cell-based Hematotherapy

Traditionally, in bone marrow transplantation, the entire hematopoietic system of the recipient, including the most primitive multipotent stem cells, is ablated and restored with cells from the donor. However, using stem cell-based 'hematotherapy', only the specific committed stem cells are transplanted that develop along specific lineages into the mature cells that are nonfunctional in a patient with a particular disease. The healthy portion of the patient's hemopoietic system is thus kept intact (Fig. 1.30).

- Platelet progenitors may be used in patients with inborn or acquired thrombocytopenia.
- Treatment of some of the most common degenerative diseases such as Alzheimer's disease, Parkinson's disease, muscular dystrophy, spinal cord injury, stroke, and various liver and cardiac diseases.

Role of molecular biology: The clinical potential of stem cell therapy can be enhanced by combining traditional stem cell harvesting methods with modern molecular biology methods. Therapeutic cloning might enable the creation of embryonic stem cells that are genetically identical to the patients' cells. Embryonic stem cells are highly desirable to work with because they have the capacity to become any mature cell (totipotency). Existing stem cells can be genetically manipulated by replacing a defective or missing gene.

Demerits of stem cell therapy: One limitation for the use of stem cells lies in the problem of avoiding tumor growth because stem cells are naturally programmed to divide. Additionally, the benefits of stem cell therapy must be carefully balanced with ethical and social concerns.

1

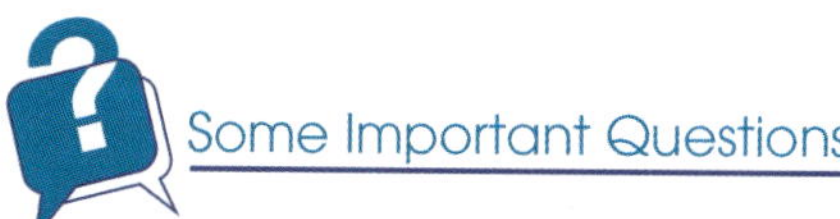

Some Important Questions

1. **Describe structure, functions, isolation and biochemical markers of various subcellular entities of a eukaryotic cell.**
2. **Discuss composition of a biological membrane.**
3. **Biomedical importance of stem cells.**
4. **Explain:**
   i. Mitochondria as a powerhouse of the cell.
   ii. Functions of the rough endoplasmic reticulum.
   iii. Differences between nuclear and mitochondrial DNA.
   iv. Molecular organization of a cell.
   v. Differences between primary and secondary active transport.
5. **Describe:**
   i. Fluid-mosaic model of cell membrane
   ii. Important functions of a biological membrane
   iii. Ion channels
   iv. Carrier-mediated transport
   v. Amino acid transport systems
   vi. Transport disorders
6. **Write notes on:**
   i. The nucleus
   ii. Ribosomes
   iii. The Golgi apparatus
   iv. Matrix
   v. Micelles
   vi. Lipid bilayer
   vii. Liposomes
   viii. Integral membrane proteins
   ix. Peripheral proteins
   x. Nonmediated transport
   xi. Channelopathies
   xii. Nephrogenic diabetes insipidus
   xiii. Endocytosis
   xiv. Suicide bags
   xv. Age pigments
   xvi. Lysosomal disorders
   xvii. Ionophores
   xviii. Facilitated diffusion
   xix. Group translocation
   xx. Exocytosis
   xxi. Pinocytosis
   xxii. Gibbs-Donnan equilibrium

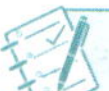

Multiple Choice Questions

1. **The following is not a true organelle:**
   A. Ribosome
   B. Mitochondrion
   C. Lysosome
   D. Nucleus
2. **Galactosyltransferase is the biomarker for the following subcellular entity:**
   A. Cell membrane
   B. Cytoplasm
   C. Golgi apparatus
   D. Endoplasmic reticulum
3. **Protein synthesis occurs in:**
   A. Ribosomes only
   B. Mitochondria only
   C. Ribosomes and mitochondria
   D. Smooth endoplasmic reticulum and mitochondria
4. **Protein sorting occurs in:**
   A. Golgi apparatus
   B. Endoplasmic reticulum
   C. Cell membrane
   D. Mitochondria
5. **Mitochondrial DNA is:**
   A. Paternally inherited and more prone to mutations than nuclear DNA
   B. Paternally inherited and less prone to mutations than nuclear DNA
   C. Maternally inherited and more prone to mutations than nuclear DNA
   D. Maternally inherited and less prone to mutations than nuclear DNA

6. **Zellweger syndrome is due to absence or loss of functions of:**
   A. Lysosomes
   B. Peroxisomes
   C. Ribosomes
   D. Endoplasmic reticulum

7. **The ideal source for obtaining stem cells is:**
   A. Adult peripheral blood
   B. Adult bone marrow
   C. Neonatal peripheral blood
   D. Umbilical cord blood

8. **In the myelin sheath, lipid:protein ratio is nearly:**
   A. 4:1 B. 1:4
   C. 1:1 D. 3:2

9. **In the renal collecting tubules, expression of aquaporin 2 (AQP2) is increased by:**
   A. ADH B. ANP
   C. Aldosterone D. Angiotensin II

10. **Valinomycin and nigericin translocate:**
   A. K^+ B. Na^+
   C. Ca^{2+} D. Cl^-

CHAPTER

2

Enzymes

Competency Achievement: The student should be able to:

BI2.1 Explain fundamental concepts of enzyme, isoenzyme, alloenzyme, coenzyme and cofactors. Enumerate the main classes of IUBMB nomenclature

BI2.3 Describe and explain the basic principles of enzyme activity

BI2.4 Describe and discuss enzyme inhibitors as poisons and drugs and as therapeutic enzymes

BI2.5 Describe and discuss the clinical utility of various serum enzymes as markers of pathological conditions

BI2.6 Discuss use of enzymes in laboratory investigations (enzyme-based assays)

BI2.7 Interpret laboratory results of enzyme activities and describe the clinical utility of various enzymes as markers of pathological conditions

Enzymes are biological catalysts, nondialyzable, colloidal, organic macromolecules which are produced in the living organisms and catalyze biochemical reactions without being utilized in the process. They are so called since they were discovered as the substances found in yeast (Greek *en* = in, and *zyme* = yeast) and were capable of catalyzing the reactions of fermentation. Most of them are proteins (except ribozymes), thermolabile, and accelerate the rate at which a reaction proceeds towards equilibrium, by lowering the free energy barrier that separates the substrates (reactants) from the products.

CHEMICAL NATURE OF ENZYMES

Most of the enzymes are protein in nature with large molecular weight though certain RNAs, called ribozymes, also show highly substrate specific catalytic activity.

Multimeric proteins: Most of the enzymes though are simple proteins having a single polypeptide chain, there are several enzymes which have more than one polypeptide chain. These are called multimeric proteins which may be found as either oligomeric enzymes or as multienzyme complexes.

Oligomeric enzymes: Enzymes with two or more subunits are called oligomeric enzymes, e.g. phosphorylase, hexokinase, lactate dehydrogenase, etc. These occur as tetramers, i.e. each enzyme has four protein subunits. Others like phosphofructokinase, fructose-1,6-bisphosphatase and creatine phosphokinase are dimers, i.e. each has two protein subunits.

Multienzyme complexes: Several enzymes occur in the form of a multienzyme complex, i.e. they have more than one enzyme activity. Such a complex catalyzes the conversion of a substrate, in a sequential series of reactions, to different products, e.g. pyruvate dehydrogenase complex, α-ketoglutarate dehydrogenase complex, etc. Each of these complexes contain three enzymes. Fatty acid synthase is a multienzyme complex with six different enzyme activities.

LOCATION OF ENZYMES IN THE CELL

Most of the enzymes are produced by the cells of a particular tissue and function within the cell. Such enzymes are called **intracellular enzymes**, e.g. the enzymes of glycolysis, TCA cycle and fatty acid synthesis. On the other hand, there are certain enzymes which are produced by the cells of a particular tissue and liberated from there for use in the other tissues. Such enzymes are called **extracellular enzymes**, e.g. various proteolytic enzymes like trypsin, chymotrypsin, etc. These are secreted by the pancreas for their action in the small intestine.

PROENZYMES

Most of the intracellular enzymes are secreted in their active forms called **'zymases'**. Proteolytic enzymes, on the other hand, are usually synthesized as somewhat larger inactive precursors, known as **zymogens** or **proenzymes** (Chemistry to Clinics 2.1).

> **Chemistry to Clinics 2.1: Acute Pancreatitis**
>
> The inactivity of zymogens is crucial because if these enzymes were synthesized in their active forms within the cell, this situation would be potentially self-destructing. Acute pancreatitis, a painful and sometimes fatal condition is characterized by the premature activation of the digestive enzymes synthesized by this organ. The enzymes damage the pancreas and spill over into the circulation. Pancreatic amylase and lipase are significantly raised in the serum of these patients and help to establish the diagnosis.

These molecules are stored in the storage vesicles known as zymogen granules, secreted as zymogens and undergo modifications in structure, after coming in contact with certain activating agents (Table 2.1).

An activating agent can be H^+, another enzyme or an active form of the zymogen itself. For example, gastric juice contains pepsin which is secreted as pepsinogen (a zymogen). Pepsinogen is transformed to its active form pepsin by the H^+ of the gastric juice. Once formed, pepsin itself also acts on pepsinogen and catalyzes its own conversion into pepsin. This process is called **autocatalysis** (Fig. 2.1).

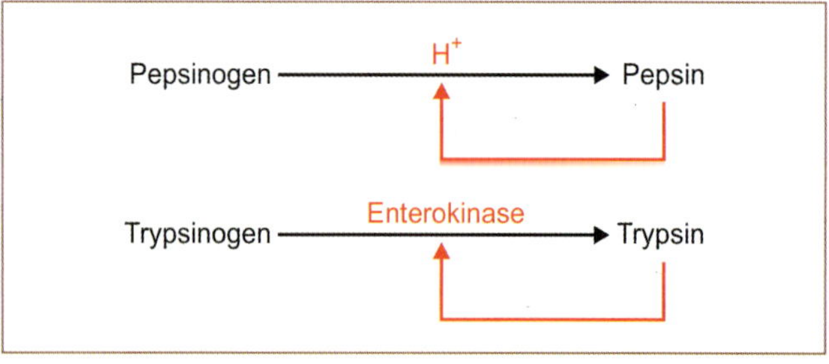

Fig. 2.1: Activation of zymogens

ISOENZYMES

Isoenzymes (isozymes) are the physically distinct forms of an enzyme, which have the same specificity, but may be present in different tissues of the same organism, in different cell types, or subcellular compartments. Besides the source, they also differ, from each other, with respect to their structure, electrophoretic mobility and immunological properties. The most common mechanism for the formation of isoenzymes involves arrangement of the subunits which arise from different genetic loci and assemble in different combinations, to form the active polymeric enzyme. Various enzymes, whose isoenzymes have wide clinical utility, include lactate dehydrogenase, creatine phosphokinase and alkaline phosphatase (Table 2.2).

Lactate Dehydrogenase

Lactate dehydrogenase (LDH or LD) catalyzes a reversible reaction between pyruvic acid and lactic acid. It is found in cardiac and skeletal muscles, liver, kidneys, erythrocytes, leukocytes, lungs, lymph nodes, spleen and brain.

LDH is a **tetrameric protein**, i.e. it has four polypeptide subunits. Each subunit may be one of the two types, designated as the **H type** (heart type) or the **M type** (muscle type), and thus, LDH exists in serum in **five** distinct forms (**isoenzymes**), which have different proportions of the H and M subunits.

LDH1 has all the 4 subunits of the H type, i.e. as $\mathbf{H_4}$ (HHHH) and is, predominantly, found in myocardium. **LDH2** consists of 3H and 1M subunits, i.e. as $\mathbf{H_3M}$ (HHHM) and is primarily associated with the system that defends the body against infections. **LDH3** consists of 2H and 2M subunits, i.e. as $\mathbf{H_2M_2}$ (HHMM) and is, mainly, found in lungs. **LDH4** consists of 3H and 1M subunits, i.e. as $\mathbf{HM_3}$ (HMMM) and is found in the kidneys, placenta and pancreas. LDH5 consists of all the 4 subunits of the M type, i.e. as M_4 (MMMM) and is found in the liver and skeletal muscle. Recently,

Table 2.1: Gastric and pancreatic proenzymes/zymogens

Proenzyme/zymogen	Site of synthesis	Activator	Active enzyme
Pepsinogen	Chief cells of stomach	H^+, pepsin	Pepsin
Trypsinogen	Pancreatic acinar cells	Trypsin	Trypsin
Chymotrypsinogen	Pancreatic acinar cells	Trypsin	π- or α-chymotrypsin
Procarboxypeptidase A	Pancreatic acinar cells	Trypsin	Carboxypeptidase A
Procarboxypeptidase B	Pancreatic acinar cells	Trypsin	Carboxypeptidase B
Proelastase	Pancreatic acinar cells	Trypsin	Elastase

Table 2.2: Diagnostic importance of some isoenzymes

Enzyme	Isoenzymes	Predominant location	Diagnostic significance (↑serum levels)
Creatine kinase (CK, a dimer with 2 polypeptide chains, B [brain] and M [muscle])	CK-1 (BB)	Brain	Cerebrovascular accidents
	CK-2 (MB)	Myocardium	Myocardial infarction
	CK-3 (MM)	Skeletal muscle	Muscular dystrophies
Lactate dehydrogenase (LD, a tetramer with 4 polypeptide chains, H [heart] and M [muscle])	LD-1 (H_4)	Myocardium	Myocardial infarction
	LD-2 (H_3M)	Erythrocytes	Hemolytic anemia
	LD-3 (H_2M_2)	Brain	Cerebrovascular accidents
	LD-4 (HM_3)	Liver	Hepatocellular damage
	LD-5 (M_4)	Skeletal muscle	Muscular dystrophies
Alkaline phosphatase (ALP, monomeric isoenzymes because of differences in carbohydrate contents [sialic acid residues])	α_1-ALP	Liver	Obstructive jaundice
	α_2-ALP: Heat labile	Liver	Hepatitis
	: Heat stable	Placenta	Pregnancy
	Pre-β-ALP	Bones	Osteoblastic bone diseases
	γ-ALP	Colon	Ulcerative colitis
	Regan ALP	Some primary tumors	Bronchogenic carcinoma

LDH6 and LDH7 have also been reported. Normally, levels of LDH2 are higher than those of the other isoenzymes.

Creatine Kinase

Creatine kinase (CK), also referred to as creatine phosphokinase (CPK), catalyzes reversible transfer of a phosphate group between creatine and ATP. Most of the CPK resides in skeletal and cardiac muscles. The enzyme enters the blood rapidly, following damage to the muscle cells, and has been suggested as an excellent marker for acute myocardial infarction (heart damage) or skeletal muscle damage. Besides, CPK levels also rise and fall rapidly, and coincide with a variety of other conditions including surgical procedures and vigorous exercise.

CPK is a **dimeric protein**, i.e. it has two polypeptide subunits. Each subunit may be one of the two types, designated as the **M type** (muscle type) or the **B type** (brain type), and thus, CPK exists in serum in **three** distinct forms (**isoenzymes**), which have different proportions of the M and B subunits.

CK-1 has both the subunits of the B type, i.e. as **BB** and is, predominantly, found in brain. CK-**2** consists of one M and one B subunit, i.e. as **MB** and is found in the myocardium. CK-**3** consists of both the subunits of M type, i.e. as **MM** and is, mainly, found in skeletal muscle. Recently, LDH6 and LDH7 have also been reported. Normally, levels of LDH2 are higher than those of the other isoenzymes.

Alkaline Phosphatase

Alkaline phosphatase, also referred to as ALP, catalyzes the hydrolysis of various phosphomonoesters in alkaline pH. Highest concentration of ALP is found in bone, liver, spleen, intestine, placenta and kidneys.

Different tissues contain different forms of the alkaline phosphatase. A major portion of the alkaline phosphatase, in serum, is derived **from liver** and its level rises in post-hepatic jaundice. In growing children the major isoenzyme is from **bone**, which is related to increased osteoblastic activity. During the last trimester of pregnancy there is increase in alkaline phosphatase activity, which is of **placental origin.** Since this isoenzyme is heat stable, it is also called **heat stable alkaline phosphatase**.

ALLOENZYMES

Alloenzymes (also called **allozymes**) are variant forms of an enzyme which differ structurally but not functionally from other allozymes coded for by different alleles at the same locus. These are opposed to isozymes, which are enzymes that perform the same function, but are coded by genes located at different loci.

Alloenzymes are common biological enzymes that exhibit high levels of functional evolutionary conservation throughout specific phyla and kingdoms. They are used by phylogeneticists as molecular markers to gauge evolutionary histories and relationships between different species. They can be separated by capillary electrophoresis. These enzymes generally perform very basic functions found commonly throughout all life forms, such as DNA polymerase, the enzyme that repairs and copies DNA. Significant changes in this enzyme reflect significant events in evolutionary history of organisms. As expected, DNA polymerase shows relatively small differences in its amino acid sequence between phyla and even kingdoms.

The various forms of an alloenzyme can be separated by capillary electrophoresis.

COENZYMES AND COFACTORS

Some of the enzymes require the presence of certain small nonprotein factors, such as an organic molecule (coenzyme) or a metal ion (cofactor) for their activity.

COENZYMES

Organic cofactors which are dialyzable, thermostable and of low molecular weight are called coenzymes. Some of them are only transiently associated with the enzyme and function as cosubstrates. Others, known as **prosthetic groups**, are tightly associated with their proteins, often by covalent bonds. For example, heme, the prosthetic group of cytochromes. It is tightly bound to the protein through extensive hydrophobic and hydrogen bonding interactions, together with the covalent bonds.

The catalytically active form of an enzyme is the **apoenzyme–coenzyme complex**, called the **holoenzyme**. The inactive enzyme resulting from the removal of a cofactor from the holoenzyme is referred as **apoenzyme,** while the nonprotein component of the holoenzyme is called **coenzyme**.

Holoenzyme = Apoenzyme + Coenzyme
(active) (inactive)

Vitamins as coenzymes: Coenzymes are the derivatives of the B complex group of vitamins (*see* Chapter 8 for details). These are chemically changed by the enzymatic reaction in which they participate but regenerated to their original state after the completion of the catalytic cycle. For example, NAD^+ is reduced to NADH in alcohol dehydrogenase reaction, but is oxidized back, may be by a different enzyme (Table 2.3).

COFACTORS

The inorganic ions, such as Mg^{2+}, Zn^{2+} or Cl^- required for the catalytic activity of an enzyme are called **'inorganic cofactors'**. Sometimes, a metal ion is loosely associated with the enzyme and forms a metal-enzyme complex. Such enzymes are called **metal-activated enzymes** (Table 2.4).

On the other hand, a metal ion may form an integral part of the enzyme. Such enzymes are called **metallo-**

Table 2.3: Lists various coenzymes, their precursor vitamins, along with the type of reaction in which the coenzyme participates

Vitamin	Coenzyme form(s)	Reactions catalyzed
Thiamin	TPP	Pyruvate ⟶ Acetyl-CoA α-Ketoglutarate ⟶ Succinyl-CoA
Riboflavin	FMN FAD	L-Amino acids ⟶ α-Keto acids Succinate ⟶ Fumarate
Niacin	NAD^+ $NADP^+$	Lactate ⟶ Pyruvate Glucose-6-P ⟶ 6-P-Gluconolactone
Pyridoxine	Pyridoxal-5-P	Alanine + α-Ketoglutarate ⟶ Pyruvate + Glutamate Tyrosine ⟶ Tyramine
Pantothenic acid	CoA	Pyruvate ⟶ Acetyl-CoA Fatty acid ⟶ Fatty acyl-CoA
Biotin	Carboxybiotin	Acetyl CoA ⟶ Malonyl-CoA Pyruvate ⟶ Oxaloacetate
Folate	Tetrahydrofolic acid	Glycine ⟶ Serine Homocysteine ⟶ Methionine
B_{12}	Deoxyadenosylcobalamin Methylcobalamin	Methylmalonyl-CoA ⟶ Succinyl-CoA Homocysteine ⟶ Methionine
Lipoic acid	Lipoic acid	Pyruvate ⟶ Acetyl-CoA α-Ketoglutarate ⟶ Succinyl-CoA

Table 2.4: Metal-activated enzymes

Enzymes	Ion required for activity
Lipase, ATPase, succinate dehydrogenase	Ca^{2+}
Phosphorylase, enolase, DNA polymerase	Mg^{2+}
Arginase, phosphoglucomutase, choline esterase	Mn^{2+}
Salivary amylase	Cl^-
Pyruvate kinase	K^+

enzymes. Transition metal ions, such as Fe, Cu, Zn or Mn may form an integral part of several metalloenzymes (Table 2.5).

Table 2.5: Metalloenzymes

Enzymes	Integrated metal
Cytochromes, peroxidases, catalase	Fe
Ascorbic acid oxidase, cytochrome oxidase, tyrosinase	Cu
Aldehyde oxidase, xanthine oxidase, nitrate reductase	Mo
Carbonic anhydrase, lactate dehydrogenase, carboxypeptidase	Zn
Glutathione peroxidase	Se

NOMENCLATURE AND CLASSIFICATION OF ENZYMES

Enzymes are commonly named by putting the suffix '-ase' to the name of the substrate or with the catalytic action of the enzyme, e.g. a lipase is an enzyme which catalyzes the hydrolysis of a lipid, a fatty acid synthase is an enzyme that catalyzes the synthesis of a fatty acid. These names of the enzymes are called the trivial names for which no systematic rules are followed.

IUBMB NOMENCLATURE OF ENZYMES

For the rational naming of each enzyme, International Union of Biochemistry and Molecular Biology (IUBMB) adopted a scheme and suggested functional classification of enzymes. As per IUBMB, enzymes are named with the suffix '-ase' with the name of the substrate and/or the type of the reaction it catalyzes. Each enzyme is assigned a name and a systematic four-digit enzyme code, commonly known as **Enzyme Commission number** (EC number):

- Its first digit denotes the main class which is according to the general type of a chemical reaction that an enzyme catalyzes.
- The second digit characterizes the subclass, based on the nature of a chemical group removed or transferred, or any bond split or formed.
- The third digit indicates the subsubclass and is used for more detailed subdivision of the subclass.
- The last digit of the EC number indicates an arbitrarily assigned serial number to each enzyme in a subsubclass.
- For example, 1.1.1.1 is the enzyme code for alcohol dehydrogenase that catalyzes the oxidation of an alcohol to yield an aldehyde. It removes $2e^-$ and $2H^+$, and in turn reduces NAD^+. It is the first enzyme of the subsubclass 1 (NAD^+ utilizing), of the subclass 1 (dehydrogenases) and belongs to class 1 (oxidoreductase).

CLASSIFICATION OF ENZYMES

Enzymes are thus classified according to the nature of a chemical reaction they catalyze. Accordingly, there are six major classes of enzymatic reactions (Table 2.6).

1. ***Oxidoreductases***: These are enzymes involved in the oxidation and reduction of their substrates, i.e. they catalyze addition of oxygen or removal of hydrogen or electrons. Accordingly, several subclasses include dehydrogenases, oxidases, oxygenases, etc. Examples of oxidoreductases are alcohol dehydrogenase, xanthine oxidase, glutathione reductase, etc.
2. ***Transferases***: These are enzymes which catalyze the transfer of a functional group from one substrate (donor) to another (acceptor). On the basis of the transferring group, transferases are further subclassified as aminotransferases, phosphotransferases, etc. Glutamate oxaloacetate transaminase, hexokinase, glucose-1-phosphate uridyltransferase are some of the examples of the class transferases.
3. ***Hydrolases***: These enzymes bring about cleavage of a substrate by the addition of a molecule of water, termed hydrolysis. According to the nature of the group or the bond being hydrolyzed, hydrolases are subclassified as peptidases, glycosidases, etc. Examples include glucose-6-phosphatase, amylase, pepsin, etc.
4. ***Lyases***: These enzymes catalyze the removal of a small molecule such as water, ammonia or CO_2, from a large substrate, i.e. they bring about the cleavage without the addition of water. These enzymes are further subclassified on the basis of the linkage they

Table 2.6: Classification of enzymes

Enzyme class	Examples
Oxidoreductases	Alcohol dehydrogenase, xanthine oxidase, catalase
Transferases	Glutamate pyruvate transaminase, serine hydroxymethyl transferase, hexokinase
Hydrolases	Glucose-6-phosphatase, carboxypeptidase, pepsin
Lyases	Pyruvate decarboxylase, aldolase, histidase
Isomerases	Phosphotriose isomerase, phosphoglucomutase, alanine racemase
Ligases	Glutamine synthetase, acetyl-CoA carboxylase, glutathione synthetase
Translocase	Ornithine translocase, carnitine-acylcarnitine translocase

attack. Examples include aldolase, argininosuccinase, histidase, etc.

5. ***Isomerases***: These are involved in the isomerization of a substrate and catalyze the interconversion of one isomeric form to the other. Racemases, epimerases and mutases are some of the subclasses of this class. Examples of isomerases include phosphohexose isomerase, phosphoglucomutase, alanine racemase, etc.
6. ***Ligases***: These are also called synthetases (ligate means to bind), as they are involved in the synthesis of a molecule, by joining two different compounds together, at the expense of a high energy phosphate bond of ATP. Various subclasses include the ligases forming a C–C, C–N or C–S bond. Examples of ligases are glutamine synthetase, glutathione synthetase, etc.
7. ***Translocases:*** These enzymes have a role in moving ions or molecules across the cell membrane against a concentration gradient. They play important roles in biological membranes, e.g. translocase of the outer membrane of mitochondria work in conjunction with translocase of the inner membrane to transport proteins in the mitochondria.

RIBOZYMES

Structure and properties: These are certain ribonucleic acids (RNAs) which exhibit highly substrate specific catalytic activity. They catalyze hydrolysis of phosphodiester bonds within the RNA molecule and play a key role in the intron splicing events, which are essential in the conversion of pre-mRNAs to mature mRNAs. Many ribozymes have a hair-pin or hammerhead shaped active center and require divalent metal ions (e.g. Mg^{2+}) as cofactors. They obey simple Michaelis-Menten kinetics and some of them can be allosterically modulated.

2

Examples: RNAse-P from *E. coli*, self-splicing RNA introns, telomerase and eukaryotic peptidyl transferase.

Applications: Synthetic ribozymes have been developed that possess better catalytic activity than the natural ones and their biomedical applications include:

1. Tools for RNA cleavage *in vitro.*
2. Designing of specific catalytic RNA molecules to cleave nucleic acids of infectious viruses (HIV, hepatitis C, herpes simplex, etc.) and malignant cells.
3. Study of gene expression, function and use in gene therapy.

Protein versus RNA catalysts: Compared with protein catalysts, ribozymes have the following drawbacks:

1. Ribozymes are not as efficient and versatile as protein catalysts since there are only four different nucleotide building blocks for RNA rather than the twenty amino acids available for proteins.
2. Ribozymes generally act only once in a chemical event, whereas protein enzymes are reused after each round of catalysis.
3. Rate of catalysis is slower for ribozymes because for substrate binding, they rely mostly on H-bonding and less on hydrophobic plus electrostatic interactions exploited by protein catalysts.

ABZYMES

Abzymes are the artificially synthesized catalytic antibodies against the enzyme-substrate complex in the transition state of the reaction. They are also called 'catmab' (catalytic monoclonal antibody) since they are monoclonal antibodies possessing catalytic activity. However, sometimes natural abzymes may be found in the blood, e.g. anti-vasoactive intestinal peptide autoantibodies, DNA-hydrolyzing abzymes seen in systemic lupus erythematosus, etc. Abzymes exhibit the same kind of substrate specificity as do enzymes and yield products with defined stereochemistry. Abzymes can be useful in the treatment of various diseases, e.g. abzymes against the gp120 envelope protein of HIV may potentially prevent the virus entry into the host cell.

BASIC PRINCIPLES OF ENZYME ACTIVITY

An enzyme binds to a substrate and forms an **enzyme-substrate complex** which is subsequently transformed into a product and releases the enzyme.

$$E + S \rightarrow ES \rightarrow P + E$$

Enzymes are highly specific catalysts, both with regard to their substrates as well as to the type of reaction.

Some of the enzymes show **absolute specificity for substrate**, e.g. L-amino acid oxidase. The enzyme binds only to L-amino acids and not to D-amino acids (Fig. 2.2).

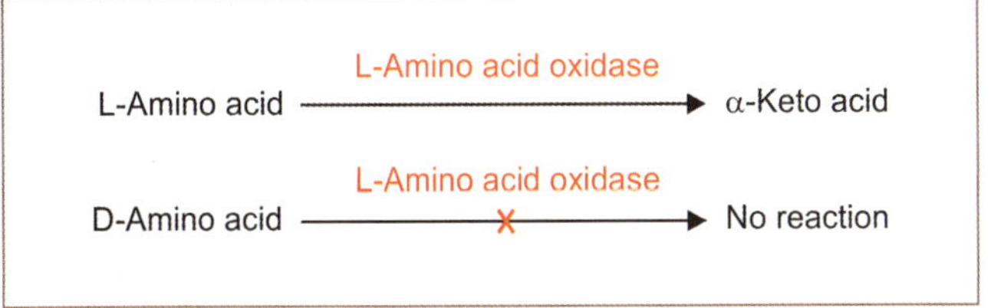

Fig. 2.2: Absolute specificity of an enzyme

Others have **broader specificity**. Such an enzyme can accept several analogs of the specific substrate. For example, hexokinase can catalyze phosphorylation of glucose, fructose or mannose (Fig. 2.3).

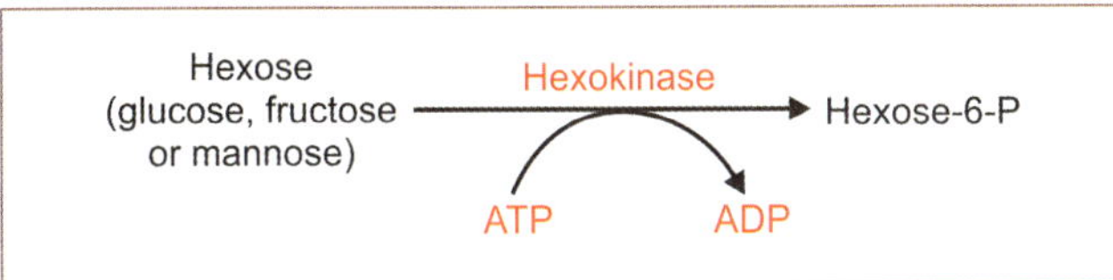

Fig. 2.3: Reaction specificity of an enzyme

Hexokinase, thus, has a broader specificity and is **reaction specific**. On the other hand, glucokinase is specific for its substrate, i.e. glucose only.

The specificity of an enzyme is located in a particular region on the enzyme surface that is designated as the active site/center.

ACTIVE SITE OF AN ENZYME

The specificity of an enzyme is located in a particular region called the active site or active center (Fig. 2.4).

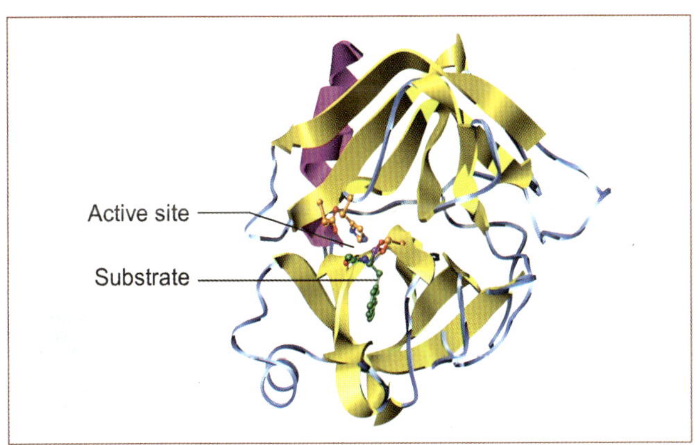

Fig. 2.4: Active site/center of an enzyme is a small cleft in the tertiary structure

Salient features of the active site are that:

1. It has a small cleft in the tertiary structure of an enzyme molecule, which is made up of:
   i. **Substrate binding site:** A substrate binds to the enzyme through various noncovalent forces, such as van der Waals forces, electrostatic forces, hydrogen bonds and hydrophobic interactions.
   ii. **Catalytic site**
      - Lined by specific amino acids called catalytic residues, most commonly serine (others include cysteine, aspartate, histidine, tyrosine, arginine, lysine, etc.).
      - Catalytic residues are spatially close but actually distant from each other in the primary structure.
      - Cofactors are a part of the catalytic site.
      - Specific nucleotides are present in ribozymes.
2. Binding of the substrate with the active site is explained by **'lock-and-key' model** (assumes a rigid character of active site) or **'induced-fit' model** (assumes a flexible character of active site).
3. It may be inactivated by alterations in temperature and pH.
4. It may be blocked by various compounds resembling the substrate (reversible competitive enzyme inhibition) or by unrelated substances (irreversible enzyme poisoning).
5. Identification and analysis of active site is crucial in the process of drug discovery (Chemistry to Clinics 2.2).
6. A software-based technology, called comparison of protein active site structures (CPASS), helps to compare active sites and hence, in new drug designing.

Chemistry to Clinics 2.2: HIV Protease Inhibitors

Proteases play an important role in the pathogenesis of diseases caused by retroviruses such as HIV. The 3-dimensional characterization of HIV protease and identification of its active site helped to develop a popular antiretroviral drug called ritonavir. It is a tetrapeptide resembling the protein that is the substrate of HIV protease. Thus, it inhibits protease through competitive inhibition.

FORMATION OF ENZYME-SUBSTRATE COMPLEX

Interaction of the enzyme with the substrate results in the formation of the enzyme-substrate complex. There are two mechanisms by which enzyme-substrate complex can be formed. These include:

Lock-and-key Model

- The first proposal, by Emil Fischer, to explain the interaction of substrate with the active site of an enzyme and the formation of enzyme-substrate complex.
- Also called the **rigid** template model.
- It is based on the complementarity between the enzyme and its substrate. In other words, a pocket or cleft on the surface of the enzyme contains a 'negative impression' of the molecular features of the substrate, thus allowing specificity of the enzyme for a particular substrate (Fig. 2.5).

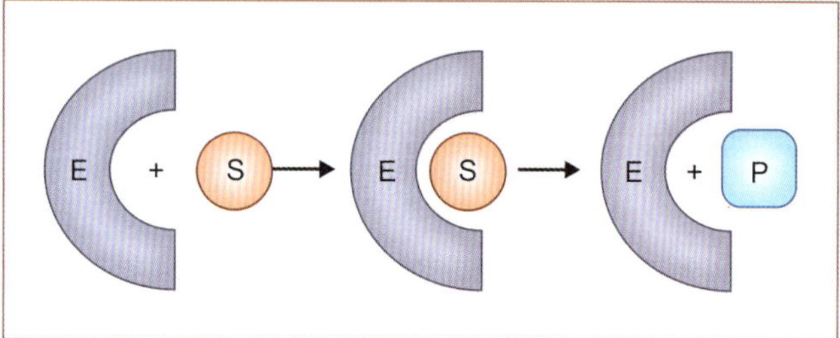

Fig. 2.5: Lock-and-key theory

- The amino acid residues that form the binding site are so arranged that they interact specifically with the substrate. During the process of formation of an enzyme-substrate complex, the substrate attaches itself onto the specific amino acid residues in the active site on the enzyme molecule like a key fits into its lock.
- The model implies rigidity of the enzyme's active site; explains enzyme specificity but fails to explain alteration in the structure of active site in the presence of allosteric modulators.

Induced-fit Model

- A **flexible** model, proposed by Koshland, to explain the interaction of substrate with the active site of an enzyme and the formation of enzyme-substrate complex.
- The substrate binding site of enzyme undergoes some conformational change on its binding with the substrate. That is to say, during its binding with the enzyme, a substrate induces conformational changes in the enzyme's active site, so as to attain a desired shape, in such a way that the substrate can fit the active site conveniently (Fig. 2.6).
- The model implies flexibility of the enzyme's active site; explains enzyme specificity plus alteration in the structure of active site in the presence of allosteric modulators.

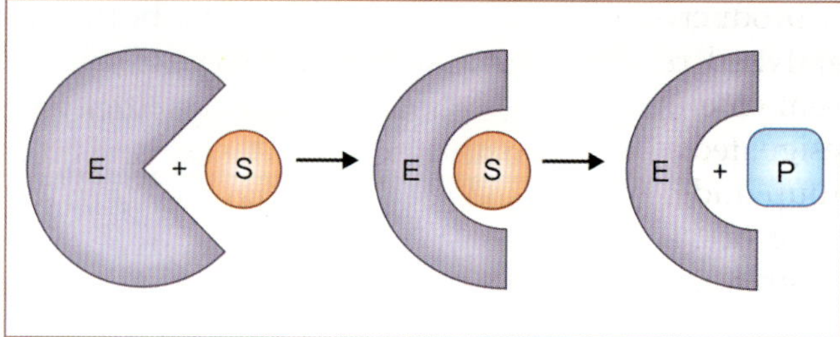

Fig. 2.6: Induced-fit theory

- Explains competitive inhibition and enzyme inactivation.

MULTISUBSTRATE REACTIONS

If an enzyme utilizes more than one substrate or acts upon a substrate and a coenzyme together to generate one or more products, such a reaction is called a multisubstrate reaction which may proceed by any of the following two mechanisms, i.e. the ping-pong mechanism or the sequential mechanism.

Ping-pong Mechanism

A substrate (S1) reacts with an enzyme (E) forming an enzyme-substrate complex (ES1) to produce a product (P1). The release of product (P1) in turn results in some modification in the enzyme structure, e.g. E to E1. The second substrate (S2) thereafter binds to the modified enzyme (E1) and is converted to the second product (P2). After the release of P2, the enzyme (E1) is regenerated in its original form (E). For example, in a transaminase catalyzed reaction, the enzyme-bound pyridoxal phosphate accepts α-amino group from an amino acid and releases the amino acid as α-keto acid. Another α-keto acid then binds to the modified enzyme from where the amino group is transferred onto the α-keto acid resulting in the formation of a new amino acid. With the release of this amino acid, the enzyme is regenerated in its original form (Fig. 2.7).

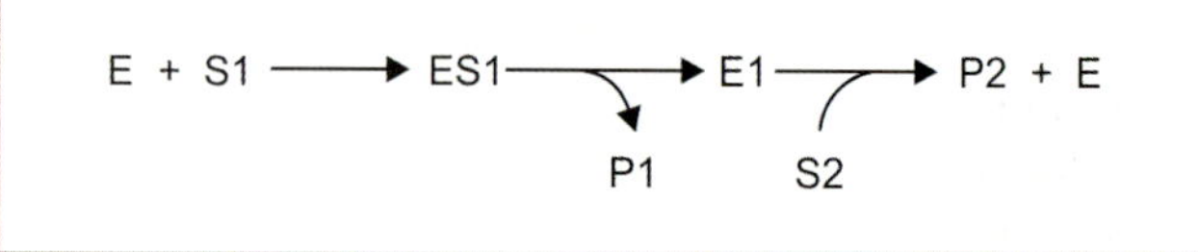

Fig. 2.7: Ping-pong mechanism of enzyme catalyzed reaction

Sequential Mechanism

In sequential mechanism, the reaction is bimolecular, i.e. if there are two substrates (S1 and S2), both of them bind with the enzyme before the reaction occurs and

2

the product is released. An example is a dehydrogenase catalyzed reaction where the second substrate is a coenzyme (NAD^+ or FAD). These reactions are also designated as single displacement reactions because the group undergoing transfer is directly passed from the donor (the first substrate) to the acceptor (the second substrate).

MECHANISMS OF ENZYME CATALYSIS

In the initial stage of the reaction, the reactants and the products are in states of minimum free energy, whereas the transition state corresponds to the point of highest free energy. The difference in free energy between the reactants and the transition state is known as the **free energy of activation** (ΔG°). A catalyst such as an enzyme acts by lowering the transition state free energy for the reaction it catalyzes. The enzyme-substrate complex, in the transition state, can breakdown to products or go back to reactants. Since the overall energy difference between the reactants and the products is the same, the enzyme equally accelerates the forward and the backward reaction (Fig. 2.8).

Enzymatic catalysis may take place by several processes (Table 2.7).

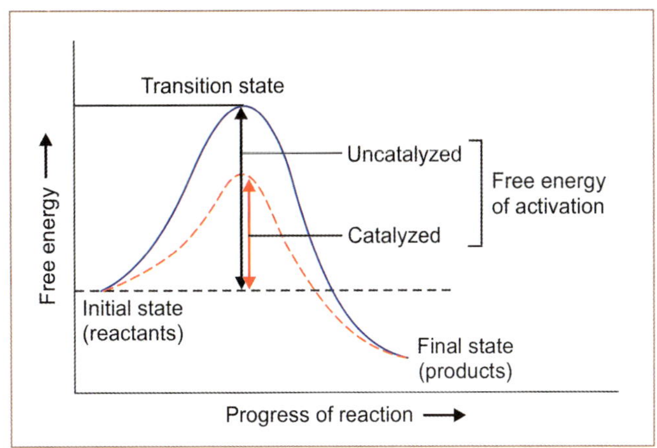

Fig. 2.8: Energy state for a catalyzed versus a noncatalyzed reaction

Table 2.7: Mechanisms of enzyme catalysis

Mechanism	Example
Acid–Base Catalysis: The catalytic activity of an enzyme may be sensitive to pH, since pH can influence the state of protonation of the side chain at the active site. At physiological pH, the protonated form of histidine is the most important general acid while its conjugate base is an important general base. Besides, the imidazole group of histidine, the –SH group of cysteine, the –OH group of tyrosine, and the ε-amino group of lysine can also act as acids. The general bases are carboxylic acid anions and the conjugate bases of the general acids.	**Ribonuclease A** (RNase-A, a digestive enzyme secreted by the pancreas into the small intestine) hydrolyzes RNA to its component nucleotides with the formation of 2′,3′-cyclic nucleotides as the intermediates. The enzyme has two His residues, His-12 and His-119, which act in a concerted manner as a general base and general acid, respectively.
Covalent Catalysis: It accelerates the reaction rate through the transient formation of a catalyst-substrate covalent bond, by the reaction of a nucleophilic group (negatively charged) on the catalyst with an electrophilic group (positively charged) on the substrate. Hence, this form of catalysis is also called nucleophilic catalysis.	**Functional groups in proteins,** such as the ε-amino group of Lys, the imidazole group of His, the –SH group of Cys, the –COOH group of Asp and the –OH group of Ser, which have high polarity, are good covalent catalysts. In addition, several coenzymes, such as TPP and pyridoxal phosphate, also function in association with their apoenzymes, as covalent catalysts. Serine proteases, such as trypsin, chymotrypsin and thrombin are some other examples.
Metal Ion Catalysis: Metalloenzymes require the presence of a metal ion (Fe^{2+}, Fe^{3+}, Cu^{2+}, Zn^{2+}, etc.) for their catalytic activity. Metal ions facilitate substrate binding and thus catalysis, by forming several kinds of bridge complexes of the enzyme, the metal and the substrate.	**Carbonic anhydrase** contains Zn^{2+} which is implicated in the catalytic mechanism of the enzyme.
Transition State Stabilization: In an enzyme catalyzed reaction, the point of highest free energy is called the transition state of the system. An enzyme binds in the transition state of the reaction it catalyzes with greater affinity than either of its substrate or the product.	By taking the **enzyme-substrate complex in the transition state** as an antigen, antibodies can be synthesized artificially. These antibodies have catalytic activity and are called abzymes. The potential applications of catalytic antibodies are discussed later.

FACTORS AFFECTING ENZYME ACTIVITY

Enzymes exhibit maximum activity under optimal conditions. The activity of an enzyme is markedly affected by several factors as discussed below.

1. Temperature

Rate of an enzyme-catalyzed reaction increases with the increase in temperature of the reaction mixture, because a rise in temperature increases the energy of activation of the system which in turn increases reaction velocity. But it is possible only up to an **'optimum temperature'** which is defined as the temperature at which enzyme activity is maximum. For most of the enzymes, optimum temperature is near the body temperature, i.e. 37°C. With further rise in the temperature, the enzyme (protein) is denatured and results in a loss of its activity. The relationship of the enzyme activity to a change in temperature is usually represented by a bell-shaped curve, the peak of which denotes optimum temperature (Fig. 2.9).

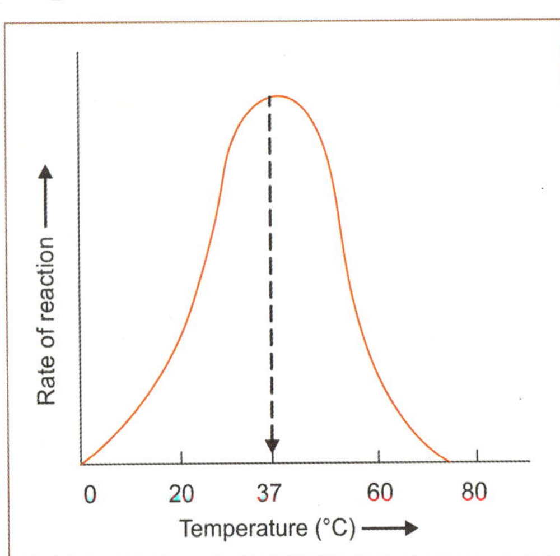

Fig. 2.9: Effect of temperature on enzyme activity

2. pH

The relationship between enzyme activity and pH of the reaction medium is also represented by a bell-shaped curve which has its peak at the **optimum pH**. This pH is characteristic for each enzyme (Fig. 2.10).

Optimum pH for most of the intracellular enzymes is in the neutral range, i.e. around 7.0. The optimum pH for pepsin, however, is about 2.0 while for the enzymes of the pancreatic juice, optimum pH is nearly 8.0. The optimum pH of an enzyme depends upon the ionization of the enzyme as well as of the substrate. A change in pH affects ionization of the protein molecule thereby decreasing the number of active sites. At an

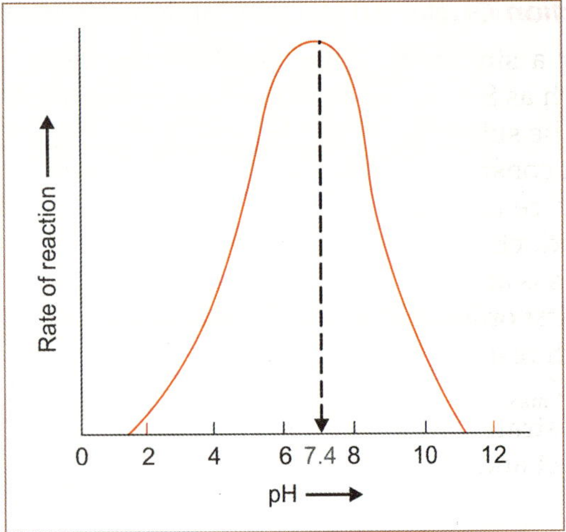

Fig. 2.10: Effect of pH on enzyme activity

extremely low or high pH, enzyme (protein) gets denatured.

3. Substrate Concentration

For an enzyme catalyzed reaction (with a single substrate and a single product), the reaction rate is directly proportional to substrate concentration. If the concentration of a substrate (S) is increased while all other conditions are kept constant, the measured initial velocity (V_0), i.e. the reaction velocity at zero time, increases as the substrate concentration increases, up to a point where the enzyme is said to be saturated with the substrate. The measured initial velocity reaches a maximal value and is unaffected by a further increase in the substrate concentration. This, however, is true only up to a certain point, i.e. the point at which the enzyme will be working at its maximum velocity (V_{max}). Any further increase in substrate concentration, thereafter, does not increase the reaction rate (Fig. 2.11).

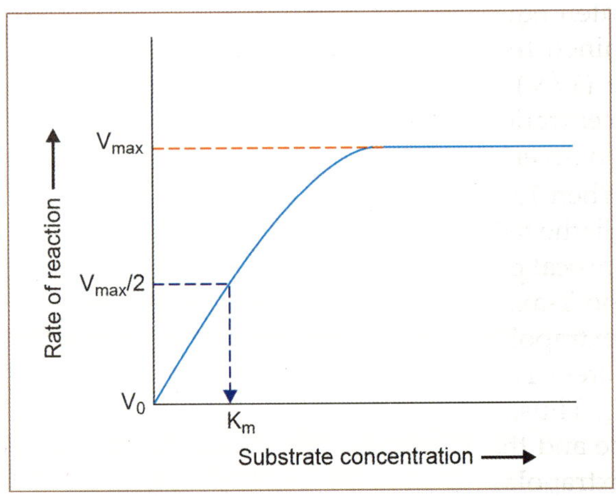

Fig. 2.11: Effect of substrate concentration on enzyme activity

2

Reaction Order

- For a simple one-substrate/one-product reaction such as $S \rightarrow P$, the reaction velocity is proportional to the substrate concentration, i.e. $V = k[S]$ where k is a constant. This is a **first order reaction**.
- For reactions involving multiple substrates/products such as $S1 + S2 \rightarrow P1 + P2$, $V = k[S1][S2]$. This is an overall **second order reaction** although it is first order with respect to S1 as well as first order with respect to S2.
- If V_{max} (maximum velocity) is independent of substrate concentration, it indicates a saturation effect and the reaction is **zero order**.

Michaelis-Menten Equation

The relationship between substrate concentration and reaction velocity can be derived by Michaelis-Menten equation. Michaelis-Menten proposed that an enzyme (E) forms enzyme-substrate complex (ES), with a single substrate (S). The complex (ES) is broken down, relatively slowly, into free enzyme (E) and the product (P). Accordingly, Michaelis-Menten derived an equation called **Michaelis-Menten equation**, where V_0 is the initial reaction velocity, V_{max} is the maximum velocity of a reaction [S], is concentration of the substrate and $\mathbf{K_m}$ is a constant, called **Michaelis constant**.

MICHAELIS CONSTANT

Michaelis constant **(K_m)** is defined as the concentration of the substrate at which the reaction velocity is half of the maximum velocity ($V_{max/2}$). It is independent of the enzyme concentration. Therefore, if an enzyme has a small value of K_m, it achieves maximal catalytic efficiency at low substrate concentration.

For convenience, a linear form of the Michaelis-Menten equation is used to determine K_m and V_{max} obtained from a plot of the reciprocal of the reaction rate (1/V) against the reciprocal of the substrate concentration, 1/[S]. The Michaelis-Menten equation, when inverted, can be written as shown in Fig. 2.12.

When $1/V_0$ (the reciprocal of V_0) is plotted against 1/[S] (the reciprocal of [S]), such a plot is called a double reciprocal plot or Lineweaver-Burk plot. The intercept at the Y-axis is given by $1/V_{max}$. On the other hand, the extrapolation at the X-axis (the negative X intercept) denotes $-1/K_m$. The slope of the plot represents $-K_m/V_{max}$. Thus, K_m can be calculated by using either the slope and the Y intercept, or the negative X intercept. Its extrapolation intercepts the 1/[S] line and gives the value of $-1/K_m$, from which K_m can be calculated (Fig. 2.13).

$$E + S \underset{K_2}{\overset{K_1}{\rightleftharpoons}} ES \xrightarrow{K_3} P + E$$

$$V_0 = \frac{V_{max}[S]}{K_m + [S]}$$

$$\frac{1}{V_0} = \frac{K_m + [S]}{V_{max}[S]} \quad \text{Or}$$

$$\frac{1}{V_0} = \frac{K_m}{V_{max}} \times \frac{1}{[S]} + \frac{[S]}{V_{max}[S]} \quad \text{Or}$$

$$\frac{1}{V_0} = \frac{K_m}{V_{max}} \times \frac{1}{[S]} + \frac{1}{V_{max}}$$

Fig. 2.12: Michaelis-Menten equation (linear and reciprocal forms)

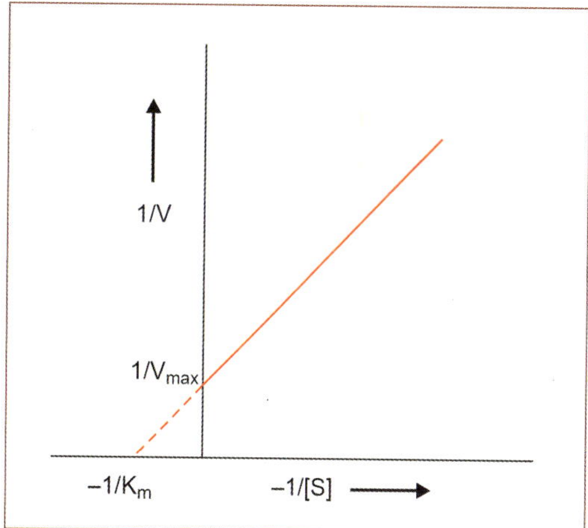

Fig. 2.13: Lineweaver-Burk plot (double-reciprocal plot)

Significance of K_m

- **Physiological significance:** Glucose can be phosphorylated to glucose-6-phosphate by glucokinase (present in the liver and is specific for glucose) or hexokinase (nonspecific for hexoses except galactose and present in all tissues). Glucokinase has a high K_m (i.e. low affinity for glucose), hence, it is important during the fed state when glucose is in excess and needs to be stored as glycogen. On the other hand, under post-absorptive/fasting conditions, hexokinase having a low K_m (i.e. high affinity for glucose) is important so that glycolysis continues to provide energy to the vital organs even at comparatively lower blood glucose levels.
- **Laboratory significance:** During enzyme assays in the laboratory, the substrate concentration is kept at saturating amounts (at least 10 times the K_m) so that the reaction proceeds to completion.

- **Clinical significance:** The K_m value for a given enzyme may differ from person to person and explains the varied response to drugs/chemicals (Chemistry to Clinics 2.3).

Chemistry to Clinics 2.3: Aldehyde Dehydrogenase

This enzyme oxidizes acetaldehyde (formed from alcohol) into acetic acid. People having a low K_m (i.e. high affinity) variant of the enzyme metabolize acetaldehyde rapidly and are less susceptible to its adverse effects such as headache and flushing. On the other hand, people having the high K_m variant are more prone to these side effects of alcohol.

4. Enzyme Concentration

The rate of an enzyme catalyzed reaction is proportional to the concentration of the enzyme presents in a reaction mixture. When concentration of the enzyme is doubled, it combines with twice the amount of substrate and the amount of product formed will also be twofold. This relationship holds good for low concentration of enzyme but with adequate substrate concentration (Fig. 2.14).

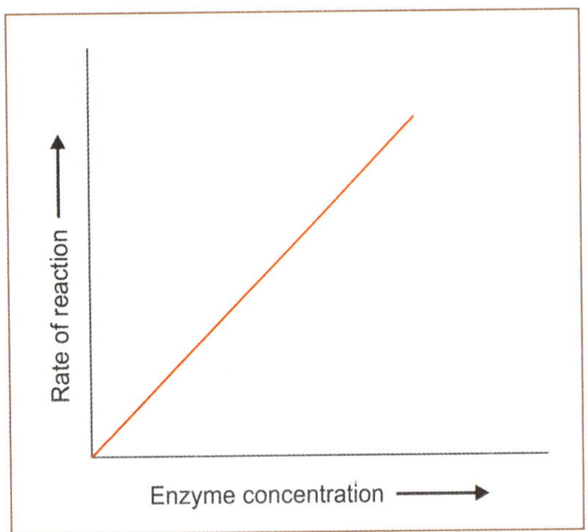

Fig. 2.14: Effect of enzyme concentration on enzyme activity

5. Enzyme Inhibition

Chemical substances which inhibit enzyme activity and reduce the velocity of an enzyme catalyzed reaction are called inhibitors, and the phenomenon is called enzyme inhibition. There are several classes of inhibitors.

Competitive Inhibitors

A substance that competes directly with a normal substrate for an enzyme's substrate-binding site is known as a competitive inhibitor. Competitive inhibition thus occurs when both substrate and inhibitor can fit into the active site and compete with each other to occupy the same. Chemical structure of the competitive inhibitor closely resembles with that of the substrate. It is called a **structural analog**. For example, in a reaction catalyzed by the enzyme succinate dehydrogenase, that converts succinate to fumarate, malonate, a structural analog of succinate, acts as a competitive inhibitor for the enzyme (Fig. 2.15).

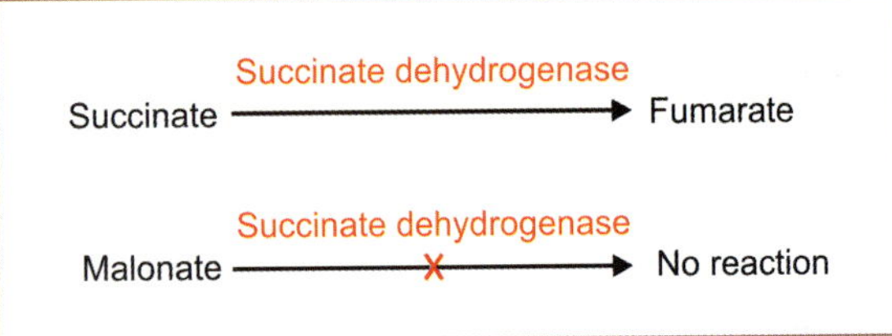

Fig. 2.15: Inhibition of succinate dehydrogenase by malonate

The inhibitor forms a complex with the enzyme called **enzyme-inhibitor** (EI) **complex**, instead of the enzyme substrate (ES) complex, and inhibits the enzyme from acting on the substrate (Fig. 2.16).

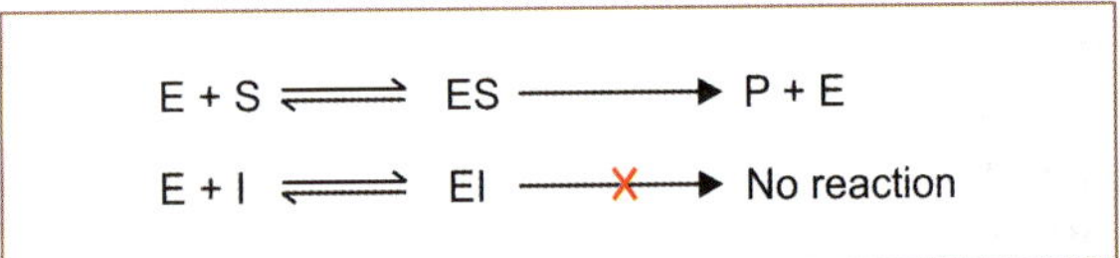

Fig. 2.16: Competitive inhibition

A competitive inhibitor, thus, reduces concentration of free enzyme available for the substrate binding. The binding of the enzyme with the inhibitor or with the substrate depends upon the relative concentrations of the substrate as well as the inhibitor. It is, therefore, usually a reversible process, as the degree of inhibition can be reduced by increasing the concentration of the substrate. The presence of a competitive inhibitor therefore increases the apparent K_m for the substrate, without any change in V_{max} (Fig. 2.17).

Some of the competitive inhibitors are given in Table 2.8.

Table 2.8: Some enzymes, their substrates and competitive inhibitors

Enzyme	Substrate	Competitive inhibitor
Succinate dehydrogenase	Succinate	Malonate
Carbonic anhydrase	Carbonate	Acetazolamide
Dihydrofolate reductase	Dihydrofolate	Amethopterin (methotrexate)
L-Histidase	L-Histidine	D-Histidine
Xanthine oxidase	Hypoxanthine	Allopurinol
HMG-CoA reductase	HMG-CoA	HMG

2

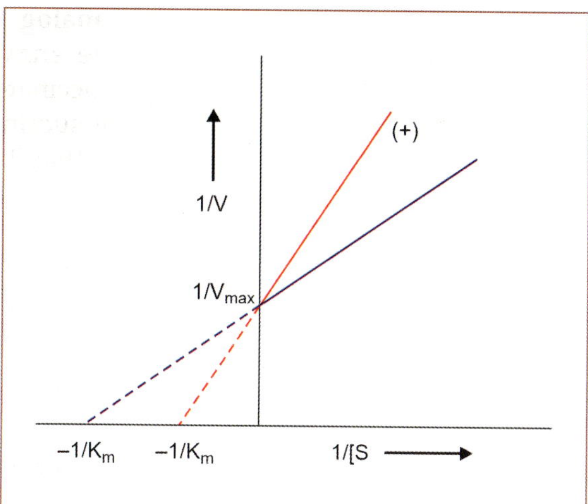

Fig. 2.17: Lineweaver-Burk plot for a competitive inhibitor (+); V_{max} unaltered, apparent K_m increased

Noncompetitive Inhibitors

The inhibitor (I) usually bears no structural similarity to the substrate (S) and thus there occurs no competition between I and S. A noncompetitive inhibitor binds at a site other than the substrate binding site, hence, the enzyme as well as the enzyme-substrate complex can bind to inhibitor. Therefore, both binary (EI) and ternary (ESI) complexes can be formed. Since, ESI may break down to form a product but at a slower rate, a reversible noncompetitive inhibitor decreases V_{max} but does not change K_m (Fig. 2.18).

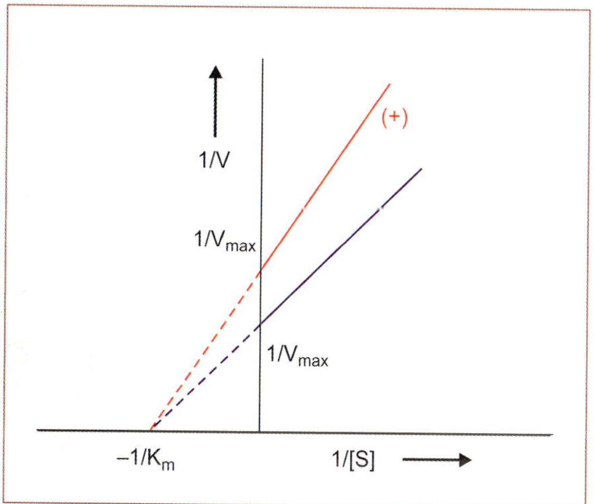

Fig. 2.18: Lineweaver-Burk plot for a noncompetitive inhibitor (+); V_{max} reduced, K_m unaltered

Antimetabolites, such as 5-fluorouracil (5-FU), act as noncompetitive inhibitors.

Uncompetitive Inhibitors

Uncompetitive inhibition occurs when the inhibitor binds after the substrate has bound to the enzyme, and then stops the reaction. The uncompetitive inhibitor affects catalytic function of the enzyme but not the substrate binding. Both K_m and V_{max} are decreased (Fig. 2.19).

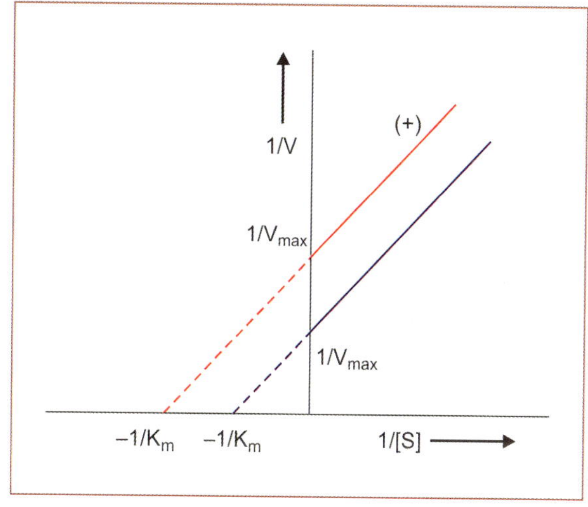

Fig. 2.19: Lineweaver-Burk plot for an uncompetitive inhibitor (+); both V_{max} and apparent K_m are reduced

Irreversible Inhibitors

Several oxidizing agents, e.g. enzyme poisons and heavy metals, cause irreversible inhibition of the enzyme activity. As these inhibitors bear no structural similarity to the substrate, the inhibition cannot be reversed by the increasing concentration of the substrate. These inhibitors result in chemical modification of the enzyme molecule and inactivate it, e.g. aspirin.

Some of the reagents that chemically modify specific amino acid residues also act as inactivators, e.g. di-isopropyl-phosphofluoridate. It is used for the detection of the active site, Ser of serine protease, and irreversibly inactivates the enzyme. These inactivators reduce V_{max} at all levels of [S], without changing K_m.

Table 2.9 summarizes the effect of various types of inhibitors on K_m and V_{max} of an enzyme catalyzed reaction.

Table 2.9: Effect of various types of inhibitors on V_{max} and K_m of an enzyme catalyzed reaction

Type of inhibition	Effect of inhibition on	
	V_{max}	K_m (Apparent change)
Reversible		
Competitive	Unaltered	↓
Noncompetitive	↓	Unaltered
Uncompetitive	↓	↓
Irreversible	↓	Unaltered

Suicide Inhibition

A special class of irreversible enzyme inhibition is referred to as suicide inhibition, where an inhibitor, such as allopurinol, binds to the active center of the enzyme xanthine oxidase and, through the catalytic action of the enzyme, is converted to a reactive compound oxypurinol that binds tightly with the functional group at the active center of the enzyme, thereby irreversibly inactivating the enzyme. This type of inhibition is also known as **mechanism-based enzyme inactivation** (the inhibitor is called a **suicide substrate** or **Trojan horse substrate**).

ENZYME INHIBITORS AS METABOLIC POISONS

Many compounds act as poisons, since they bind, covalently, to a particular enzyme or kind of enzymes, and inactivate them. For example:

- **Di-isopropylfluorophosphate:** The nerve gases, such as di-isopropylfluorophosphate (DIFP, a nerve poison), irreversibly inhibits biological systems by forming an enzyme-inhibitor complex with a specific –OH group of serine situated at the active site of certain enzymes.
- **Inhibitors of glycolysis:** Arsenate inhibits glyceraldehyde-3-phosphate dehydrogenase, whereas iodoacetate inhibits triose phosphate dehydrogenase, etc.
- **Inhibitors of the electron transport chain:** Potassium cyanide (KCN) is an irreversible inhibitor of the enzyme cytochrome C oxidase, which takes part in respiration reactions in the cells. If this enzyme is inhibited, ATP cannot be made since use of oxygen is decreased. This means that cells can only respire anaerobically, leading to a build up of lactic acid in the blood. This is potentially fatal. Malonate binds to active site of the enzyme succinate dehydrogenase competing with succinate, which is important in respiration.

ENZYME INHIBITORS AS MEDICINES

Some **enzyme inhibitors** are used as **medicines,** i.e. in the treatment of certain pathological **conditions.** For example, infections by the virus can be treated by the inhibitors of the viral enzyme protease. As a result of it, the virus cannot buildup the new protein coat and therefore, cannot replicate. **Chemotherapy** is also based on the strategic use of chemicals (the drugs) to destroy the cancer cells. Penicillin, one of the most widely used antibiotics, also functions by interfering with the synthesis of the cell walls of the reproducing bacteria. It does so by inhibiting the enzyme transpeptidase that is essential in bacterial cell wall biosynthesis, as a result of which bacterial cells burst. Human cells are not affected by it, because they have cell membranes and not the cell wall. Several types of enzyme inhibitors can be used as medicines. These include:

- **Competitive inhibitor:** Some of the **enzyme inhibitors** (competitive inhibitors) are used **as medicines** (Table 2.8).

  Besides, ethanol, a competitive inhibitor of the enzyme alcohol dehydrogenase, can be used in the treatment of methanol poisoning (Chemistry to Clinics 2.4).

Chemistry to Clinics 2.4: Ethanol in the Treatment of Methanol Poisoning

Methanol as such is only mildly toxic, in the liver. However, when acted upon by the enzyme alcohol dehydrogenase, methanol is converted into a highly toxic compound, i.e. formaldehyde.

In methanol poisoning, the toxicity of methanol can be overcome by giving ethanol. Since ethanol competes with methanol for binding to the active site of the enzyme and slows down the conversion of methanol to formaldehyde, this in turn facilitates the excretion of methanol from the body in the urine, without being converted into formaldehyde. Ethanol thus is used in the treatment of methanol poisoning due to its competitive inhibition of the enzyme alcohol dehydrogenase.

- **Antimetabolites:** Many antimetabolites, such as 5-fluorouracil (5-FU), are used as medicines (Chemistry to Clinics 2.5).

Chemistry to Clinics 2.5: Antimetabolites

Certain analogs of purines and pyrimidines (called antimetabolites) are noncompetitive inhibitors of some of the enzymes of purine/pyrimidine biosynthetic pathways. This blocks DNA synthesis hence these antimetabolites are used as anticancer drugs. For example, 5-fluorouracil, an analog of thymine inhibits thymidylate synthetase, noncompetitively (Fig. 2.20).

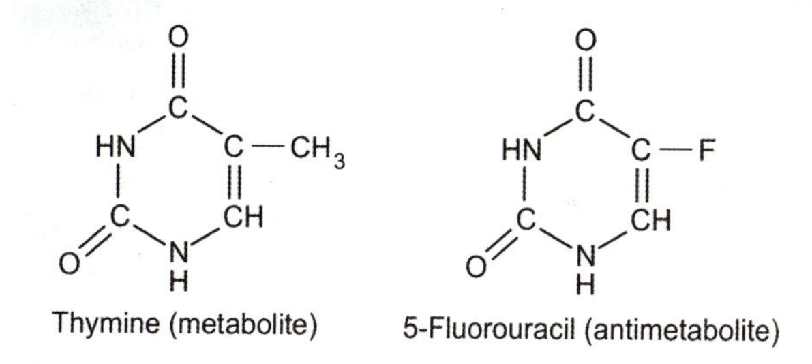

Fig. 2.20: Thymine and its structural analog 5-fluorouracil

- **Structural analogs:** A class of the enzyme inhibitors which are structural analogs of the substrate cause inhibition (suicide inhibition) of the enzyme and are used as medicines (Chemistry to Clinics 2.6).

Chemistry to Clinics 2.6: Allopurinol and Hyperuricemia

Allopurinol, a structural analog of hypoxanthine, is a competitive inhibitor as well as a substrate for xanthine oxidase. By itself, it is not capable of inhibiting the enzyme; however, when transformed to alloxanthine (oxypurinol) by the host enzyme (xanthine oxidase), it becomes a competitive inhibitor. Allopurinol, which affects both the penultimate and ultimate steps in the formation of uric acid, is used to lower plasma uric acid levels in clinical conditions associated with excessive uric acid production and hyperuricemia (e.g. gout, hematological disorders and antineoplastic therapy).

- **Uncompetitive inhibitors:** They bind directly to the enzyme-substrate complex and do not resemble the substrate (Chemistry to Clinics 2.7).

Chemistry to Clinics 2.7: Lithium in the Treatment of Manic Depressive Psychosis

Lithium (as lithium carbonate) is commonly used in the treatment of a psychiatric disorder called manic depressive psychosis (MDP), characterized by alternating periods of mania and depression. Normally, inositol monophosphatase (IMPase) catalyzes the hydrolysis of myo-inositol monophosphate to myo-inositol, which is important in stabilizing mood and behaviour through a complex mechanism. In MDP, there is altered metabolism of phosphatidylinositol in the brain. Lithium prevents inositol recycling through uncompetitive inhibition of IMPase.

- **Irreversible inhibitors:** Several oxidizing agents, e.g. enzyme poisons and heavy metals, cause irreversible inhibition of the enzyme activity. These inhibitors result in chemical modification of the enzyme molecule and inactivate it (Chemistry to Clinics 2.8).

Chemistry to Clinics 2.8: Aspirin

Eicosanoid is an important group of compounds, which are synthesized in the body from the unsaturated fatty acids. Their concentration increases during acute inflammation. For example, aspirin (acetylsalicylic acid) is a very popular nonsteroidal anti-inflammatory drug (NSAID). Aspirin irreversibly acetylates and inactivates the enzyme cyclo-oxygenase which is essential in eicosanoid biosynthesis.

Besides, reagents that chemically modify specific amino acid residues also act as inactivators, e.g. di-isopropylphosphofluoridate, used for the detection of active site Ser of serine protease, irreversibly inactivates the enzyme.

ENZYMES AS THERAPEUTIC AGENTS

Enzymes are widely used as drugs in the therapy of specific medical problems:

In the treatment of inherited disorders

1. **Adenosine deaminase (ADA):** Adenosine deaminase (ADA) is used in severe combined immuno-deficiency (SCID, due to lack of ADA); the first successful application of enzyme replacement therapy for an inherited disease.
2. **Glucocerebrosidase:** As enzyme replacement therapy for Gaucher's disease.

In treatment of acquired disorders

1. **Streptokinase:** It is obtained from streptococci and is used in blood clot-dissolution during myocardial infarction or in deep vein thrombosis. Tissue plasminogen activator (tPA) serves the same purpose.
2. **Asparaginase:** It is used for some types of leukemias based on the rationale that the tumor cells are asparagine-dependent for their multiplication and survival.
3. **Deoxyribonuclease (DNase):** It is administered by the respiratory route to clear up the viscid secretions in patients of cystic fibrosis.
4. **Serratiopeptidase**: It is used to minimize the edema that accompanies a physical trauma or an acute inflammation of the skin.
5. **Hyaluronidase:** It is used for hypodermoclysis, to facilitate the subcutaneous administration of water/electrolyte solutions in patients with hypovolemic shock where the collapsed veins are difficult to locate.
6. **Hemocoagulase:** It is used as a hemostat.
7. **Fungal diastase (amylase) and pepsin:** They are used in digestive preparations.

CLINICAL UTILITY OF SERUM ENZYMES AS MARKERS OF PATHOLOGICAL CONDITIONS

PRINCIPLES OF CLINICAL UTILITY OF SERUM ENZYMES AS MARKERS OF PATHOLOGICAL CONDITIONS

1. **Functional plasma enzymes:** These are normally present at all times in the circulation, where each one of it performs a physiological function. They are, generally, synthesized in the liver but are present in blood, in equivalent or higher concentrations than in the tissues, e.g. lipoprotein lipase, pseudocholine esterase and the enzymes of blood coagulation.
2. **Nonfunctional plasma enzymes:** These are present in very low concentrations in blood, where they perform no physiological function. Elevation in the levels of these enzymes suggests an increased rate of tissue destruction and thus, provides valuable diagnostic information to the physician.
3. **Isoenzymes:** Whenever possible, the specific isoenzyme, relevant to the clinical condition, should be estimated.
4. **Enzyme clearance:** Besides the release of the enzyme from the damaged or dying cells (resulting in increased enzyme activity in the serum), clearance of the enzyme from circulation can also influence its concentration in serum and other body fluids. For example, increased level of serum amylase after acute pancreatitis is accompanied by its increased excretion in urine.
5. **Serial analysis:** It is often clinically useful to measure the level of an enzyme activity on more than one occasion, as the time course over which enzyme activity changes is a characteristic of the condition. Further, it also helps to assess response to treatment.
6. **Supporting parameters:** Results of the enzyme analysis should always be assessed along with the results of some other nonenzymatic parameters (such as bilirubin in acute hepatitis) and the clinical findings of the patient.

SOME SERUM ENZYMES AS MARKERS OF VARIOUS PATHOLOGICAL CONDITIONS

Several enzymes are extensively used as markers of various pathological conditions. For example, creatine kinase (CK or CPK), alanine transaminase (ALT or GPT), aspartate transaminase (AST or GOT), acid phosphatase (ACP), alkaline phosphatase (ALP), etc. are used as markers in various pathological conditions such as myocardial infarction, jaundice, pancreatitis, cancer, neurodegenerative disorders, etc. They provide insight into the disease process in diagnosis, prognosis and assessment of response to therapy (Table 2.10).

Alkaline phosphatase: The reference range for serum ALP varies with age and sex, where higher levels are found in young individuals compared to the older ones, and for men compared to women. Serum ALP level is, normally, increased during pregnancy and in growing children. This increase in ALP is of placental and the bone fractions, respectively.

ALP activity is significantly **increased** in **hepatobiliary** and **bone disorders**. ALP activity is also increased in **disorders of the digestive tract** and the **liver**. On the other hand, ALP activity is **decreased** in inherited **hyperphosphatasia**.

Amylase: Estimation of amylase activity in **serum as well as urine** is of significance in the diagnosis of diseases of the pancreas (**P-type amylase**) and the salivary glands (**S-type amylase**). In **acute pancreatitis,** a transient **rise in serum amylase** activity **(P-type)** occurs within 2 to 12 hours of onset of the disease (4–6 folds) and the level returns towards normal by 3rd to 5th day. **Diseases of the salivary glands**, e.g. mumps, also cause **increase in serum amylase** activity (S-type).

Aldolase: Aldolase is present mostly in the skeletal and cardiac muscles. Damage to skeletal muscle produces high serum level of aldolase, particularly, in progressive muscular dystrophy. Serum aldolase activity is also slightly increased in early stage of viral hepatitis and advanced cancer of the prostate.

Lipase: Lipase is an enzyme secreted by the pancreas into the duodenum. Damage to the pancreas, such as in acute pancreatitis, results in the secretion of lipase in serum, from the secretory cells. Serum lipase activity increases within 4 to 8 hours of acute pancreatitis and returns towards normal in 7 to 14 days, post-treatment.

Gamma-glutamyl transpeptidase: Gamma-glutamyl transpeptidase, also referred to as gamma-glutamyl transferase or GGT (γ-GT) catalyzes the transfer of the γ-glutamyl residue from γ-glutamyl peptides to amino acids. This epithelial enzyme is also responsible for the catabolism of extracellular glutathione. It is present in the kidneys, brain, prostate, pancreas and liver. The reference range for serum GGT is 6 to 55 U/L for men and 5 to 38 U/L for women. Values are slightly lower in females due to higher levels of estrogen and progesterone.

Table 2.10: Diagnostic significance of enzymes

Enzyme	Principle source	Clinical situation in which altered
Acid phosphatase	Prostate, RBC	**Increases** in carcinoma of prostate
Alkaline phosphatase	Liver, bone, placenta, kidney	**Increases** in obstructive jaundice, rickets, Paget's disease, hyperparathyroidism
Aldolase	Skeletal muscle, heart	**Increases** in muscular dystrophies, acute liver disease
Amylase	Salivary glands, pancreas, ovaries	**Increases** in acute pancreatitis, intestinal obstruction, acute parotitis **Decreases** in acute liver diseases
Ceruloplasmin	Liver	**Increases** in cirrhosis **Decreases** in Wilson's disease
Choline esterase	Liver	**Increases** in nephrotic syndrome, organophosphorus poisoning **Decreases** in acute liver diseases
Creatine phosphokinase	Skeletal muscle, brain, heart	**Increases** in myocardial infarction, muscular dystrophies
Glutamate oxaloacetate transaminase (GPT)	Liver, skeletal muscle, heart, kidney, RBCs	**Increases** in myocardial infarction, toxic liver cell necrosis, acute liver disease, muscle disease
γ-Glutamyltransferase	Liver, kidney	**Increases** in alcoholism, hepatobiliary disease
Lactate dehydrogenase	Heart, liver, skeletal muscle, RBCs, platelets	**Increases** in acute myocardial infarction, acute hepatitis, muscle disorders
Lipase	Pancreas	**Increases** in acute pancreatitis, pancreatic carcinoma **Decreases** in liver disease, diabetes mellitus
5′-Nucleotidase	Hepatobiliary tract	**Increases** in liver disease, obstructive jaundice, hepatic carcinoma
Trypsin	Pancreas	**Increases** in acute pancreatic disease

Serum GGT activity increases in obstructive diseases of the biliary tract and in liver cancer. The estimation of serum enzyme activity is, especially, useful in assessing liver functions associated with the alcohol-induced liver disease. Its levels are also increased in chronic alcoholics, in patients who take enzyme-inducing drugs such as warfarin and phenytoin, as well as in conditions like pancreatitis and diabetes mellitus. High serum GGT levels are also associated with high rates of all-cause mortality.

Creatine phosphokinase: Total creatine phosphokinase (CPK) activity has been suggested as an excellent marker for acute myocardial infarction (heart damage) as well as skeletal muscle damage. Besides, CPK activity also rises and falls rapidly, and coincides with a variety of other conditions including surgical procedures and vigorous exercise.

As discussed earlier, CPK exists in three isomeric forms and that the estimation of its serum isoenzymes activity is of more clinical utility than the total enzyme activity. Serum CK-1 activity increases in patients with cerebrovascular diseases and head injury. Serum CK-2 isoenzyme activity is present in very small amount in normal individuals, but the activity rises within 4–6 hours of myocardial infarction, reaching to maximum within 1 day of the infarction. CK-3 activity is greatly elevated in all types of muscular dystrophies.

Lactate dehydrogenase: The reference range for total LDH activity in serum is 125 to 220 U/L. As discussed earlier, LDH exists in five isomeric forms and that the estimation of its isoenzymes in serum is of more clinical utility than its total activity. Normally, serum level of LDH-2 is higher than those of the other isoenzymes.

Certain diseases have classic patterns of elevated LDH isoenzyme levels. For example, an LDH-1 level higher than that of LDH-2 is indicative of heart attack or injury; elevations of LDH-2 and LDH-3 indicate lung injury or lung disease; elevations of LDH-4 and LDH-5 indicate liver or muscle disease, or both. A rise of all the isoenzymes at the same time is diagnostic of injury to multiple organs. One of the most important diagnostic uses for serum LDH isoenzymes is in differential diagnosis of myocardial infarction (or heart attack).

Total LDH activity in serum is increased within 24–48 hours after a heart attack, with a peak in 2–3 days, and the serum LDH activity returns to normal in, approximately, 5–10 days. This pattern is a useful tool for the delayed diagnosis of heart attack. The LDH-1 isoenzyme activity in serum, however, is a more sensitive index than total LDH activity. Normally, the level of LDH-2 is higher than LDH-1. Higher serum LDH-1 activity than LDH-2, a phenomenon known as **flipped ratio**, is strongly indicative of heart attack (Chemistry to Clinics 2.9).

Chemistry to Clinics 2.9: Flipped Ratio

LDH-1 and LDH-2 predominate in myocardium and RBC, respectively. Normally, serum LDH-1 concentration is less than that of LDH-2, i.e. LDH-1/LDH-2 ratio is <1. Serum LDH-1 activity becomes greater than LDH-2 (known as a flipped LDH ratio) between 12–24 hours following myocardial infarction.

Transaminases: Transaminases (aminotransferases) are a group of enzymes that catalyzes the conversion of amino acids to alpha-keto acids, by the transfer of the alpha-amino group. Two of these transaminases, referred to as aspartate aminotransferase (**AST**), also referred to as glutamic-oxaloacetic transaminase (**GOT**), and alanine aminotransferase (**ALT**), also called serum glutamate pyruvate transaminase (**GPT**) have clinical utility. They are present in the liver, cardiac tissue and skeletal muscle, with smaller amounts in the kidneys, pancreas and erythrocytes. The reference range for ALT is 7–45 U/L and that of AST is 5–35 U/L.

Serum activities of both (ALT and AST) the enzymes are used as markers of a liver disease, however, ALT is more specific than AST. So, when liver cells are damaged, serum activities of both the enzymes, i.e. ALT and AST, are increased. In hepatitis, transaminases levels rise several days before the jaundice begins. The enzyme levels are also useful in assessing subtle and early changes in biliary obstruction and active cirrhosis. Besides, serum AST levels are also significantly increased in skeletomuscular disorders and pulmonary embolism. Estimation of serum AST activity is used to diagnose myocardial infarction within 10–48 hours. Other conditions with elevated AST include arrhythmias and severe angina.

INTERPRETATION OF LABORATORY RESULTS OF ENZYME ACTIVITIES

Interpretation of laboratory results of several enzyme activities are of clinical utility, particularly, in the diagnosis of liver and cardiac disorders (Chemistry to Clinics 2.10 and 2.11).

Chemistry to Clinics 2.10: Liver Enzyme Panel

Liver enzyme panel includes the estimation of serum transaminases (**ALT** and **AST**), alkaline phosphatase (**ALP**) and γ-glutamyl transpeptidase (**γ-GT**).

- **Transaminases:** Both, serum AST and ALT levels are raised, even before the clinical signs and symptoms of the disease appear, in the liver. However, ALT is more specific, where the levels may show multi-fold increases. Duration of the illness is variable and that the serum enzyme activity is increased for sometime even after clinical recovery (Fig. 2.21).

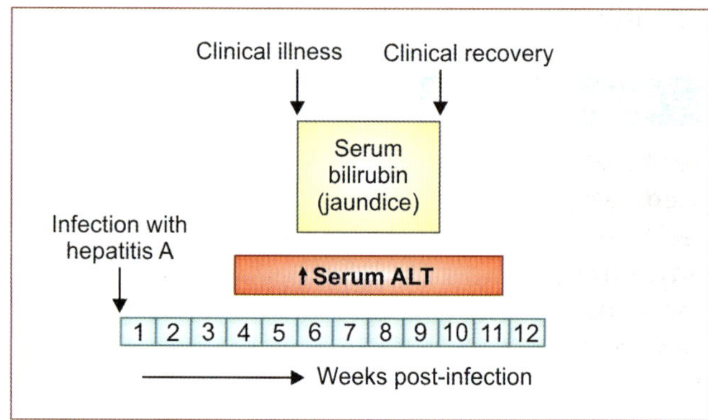

Fig. 2.21: Serum alanine transaminase (ALT) is raised prior to serum bilirubin in viral hepatitis. High levels persist for sometime even after clinical recovery and clearance of jaundice

- **Alkaline phosphatase:** Intrahepatic obstruction of the bile flow raises serum ALP to a lesser extent, i.e. up to 2–3 times of the upper normal limit only. However, a marked rise (up to 10 times or more) occurs in **post-hepatic obstruction**.
- **γ-Glutamyl transpeptidase:** Serum γ-GT, primarily, originates from the hepatobiliary system. Its activity is increased in all forms of liver diseases. Elevated level of the enzyme, however, is of special significance in detecting **alcohol-induced liver disease**. Its levels are increased not only in patients with alcoholic cirrhosis but also in majority of people who are heavy drinkers.

Chemistry to Clinics 2.11: Cardiac Enzyme Panel

Cardiac enzyme panel includes the estimation of serum creatine phosphokinase (**CPK**, CPK-2), lactate dehydrogenase (**LDH**) and transaminases (ALT and AST).

- **CPK:** The measurement of serum CPK-2 (CK-MB) is the most commonly used enzymatic test for the diagnosis of myocardial infarction. An initial rise occurs in 4–6 hours. Peak levels are found at approximately 24 hours while return to normal occurs within 48–72 hours.
- **LDH:** Rise in LDH starts 12–18 hours after the onset of myocardial infarction, with peak at 48–72 hours. The levels return to below the upper normal level after 6–10 days. Rise in total LDH parallels LDH-1 isozyme.
- **AST and ALT:** Increased AST activity appears in serum as its concentration is highest in the cardiac muscle. Since ALT concentration is much less than AST in the cardiac muscle, it is only marginally increased. Peak level of AST is reached after 18–24 hours and falls to within normal limit by the fourth or fifth day (Fig. 2.22).

ENZYMES IN LABORATORY INVESTIGATIONS

Use of enzymes in laboratory investigations (in **enzyme-based assays**) is very common because of their high specificity and sensitivity, which permits quantitative assays on crude materials under controlled, mild reaction conditions. Applications involve determining enzyme amounts in analyses for inborn errors of metabolism, nongenetically associated diseases and in quality control of foods. Enzymes are also used to determine isomeric configuration of compounds, the primary structures of complex molecules such as proteins, nucleic acids, carbohydrates and triglycerides, the conformation of complex molecules, and the structures of cells and subcellular organelles.

COMMONLY USED ENZYMES IN LABORATORY INVESTIGATIONS

Commonly used enzymes in laboratory investigations include:

- Alcohol dehydrogenase which oxidizes alcohols
- Arginase for determination of L-arginine in plasma and urine
- Cholesterol esterase for the determination of serum cholesterol levels
- Creatine kinase in diagnosis of cardiac and skeletal malfunction
- Glycerol-3-phosphate dehydrogenase in determination of serum triglycerides
- Uricase for determination of uric acid
- Glucose oxidase for glucose estimation
- Horseradish peroxidase for the oxidation of a wide variety of substrates.

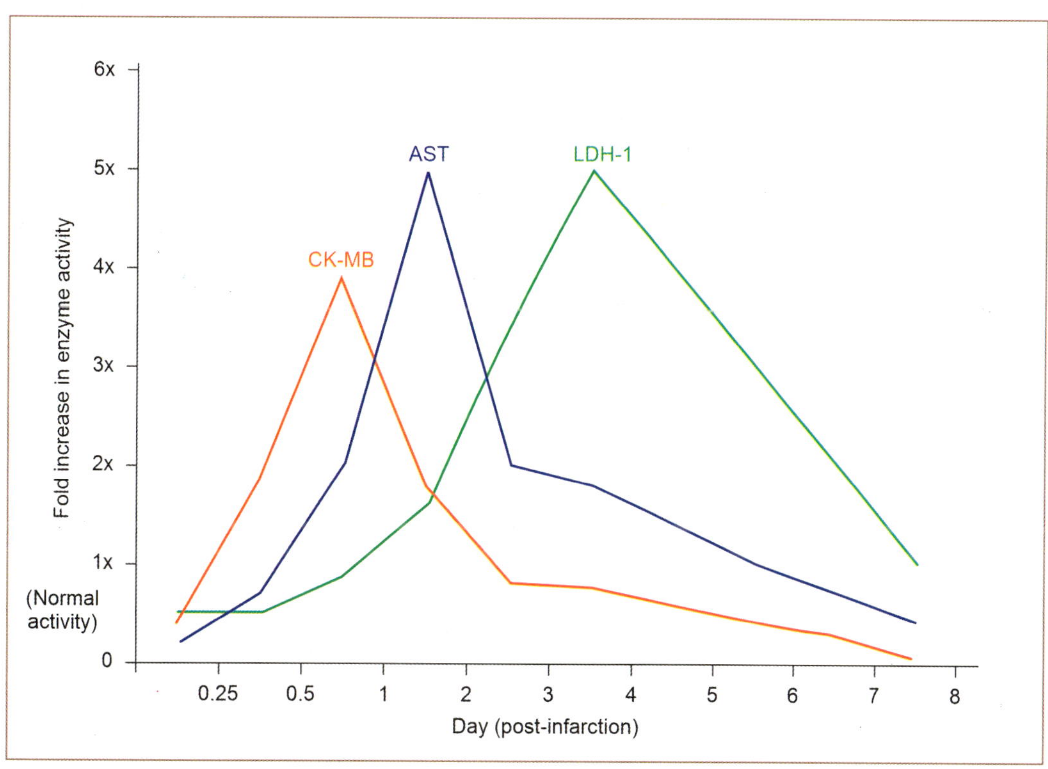

Fig. 2.22: Serum enzyme profile in myocardial infarction

2

ENZYME-BASED ASSAYS

Enzyme-based assays are routinely being used in laboratory investigations in procedures such as dipsticks, immobilized enzymes, enzyme-linked immunosorbent assays and enzyme biosensors.

Dipsticks

A dipstick is one of several measurement devices, which are dipped into a liquid to perform a chemical test. In medicine, dipsticks are used to test for a variety of liquids for the presence of a given substance, known as an analyte. For example, urine dipsticks are used to test urine samples for hemoglobin, nitrite (produced by bacteria in a urinary tract infection), protein, glucose and occasionally urobilinogen or ketones.

The dipstick is a point of care testing (POCT) technology that has stood the test of time and is used frequently by patients, nurses and doctors. In its simplest form a urine sample is applied to a porous pad containing reagent(s) and reflectance technology is used to provide a semi-quantitative estimate of the analyte. Dipsticks can detect one or up to 10 analytes and can be used in conjunction with a small reading device in order to reduce potential operator error. Dipsticks for glucose contain the enzyme glucose oxidase immobilized onto the paper pad at the end of the stick. This enzyme oxidizes glucose to yield gluconic acid and hydrogen peroxide. Peroxidase is also immobilized on the paper pad and it uses the hydrogen peroxide to oxidize a colored dye to a form with a different color (or no color). The degree of color change is proportional to the amount of glucose.

Immobilized Enzymes

Immobilized enzymes are chemically bonded to a solid support, e.g. agarose. When a sample containing substrate (the analyte to be estimated) is passed through the preparation, the product is retrieved and analyzed, whereas the enzyme (being a recoverable reagent) becomes free to react with more substrate. Immobilized enzymes are more stable than enzymes in solution and are suited for batch analysis. Immobilized enzyme technology has been used in the assay of blood urea nitrogen (BUN), glucose, uric acid, amino acids, ethanol and other metabolites.

An immobilized enzyme is an enzyme chemically bonded to a solid support, e.g. agarose. This can provide increased resistance to changes in conditions such as pH or temperature. It also lets enzymes be held in place throughout the reaction, following which they are easily separated from the product and may be used again, a far more efficient process and so is widely used in industry for enzyme catalyzed reactions.

Enzyme Biosensors

An enzyme biosensor is an analytical device that combines an enzyme with a transducer to produce a signal proportional to target analyte concentration. This signal can result from a change in proton concentration, release or uptake of gases, such as ammonia or oxygen, light emission, absorption or reflectance, heat emission and so forth, brought about by the reaction catalyzed by the enzyme. The transducer converts this signal into a measurable response, such as current, potential, temperature change, or absorption of light through electrochemical, thermal, or optical means. This signal can be further amplified, processed, or stored for later analysis.

Biosensors offer many advantages in comparison to many conventional analytical approaches in terms of simplicity, lower limits of detection and sensitivity. These are used to carry out ultramicroanalysis of the analyte in the fluid. At present, more and more factories in the world are developing point of care testing (POCT) devices, including hematology analyzer, electrolysis analyzer and blood gas analyzer, etc.

Enzyme-linked Immunosorbent Assays

The enzyme-linked immunosorbent assay (**ELISA**) is a commonly used analytical biochemistry assay which uses a solid-phase **enzyme immunoassay** (**EIA**) to detect the presence of a ligand (commonly a protein) in a liquid sample using antibodies directed against the protein to be measured. The sample with an unknown amount of antigen is immobilized on a solid support (usually a polystyrene microtiter plate) either non-specifically (via adsorption to the surface) or specifically (via capture by another antibody specific to the same antigen, in a sandwich ELISA). After the antigen is immobilized, the detection antibody is added, forming a complex with the antigen. The detection antibody can be covalently linked to an enzyme or can itself be detected by a secondary antibody that is linked to an enzyme through bioconjugation. Between each step, the plate is typically washed with a mild detergent solution to remove any proteins or antibodies that are non-specifically bound. After the final wash step, the plate is developed by adding an enzymatic substrate to produce a visible signal, which indicates the quantity of antigen in the sample. Enzymes such as horseradish peroxidase, alkaline phosphatase, glucose-6-phosphate dehydrogenase, β-galactosidase, etc. are commonly employed as reagents in ELISA to measure HIV antibodies, therapeutic agents, tumor antigens, etc.

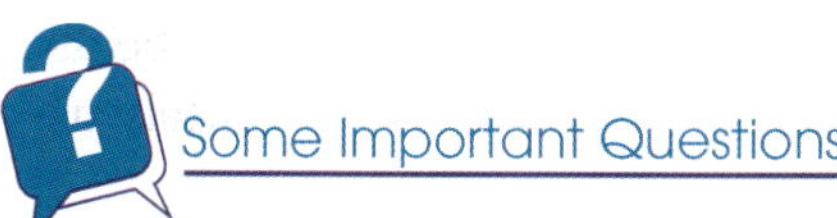

1. What are enzymes? Classify them. Discuss factors affecting enzyme activity.

2. Define enzyme, coenzyme and cofactor. Discuss the role of B-complex group of vitamins as coenzymes.

3. What are isoenzymes? Discuss the importance of enzymes in clinical diagnosis.

4. Give a brief account of factors affecting enzyme activity.

5. Discuss briefly:

i. Mechanisms of enzyme action.
ii. Various types of enzyme inhibition, giving examples.
iii. Apoenzyme, holoenzyme and coenzyme.
iv. Classification of enzymes with suitable examples.
v. Michaelis-Menten equation

6. Write notes on:

i. Diagnostic significance of enzymes
ii. Noncompetitive inhibition of enzyme activity
iii. K_m
iv. Isoenzymes and their clinical importance
v. Zymogens
vi. Competitive inhibitors
vii. Specificity of enzyme action
viii. Coenzymes
ix. Classification of enzymes
x. Ribozymes
xi. Abzymes

Multiple Choice Questions

1. The following is not a lyase:

A. Glucose-6-phosphatase
B. Aldolase
C. Argininosuccinase
D. Histidase

2. Hexokinase does not phosphorylate:

A. Glucose B. Fructose
C. Mannose D. Galactose

3. In enzyme catalysis, the following is reduced:

A. Free energy of substrate
B. Free energy of transition state
C. Free energy of product
D. All of the above

4. K_m is:

A. Directly proportional to enzyme concentration
B. Inversely proportional to enzyme concentration
C. Half of enzyme concentration
D. Independent of enzyme concentration

5. 5-Fluorouracil inhibits thymidylate synthetase by:

A. Competitive inhibition
B. Noncompetitive inhibition
C. Uncompetitive inhibition
D. Allosteric inhibition

6. Isoenzymes may be present in:

A. Different tissues
B. Different cell types of a tissue
C. Different subcellular compartments of a cell
D. All of the above

7. In myocardial infarction, the marker to rise earliest in serum is:

A. CPK-MM B. LDH-1
C. CPK-MB D. ALT

8. The following serum analyte is a good index of recent alcohol intake:

A. ALT B. γ-GT
C. LDH-5 D. Ceruloplasmin

9. Ribozymes may function in/as:

A. Intron splicing
B. Peptidyl transferase
C. Both
D. None of the above

10. Abzymes are directed against:

A. Substrate
B. Enzyme
C. Enzyme-substrate complex in transition state
D. Product

2

CHAPTER

3

Chemistry and Metabolism of Carbohydrates

Competency Achievement: The student should be able to:

BI3.1 Discuss and differentiate monosaccharides, disaccharides and polysaccharides giving examples of main carbohydrates as energy fuel, structural element and storage in the human body

BI3.2 Describe the processes involved in digestion and assimilation of carbohydrates and storage

BI3.3 Describe and discuss the digestion and assimilation of carbohydrates from food

BI3.4 Define and differentiate the pathways of carbohydrate metabolism (glycolysis, gluconeogenesis, glycogen metabolism, HMP shunt)

BI3.5 Describe and discuss the regulation, functions and integration of carbohydrate along with associated diseases/disorders

BI3.6 Describe and discuss the concept of TCA cycle as an amphibolic pathway and its regulation

BI3.7 Describe the common poisons that inhibit crucial enzymes of carbohydrate metabolism (e.g. fluoride, arsenate)

BI3.8 Discuss and interpret laboratory results of analytes associated with metabolism of carbohydrates

BI3.9 Discuss the mechanism and significance of blood glucose regulation in health and disease

BI3.10 Interpret the results of blood glucose levels and other laboratory investigations related to disorders of carbohydrate metabolism

PY4.4 Describe the physiology of digestion and absorption of nutrients

Carbohydrates, also called saccharides (Greek *Sakcharon*: Sugar), are aldehyde or ketone derivatives of polyhydroxy alcohols. They are the most abundant biological molecules containing three elements, i.e. C, H and O, which are combined as $(CH_2O)n$, where $n \geq 3$.

CLASSIFICATION OF CARBOHYDRATES

Depending upon the number of monomeric units present in the molecule, carbohydrates are classified as monosaccharides, disaccharides and polysaccharides (Fig. 3.1).

MONOSACCHARIDES

Simple sugars are called monosaccharides. They join together in various ways to form disaccharides and polysaccharides. Monosaccharides are further subdivided into different groups according to either

i. chemical nature of their carbonyl group, or

ii. number of carbon atoms in a chain (Table 3.1).

According to chemical nature of the carbonyl group monosaccharides are divided into two groups, as aldoses and ketoses:

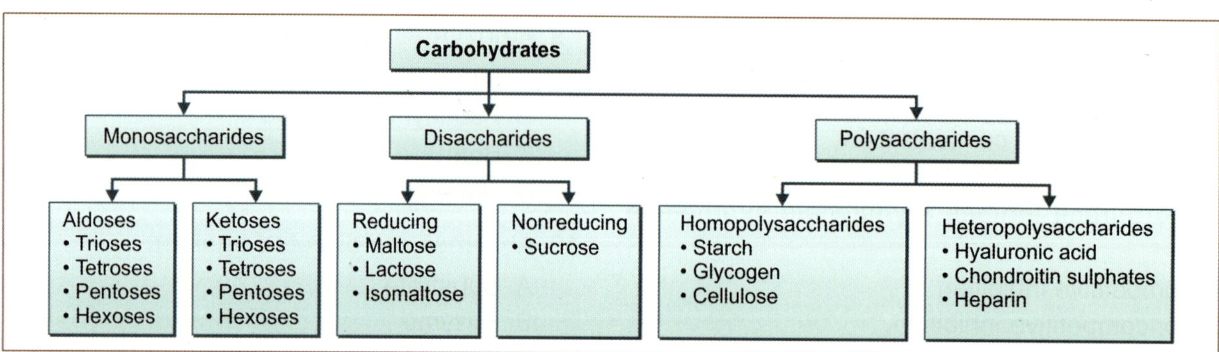

Fig. 3.1: Classification of carbohydrates

Table 3.1: Classification of monosaccharides

Monosaccharides	Number of C-atoms	Aldoses	Ketoses
Trioses	3	Glyceraldehyde	Dihydroxy-acetone
Tetroses	4	Erythrose	Erythrulose
Pentoses	5	Ribose	Ribulose
Hexoses	6	Glucose	Fructose

Aldoses: A sugar is an aldose when it contains an aldehyde (–CHO) group on C1, e.g. glucose.

Ketoses: The sugar is a ketose when it has a ketone (–CO) group at C2, e.g. fructose.

Some of the ketoses are named by inserting '-ul-' before the suffix '-ose' in the name of the corresponding aldose, e.g. erythrulose, from erythrose (an aldose).

According to the number of carbon atoms monosaccharides are designated as trioses, tetroses, pentoses, etc.

Trioses: The smallest monosaccharides with three carbon atoms, include glyceraldehyde (an aldotriose) and dihydroxyacetone (a ketotriose). Both of these molecules are of physiological significance since the phosphate esters of these sugars, i.e. glyceraldehyde-3-phosphate and dihydroxyacetone phosphate, are important intermediates in glycolysis.

Tetroses: These are compounds with four carbon atoms, e.g. erythrose (an aldotetrose) and erythrulose (a ketotetrose). Erythrose, as erythrose-4-phosphate, is an intermediate in hexose monophosphate (HMP) shunt.

Pentoses: These are sugars containing five carbon atoms such as ribose (an aldopentose) and xylulose (a ketopentose) both of which are intermediates in the HMP shunt.

Ribose is also an important constituent of nucleotides present in RNA.

Hexoses: They contain six carbon atoms, e.g. glucose (an aldohexose) and fructose (a ketohexose). Glucose, commonly known as dextrose, is an important source of energy in the body. Fructose is an important constituent of the common sugar sucrose.

Some of the monosaccharides of biological significance are given in Fig. 3.2.

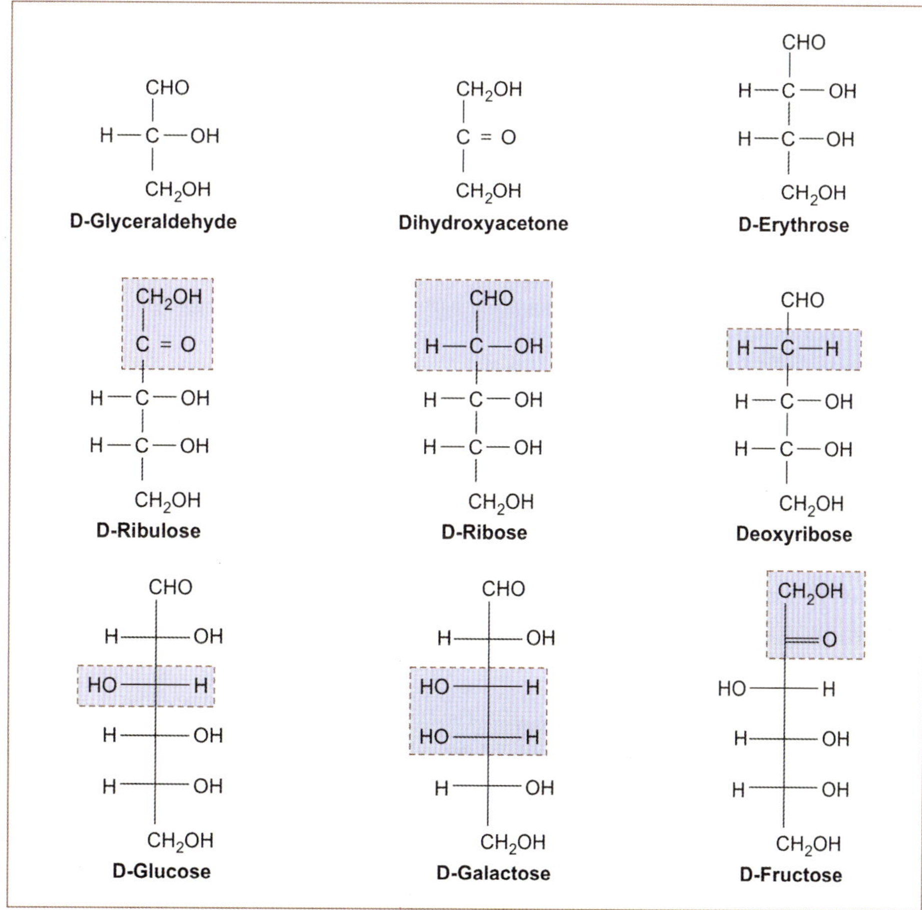

Fig. 3.2: Some monosaccharides of biological significance

DISACCHARIDES

Disaccharides consist of two similar or dissimilar units of monosaccharides linked by a glycosidic bond. Maltose, lactose and sucrose are the disaccharides of biological significance.

Maltose

Maltose consists of **two glucose** (α-D-glucopyranose) units which are linked together by α-1,4-glycosidic linkage. The symbol (1→4) indicates that the glycosidic bond links C1 of a glucose molecule to C4 of the other molecule of glucose. Accordingly, in maltose –OH group at C4 of a glucose molecule is linked to the –OH group at C1 (the anomeric carbon) of another glucose molecule. This leaves a free –OH group at the anomeric carbon (C1) of the first glucose molecule, which can form a reducing aldehyde group if the ring opens. Thus, maltose is a reducing disaccharide (Fig. 3.3).

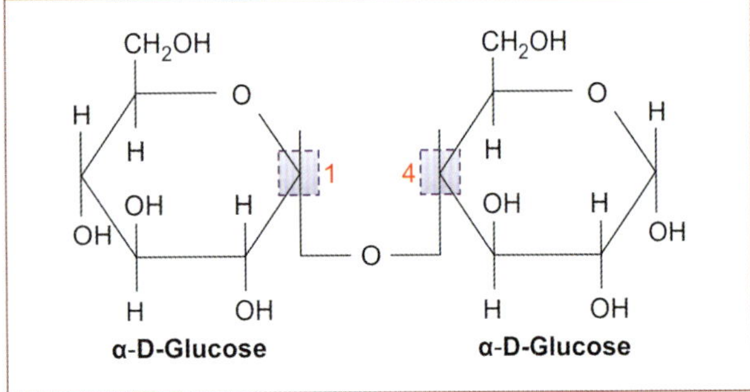

Fig. 3.3: Maltose

Maltose is usually obtained as a hydrolyzed product of polysaccharides such as starch, glycogen and dextrins. It is hydrolyzed to its component monosaccharides, i.e. the two glucose units, by the enzyme maltase in the intestinal lumen.

Lactose

Lactose (**milk sugar**) consists of galactose (β-D-galactopyranose) and glucose (β-D-glucopyranose) which are linked together by the β-1,4-glycosidic linkage. The glycoside bond links C1 of galactose to C4 of glucose residue. There is a free –OH group at the anomeric carbon (C1) of β-D-glucose, which can form a reducing aldehyde group if the ring opens. Thus, lactose is a reducing disaccharide (Fig. 3.4).

Lactose occurs naturally in milk hence, it is also called as milk sugar. In females, lactose is synthesized during lactation and is secreted in milk. During late pregnancy and lactation, lactose may be excreted in the urine of these females (physiological lactosuria). Lactose is hydrolyzed by the intestinal enzyme lactase (β-D-galactosidase) to its component monosaccharides, i.e. glucose and galactose.

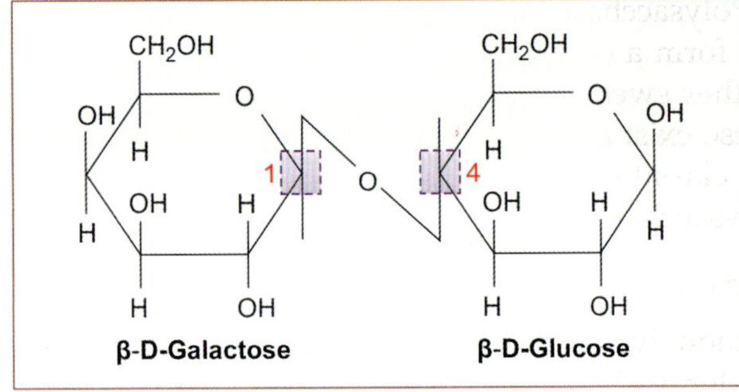

Fig. 3.4: Lactose

Sucrose

Sucrose, also called **table sugar, cane sugar** or **invert sugar**, consists of glucose (α-D-glucopyranose) and fructose (β-D-fructofuranose), which are linked by β-1, 2-glycosidic linkage (Fig. 3.5).

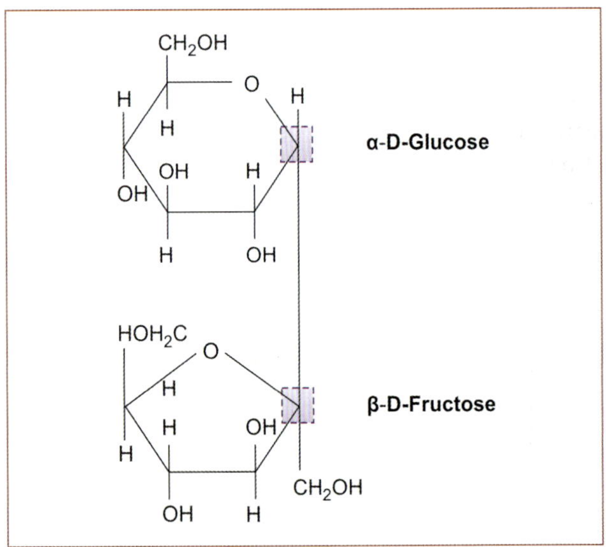

Fig. 3.5: Sucrose

Since the carbonyl groups of both the monosaccharides, i.e. the C1 in glucose and C2 in fructose participate in the glycosidic bond, there is no free carbonyl carbon on any of its monosaccharides. Thus, sucrose is a non-reducing sugar. Sucrose is the most abundant disaccharide found in plants and is familiar to human beings as table sugar. It is hydrolyzed to its monosaccharide components, i.e. glucose and fructose, by the intestinal sucrase (also called invertase).

POLYSACCHARIDES

Polysaccharides are also called glycans. These are polymers of large number of monosaccharides which are linked together by the glycosidic bonds. Where the number of monosaccharide units is <10, these are termed **oligosaccharides**.

Polysaccharides are sparingly soluble in cold water but form a colloidal solution in hot water. These are neither sweet in taste nor have reducing properties. These exist as linear and/or branched polymers, and are classified as homopolysaccharides and heteropolysaccharides.

Homopolysaccharides

Homopolysaccharides (homoglycans) are the polymers of identical monosaccharide units. Common homopolysaccharides of biological significance are starch, glycogen and cellulose (the homopolymers of glucose, also called glucosans), and inulin (the homopolymer of fructose, also called fructosan).

Starch

Starch is stored as a reservoir of food in cereals and tubers of plants. Starch consists of two polysaccharides, i.e. α-amylose and amylopectin.

The α-amylose is a linear polymer of glucose residues linked by α-(1→4) glycosidic bonds. Amylopectin is a branched molecule with, both, α-1, 4 straight chain and α-(1→6) branch points, which occur after every 24–30 glucose residues (Fig. 3.6).

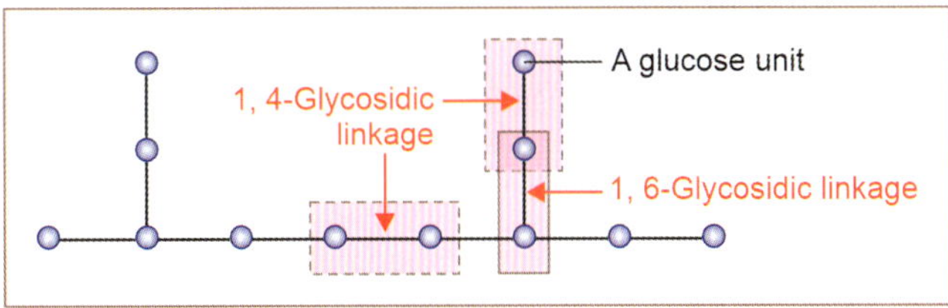

Fig. 3.6: Starch

Starch is a main source of carbohydrate in the human diet. Amylase presents in the saliva and in the pancreatic juice randomly hydrolyses α-(1→4) glycosidic bonds of starch and degrades it to a mixture of maltose, maltotriose and dextrins.

Glycogen

Glycogen is the storage polysaccharide of animals and is, therefore, also called **animal starch**. It is present in all cells but is most prevalent in the skeletal muscle and the liver. Structure of glycogen is similar to amylopectin with a linear chain of α-(1→4) glycosidic bonds and α-(1→6) branch points, but branching occurs more frequently, i.e. after every 10–12 glucose residues. Glycogen is, thus, highly branched with a tree-like structure (Fig. 3.7).

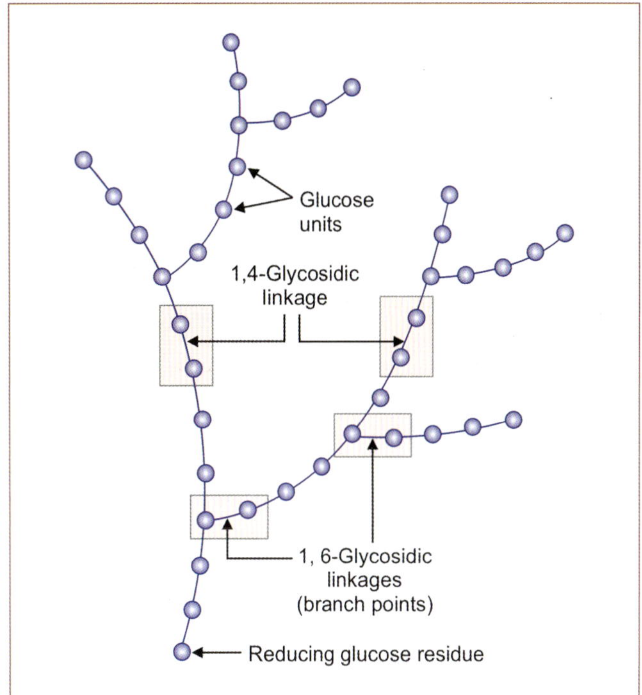

Fig. 3.7: Glycogen

In the liver, glycogen serves as a readily available source of glucose, especially, during the initial 18–24 hours of fasting.

Table 3.2 lists various differences between starch and glycogen.

Table 3.2: Differences between starch and glycogen

Starch	Glycogen
• It is a plant reserve food that is mostly stored in seeds	• It is an animal reserve food that is mainly stored in the liver and muscle
• It is less branched. Branching occurs after nearly 20–30 glucose units	• It is highly branched. Branching occurs after nearly 10–12 glucose units
• It consists of two structural units referred to as amylose and amylopectin	• No amylose and amylopectin-like structures are present
• It is sparingly soluble in cold water and forms a paste in hot water	• It forms an opalescent solution in water
• It gives violet color with iodine	• It gives brown to red color with iodine

Cellulose

Cellulose is the primary structural component of the plant cell wall. It is a linear polymer of [-β-D-glucosyl-(1→4)-α-D-glucosyl-] repeating units (Fig. 3.8).

3

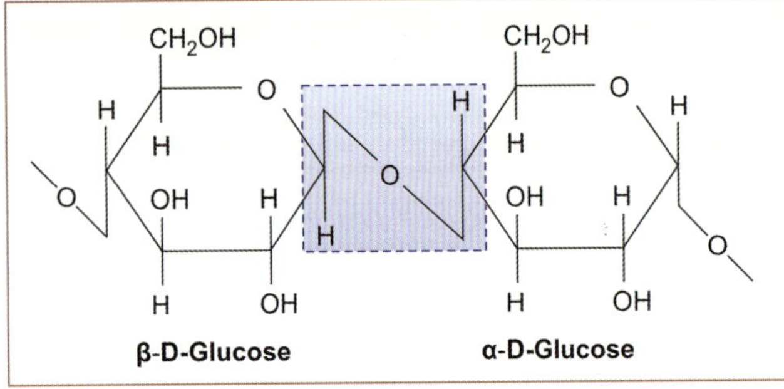

Fig. 3.8: Cellulose

Cellulose cannot be digested by human beings because of lack of cellulases, the enzymes which are capable of hydrolyzing β-(1→4)-glycosidic linkages present in cellulose. Cellulose though cannot be utilized by the human body, it still forms a considerable part of the vegetable food and adds to the bulk of the feces.

Inulin

Inulin is a linear polymer of β-D-fructose. It occurs in bulbs of dahlia, onion and garlic. Though, inulin is not utilized by human beings, it is of biological significance as it is used for determining the glomerular filtration rate (GFR).

Dextrans

Dextrans are highly branched homopolymers of glucose units with 1–6, 1–4 and 1–3 linkages. They are produced by various microorganisms growing in sucrose media. They have high molecular weight. They are used in:

1. Intravenous infusion as plasma volume expanders in the treatment of hypovolemic shock.
2. Food additives and as cryopreservatives.

Chitin

Chitin is present in the exoskeleton of insects and is composed of units of N-acetyl-glucosamine joined by β-1,4-glycosidic linkages.

Heteropolysaccharides

Heteropolysaccharides (heteroglycans) are the polymers of nonidentical monosaccharide units, also referred to as glycosaminoglycans (GAGs). The GAGs (originally designated as mucopolysaccharides) are large complexes of negatively charged heteropolysaccharides associated with a small amount of protein, forming proteoglycans, which are the gel forming components of the extracellular matrices. The GAGs are unbranched polysaccharides and consist of alternating uronic acid and hexosamines residues. Solutions of GAGs have slimy, mucus-like consistency due to their high viscosity and elasticity. Most important glycosaminoglycans are hyaluronic acid, chondroitin sulfates, heparin, etc. (Fig. 3.9).

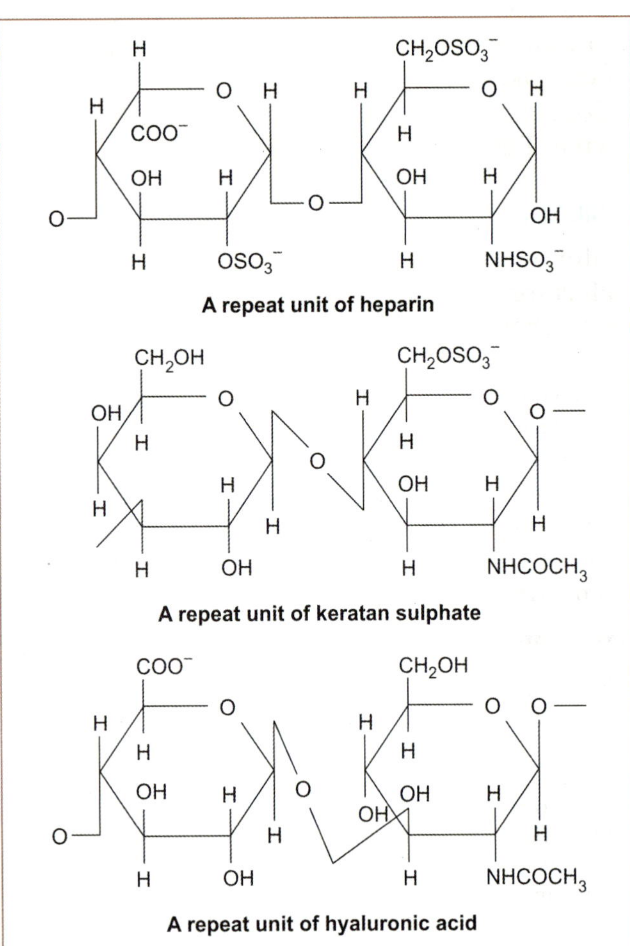

Fig. 3.9: Some of the heteropolysaccharides

Functions of Glycosaminoglycans

1. Provide structural support to tissues, especially cartilage and connective tissue.
2. Enable the tissues to withstand torsion and shock.
3. Provide a balance between integrity and flexibility.
4. Perform specific functions in certain organs such as liver, kidney, cornea, etc.

Structure and Classification of Glycosaminoglycans

Each glycosaminoglycan chain is composed of a repeating disaccharide unit which comprises an acidic sugar and an amino sugar, i.e. it has the structure as:

$$[\text{Acidic sugar} - \text{Amino sugar}]_n$$

The acidic sugar is either D-glucuronic acid or its carbon-5 epimer, called L-iduronic acid. The amino sugar is either D-glucosamine or D-galactosamine in which the amino group is usually acetylated. It may also be sulfated on carbon-4 or -6, or on nonacetylated nitrogen.

The GAGs are divided into six major classes according to monomeric composition, type of glycosidic linkage and degree and location of sulfate units.

Composition of GAGs and their distribution are given in Table 3.3.

Hyaluronic Acid

Hyaluronic acid is composed of repeating units of D-glucuronic acid and N-acetyl-D-glucosamine. This polysaccharide chain is the longest of the GAGs and is the only one which is non-sulfated. It is not covalently attached to protein and is not limited to animal tissues but also found in bacteria. It is an important component of synovial fluid and the vitreous humor. The viscoelastic behavior of hyaluronate solution makes them excellent biological shock absorbers and lubricants. Its concentration is decreased in osteoarthritis (Chemistry to Clinics 3.1).

Chemistry to Clinics 3.1: Osteoarthritis

Degenerative disorders of large weight-bearing joints, e.g. knee joints, are common in old age. However, obesity may result in premature osteoarthritis. The condition is characterized by reduced joint space, damage to articular cartilage and limitation of movement associated with reduced content of hyaluronic acid in synovial fluid. Commercially available hyaluronic acid is sometimes required to be injected intra-articularly.

Chondroitin Sulfates

Chondroitin sulfates contain glucuronic acid and N-acetylgalactosamine with sulfate on the hydroxyl group of either carbon-4 (chondroitin-4-sulfate) or carbon-6 (chondroitin-6-sulfate). They are the major components of cartilage where they bind collagens and hold fibers in a tight, strong network. They are also found in aorta, tendons and ligaments.

Dermatan Sulfate

Dermatan sulfate is derived from chondroitin by enzymatic epimerization of carbon-5 of glucuronate residues to form iduronate residues. Thus, dermatan sulfate contains L-iduronic acid (with variable amounts of glucuronic acid) and N-acetylgalactosamine. It is found in skin, blood vessels, tendons and heart valves.

Heparan Sulfate

Heparan sulphates are not constructed of identical disaccharides but exhibit structural diversity. They consist of glucuronic or iduronic acid and glucosamine. Some glucosamines are acetylated and may have N- and O-sulfate groups. It is a ubiquitous cell-surface component as well as extracellular substance in blood vessel walls and brain. Heparan sulfates which function directly at the cell surface interact with a variety of proteins including growth factors and their receptors (such as fibroblast growth factors and their receptors) to initiate signaling processes.

Heparin

Heparin consists of glucuronic or iduronic acid and glucosamine. Most of its glucosamine units are N-sulfated. Sulfate is also bound to the hydroxyl group on carbon-2 of the uronic acid residues and the carbon-2 and/or -6 of glucosamine. It is a highly charged polymer found in the intracellular granules of the mast cells that occur in arterial walls, especially in liver, lungs and skin. Heparin is clinically important (Chemistry to Clinics 3.2).

Table 3.3: Composition and functions of glycosaminoglycans

Glycosaminoglycan	Repeating disaccharide unit	Tissue location	Major functions
Hyaluronic acid	[GlcUA-GlcNAc]	Joint and ocular fluids	Serves as excellent biological shock absorber and lubricant
Chondroitin sulfates	[GlcUA-GalNAc]	Cartilage, tendons, bone	Bind collagen and give it strength
Dermatan sulfate	[IdUA-GalNAc]	Skin, valves, blood vessels	Valve integrity
Heparan sulfate	[IdUA-GlcNAc]	Cell surfaces	Initiation of signaling processes
Heparin	[IdUA-GlcNAc]	Mast cells, liver	Serves as an anticoagulant
Keratan sulfates	[Gal-GlcNAc]	Cartilage, cornea	Corneal transparency

Chemistry to Clinics 3.2: Clinical Applications of Heparin

Heparin inhibits clotting of blood and is thus widely used to inhibit blood clotting after sample collection from a patient. It is also used to periodically flush intravenous lines/cannulas to keep them clot-free. Suitably modified low-molecular weight heparin is used in the prophylaxis and treatment of deep vein thrombosis (Fig. 3.10).

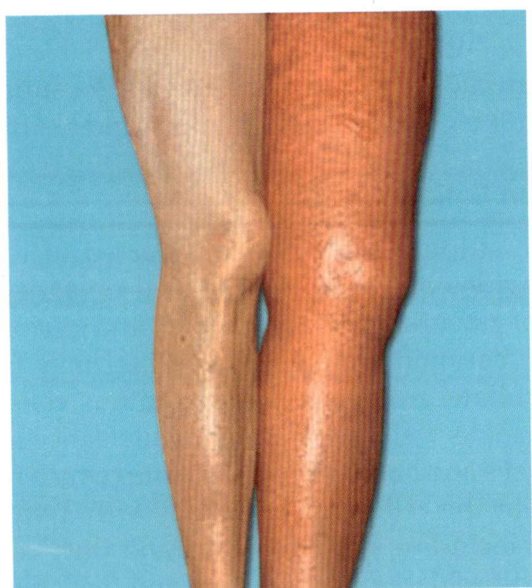

Fig. 3.10: Deep vein thrombosis caused by a thrombus in the deep veins (ileofemoral veins) in the left groin. The affected limb has all the cardinal signs of acute inflammation, swelling, heat, redness, pain and loss of function. The condition mandates urgent treatment with intravenous heparin

Keratan Sulfates

Keratan sulfate is the most heterogeneous group of GAGs as its sulfate content is variable and it contains small amounts of fucose, mannose, N-acetylglucosamine and sialic acid. The repeating disaccharide generally is N-acetylglucosamine and galactose. Keratan sulfates are linked to protein either by an N-linked (keratan sulfate I) or O-linked (keratan sulfate II) oligosaccharide. Keratan sulfate I is found in cornea while keratan sulfate II occurs in loose connective tissue proteoglycan aggregates with chondroitin sulfate. Corneal clouding in macular corneal dystrophy is associated with undersulfation of keratan sulfate I.

DIGESTION AND ASSIMILATION OF CARBOHYDRATES

3

Metabolism of carbohydrates involves **digestion, absorption and transportation to various cells of the body for its utilization** (i.e. **assimilation**).

Digestion refers to the process of breakdown of food by mechanical and chemical means. It requires several enzymes that help in breaking down complex food materials into simpler end products. Digestion is a stepwise process, occurring in stages in different parts of the alimentary canal.

Assimilation is utilizing the absorbed materials by the body. It is the delicate process where the nutrients must pass through the cellular membrane into our cells. Assimilation helps in utilizing the digested food for obtaining energy, building up new tissues and repair of old tissues.

Digestion of Carbohydrates from Food

Carbohydrates are most commonly consumed as polysaccharides (e.g. starch, fiber or cellulose) or disaccharides (e.g. lactose, sucrose, galactose) and therefore need to be broken down into their simpler monosaccharides, which are utilized by the body.

- Digestion of dietary carbohydrates starts **in the mouth** when food comes in contact with the saliva. Salivary amylase (**S-type amylase**) hydrolyzes 1,4α-glycosidic linkages randomly, within the polysaccharide chain of starch or glycogen and produces maltose and various oligosaccharides. After food reaches the stomach, salivary amylase becomes inactive in the acidic environment.
- **In the duodenum**, pancreatic amylase (**P-type amylase**), present in the pancreatic juice, helps in further hydrolysis of the remaining polysaccharide units. Pancreatic amylase is similar in action to salivary amylase and hydrolyzes the partially hydrolyzed products of starch and glycogen to maltose, isomaltose, maltotriose, limit dextrin and glucose (Table 3.4).
- Digestion continues **in the small intestine** as the intestinal juice also contains **oligosaccharidases** which hydrolyze the terminal 1,4α-glycosidic linkage from the oligosaccharides. At the same time, various **disaccharidases** (maltase, lactase and sucrase) hydrolyze disaccharides, i.e. maltose, lactose and sucrose respectively, to their constituent monosaccharide units (Table 3.4).

Lack of the enzyme lactase results in **lactose intolerance.**

Congenital sucrase deficiency results in symptoms similar to those of lactase deficiency.

Table 3.4: Effect of various digestive ennzymes on dietary carbohydrates

Enzyme	Site of action	Catalytic action
Salivary amylase	Mouth	Starch/glycogen → partially hydrolyzed dextrins, oligosaccharides, isomaltose and maltose
Pancreatic amylase	Small intestine	Partially hydrolyzed dextrins/oligosaccharides → dextrins, maltose, isomaltose and maltotriose
α-Dextrinase	Small intestine	α-Limit dextrins → maltotriose and glucose
Disaccharidases	Small intestine	
Sucrase		Sucrose → glucose and fructose
Lactase		Lactose → glucose and galactose
Maltase		Maltose/maltotriose → glucose
Isomaltase		Isomaltose → glucose

Assimilation of Carbohydrates

After digestion by the action of various enzymes, polysaccharides and disaccharides from food are released as monosaccharides, i.e. glucose, galactose and fructose. These are, almost, completely absorbed and transported through the wall of the small intestine into the portal vein, which then takes them straight to the liver. The mode of transport varies between the three monosaccharides and is described in brief below:

Glucose, at low concentrations is transported through the mucosal lining into the epithelial cells of the intestine by active transport, via a sodium-dependent transporter (**sodium-glucose transporter 1, SGLT-1**). At higher concentrations, a second facilitative transporter becomes involved. From the epithelial cells glucose is moved into the surrounding capillaries by facilitated diffusion (*see* Fig. 1.20).

Galactose is transported in the same way, as glucose, utilizing the same transporters.

Fructose moves entirely via facilitated diffusion. The process utilizes a different transporter to glucose when entering the enterocytes, however, both fructose and glucose utilize the same transporter to exit the enterocyte into the capillaries. The absorption of fructose is much slower than that of glucose and is quantitatively limited.

Once in the liver, galactose and fructose are removed from the blood and converted into other metabolites. When eaten in moderate quantities, most of the fructose is taken up by the liver and is converted to glucose, glycogen and lactate. A fraction may also be oxidized or converted into fatty acids. Only a small amount of fructose reaches the bloodstream. Thus, blood fructose concentration is always low. Galactose is primarily converted into glucose and stored as glycogen.

On the other hand, most of the glucose, derived from food, is transported via bloodstream to the peripheral tissues, where under normal circumstances, the hormone insulin enables it to be taken up by the cells and used as an energy source via the glycolysis pathway.

The most notable exception to the carbohydrate metabolism is **dietary fiber**. Dietary fiber is a type of polysaccharide, which can be classed as either soluble (dissolves in water) or insoluble (cannot be dissolved in water). The body cannot digest or absorb dietary fiber like other carbohydrates. Instead, a portion of it is fermented by colonic gut bacteria. As a result, it passes relatively untouched through the digestive system and is removed in stools.

Storage of Dietary Carbohydrates

Surplus glucose is initially stored as **glycogen in the liver and muscle**. The liver can store approximately 100 g of glycogen, which i s used to maintain basal blood glucose levels between meals, while the muscles typically store 400–500 g of glycogen, which is often used during movement. Once these reserves are saturated, excess of glucose is converted to **fat** for long-term storage.

PATHWAYS OF CARBOHYDRATE METABOLISM

Various metabolic pathways of carbohydrate metabolism include glycolysis, gluconeogenesis, glycogenesis, glycogenolysis and hexose monophosphate shunt (HMP shunt). Out of these, glycolysis, glycogenesis and HMP shunt are glucose utilizing pathways while gluconeogenesis and glycogenolysis are glucose generating pathways (Fig. 3.11).

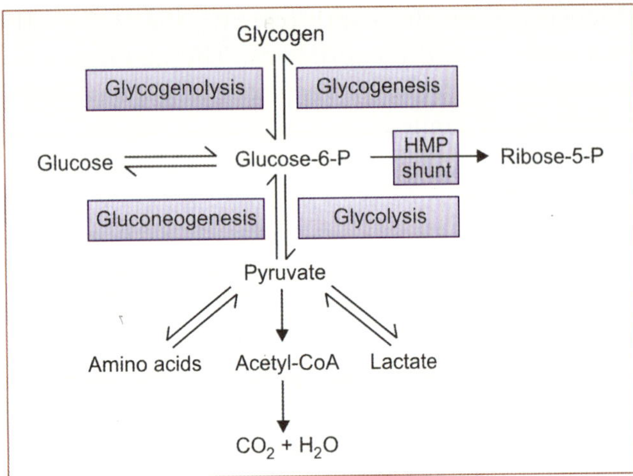

Fig. 3.11: Overview of glucose metabolism

GLYCOLYSIS

Glycolysis, also called **Embden-Meyerhof-Parnas pathway**, is the process of catabolism of glucose either in the presence of oxygen, such as in the liver, to pyruvic acid (called **aerobic glycolysis**), or in the absence of oxygen, such as during exercise in the skeletal muscle and in the erythrocytes, to lactic acid (referred to as **anaerobic glycolysis;** Fig. 3.12).

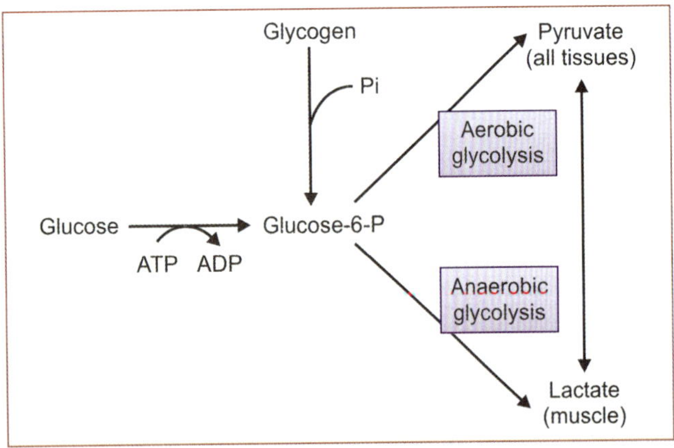

Fig. 3.12: Aerobic and anaerobic glycolysis

Glycolytic enzymes are present in the **cytosol of all the cells of the body.** Various reactions of the glycolytic pathway are shown in Fig. 3.13.

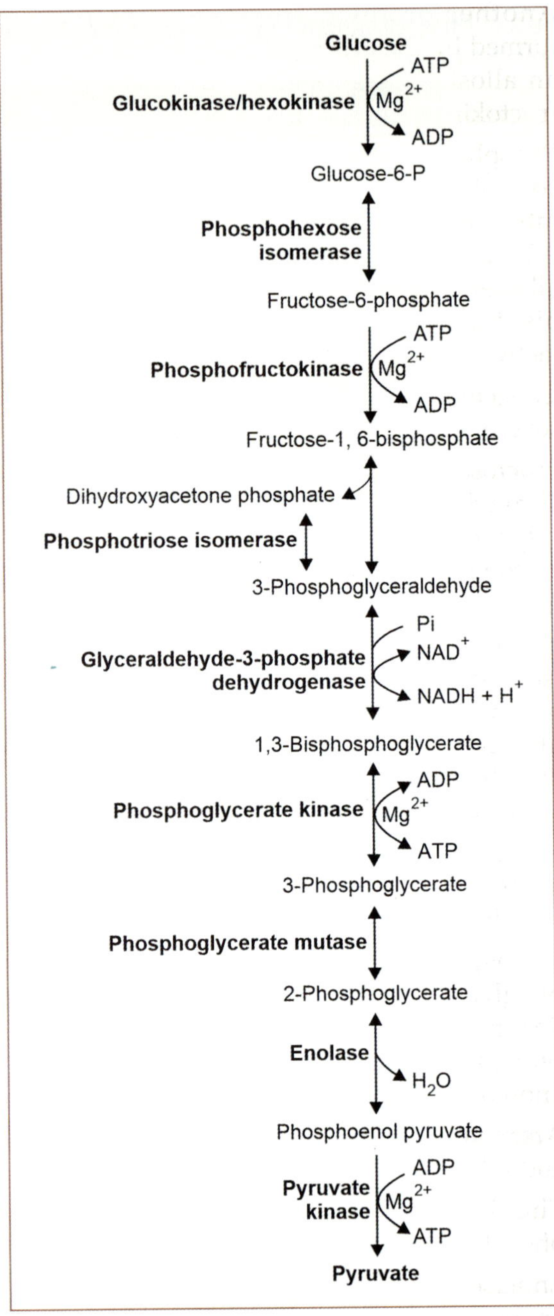

Fig. 3.13: The process of glycolysis

These are discussed below

1. **Activation of glucose:** Glucose is activated **irreversibly**, to glucose-6-phosphate by glucokinase or hexokinase, in the presence in ATP and Mg^{2+}. Hexokinase is allosterically inhibited by glucose-6-phosphate and has a high affinity (low K_m) for glucose. The enzyme is present in all extra-hepatic tissues. In the liver, this reaction is also carried out by glucokinase, which is actually an isoenzyme of hexokinase.
2. Glucose-6-phosphate is **isomerized**, in a freely reversible reaction, to fructose-6-phosphate by the enzyme phosphohexose isomerase.
3. Fructose-6-phosphate is **phosphorylated** by an allosteric enzyme phosphofructokinase (phosphofructokinase 1) to form fructose-1,6-bisphosphate. This is an **irreversible** reaction and requires ATP, which acts as a co-substrate as well as an allosteric inhibitor of the enzyme.

3

Another product, fructose-2,6-bisphosphate, formed by the action of phosphofructokinase-2, is an allosteric regulator of the enzyme phosphofructokinase 1.

Phosphofructokinase 1 plays a central role in the control of glycolysis because it catalyzes **one of the rate determining reactions** of the pathway. Citrate, ATP and hydrogen ions (low pH) are negative allosteric effectors whereas AMP and fructose-2,6-bisphosphate are positive allosteric effectors (activators) of the enzyme.

Congenital phosphofructokinase 1 deficiency causes severe muscular weakness.

4. Fructose-1,6-bisphosphate (the hexose molecule) is **cleaved,** by aldolase, to 3-phosphoglyceraldehyde (glyceraldehyde-3-phosphate) and dihydroxyacetone phosphate, i.e. the two trioses.
5. Since only 3-phosphoglyceraldehyde enters the pathway, dihydroxyacetone phosphate is also **isomerized** to 3-phosphoglyceraldehyde, catalyzed by phosphotriose isomerase. Glycerol also enters glycolytic pathway through this reaction, i.e. via dihydroxyacetone phosphate.
6. In the presence of NAD^+ and inorganic phosphate, glyceraldehyde-3-phosphate dehydrogenase **oxidizes** 3-phosphoglyceraldehyde to 1,3-bisphosphoglycerate.
7. 1,3-bisphosphoglycerate is converted to 3-phosphoglycerate. This reaction is catalyzed by Mg^{2+}-dependent phosphoglycerokinase (phosphoglycerate kinase) and generates one ATP. This is also known as **substrate level phosphorylation**.

   Arsenate results in **uncoupling of phosphorylation** and inhibits ATP production.
8. The 3-phosphoglycerate is **isomerized** to 2-phosphoglycerate by phosphoglycerate mutase.
9. Enolase converts 2-phosphoglycerate to a **high energy compound,** called phosphoenolpyruvate. Enolase is inhibited by fluoride.
10. Phosphoenolpyruvate is converted to pyruvate, **irreversibly**. The reaction is catalyzed by pyruvate kinase, which transfers high energy phosphate group from phosphoenolpyruvate to ADP and generates ATP.

    Deficiency of pyruvate kinase leads to **hemolytic anemia** (Chemistry to Clinics 3.3).

Chemistry to Clinics 3.3: Pyruvate Kinase Deficiency

It results in reduced glycolytic activity, reduced ATP synthesis in RBC, failure to maintain membrane integrity and functions, leading to hemolysis. There is an accumulation of 2,3-BPG which partially compensates for the anemia, however, it also inhibits hexokinase and phosphofructokinase thereby further reducing the rate of glycolysis.

11. Pyruvate is either converted to acetyl-CoA (aerobic glycolysis) or to lactate (anaerobic glycolysis).

Under aerobic condition: Pyruvate is transported into mitochondria via pyruvate transporter and is oxidatively decarboxylated to **acetyl-CoA,** by pyruvate dehydrogenase complex (Fig. 3.14).

Subsequently, acetyl-CoA is coupled with oxaloacetate and is utilized in the **Krebs cycle**.

Pyruvate dehydrogenase complex: It is a **multienzyme complex** consisting of **three enzymes**, i.e. pyruvate dehydrogenase, dihydrolipoyl transacetylase and dihydrolipoyl dehydrogenase. In addition to Mg^{2+}, the complex requires **five coenzymes**, i.e. TPP, CoA, NAD^+, FAD and lipoic acid. It is regulated by phosphorylation-dephosphorylation involving an ATP-specific kinase. While **insulin stimulates** its activity, the enzyme is inhibited by:

- Its products, i.e. acetyl-CoA and NADH.
- Dietary deficiency of thiamin (as observed in nutritionally deprived alcoholics).
- Increased acetyl-CoA/CoA, NADH/NAD^+ and ATP/ADP ratios.
- Arsenite and mercuric ions (which complex –SH groups of enzyme-bound lipoic acid).

Inhibition of the enzyme results in accumulation of pyruvate and lactate, and causes lactic acidosis. It also manifests in neurological disturbances.

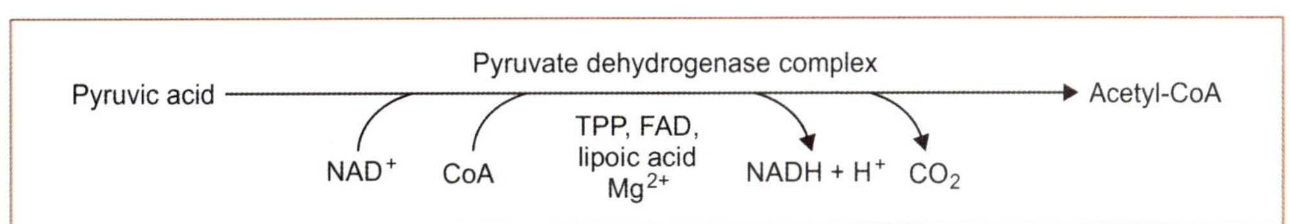

Fig. 3.14: Fate of pyruvate under aerobic condition

3

Under anaerobic condition: Pyruvate is reduced to **lactate**. This reaction is catalyzed by lactate dehydrogenase, which also requires NADH + H^+ (Fig. 3.15).

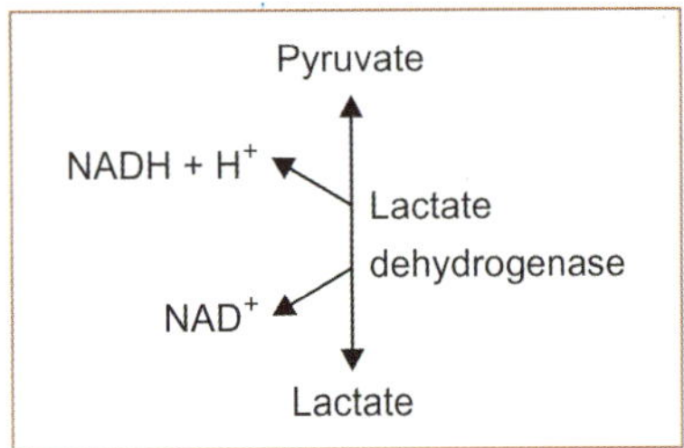

Fig. 3.15: Fate of pyruvate under anaerobic condition

Tissues such as skeletal muscle, when function under hypoxic condition, produce large amount of lactic acid. Pathological causes of sustained hypoxia lead to lactic acidosis (Chemistry to Clinics 3.4).

Chemistry to Clinics 3.4: Lactic Acidosis

Elevated concentration of lactate in the blood is termed lactic acidosis or lactacidosis. It occurs when there is reduced supply of oxygen to the tissues (hypoxia) such as in myocardial infarction, pulmonary embolism and hypovolemic shock. Hypoxia results in inadequate oxidative phosphorylation and decreased ATP synthesis, because oxygen is the terminal electron acceptor in the mitochondrial electron transport chain. To survive, cells rely on anaerobic glycolysis for generating ATP and thus produce lactic acid as the end product. The excess oxygen required to recover from a period of hypoxia is termed the **'oxygen debt'**. It is related to the patient's morbidity or mortality. To assess the presence and severity of shock, measuring the blood levels of lactic acid helps in the rapid and early detection of oxygen debt.

Energy Production during Glycolysis

Under anaerobic condition: Since each of the energy yielding steps, i.e. the conversion of 1,3-bisphosphoglycerate to 3-phoshoglycerate and phosphoenolpyruvate to pyruvate, produces one ATP, a total of 2 ATP are produced for each molecule of the triose oxidized, i.e. 4 ATP per hexose (Fig. 3.16).

As 2 ATP are used in the initial reactions of the process, i.e. in the conversion of glucose to glucose-6-phosphate and fructose-6-phosphate to fructose-1,6-bisphosphate, the **net yield per molecule of glucose, is only 2 ATP**.

In the erythrocytes, when glycolysis occurs via 2,3-bisphosphoglycerate, the net energy yield is zero.

Under aerobic condition: In this process, since NADH produced during the conversion of 3-phosphoglycerate to 1,3-bisphosphoglycerate enters the electron transport chain and releases 2.5 ATP (by oxidative phosphorylation), additionally 5 ATP are produced per molecule of glucose. The total yield under these conditions is therefore 9 ATP. The **net yield thus becomes 7 ATP, per molecule of glucose.**

Regulation of Glycolysis

The **three irreversible steps** catalyzed by various kinases, i.e. hexokinase, phosphofructokinase 1 (PFK-1) and pyruvate kinase are the sites of regulation of glycolysis:

- **Hexokinase** is under the feedback inhibition of its product, glucose-6-phosphate. When energy charge of the cell is adequate and ATP level is high, it causes inhibition of glycolysis at PFK-1 and pyruvate kinase step. PFK-1 is an allosterically regulated enzyme. ATP, low pH and citrate inhibit it while AMP and fructose 2,6-bisphosphate are potent activators.
- **Fructose-2,6-bisphosphate** concentration is regulated by a different enzyme, referred to as phosphofructokinase 2 (PFK-2). It is a bifunctional enzyme with kinase and phosphatase activities. It acts on fructose-6-phosphate and converts it to fructose-2,6-bisphosphate by its kinase activity and vice versa, when the phosphatase activity is dominant. PFK-2 is under allosteric and covalent

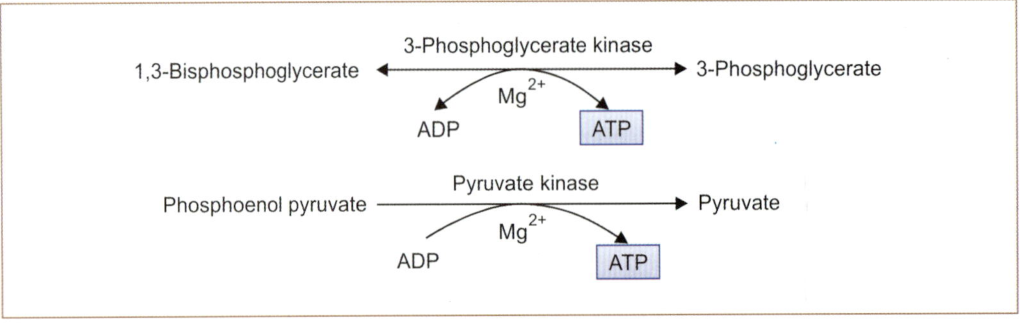

Fig. 3.16: Energy yielding steps in aerobic condition

3

regulation. Kinase is active in the dephosphorylated state (which occurs when insulin is present) and phosphatase is active in phosphorylated form (which occurs in glucagon excess) under condition of fasting and hypoglycemia. Fructose-6-phosphate is the allosteric activator for PFK-2. So, under fed condition concentration of fructose-2,6- bisphosphate increases due to allosteric stimulation of PFK-2 kinase activity by fructose-6-phosphate. But under hypoglycemia concentration of fructose-2,6-bisphosphate decreases, which ultimately inhibits PFK-1. It is important to note that PFK-1 is only allosterically regulated (Fig. 3.17).

- **Pyruvate kinase** is, both, under allosteric control and covalent modification. It is stimulated by fructose-1,6-bisphosphate and inhibited by ATP. Under starvation, pyruvate kinase is phosphorylated by glucagon and becomes inactive. Insulin favors its dephosphorylated state and hence, the enzyme is activated after meals. Insulin also induces glucokinase, however, it does not affect the activity of hexokinase.

Several factors regulate activities of the key enzymes of glycolysis (Table 3.5.)

GLUCONEOGENESIS

Gluconeogenesis (neoglucogenesis) is the process of the **formation of glucose** from various **noncarbohydrate sources,** i.e.:

- Glucogenic amino acids
- Lactate
- Glycerol
- Propionate

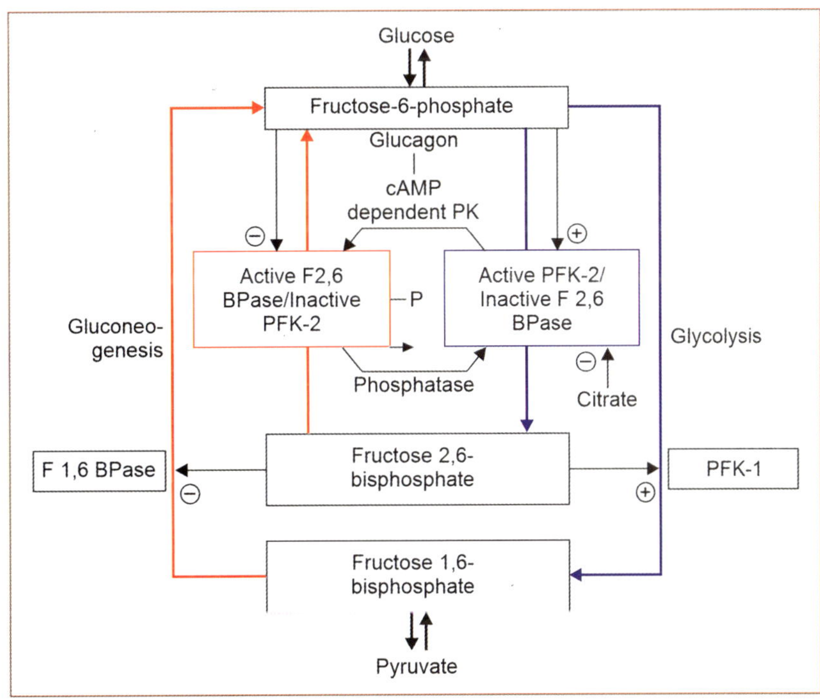

Fig. 3.17: Allosteric regulation of phosphofructokinase-1 by fructose-2,6-bisphosphate

Table 3.5

Enzyme	Acitvity		Allosteric		Inducer	Repressor
	After meal	Starvtion	Acivity	Inhibition		
Hexopinse				G–6–P		
Glucokinase	↑	↓			Insulin	Glucagon
PFK-1	↑	↓	AMP, F-6-P F2,6 Bis PO_4	Citrate, Fatty acid, ATP	Insulin	Glucagon
Pyruvate kinase	↑	↓	F 1,6 Bis PP4	ATP, Alanine	Insulin	Glucagon

Formation of Glucose from Pyruvate

As discussed earlier, all the glycolytic reactions are reversible except the three steps of the pathway.

Gluconeogenesis is, actually, the reversal of these three irreversible reactions (Fig. 3.18).

1. **Reversal of pyruvate to phosphoenolpyruvate:**
   i. Firstly, pyruvate is changed to oxaloacetate by **pyruvate carboxylase** in the mitochondria. Active biotin or biocytin is used as a coenzyme. The enzyme is regulated by induction, repression as well as allosteric regulation.
   ii. Oxaloacetate is then reduced to malate via citric acid cycle in the mitochondria, from where it comes out to the cytoplasm and is re-oxidized to oxaloacetate. Oxaloacetate, thus, is formed from pyruvate by the reaction which occurs in the mitochondria, whereas the enzymes which convert phosphoenolpyruvate to glucose are present in the cytoplasm. Oxaloacetate, therefore, has to be transported across the mitochondrial membrane.
   iii. For the transport of oxaloacetate across the mitochondrial membrane, the enzyme malate dehydrogenase converts mitochondrial oxaloacetate to malate, which is readily transportable.
   iv. In the cytosol, malate is reconverted back to oxaloacetate and, in turn, reduces NAD^+. The enzyme, thus, not only transports oxaloacetate (via malate) but also transports reducing equivalents from mitochondria to the cytosol.

   Reactions of gluconeogenesis, thus, occur both, in the cytosol as well as in the mitochondria.
   v. In the cytoplasm, oxaloacetate is converted to phosphoenolpyruvate by **phosphoenolpyruvate carboxykinase** (PEP carboxykinase), which requires GTP as a coenzyme.
2. **Reversal of fructose-1,6-bisphosphate to fructose-6-phosphate:**
   Fructose-1,6-bisphosphate is converted to fructose-6-phosphate by **fructose-1,6-bisphosphatase**. Deficiency or inhibition of fructose-1,6-bisphosphatase can impair synthesis of glucose from pyruvate.
3. **Reversal of glucose-6-phosphate to glucose:** Glucose-6-phosphate is converted to glucose by **glucose-6-phosphatase**. This enzyme is not found in the muscle and adipose tissue.

Formation of Glucose from Amino Acids

In the liver, various glucogenic amino acids transfer the α-amino group and release carbon skeletons which form certain intermediates of the citric acid cycle. These intermediates can enter gluconeogenic pathway and from glucose (Table 3.6).

Table 3.6: Conversion of glucogenic amino acids to the citric acid cycle intermediates

Amino acid	Citric acid cycle intermediate formed
Gly, Ala, Ser, Thr, Cys, Trp and HO-Pro	Pyruvate
Arg, His, Glu, Gln and Pro	α-Ketoglutarate
Phe and Tyr	Fumarate
Val, Ile and Met	Succinyl-CoA

Glucose-alanine cycle: During starvation, amongst the several amino acids which are transported from the muscle to the liver, alanine predominates. It is synthesized in the muscle by transamination of pyruvate (derived from glucose) and is transported via blood to the liver. In the liver, the carbon skeleton of

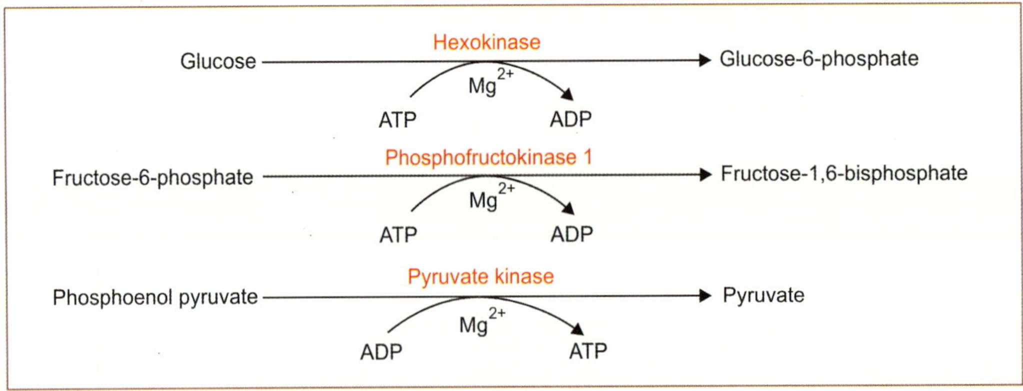

Fig. 3.18: Irreversible steps in glycolysis

3

alanine, i.e. pyruvate, is reconverted to glucose and released to the bloodstream. It is then taken up by the muscle and used as a source of energy. The pyruvate so formed is again transaminated and is used to resynthesize alanine. This is called glucose-alanine cycle (Fig. 3.19).

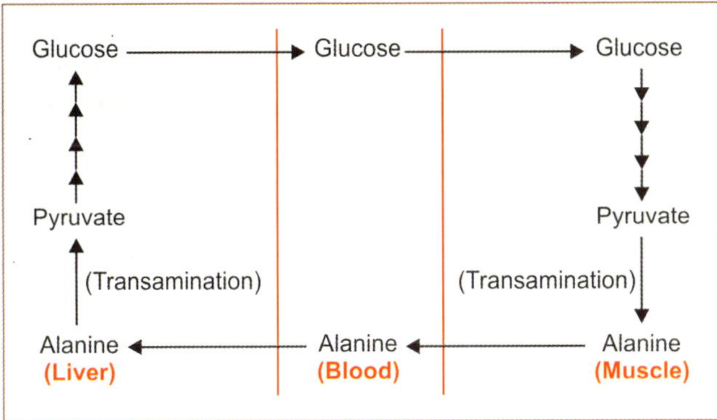

Fig. 3.19: Glucose-alanine cycle

Formation of Glucose from Lactate

Lactate produced during anaerobic glycolysis is also converted to glucose. To achieve this, lactate is first oxidized to pyruvate. The reaction is catalyzed by lactate dehydrogenase and requires NAD^+. Subsequently pyruvate is converted to glucose by the reversal of the glycolytic reactions.

Cori cycle: The end product of glycogen breakdown in the muscle is glucose-6-phosphate, and not free glucose, due to the absence of glucose-6-phosphatase. Glucose-6-phosphate so produced is used for energy production, particularly, during exercise (anaerobic glycolysis) and results in the production of lactic acid. Lactic acid is transported to the liver and reforms glucose by the process of gluconeogenesis. Glucose via circulation again becomes available for its oxidation in the muscle and other tissues. This is called **lactic acid cycle** or Cori cycle. It results in the net exchange of glycogen (via glucose-6-phosphate) and lactic acid in the two tissues, i.e. the muscle and the liver (Fig. 3.20).

Formation of Glucose from Glycerol

Glycerol is produced as a result of lipolysis in the adipose tissue. Glycerol kinase converts it to α-glycerol-phosphate in the liver which is later reduced by a dehydrogenase to dihydroxyacetone phosphate and enters glycolysis (Fig. 3.21).

Due to the absence of glycerol kinase, adipose tissue cannot utilize glycerol.

Formation of Glucose from Propionate

Oxidation of **fatty acids containing odd number of carbon atoms**, in addition to acetyl-CoA, also produces propionate. The latter is converted to propionyl-CoA, by acyl-CoA synthetase, which is further converted to D-methylmalonyl-CoA by propionyl-CoA carboxylase. D-Methylmalonyl-CoA is then changed to L-methyl-malonyl-CoA and finally, by an isomerase, to succinyl-CoA (an intermediate of the citric acid cycle). Succinyl-CoA enters the gluconeogenic pathway. **Vitamin B_{12}** is required as a coenzyme for the synthesis of glucose from propionyl-CoA. This mode of gluconeogenesis, however, is more important in ruminants (Fig. 3.22).

Regulation of Gluconeogenesis

The two opposing pathways, i.e. **gluconeogenesis and glycolysis are 'reciprocally' regulated** to meet the glucose needs of the organism. Gluconeogenesis is regulated by the enzymes (pyruvate carboxylase, PEP carboxykinase, fructose-1,6-bisphosphatase and glucose-6-phosphatase) which catalyze to bypass the irreversible steps of glycolysis (hexokinase, phosphofructokinase 1 and pyruvate kinase). Turning-on

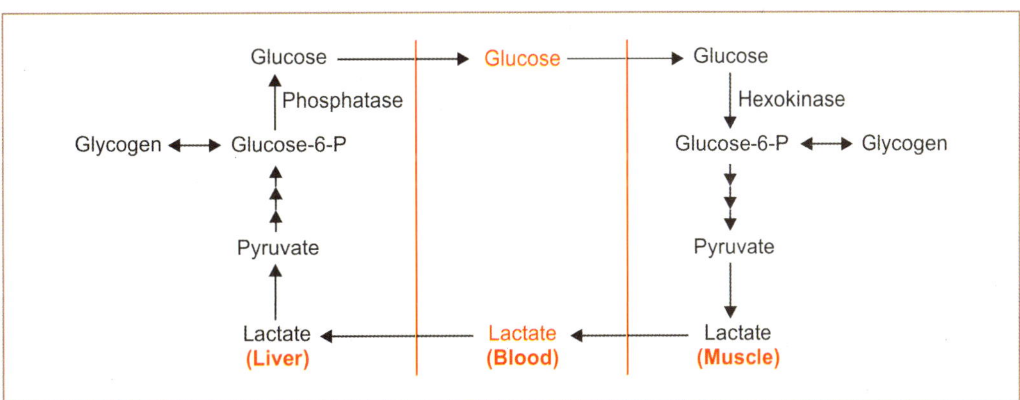

Fig. 3.20: Glucose-lactate cycle (Cori cycle)

3

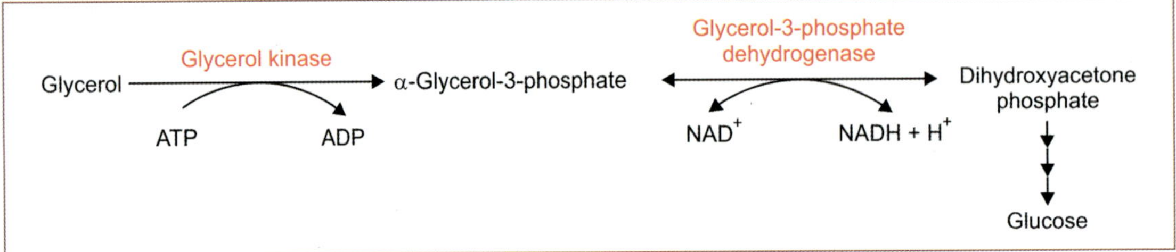

Fig. 3.21: Conversion of glycerol to glucose

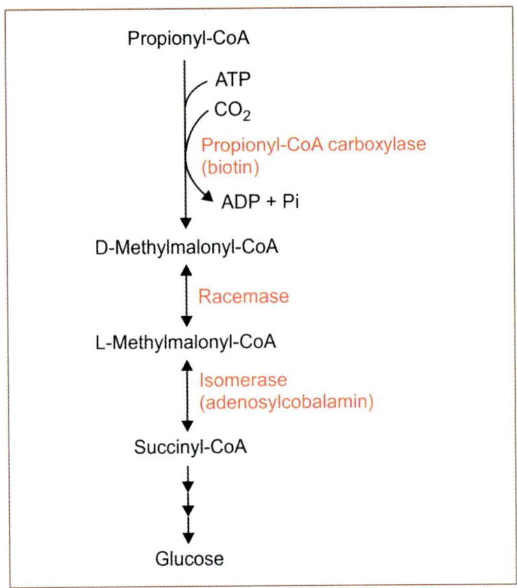

Fig. 3.22: Coversion of propionyl-CoA to glucose

gluconeogenesis is thus accomplished by shutting-off glycolysis (Fig. 3.23).

Glucagon and insulin also regulate gluconeogenesis by influencing the state of phosphorylation/dephosphorylation of the hepatic enzymes.

Importance of Gluconeogenesis

Gluconeogenesis occurs in the **fasting state or on a low carbohydrate diet**, particularly in the **liver** and some other tissues which are solely dependent on glucose for their energy demand but not in the muscle. Gluconeogenesis thus enables the **maintenance of blood glucose** when all the dietary glucose has been absorbed and oxidized, and liver glycogen is nearly depleted. The process is essential since blood glucose level has to be maintained to support metabolism of the **tissues that use glucose as the primary substrate, such as the brain, the red blood cells and the lens**.

METABOLISM OF GLYCOGEN

Glycogen is the major form of carbohydrate present in the body. It corresponds to starch in plants but is comparatively more branched. It is stored in the body mainly in the **liver** and the **muscle**.

The process of glycogen synthesis is called **glucogenesis** while the process of glycogen breakdown is referred to as **glycogenolysis**.

Glycogenesis

Glycogenesis (**glycogen synthesis**) is the process of the conversion of **glucose to glycogen**. Although it is operative in several tissues, the liver and the muscle are the main organs for the synthesis of glycogen. Glycogenesis is **increased by insulin**. Glucose is converted to glycogen as follows (Fig. 3.24):

1. Glucose is first activated (phosphorylated) to form glucose-6-phosphate. The reaction is catalyzed by hexokinase in the extrahepatic tissues. The enzyme is allosterically inhibited by glucose-6-phosphate. In the liver, in the fed state, another enzyme, glucokinase converts most of the glucose into glucose-6-phosphate. This is an inducible enzyme and has greater specificity for its substrate.
2. Glucose-6-phosphate is epimerized to form glucose-1-phosphate by phosphoglucomutase.
3. Glucose-1-phosphate reacts with UTP (a high energy compound) and is converted to uridine diphosphate glucose (UDP-glucose). The reaction is catalyzed by UDP-glucose pyrophosphorylase (glucose-1-phosphate uridyltransferase). The pyrophosphate so released is immediately hydrolyzed to two molecules of inorganic phosphate by the enzyme pyrophosphatase.
4. From UDP-glucose, the glucose moiety (a molecule of glucose) is transferred by the enzyme glycogen synthase to the pre-formed glycogen molecule, called **glycogen primer**. The glycogen primer is formed on a protein known as **glycogenin**.

   The incoming glucose is linked to the primer at the non-reducing end by 1,4-α-glycosidic linkage, resulting in elongation of the pre-existing branches. This results in the formation of an unbranched glycogen (Fig. 3.25).

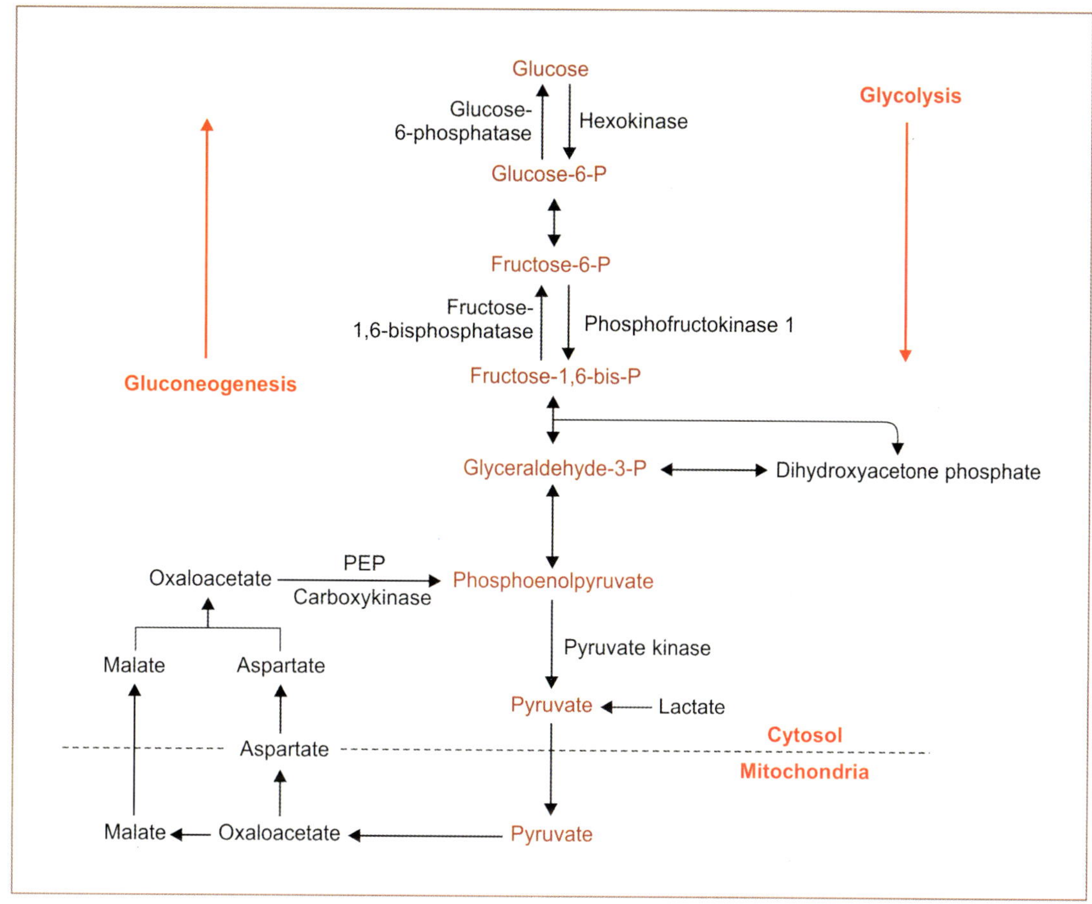

Fig. 3.23: Gluconeogenesis versus glycolysis: Reciprocal regulation

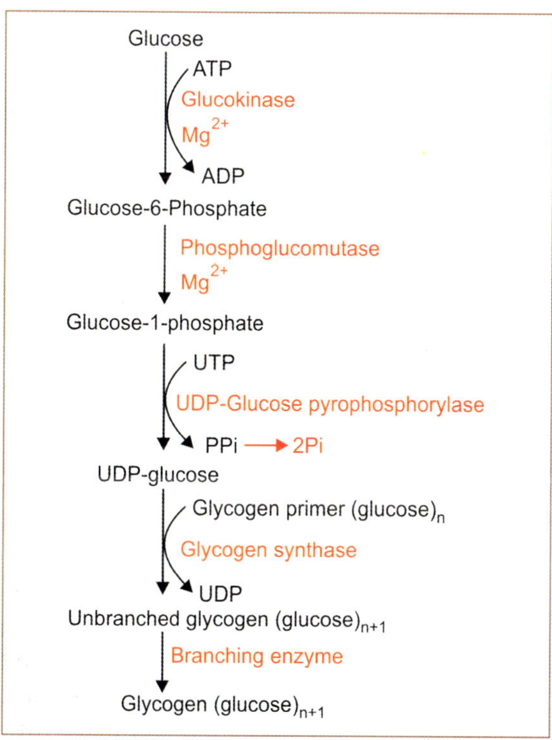

Fig. 3.24: Glycogenesis

Both glycogen primer and UDP-glucose are the substrates for **glycogen synthase**. This is a **key enzyme** of glycogenesis. Muscle glycogen synthase is a homotetramer. The enzyme exists in two interconvertible forms, i.e. glycogen synthase a and glycogen synthase *b*. Glycogen synthase *b* is phosphorylated and is the inactive form. On the other hand, glycogen synthase a (dephosphorylated enzyme) is active (Fig. 3.26).

The enzyme is under allosteric control. It is strongly inhibited by physiological concentrations of ATP, ADP and Pi and is activated by glucose-6-phosphate.

4. Once a straight chain of about 11 residues has been formed, a branching enzyme (1,4-α-glucan branching enzyme) removes a block of about 7 glucosyl residues from a growing chain and transfers it to the neighboring chain, to produce an α-1,6-glycosidic linkage (Fig. 3.27).

The branch again grows by addition of the glucose molecules at the α-1→4 linkage and with further branching, it results in the formation of a highly branched polymer of glucose called glycogen.

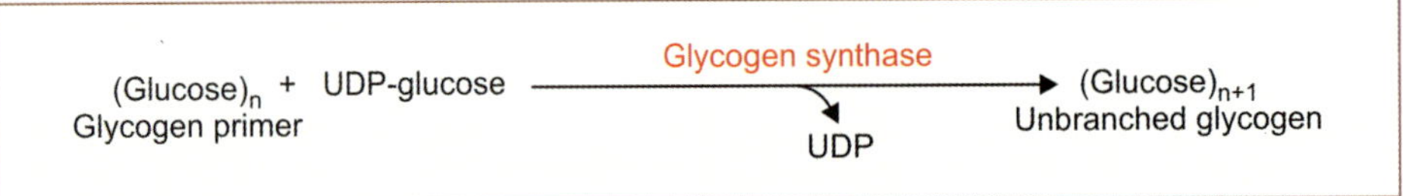

Fig. 3.25: Synthesis of unbranched glycogen

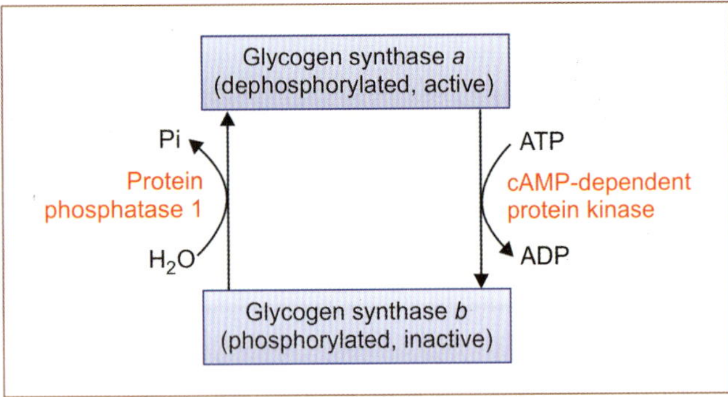

Fig. 3.26: Active and inactive glycogen synthase

Since one ATP and one UTP molecule is used in the incorporation of each glucose unit in glycogen synthesis, the energy spent for the addition of each glucose unit onto the glycogen primer is equivalent to two ATP.

Glycogenolysis

Glycogenolysis is the process of **breakdown of glycogen either to glucose-6-phosphate in the muscle or to free glucose in the liver and the kidney** (Fig. 3.28).

In the liver, glycogenolysis is stimulated by glucagon. Glycogen is broken down to glucose as follows:

1. Glucose molecules are sequentially removed from glycogen as glucose-1-phosphate (Fig. 3.29). This is catalyzed by the enzyme **phosphorylase**, with **pyridoxal phosphate** as a **coenzyme**. The enzyme hydrolyzes α-1,4-glycosidic bonds until nearly four glucose residues are left on either side of the branch. After the action of phosphorylase, glycogen is partially hydrolyzed leaving a limit branch (**limit dextrin**).

Glycogen phosphorylase is subjected to allosteric activation by AMP and is allosterically inhibited by ATP, glucose-6-phosphate and glucose. The enzyme is a dimer and has two identical subunits. It is regulated both allosterically and by covalent modification (phosphorylation/dephosphorylation). The phosphorylated form of the enzyme is called phosphorylase *a*, the active form of the enzyme. The dephosphorylated form is called phosphorylase *b*, the inactive form.

The two forms of the enzyme are interconvertible by the actions of phosphorylase kinase and phosphoprotein phosphatase. Phosphorylase kinase is also subjected to regulation by a cyclic phosphorylation-dephosphorylation mechanism. Protein kinase A phosphorylates and activates phosphorylase kinase while phosphoprotein phosphatase in turn dephos-

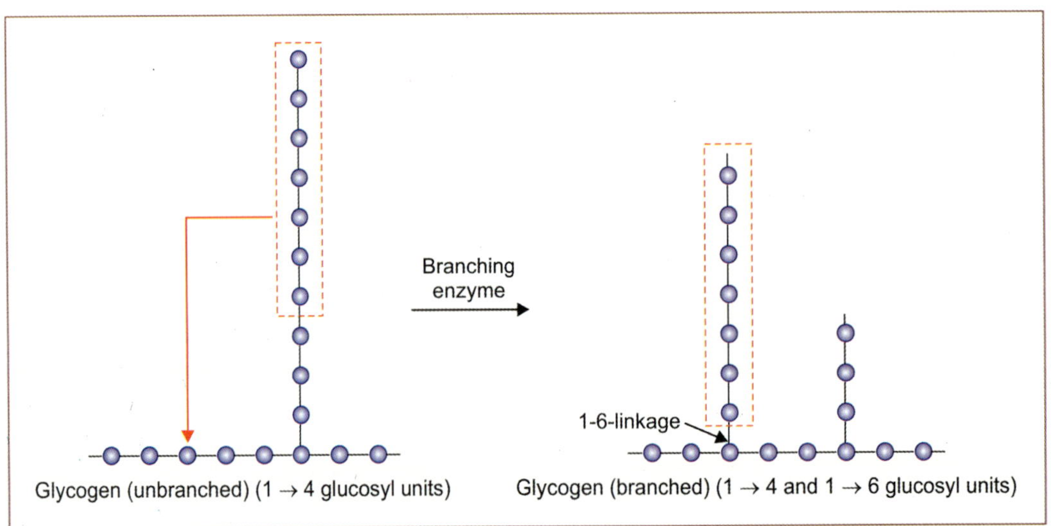

Fig. 3.27: Branching of glycogen

3

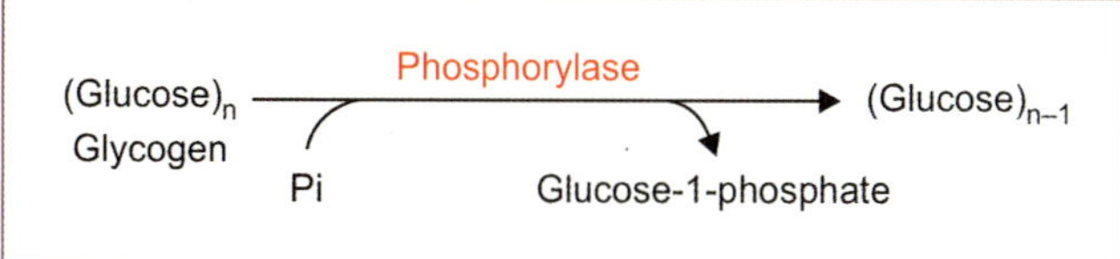

Fig. 3.29: Reaction catalyzed by phosphorylase

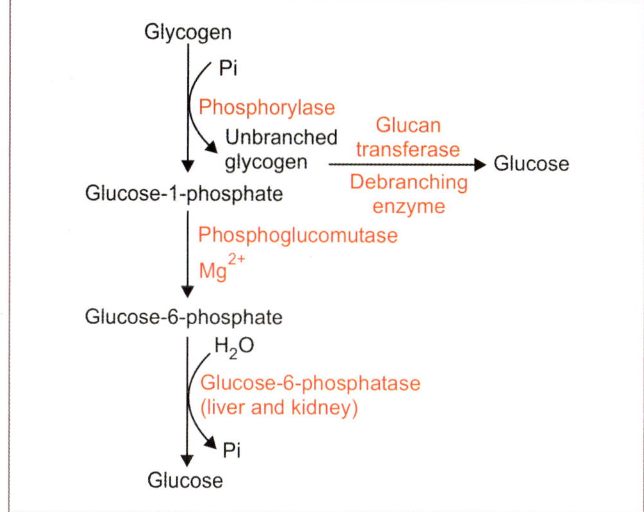

Fig. 3.28: Glycogenolysis

phorylates and inactivates phosphorylase kinase (Fig. 3.30).

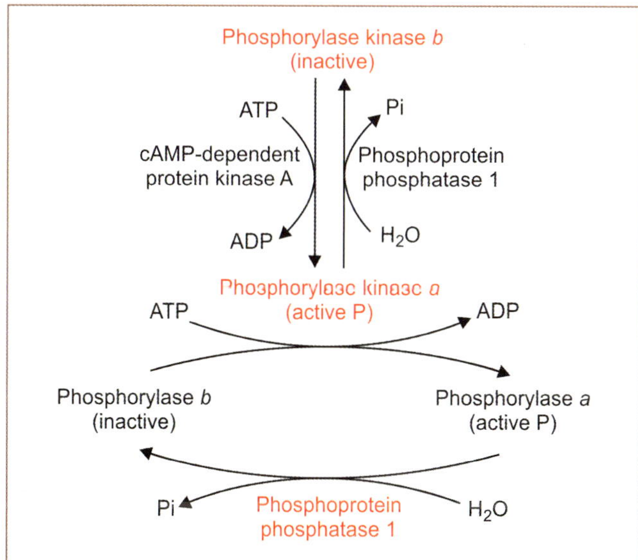

Fig. 3.30: Activation-inactivation of glycogen phosphorylase

2. Debranching enzyme is a bifunctional enzyme that catalyzes two reactions necessary for the debranching of glycogen.

   The **first unit of the enzyme** 1→ 4-α-D-glucan-transferase has glycosyltransferase activity in which a strand of three glucosyl residues is removed from a four glucosyl residue branch of the glycogen molecule to the nonreducing end of another branch. This reaction forms a new α(1→4) linkage with three more units available for the phosphorylase reaction.

   The α(1→ 6) bond linking the remaining glucosyl residues in the branch to the main chain, is hydrolyzed by the **second enzyme activity** of the debranching enzyme, i.e. amylo-α-1,6-glucosidase. This glucosyl residue is released as glucose (rather than glucose-1-phosphate) leaving unbranched glycogen (Fig. 3.31).

   The cooperative and repetitive actions of phosphorylase and debranching enzyme result in complete phosphorolysis of glycogen. During glycogenolysis, glucose-1-phosphate and glucose are liberated in the ratio of approximately 10:1.

3. Glucose-1-phosphate, produced as a result of the action of phosphorylase, is converted to glucose-6-phosphate by phosphoglucomutase.

   In the **muscle**, this is the end product of glycogen breakdown and is used by the glycolytic pathway to give energy during exercise. Since glucose-6-phosphatase is absent in the muscle, glycogenolysis is immediately followed by glycolysis.

   In the **liver and the kidneys**, glucose-6-phosphatase further hydrolyzes glucose-6-phosphate and produces glucose.

   Thus, glycogen stored in the liver is used to maintain blood glucose during fasting so as to prevent a hypoglycemic state, whereas glycogen stored in the muscle is used to provide energy during exercise.

Regulation of Glycogen Metabolism

Regulation of glycogen metabolism involves allosteric as well as hormonal control by covalent modification of the regulatory enzymes.

Allosteric Control

Both glycogen phosphorylase and glycogen synthase are under allosteric control by effectors that include ATP, glucose-6-phosphate and AMP.

As mentioned earlier, muscle glycogen phosphorylase is activated by AMP while inhibited by ATP and glucose-6-phosphate. On the other hand, glycogen synthase is activated by glucose-6-phosphate.

Hormonal Control

Glycogen metabolism in the liver is controlled by **glucagon** while in the muscles and various other tissues this control is exerted by **insulin and epinephrine/**

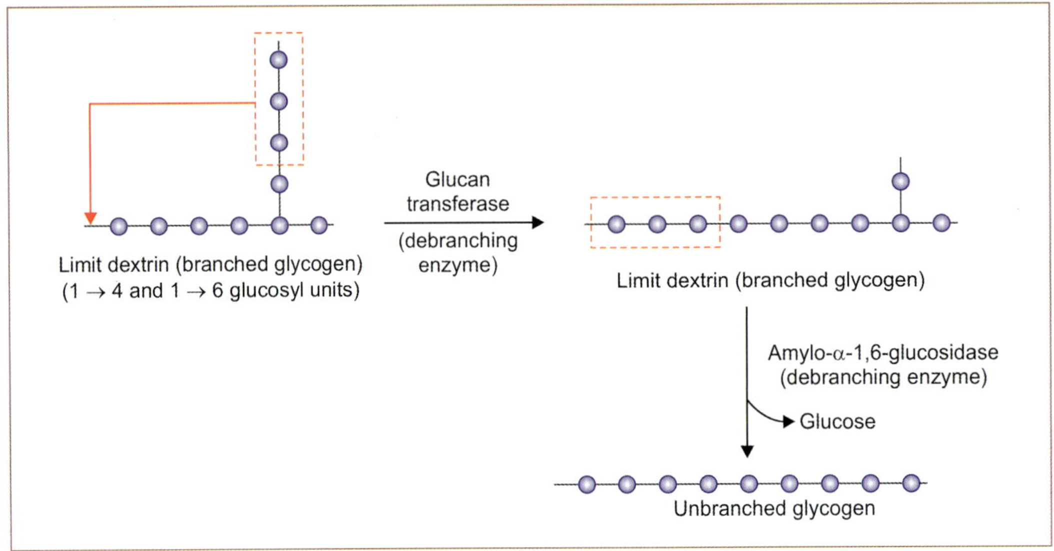

Fig. 3.31: Debranching of glycogen molecule

norepinephrine. Hormones bind to the transmembrane receptors on surface of the cells and result in the release of second messengers, i.e. cAMP/Ca^{2+}.

Glucagon binds to its receptors in the liver cells and increases intracellular cAMP concentration. This, in turn, promotes degradation of glycogen to glucose. Muscle cells, however, do not have receptors for glucagon.

There are two types of receptors for **epinephrine:**

- Epinephrine binds to α-adrenergic receptors on the **liver cells** and leads to increased cytosolic concentration of Ca^{2+} which promotes glycogenolysis and increases blood glucose concentration.
- Epinephrine binds to β-adrenergic receptors on the **liver and muscle cells**, and increases intracellular cAMP concentration. cAMP, in turn, promotes glycogen breakdown to glucose-6-phosphate for glycolysis in the muscle or to free glucose in the liver (Fig. 3.32).

  When circulating glucose concentration is high, insulin increases the rate of glucose transport into many types of cells that have insulin receptors, such as the muscle cells and the fat cells (adipocytes). This, in turn, decreases cAMP concentration, promotes inactivation of glycogen phosphorylase and stimulates glycogen synthesis and thus stores excess of glucose as glycogen.

Covalent Modification of the Regulatory Enzymes

The key enzymes of glycogen metabolism, i.e. glycogen synthase and phosphorylase, as discussed earlier, exist in two different forms, designated as a and b. Interconversion of the a and b forms of these two enzymes is accomplished through enzyme-catalyzed phosphorylation and dephosphorylation under the control of various hormones, e.g. glucagon and epinephrine. **Glycogen phosphorylase is activated by phosphorylation, whereas glycogen synthase is inactivated by phosphorylation**. On the other hand, dephosphorylation inactivates phosphorylase and activates glycogen synthase.

Phosphorylation of glycogen phosphorylase is under the control of three enzymes, i.e. phosphorylase kinase, cAMP-dependent protein kinase and phosphoprotein phosphatase 1.

cAMP dependent protein kinase: The intracellular concentration of cAMP is regulated between its rate of synthesis from ATP by adenylate cyclase as well as its breakdown by phosphodiesterase. The binding of the hormones (glucagon as well as epinephrine) to their cell surface receptors stimulates adenylate cyclase which in turn catalyzes the synthesis of cAMP inside the cell. The cAMP is necessary for the activity of cAMP dependent protein kinase (cAMP-PK).

The enzyme consists of two regulatory subunits (R_2) and two catalytic subunits (C_2). In the absence of cAMP, the enzyme is an inactive tetramer (R_2C_2). The binding of cAMP to the regulatory subunits (R_2) causes dissociation of the active catalytic monomers (2C; Fig. 3.33).

The intracellular concentration of cAMP thus activates cAMP-PK, which stimulates activation (phosphorylation) of phosphorylase kinase. The cAMP-PK also results in the phosphorylation of phosphorylase and glycogen synthase (Fig. 3.34).

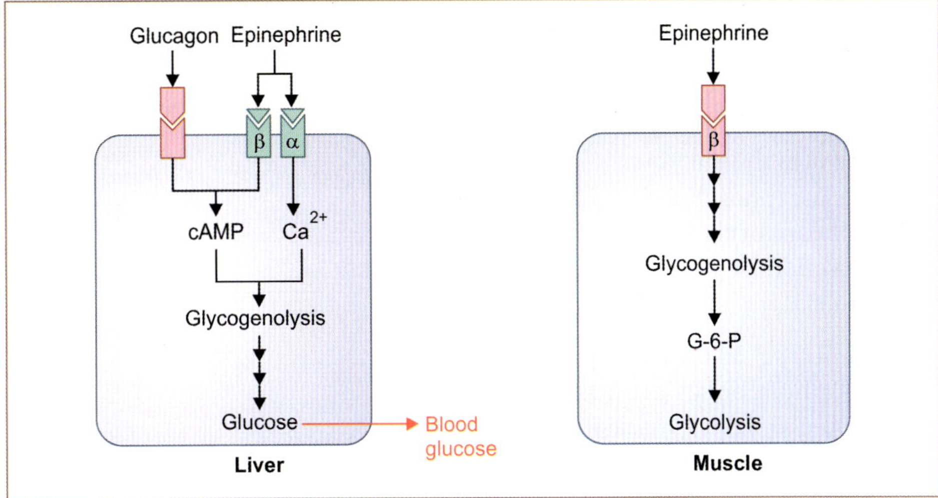

Fig. 3.32: Hormonal control of glycogen metabolism

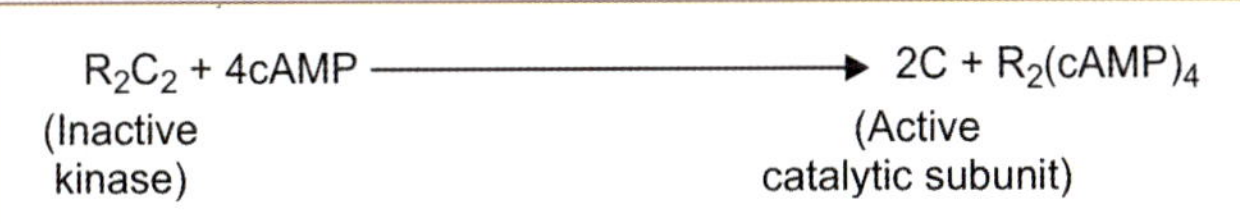

Fig. 3.33: Activation of cAMP-dependent protein kinase

The enzyme cAMP-PK also phosphorylates (activates) phosphoprotein phosphatase inhibitor 1 (Fig. 3.35).

Phosphorylase kinase: Phosphorylase kinase is a tetramer with four non-identical subunits, i.e. α, β, γ and δ. The γ subunit contains the catalytic site while

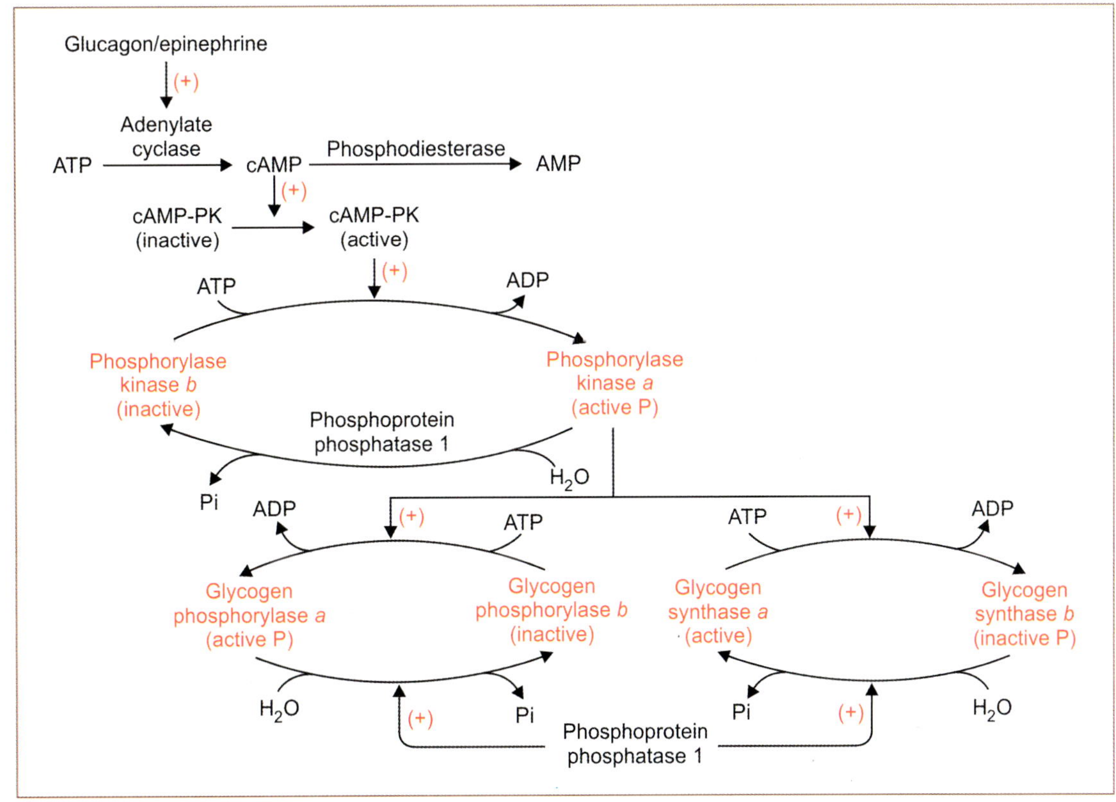

Fig. 3.34: Regulation of glycogen phosphorylase and glycogen synthase by covalent modification

the other three subunits have regulatory functions. The enzyme is activated by Ca^{2+} through its binding to the δ subunit which is also called **calmodulin**.

Phosphorylation of the α and β subunits of phosphorylase kinase also activates the enzyme.

Active phosphorylase kinase (phosphorylase kinase *a*) results in the activation (phosphorylation) of glycogen phosphorylase and inactivation of glycogen synthase (Fig. 3.34).

Phosphoprotein phosphatase 1: Phosphoprotein phosphatase 1 removes phosphoryl groups from glycogen phosphorylase *a*, glycogen synthase *b*, and from the α and β subunits of phosphorylase kinase (Fig. 3.34).

Phosphoprotein phosphatase 1 itself is also inhibited by its binding to phosphoprotein phosphatase inhibitor 1. The inhibitor 1, in turn, is activated by cAMP-PK but inactivated by the active phosphoprotein phosphatase 1 (Fig. 3.35).

The rates of phosphorylation and dephosphorylation of glycogen phosphorylase and glycogen synthase thus control glycogen synthesis as well as its breakdown.

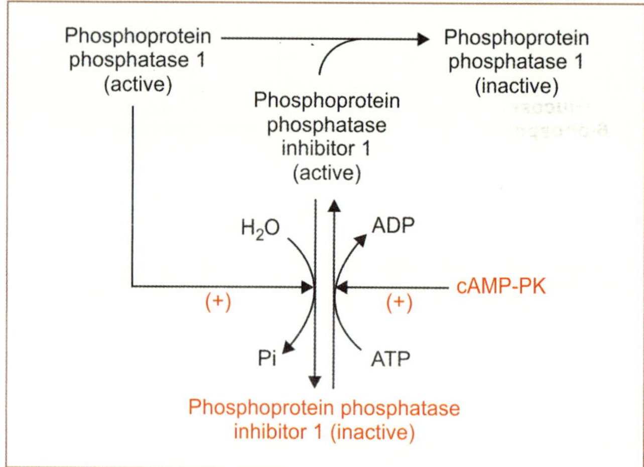

Fig. 3.35: Regulation of phosphoprotein phosphatase

Glycogen Metabolism in Liver versus Muscle

Table 3.7 shows glycogen metabolism differs in liver and skeletal muscle in several aspects.

HEXOSE MONOPHOSPHATE SHUNT

Hexose monophosphate shunt (**HMP shunt**) or **pentose phosphate pathway** is the second major pathway for the metabolism of glucose. Enzymes for this pathway are localized in the **cytosol** and the reducing equivalents are accepted by **$NADP^+$ instead of NAD^+**. This pathway is operative in many tissues, such as the liver, erythrocytes, lactating mammary gland, testes and the adipose tissue. The rate of HMP shunt reactions is **increased by insulin**. Reactions of the HMP shunt are outlined in Fig. 3.36:

1. Firstly, glucose is activated to glucose-6-phosphate by hexokinase. Thereafter, glucose-6-phosphate, by glucose-6-phosphate dehydrogenase (**G6PD, induced by insulin**), is changed to 6-phosphogluconolactone. $NADP^+$ is reduced to $NADPH + H^+$. G6PD deficiency may be associated with hemolytic anemia (Chemistry to Clinics 3.5).

   G6PD deficiency impairs the ability of RBC to form NADPH which is essential for the maintenance of reduced glutathione (GSH), a potent intracellular antioxidant (Fig. 3.37).

   This results in reduced detoxification of reactive oxygen species (free radicals such as superoxide

Table 3.7: Comparison of glycogen metabolism in liver and skeletal muscle

Parameter	Liver	Skeletal muscle
Glycogen concentration	High: 10% w/w	Low: 2% w/w
Absolute amount of glycogen in healthy adults in well-fed state	Low: ~70 g	High: ~250 g because muscle mass (~35 kg) is much greater than liver mass (~1.8 kg)
Glucose-6-phosphatase	Present, hence free glucose after glycogenolysis is released	Absent, hence glucose-6-phosphate formed in glycogenolysis directly enters glycolysis in the muscle itself
Hormonal regulation of glycogenolysis	More responsive to glucagon	More responsive to epinephrine
Purpose of glycogenolysis	To regulate blood glucose level in between meals, for use by brain, muscles, RBC	To provide glucose for its own use

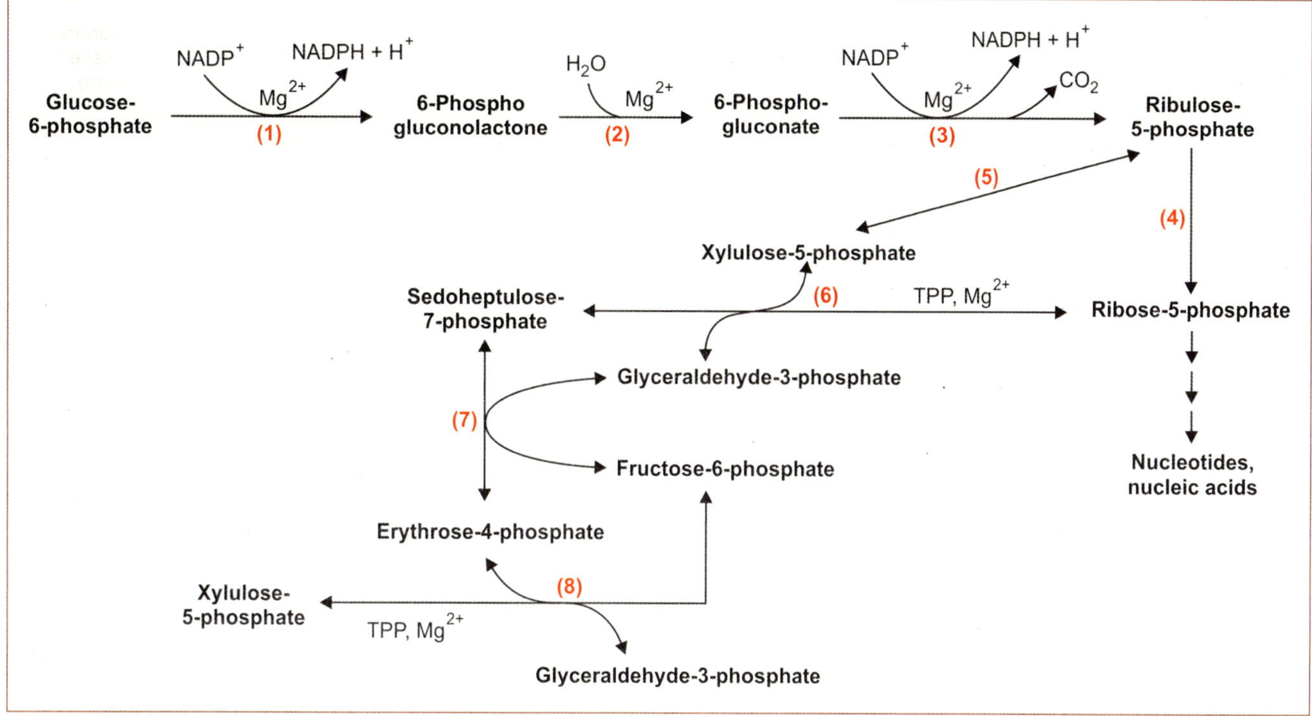

Fig. 3.36: Outline of HMP shunt: (1) Glucose-6-phosphate dehydrogenase; (2) Gluconolactone hydrolase; (3) 6-Phosphogluconate dehydrogenase; (4) Ketoisomerase; (5) Ribulose-5-phosphate epimerase; (6) Transketolase; (7) Transaldolase and ; (8) Transketolase

Chemistry to Clinics 3.5: Glucose-6-phosphate Dehydrogenase (G6PD) Deficiency

It is an X-linked inherited disease characterized by hemolytic anemia due to an inability to detoxify oxidizing agents. The molecular defect is a point mutation in the G6PD gene and >300 variants are known. Highest prevalence is seen in the Middle East, tropical Africa and Asia, and parts of Mediterranean. Babies with G6PD deficiency suffer from neonatal jaundice appearing 1–4 days after birth due to increased bilirubin production resulting from hemolysis.

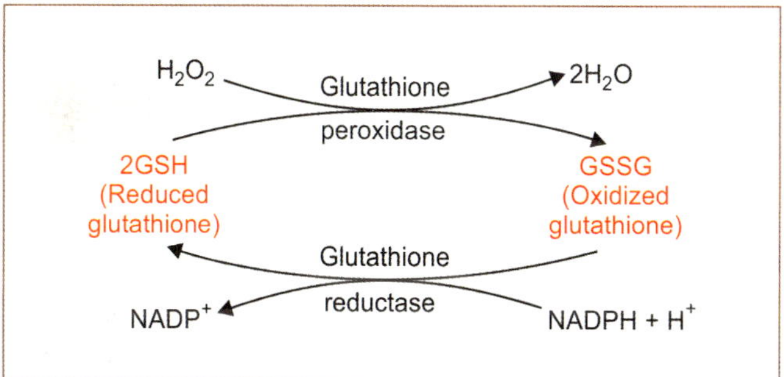

Fig. 3.37: Significance of HMP shunt in RBC

anion as well as nonradicals like hydrogen peroxide) which damage the RBC membrane with consequent hemolysis. Further, there is oxidation of sulfhydryl groups in proteins including hemoglobin and leads to the formation of denatured proteins that form insoluble masses called **Heinz bodies**, which get attached to the cell membrane. **Extreme caution** should be taken when prescribing any drug to these patients since **oxidant drugs readily trigger hemolysis**. Such drugs include antibiotics (sulfamethoxazole, chloramphenicol), antimalarials (primaquine) and antipyretics (acetanilide).

2. The 6-phosphogluconolactone is converted to 6-phosphogluconate by gluconolactone hydrolase.
3. In the next reaction, **a hexose is converted to a pentose**. 6-Phosphogluconate is oxidized by 6-phosphogluconate dehydrogenase to form an intermediate 3-keto-6-phosphogluconate. This reaction also generates NADPH + H^+. Subsequently, by the enzyme 6-phosphogluconate decarboxylase, 3-keto-6-phosphogluconate is decarboxylated (the first carbon atom is removed as CO_2) to leave a pentose, ribulose-5-phosphate.

   Both glucose-6-phosphate dehydrogenase and 6-phosphogluconate dehydrogenase are **regulatory enzymes** of the shunt.
4. In the second stage of the shunt, ribulose-5-phosphate is utilized in a multicyclic process and is converted to other pentoses. Ribulose-5-phosphate is changed to ribose-5-phosphate by ribose-5-phosphate ketoisomerase.

3

5. Ribulose-5-phosphate is also converted to xylulose-5-phosphate by ribulose-5-phosphate epimerase.
6. The carbon skeletons of these pentoses are rearranged. A **transketolase** transfers a ketol group (the first 2 carbon atoms) from xylulose-5-phosphate onto ribose-5-phosphate forming sedoheptulose-7-phosphate and glyceraldehyde-3-phosphate. Transketolase requires **TPP as a coenzyme**.
7. Dihydroxy acetone group (a 3-carbon moiety) is transferred by transaldolase from sedoheptulose-7-phosphate onto glyceraldehyde-3-phosphate forming fructose-6-phosphate and erythrose-4-phosphate. This enzyme is actually a misnomer, as it is transferring a 3-carbon ketose unit.
8. Transketolase also transfers a ketol group (2-carbon moiety) from xylulose-5-phosphate onto erythrose-4-phosphate, forming fructose-6-phosphate and glyceraldehyde-3-phosphate.

The Overall Process of HMP Shunt

Six molecules of hexoses (glucose) are utilized to give six molecules of CO_2 and six molecules of pentoses. These pentoses are rearranged to give four molecules of fructose-6-phosphate and two molecules of glyceraldehyde-3-phosphate which also forms a molecule of hexose by the reversal of glycolysis, thus regenerating five molecules of hexoses (Fig. 3.38).

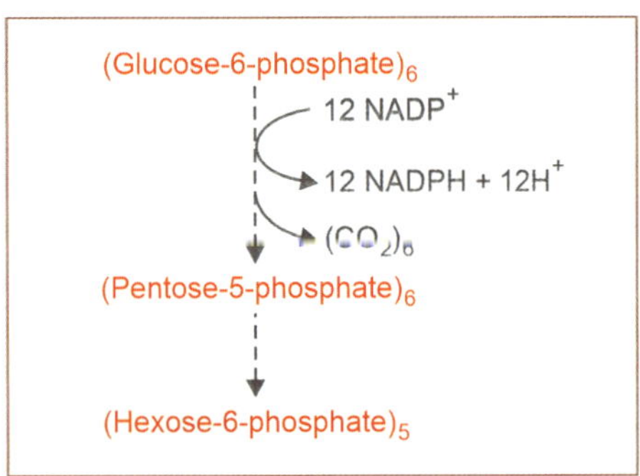

Fig. 3.38: HMP shunt—an overview

Biological Importance of HMP Shunt

1. In the liver

- The NADPH produced in the HMP shunt is used for various **anabolic reactions**, such as for the synthesis of fatty acids and cholesterol.
- The liver is an important site for the **biotransformation of xenobiotics** which take place in the smooth endoplasmic reticulum and also require NADPH.

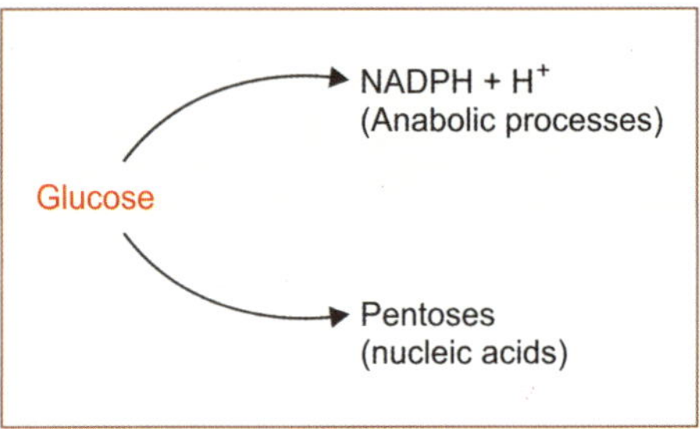

Fig. 3.39: Importance of HMP shunt in the liver

- HMP shunt is also important as a **source of pentoses** required for the biosynthesis of **nucleic acids** (Fig. 3.39).

2. In the erythrocytes

- NADPH is utilized by glutathione reductase to maintain the reduced state of glutathione, so as to **prevent RBC hemolysis**. This reaction is important for the detoxification of H_2O_2 produced in the erythrocytes since its accumulation decreases the lifespan of the erythrocytes (Fig. 3.37).
- NADPH is required for the activity of **methemoglobin reductase** that reduces the small amount of ferri-hemoglobin formed normally, back to ferrous-hemoglobin.

3. **Phagocytosis** by neutrophils and macrophages also requires NADPH.

FUNCTIONS AND INTEGRATION OF OTHER CARBOHYDRATES

Monosaccharides other than glucose, which are assimilated in the body from dietary carbohydrates, include fructose (obtained from sucrose) and galactose (obtained from milk). These are also utilized in the body, primarily in the liver. A large part of these is converted to glucose while some of these are converted to other compounds and perform specific functions.

FRUCTOSE

Fructose is obtained by the body either directly from diet or as a result of hydrolysis of sucrose in the small intestine. **Highest concentration of fructose is found in the seminal fluid**. Fructose is converted to glucose for its utilization by the body by various routes (Fig. 3.40):

1. Fructose is changed to fructose-1-phosphate by a specific enzyme fructokinase present in the liver,

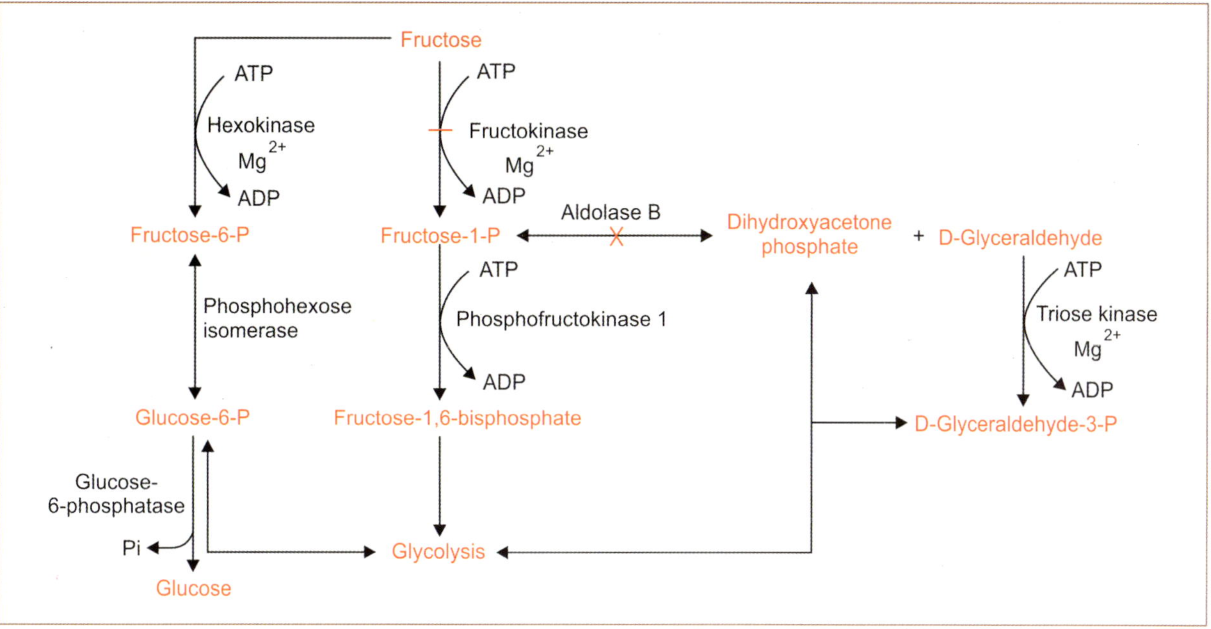

Fig. 3.40: Fructose metabolism (—: Blocked in essential fructosuria) (X: Blocked in hereditary fructose intolerance)

muscle, intestine and kidneys. Fructose-1-phosphate is cleaved by the enzyme aldolase B. This enzyme is different from aldolase A which acts on fructose-1,6-bisphosphate. Aldolase B splits fructose-1-phosphate to dihydroxyacetone phosphate and D-glyceraldehyde (Chemistry to Clinics 3.6).

Chemistry to Clinics 3.6: Disorders of Fructose Metabolism

Fructokinase deficiency results in **essential fructosuria**, due to which fructose appears in the urine, after a high fructose or sucrose diet is ingested. On the other hand, individuals with **aldolase B deficiency** suffer from **hereditary fructose intolerance**.

Subsequently, glyceraldehyde is phosphorylated by ATP in the presence of triose kinase and is changed to 3-phosphoglyceraldehyde that, in turn, can get conjugated with dihydroxyacetone phosphate and form glucose-6-phosphate, by the reversal of the glycolytic reaction.

2. Alternatively, fructose-1-phosphate may be phosphorylated to form fructose-1,6-bisphosphate by the enzyme phosphofructokinase-1. The latter can then enter the glycolytic pathway.
3. Fructose may also be changed to fructose-6-phosphate by hexokinase. The latter is isomerized to glucose-6-phosphate and either enters glycolysis or hydrolyzed to produce glucose.

GALACTOSE

Galactose is released into bloodstream by the **hydrolysis of lactose** due to the action of **lactase in the intestine**. Most of the dietary galactose is changed to glucose in the liver. This ability of the liver to utilize galactose is important in the assessment of the liver function test after a galactose load (**galactose tolerance test**).

Galactose is utilized in the liver, brain and lactating mammary gland by various routes (Fig. 3.41):

1. **In the liver**, galactose is phosphorylated by galactokinase and is converted to galactose-1-phosphate, more rapidly in children than in adults. Sub-

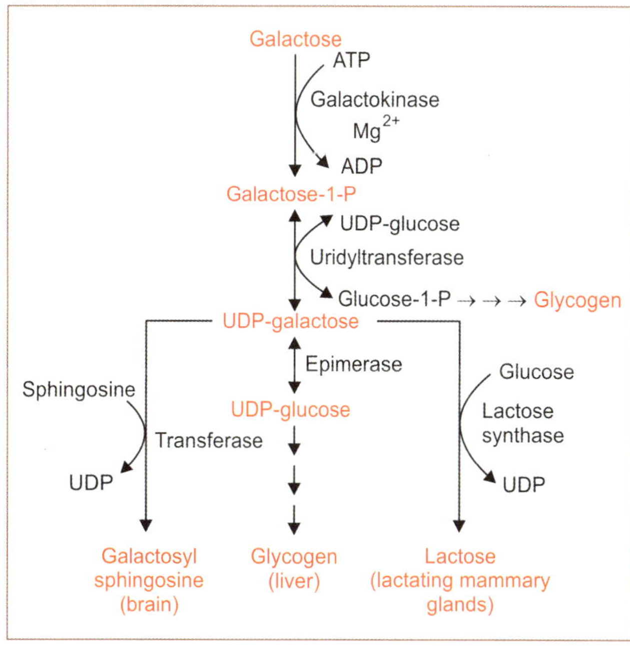

Fig. 3.41: Galactose metabolism

3

sequently, galactose-1-phosphate reacts with uridine diphosphate glucose (UDP-glucose), in the presence of galactose-1-phosphate uridyltransferase and forms glucose-1-phosphate and UDP-galactose. The latter may be changed to UDP-glucose by the enzyme UDP-galactose-4-epimerase. Both glucose-1-phosphate and UDP-glucose can be used in glycogenesis. Several enzyme deficiencies in galactose metabolism can result in galactosemia (Chemistry to Clinics 3.7).

Chemistry to Clinics 3.7: Galactosemia

It refers to increased galactose levels in blood, and is of several types:

Type 1 (classical): Deficiency of galactose-1-phosphate uridyltransferase.

Type 2: Deficiency of galactokinase.

Type 3: Deficiency of UDP-galactose-4-epimerase.

Features

1. Galactosemia, i.e. increased levels of galactose in the blood results in galactosuria (excretion of galactose in the urine).
2. Increased galactose concentration in the blood results in a higher galactose concentration in the lens of the eyes where this sugar is reduced to galactitol. This causes osmotic retention of water and damage to the lens protein (crystallin) with cataract formation.
3. In classical galactosemia, accumulation of galactose-1-phosphate inhibits glycogenolysis resulting in hypoglycemia and seizures. It also depletes the hepatic stores of inorganic phosphate (Pi) leading to liver damage and jaundice.
4. Deficiency of UDP-galactose impairs the synthesis of galactose-containing cerebral glycolipids, which, along with hypoglycemic episodes, hyperbilirubinemia and cerebral edema (due to accumulation of galactitol) may be responsible for mental retardation.

Treatment: Galactose and lactose-free diet.

2. **In the brain**, UDP-galactose reacts with sphingosine, in the presence of the enzyme galactose-sphingosine transferase and is changed to galactosyl-sphingosine for use in the synthesis of gangliosides and cerebrosides.
3. **In the lactating mammary gland**, UDP-galactose combines with glucose in the presence of lactose synthase and forms lactose, for its secretion into the milk.

TRICARBOXYLIC ACID CYCLE AS AMPHIBOLIC PATHWAY

Tricarboxylic acid cycle, also called the **citric acid cycle or Krebs cycle**, is the process of oxidation of **acetyl-CoA (active acetate) to CO_2 and H_2O**. During the process, **reducing equivalents** are produced which enter the respiratory chain and generate large amount of ATP during the process of **oxidative phosphorylation**. Enzymes of the Krebs cycle are located within the **mitochondria**. This, in turn, facilitates the transfer of reducing equivalents from the Krebs cycle to the respiratory chain, the enzymes of which are also located within the inner mitochondrial membrane.

Reactions of the Krebs cycle occur in a **cyclic manner** where two molecules of CO_2 are released and **oxaloacetate is regenerated** (Fig. 3.42).

1. In the first step, acetyl-CoA (formed from pyruvate under aerobic condition) combines with oxaloacetate and forms citric acid (a tricarboxylic acid). The reaction is catalyzed by citrate synthase (condensing enzyme).
2. Citrate is then rearranged to form *cis*-aconitate.
3. *cis*-aconitate is subsequently changed to isocitrate. Both the steps are carried out by aconitase (the enzyme requires Fe^{2+}). The conversion of citrate to isocitrate is inhibited by fluoroacetate.
4. In the presence of isocitrate dehydrogenase, isocitrate is converted to oxalosuccinate.
5. Oxalosuccinate is later decarboxylated to form α-ketoglutarate.
6. α-Ketoglutarate undergoes oxidative decarboxylation and is converted to succinyl-CoA, catalyzed by α-ketoglutarate dehydrogenase complex. The reaction is similar to the conversion of pyruvate to acetyl-CoA and also requires five coenzymes, i.e. TPP, NAD^+, FAD, coenzyme A and lipoic acid.
7. Succinyl-CoA is changed to succinate by succinate thiokinase (succinyl-CoA synthase). During this reaction, a molecule of GTP is formed. This is known as **substrate level phosphorylation** since a high energy molecule is formed at the substrate level.
8. Succinate is converted to fumarate by an FAD containing enzyme succinate dehydrogenase. Due to the structural similarity between malonate and succinate, **malonate inhibits succinate dehydrogenase competitively**. The enzyme is also inhibited by oxaloacetate but is activated by ATP, Pi and succinate.
9. With the addition of a molecule of water by fumarase (fumarate hydratase), fumarate is changed to L-malate (Chemistry to Clinics 3.8).

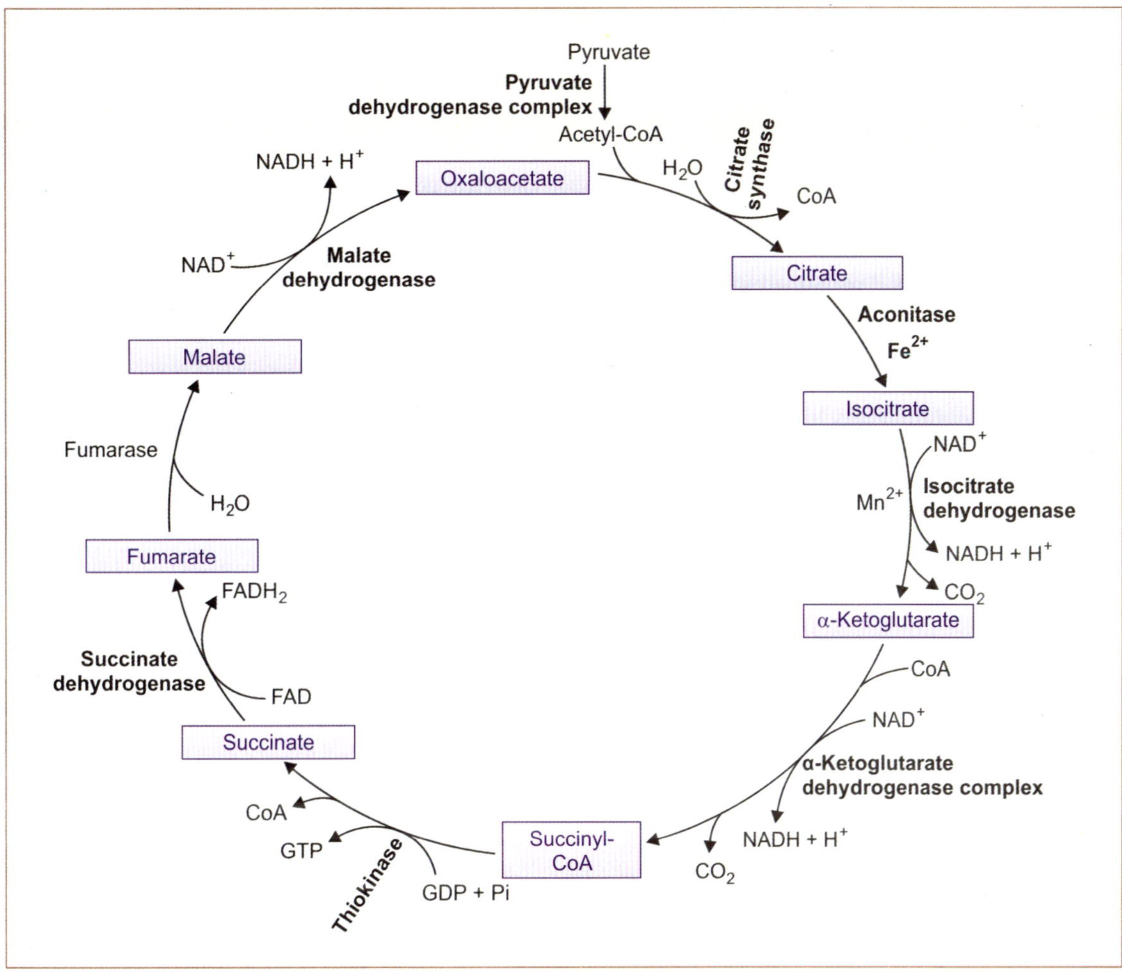

Fig. 3.42: Citric acid cycle

Chemistry to Clinics 3.8: Fumarase Deficiency

The deficiency of an enzyme of TCA cycle is generally not compatible with intrauterine life. However, fumarase deficiency has been reported. Severe deficiency of fumarase, both in the mitochondria as well as in the cytosol of certain tissues, e.g. lymphocytes is characterized by severe neurological impairment and encephalopathy. Urine of such individuals contains abnormal amounts of fumarate and one or more of, succinate, α-ketoglutarate, citrate and malate.

10. Finally, malate dehydrogenase, in the presence of NAD^+, converts malate to oxaloacetate which can then re-enter the cycle.

Energy Production during Citric Acid Cycle

As a result of oxidation of one molecule of acetyl-CoA in the Krebs cycle, three molecules of NAD^+ and one molecule of FAD are reduced. The reducing equivalents from one molecule of reduced NAD^+ ($NADH + H^+$) enter the respiratory chain and result in the production of 2.5 molecules of ATP. Similarly, reduced FAD ($FADH_2$) yields 1.5 ATP. Besides, there is a substrate level production of high energy phosphate bond as GTP. The **total energy yield, per molecule of acetyl-CoA oxidized, is thus 10 ATP** (Table 3.8).

Table 3.8: Energy production in citric acid cycle

Reaction	Reducing equivalents produced as	Number of ATP produced
Isocitrate → α-ketoglutarate	$NADH + H^+$	2.5
α-Ketoglutarate → succinyl-CoA	$NADH + H^+$	2.5
Succinyl-CoA → succinate	–	1
Succinate → fumarate	$FADH_2$	1.5
Malate → oxaloacetate	$NADH + H^+$	2.5
	Total	10

3

In addition, as mentioned earlier, conversion of pyruvate to acetyl-CoA also generates one NADH + H^+, and gives 2.5 ATP. **Total number of ATP produced from the oxidation of pyruvate is therefore 12.5.**

Since 2 molecules of pyruvate are formed from one molecule of glucose, therefore, in addition to the energy yield during aerobic glycolysis (i.e. 7 ATP), a molecule of glucose further produces 25 additional ATP via Krebs cycle. Thus, a **total of 32 ATP molecules are obtained when a molecule of glucose is completely oxidized to CO_2 and H_2O under aerobic condition**, i.e. via glycolysis and Krebs cycle.

Role of Vitamins in Citric Acid Cycle

Four vitamins of the **B complex** group, i.e. **vitamin B_1** as thiamine pyrophosphate or TPP, **vitamin B_2** as FAD, **niacin** as NAD and **pantothenic acid**, a constituent of coenzyme A, play an important role in the citric acid cycle.

Biological Significance of Citric Acid Cycle: An Amphibolic Pathway

Citric acid cycle has a **dual role**, i.e. it is important both in the oxidation as well as synthetic processes. It is thus **'amphibolic'** in nature. It is **catabolic** for the oxidation of carbohydrates, lipids and proteins as these substances are completely oxidized to CO_2 and H_2O, and release large amount of energy. It is also important for the **anabolic** reactions, as various intermediates of the cycle are used for the biosynthesis of nonessential amino acids. Various intermediates of the cycle are also potentially glucogenic and can give rise to glucose in the liver and the kidney (Fig. 3.43).

Reactions which replenish the intermediates of Krebs cycle are called **'anaplerotic reactions'** (Greek *Ana* = 'up' and *Plerotikos* = 'to fill'), whereas those which consume the intermediates are called **'cataplerotic reactions'**.

Regulation of the Citric Acid Cycle

Citrate synthase, isocitrate dehydrogenase and α-ketoglutarate dehydrogenase are the **rate limiting enzymes** of the cycle. The most crucial regulators of the cycle are its substrates, i.e. acetyl-CoA and oxaloacetate as well as NADH.

NADH, ATP and succinyl-CoA function as inhibitors while ADP and Ca^{2+} are activators of the cycle.

COMMON POISONS THAT INHIBIT CRUCIAL ENZYMES OF CARBOHYDRATE METABOLISM

Some of the common poisons inhibit enzymes of carbohydrate metabolism. These include, fluoride, arsenate, cyanide.

Fluoride

Fluoride is a competitive inhibitor of the enzyme enolase as it binds to the active site by competing with the physiological substrate 2-phosphoglycerate. This has two clinical implications:

Firstly, addition of fluoride to blood samples for the determination of blood glucose helps to maintain the true blood glucose. Otherwise, if RBC glycolysis continues, it would lead to false low blood glucose levels.

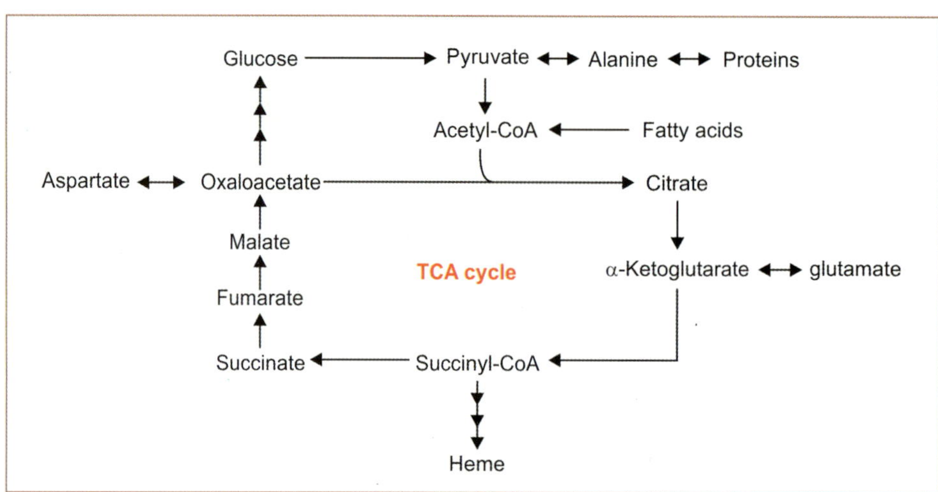

Fig. 3.43: Biological significance of Krebs cycle

Secondly, fluoridated drinking water as well as fluoridated toothpastes should provide fluoride at concentrations which inhibit the enolase activity of oral bacteria without affecting mammalian cells. Blocking the bacterial glycolytic pathway prevents fermentation and hence dental caries.

1,3-Bisphosphoglycerate is converted to 3-phosphoglycerate. This reaction is catalyzed by Mg^{2+}-dependent phosphoglycerokinase (phosphoglycerate kinase) and generates one ATP. Since this reaction does not involve O_2, it is called **substrate-level production of ATP**.

Cis-aconitate is subsequently changed to isocitrate. Both the steps are carried out by aconitase (the enzyme requires Fe^{2+}). The conversion of citrate to isocitrate is inhibited by fluoroacetate.

Arsenate

1,3-Bisphosphoglycerate is converted to 3-phosphoglycerate. This reaction is catalyzed by Mg^{2+}-dependent phosphoglycerokinase (phosphoglycerate kinase) and generates one ATP. Arsenate results in uncoupling of phosphorylation and inhibits ATP production.

Arsenate (AsO_4^{3-}) is an analog of inorganic phosphate. During an **arsenic poisoning, glycolysis** continues to produce pyruvate; however, there is no net production of ATP. That is because **arsenate** reacts with the glyceraldehyde-3-phosphate to form 1-arseno,3-phosphoglycerate (Chemistry to Clinics 3.9).

Chemistry to Clinics 3.9: Arsenic Poisoning

Both pyruvate dehydrogenase complex and α-ketoglutarate dehydrogenase complex require lipoic acid as a coenzyme. Arsenite forms a stable complex with the enzyme-bound lipoic acid and brings respiration to a halt. In arsenic poisoning, arsenic content in the hair is greatly increased which is an important observation in forensic science.

REGULATION OF BLOOD GLUCOSE

Blood glucose level is regulated by a balance between a number of factors that tend to reduce blood glucose, and others that tend to increase it. **Blood glucose homeostasis** requires tuning between:

1. Different metabolic pathways
2. Hormones
3. Kidneys.

Metabolic Pathways Regulating Blood Glucose Level

- Glycolysis, HMP shunt, and glycogenesis lower blood glucose concentration while glycogenolysis and gluconeogenesis increase blood glucose concentration.
- In the **fasting state** or on a **low carbohydrate diet** when blood glucose level is reduced, glycogenolysis and gluconeogenesis are stimulated in the liver and add glucose to the blood. Lipolysis is also stimulated and lipids serve as a source of fuel for different tissues.
- In the **fed state**, when blood glucose concentration is increased, its cellular transport in the liver and its utilization by the glycolytic reactions is also increased. Glycogenesis is also stimulated in the liver and the muscle. At the same time, lipolysis is inhibited.

Hormonal Regulation of Blood Glucose

Several hormones regulate blood glucose concentration. While insulin is the only hormone which lowers blood glucose level, various other hormones increase blood glucose level (Fig. 3.44).

Hormone with Hypoglycemic Action: Insulin

Insulin is the only hormone with hypoglycemic action. It is released into the bloodstream under the direct influence of hyperglycemia. It is a polypeptide containing 2 chains and is produced by the **β-cells of the islets of Langerhans located in the tail of the pancreas**. Insulin **lowers blood glucose concentration** by:

- Increasing the GLUT-4-mediated uptake of glucose by the extrahepatic tissues, especially muscles and adipose tissue, for its oxidation.
- Promoting glycolysis and glycogenesis, both in the liver and the muscle.
- Suppressing glycogenolysis in the liver and the kidney.
- Suppressing gluconeogenesis.

These metabolic effects are achieved because the hormone stimulates the synthesis of various enzymes,

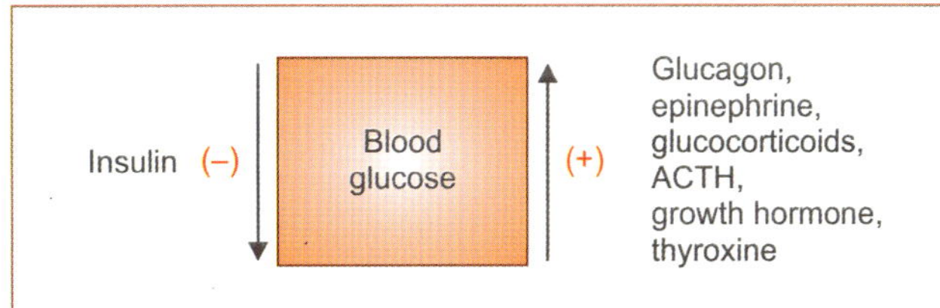

Fig. 3.44: Hormonal control of blood glucose

such as glucose-6-phosphate dehydrogenase, 6-phosphogluconate dehydrogenase, ATP-citrate lyase, etc. while represses the synthesis of pyruvate carboxylase, PEP carboxykinase and fructose-1,6-bisphosphatase.

The hormone also promotes the transport of amino acids across the cell membrane and thus **stimulates protein synthesis**. Insulin also **inhibits ketogenesis** and **promotes lipogenesis**.

Role of amylin: Amylin is a 37-amino acid peptide that is expressed within **pancreatic β-cells**, where it is **co-packaged with insulin** in secretory granules. Consequently, amylin is **co-secreted with insulin** and the plasma concentrations of the two hormones display a similar pattern of low fasting levels and rapid increases in response to meals. **Amylin complements the actions of insulin in postprandial glucose homeostasis** via several mechanisms. These include suppression of postprandial glucagon secretion and slowing of the rate at which nutrients are delivered from the stomach to the small intestine for absorption. The net effect is to control the influx of glucose into the circulation and thus to support the rate of insulin-mediated glucose clearance from the circulation. Patients with type 1 diabetes mellitus have an absolute deficiency of both insulin and amylin, whereas patients with type 2 diabetes have a relative deficiency of both hormones, including a significantly impaired amylin and insulin response to meals.

Mechanism of Insulin Secretion

- **Rising blood glucose is the most potent insulin secretagogue**. The glucose transporter GLUT2 mediates the uptake of glucose into the pancreatic β-cell. In addition to glucose, several other factors such as amino acids (arginine, lysine, leucine), incretin hormones and neural communication serve as important regulators of insulin secretion.
- In the cytosol, glycolysis converts glucose to pyruvate. The first rate-limiting step in this process is the phosphorylation of glucose to glucose-6-phosphate by the enzyme glucokinase. By determining the rate of glycolysis, **glucokinase functions as the glucose sensor of the β-cell** and this is the primary mechanism whereby the rate of insulin secretion adapts to changes in blood glucose.
- The increase in ATP synthesis from glycolysis and TCA cycle blocks the ATP-dependent K^+ channels (KATP) on the β-cell membrane. This induces membrane depolarization which activates voltage-gated Ca^{2+} channels, increasing the Ca^{2+} influx (Chemistry to Clinics 3.10).

Chemistry to Clinics 3.10: Sulfonylureas

The essential role of K_{ATP} channels in insulin secretion is the basis for sulfonylureas, a class of drugs used orally in the treatment of type 2 diabetes mellitus. The K_{ATP} channels comprise sulfonylurea receptors so that these drugs act as insulin secretagogues.

- The increase in cytosolic Ca^{2+} is the main spark for exocytosis, the process by which insulin-containing secretory granules fuse with the plasma membrane, leading to release of insulin into the circulation. The movement of insulin granules and exocytosis are also ATP-dependent processes.

Hormones with Hyperglycemic Action

Several hormones have been shown to have hyperglycemic action. These are called **'insulin counter-regulatory hormones' or 'diabetogenic principles'**, which include glucagon, epinephrine, glucocorticoids, ACTH, growth hormone and thyroxine (Table 3.9).

Insulin/Glucagon Ratio: Critical Determinant of Metabolic Status

In most instances, insulin and glucagon produce opposing effects. Therefore, the relative levels of both hormones in the plasma, the insulin/glucagon ratio **(I/G ratio)**, determine the net metabolic response. The I/G ratio varies considerably because the plasma concentration of each hormone changes rapidly in different nutritional states. In the fed state, the I/G ratio is approximately 30; after an overnight fast, it may fall to about 2 and with prolonged fasting it may fall to as low as 0.5.

A good example of the influence of I/G ratio on metabolic status is seen in type 1 diabetes mellitus. The insulin levels are low, so the insulin-stimulated metabolic pathways operate at a suboptimum level. However, insulin is also necessary for the pancreatic β-cells to sense blood glucose appropriately; in the absence of insulin, the secretion of glucagon is inappropriately elevated. The result is an imbalance in the I/G ratio and an accentuation of glucagon effects well above what would be seen in normal states of low insulin, such as in fasting.

Table 3.9: Major insulin counter-regulatory hormones

Hormone	Source	'Diabetogenic' action
Glucagon	α-Cells of the islets of Langerhans of the pancreas	Hepatic glycogenolysis and gluconeogenesis
Epinephrine/adrenaline (the first line of defense against hypoglycemia)	Adrenal medulla	• Glycogenolysis (both in liver and muscle) • Gluconeogenesis (liver) • Inhibits the release of insulin from the pancreas • Decreases the transport and utilization of glucose in different tissues • Stimulates glucagon secretion
Glucocorticoids (mainly cortisol)	Adrenal cortex	• Hepatic gluconeogenesis • Inhibit glycolysis • Facilitate other hyperglycemic hormones (permissive effects, see Chemistry to Clinics 3.16)
ACTH	Anterior pituitary	Effects are mediated through cortisol secreted from the adrenal cortex under its influence
Growth hormone	Anterior pituitary	• Decreases glucose uptake and utilization by muscle • Prolonged administration of growth hormone stimulates the secretion of insulin, exhaustion of β-cells and diabetes mellitus-like situation
Thyroxine	Thyroid gland	• Intestinal absorption of glucose • Hepatic glycogenolysis and gluconeogenesis • Destruction of insulin

Role of Kidneys in the Regulation of Blood Glucose: Renal Glucose Threshold and Tubular Maximum

At normal blood glucose levels, all of the filtered glucose is reabsorbed by the proximal convoluted tubules and none is excreted in the urine. When the blood glucose exceeds a certain value (**≈180 mg/dl**), significant quantities of glucose appear in the urine. This critical plasma concentration is called the **renal glucose threshold**. Any further increase in blood glucose leads to progressively more excreted glucose. Glucose appears in the urine because the filtered amount of glucose exceeds the capacity of the tubules to reabsorb it. At high filtered glucose loads, the rate of glucose reabsorption reaches a constant maximal value called the **tubular transport maximum** (Tm) for glucose (G), abbreviated as Tm_G. At Tm_G, the tubule glucose carriers are all saturated and transport glucose at the maximal rate.

Factors Affecting Renal Glucose Threshold

The glucose threshold is not a fixed value of blood glucose concentration. It **depends on three factors—glomerular filtration rate (GFR), Tm_G and splay:**

- A low GFR leads to an elevated threshold because the filtered glucose load is reduced and the tubules reabsorb all the filtered glucose despite elevated blood glucose.
- A reduced Tm_G lowers the threshold because the tubules have a diminished capacity to reabsorb glucose.
- Splay refers to the phenomenon that the tubular glucose reabsorption does not abruptly attain Tm_G when blood glucose is progressively elevated. One reason for splay is that not all nephrons have the same filtering and reabsorbing capacities. Thus, nephrons with relatively high filtration rates and low glucose reabsorptive rates excrete glucose at a lower blood concentration than nephrons with relatively low filtration rates and high reabsorptive rates. A second reason for splay is that the glucose carrier does not have an infinitely high affinity for glucose, so glucose escapes in the urine even before the carrier is fully saturated. An increase in splay causes a decrease in glucose threshold.

Osmotic Diuresis

In uncontrolled diabetes mellitus, the blood glucose levels are abnormally elevated, so more glucose is filtered at the glomerulus than can be reabsorbed by the tubules. The urinary excretion of glucose, called glucosuria, produces an osmotic diuresis. A diuresis is an increase in urine output. In osmotic diuresis, the increased urine flow results from the excretion of osmotically active solute. **Diabetes (from the Greek for '*syphon*') gets its name from this increased urine output**. Interestingly, glucosuria may occur even without diabetes (Chemistry to Clinics 3.11).

Chemistry to Clinics 3.11: Renal Glucosuria (Renal Diabetes)

It results from an inherited defect in the proximal tubular Na^+-glucose cotransport (due to mutated SGLT2, the membrane protein responsible for majority of tubular glucose reabsorption). It is characterized by osmotic diuresis and glucosuria despite normal blood glucose levels. It is a benign condition not warranting any treatment.

DISORDERS OF CARBOHYDRATE METABOLISM

DIABETES MELLITUS

Diabetes mellitus (DM) is the **commonest endocrine disease characterized by persistent hyperglycemia with or without glucosuria, caused by the deficiency in secretion or action of insulin**. Besides insulin, several other hormones (diabetogenic principles, as discussed above) also influence the metabolism of glucose. DM may be a result of genetic and/or environmental factors, classified into:

1. Type 1 diabetes mellitus, T1DM (formerly, insulin dependent diabetes mellitus, IDDM).
2. Type 2 diabetes mellitus, T2DM (formerly, non-insulin dependent diabetes mellitus, NIDDM).
3. DM due to miscellaneous factors, e.g. due to prolonged use of corticosteroids, cystic fibrosis, hemochromatosis (bronze diabetes), etc.
4. Gestational DM.

Type 1 Diabetes Mellitus

T1DM is also called **juvenile-onset diabetes** because it usually appears in the childhood or in younger age group (commonly <35 years of age). There is an **absolute deficiency of insulin** due to a gradual depletion of the β-cells of the pancreas which may get destroyed by an autoimmune process (Chemistry to Clinics 3.12).

3

T1DM is characterized by hyperglycemia, hyperlipoproteinemia (raised chylomicrons and VLDL) and severe **ketoacidosis**. This suggests that besides defects in carbohydrate metabolism, there are also abnormalities in lipid and protein metabolism in such patients.

Chemistry to Clinics 3.12: Type 1 Diabetes Mellitus

Type 1 diabetes is one of the most intensively studied autoimmune disorders. Although most cases of type 1 diabetes are a consequence of an inappropriate autoimmune destruction of the pancreatic β-cells, an autoimmune-independent subtype of type 1 diabetes also occurs. Recommendations have been put forth to divide type 1 diabetes into **type 1A (immune-mediated)** and **type 1B (other forms of diabetes with severe insulin deficiency)**. Type 1B appears to be a form of type 1 diabetes in which histological examination of pancreatic sections demonstrates inflammation (i.e. insulitis as in type 1A) but no anti-islet autoantibodies. Irrespective of the subtype, since the net result is the inability of the β-cells to secrete insulin, these patients must be treated with injections of insulin.

Hyperglycemia in T1DM is a result of the inability of the insulin-dependent tissues to take up glucose as well as due to the accelerated hepatic gluconeogenesis from amino acids, derived from muscle protein. Increased lipolysis in the adipose tissue and accelerated fatty acid oxidation in the liver result in ketoacidosis. Insulin deficiency, in turn, also reduces lipoprotein lipase activity thereby resulting in hyperchylomicronemia.

Patients with T1DM can usually be recognized by an abrupt appearance of **polyuria** (frequent urination), **polydipsia** (excessive thirst), and **polyphagia** (excessive hunger), often triggered by stress or an illness. These symptoms are usually accompanied by fatigue, weight loss and weakness. The diagnosis can be confirmed by high fasting blood glucose commonly accompanied by ketoacidosis.

Patients with T1DM have virtually no functional β-cells and **rely on exogenous insulin**, injected subcutaneously, in order to control hyperglycemia and ketoacidosis. Insulin injections though do not cure the disease but promote glucose uptake by the tissues and inhibit gluconeogenesis, lipolysis and proteolysis. Lifespan of the patient is reduced as a result of degenerative complications such as kidney malfunction, nerve impairment and cardiovascular disease. Hyperglycemia may also lead to blindness through retinal degeneration, and the accumulation of sorbitol along with the glycation of lens proteins causing cataract.

Type 2 Diabetes Mellitus

Majority of the diabetic patients suffer from T2DM. It is also called **maturity-onset diabetes** since this usually occurs in the middle-age group (usually ≥35 years of age), who are generally obese. The occurrence of the disease is almost completely determined by genetic factors. T2DM develops gradually without obvious symptoms. The metabolic alterations are milder than those for T1DM.

T2DM is characterized by hyperglycemia often with hypertriglyceridemia. In spite of high levels of insulin, glucose levels are poorly controlled because of **lack of normal response to insulin** (Chemistry to Clinics 3.13).

Chemistry to Clinics 3.13: Anti-incretin Theory for T2DM

'Incretins' refer to gastrointestinal hormones produced in response to the transit of nutrients through the duodenum and jejunum. The incretins enhance the sensitivity of the β-cells to glucose and thereby boost insulin secretion. It explains why the insulin secretory response is greater after oral than after intravenous glucose administration. Another set of hormones, the **'anti-incretins'**, are activated by the same nutrients but they serve to suppress the secretion and action of insulin. Healthy individuals are in a state of incretin/anti-incretin balance. An excess secretion of anti-incretins in response to a meal eventually results in T2DM. Long-acting analogs of incretins are being developed as a novel treatment strategy. A unique advantage of these drugs would be that since they augment insulin release in a glucose-dependent fashion, there would be minimum risk of drug-induced hypoglycemia.

Insulin resistance in these patients may be due to receptor downregulation caused by an increased expression of tumor necrosis factor-α in adipocytes of the obese individuals (receptor downregulation refers to a decrease in the total number of receptors of a hormone and/or a decrease in the affinity of the receptors for the hormone and/or an impairment in the post-receptor events).

Hyperglycemia is mainly a result of poor peripheral utilization of glucose, especially in the muscle. Blood glucose concentrations are much higher than normal, particularly after a meal. **Ketoacidosis does not develop** because the adipocytes remain sensitive to the effect of insulin on lipolysis. Rapid *de novo* synthesis of fatty acids and VLDL leads to hypertriglyceridemia without hyperchylomicronemia.

Weight reduction and dietary modifications often correct the hyperglycemia of T2DM. Hypoglycemic agents such as sulfonylureas may be required to achieve a satisfactory fall in blood glucose level.

Salient features of the two types of diabetes mellitus are given in Table 3.10.

Complications of Diabetes Mellitus

1. **Acute complications:** Ketoacidosis and coma (T1DM), nonketotic hyperosmolar coma (T2DM), or hypoglycemic coma (a consequence of insulin overdose or delaying/missing a meal after insulin injection).
2. **Chronic complications:** Myocardial infarction (diabetic patients often present with painless, i.e. silent myocardial infarction) due to accelerated atherosclerosis and coronary artery disease, cardiomyopathy, cerebrovascular disease, nephropathy, retinopathy, neuropathy, infections and delayed wound healing.

Biochemical Diagnosis of Diabetes Mellitus

It is based on the measurement of blood glucose or glycated hemoglobin (HbA1c, discussed later) and interpreted according to standard protocol (Table 3.11).

Table 3.10: Type 1 versus type 2 diabetes mellitus

Features	Type 1 diabetes mellitus	Type 2 diabetes mellitus
Prevalence	≈ 15%	≈ 85%
Age of onset	<35 years (juvenile-onset)	≥35 years (maturity-onset)
Primary cause	↓ Insulin production due to β-cell destruction	Insulin resistance in target tissues
Body habitus	Underweight	Overweight/obese
Plasma insulin	↓/Absent	Normal/↑
Plasma glucagon	↑, suppressible	↑, resistant
Acute complications	Ketoacidosis	Nonketotic hyperosmolar coma
Therapy	Insulin	Oral hypoglycemic agents

3

Table 3.11: Biochemical diagnosis of diabetes mellitus

	Fasting (12-hr) plasma glucose (mg/dl)	Postprandial (2-hr) plasma glucose (mg/dl)	Blood HbA1c
Normal	<100	<140	<5.7%
Pre-diabetes	100–125 (impaired fasting tolerance)	140–199 (impaired glucose tolerance)	5.7–6.4%
Diabetes mellitus	≥126	≥200	≥6.5%

- Either fasting or postprandial or casual (random) plasma glucose or blood HbA1c may be estimated.
- In case of casual plasma glucose, value ≥200 mg/dl is required for a diagnosis in patients with classical diabetic presentation of polyuria, polydipsia and unexplained weight loss.

Disease Monitoring

Once DM is diagnosed, short-term as well as long-term monitoring is essential to ensure the adequacy of glycemic control and to detect complications.

I. Short-term Monitoring

A. **Transcutaneous glucose measurement:** It is predicted that by that India may become the 'diabetic capital of the world'. Most methods of monitoring blood glucose require a blood sample, usually obtained by venepuncture or by using an automatic lancing device on a finger. Some glucometers use a blood sample from a less sensitive area such as the upper arm, forearm or thigh. Other devices use a beam of light instead of a lancet to pierce the skin.

Recent advances in insulin pump technology have created a demand for concurrent advances in the area of glucose sensing. A major reason for this is the desire to improve the quality of life of insulin pump users. When using a continuous insulin delivery system, the patients are required to check their blood glucose levels frequently throughout the day. As indicated above, many current devices rely on direct analysis of blood withdrawn from the tip of a finger. Many patients complain that these finger-sticks are painful and leave fingertips swollen and tender for many hours afterwards. The goal of many recent glucose-sensing devices is simply to minimize the pain associated with monitoring blood glucose levels.

Noninvasive blood glucose monitoring involves either radiation or fluid extraction. The most promising radiation technologies are: (1) mid-infrared radiation (mid-IR) spectroscopy; (2) near-infrared radiation (near-IR) spectroscopy; (3) radio wave impedance; and (4) optical rotation of polarized light. All of these technologies, except mid-IR spectroscopy, involve application of an external energy source to the body. The interaction between the applied radiation (or thermal emissions, in the case of mid-IR spectroscopy) and glucose in the blood is measured and converted into a blood glucose concentration.

B. **Urine glucose and ketone bodies:** This can be a bedside procedure using dipsticks.

II. Long-term Monitoring

A. **Glycated hemoglobin:** Measurement of blood glucose though is a good index of diabetes mellitus, however, it changes quickly. This mandates the need to develop better parameters for the diagnosis as well as for the long-term monitoring of these patients. Such a parameter is glycated hemoglobin. The glycation reaction is **nonenzymatic and irreversible** with **covalent** attachment of carbohydrates to the globin chains of hemoglobin, known as 'brownian reaction'. Various hemoglobin fractions may be separated and quantified by **chromatography** out of which HbA1c is of special interest as far as DM is concerned.

Advantages of glycated hemoglobin (HbA1c) measurement over blood glucose measurement

1. **Diagnostic value:** The amount of HbA1c formed is proportional to the mean blood glucose levels. Thus, increased HbA1c levels are observed in DM and may be used for its diagnosis.
2. **Glycemic control:** It is an index of blood glucose control, whether by diet restriction and/or anti-diabetic drugs. Glycation being irreversible, it leaves a record of glycemia throughout the RBC lifespan of **90–120 days**. Thus, a unique advantage of HbA1c measurement is that unlike simple blood glucose measurement, it reflects the time-average blood glucose over the preceding 2–4 months. A value >9% indicates poor glycemic control.

3. **Correlated with complications:** High HbA1c levels indicate the ongoing glycation of other body proteins forming advanced glycation end products (AGE). Loss of function of these proteins (e.g. LDL receptors, lens proteins, etc.) is associated with complications like accelerated atherosclerosis, coronary heart disease, retinopathy, cataract, nephropathy, neuropathy.
4. **Prognostic value:** Persistently high HbA1c levels indicate a poor prognosis.
5. **Low variability:** Values are fairly constant on a day-to-day basis.
6. **Convenient:** No special patient preparation is required, e.g. fasting or glucose load.

Disadvantages of Glycated Hemoglobin (HbA1c) Measurement

1. Does not give an idea of daily blood glucose fluctuations, hence difficult to adjust insulin dosage on a day-to-day basis.
2. Results influenced by RBC turnover (Chemistry to Clinics 3.14).
3. Expensive.

Chemistry to Clinics 3.14: HbA1c and RBC Turnover

All conditions that shorten the lifespan of RBC decrease HbA1c as the average time during which erythrocytes are exposed to glucose is reduced. This is observed in hemolytic anemia. Conversely, following splenectomy, RBC survival time and hence HbA1c is increased. Therefore, in patients with altered RBC turnover, it is recommended to use other tests for the determination of glycemic control, such as serum glycated albumin (turnover = 15–21 days, hence provides information on glycemic control over the past 2–4 weeks).

B. **Plasma C-peptide:** The β-cells of the pancreas secrete insulin. The product of the insulin gene is a peptide known as preproinsulin. As with other secretory peptides, the pre-peptide or signal peptide is cleaved off early in the biosynthetic process, yielding proinsulin, an 86-amino acid protein that is subsequently cleaved at two sites to yield insulin and a 31-amino acid peptide known as C-peptide. Insulin and C-peptide are therefore localized within the same secretory vesicle and are co-secreted into the bloodstream. Measurement of plasma C-peptide is gaining clinical significance (Chemistry to Clinics 3.15).

C. **Others:** Plasma lipid profile, renal function tests, uric acid, urinalysis for microalbuminuria, etc. are useful long-term monitoring parameters.

Chemistry to Clinics 3.15: C-Peptide

Measurements of circulating C-peptide levels can provide a valuable indirect assessment of β-cell insulin secretory capacity. In diabetic patients who are receiving exogenous insulin injections, the measurement of circulating insulin levels would not provide any useful information about their pancreatic function because it would primarily be the injected insulin that would be measured. However, an evaluation of C-peptide levels in such patients would provide an indirect measure of how well the β-cells were functioning with regard to insulin production and secretion.

Treatment Options for Diabetes Mellitus

Diet control, weight loss and exercise can be extremely effective in diabetes therapy and may be the only treatment necessary in the early stages. Patients are advised to switch over to foods having a low to moderate **glycemic index** (**GI**, a term that refers to the ability of a particular food to increase the blood glucose compared to 100% for an equal amount of pure glucose). Category of foods based on their GI:

- Low GI: Soybeans, apples, oranges, milk, yogurt.
- Moderate GI: Rye bread, bananas, pineapple, ice cream.
- High GI: White bread, corn flakes, potatoes, carrots, watermelon, soft drinks, honey.

For those patients who are reluctant to give up sucrose/glucose, artificial sweeteners are a good choice as a sugar substitute, their use, however, should be limited (Chemistry to Clinics 3.16).

Chemistry to Clinics 3.16: Artificial Sweeteners

Owing to the fact that diabetic patients and even those having impaired glucose tolerance are advised to avoid glucose or sucrose in their diet, 'artificial sweeteners' have become popular substitutes. The **non-nutritive sweeteners** do not yield energy, e.g. saccharin and sucralose. Their RDA is 5 mg/kg body weight. The **nutritive sweeteners**, e.g. aspartame, yield 4 kcal/g of energy that is insignificant owing to its RDA of 15 mg/kg body weight. However, aspartame also yields the amino acid phenylalanine, hence it should be avoided in patients suffering from phenylketonuria.

Commonly, however, lifestyle intervention is supplemented by treatment with **insulin injections in case of T1DM** or one or more **oral agents in case of T2DM**. Multiple classes of drugs independently address different biochemical alterations that contribute to the development of type 2 diabetes. The available oral antidiabetic agents can be divided by their mechanism of action into insulin sensitizers with primary action in the liver (e.g. biguanides), insulin sensitizers with primary action in peripheral tissues (e.g. glitazones), insulin secretagogues (e.g. sulfonylureas), agents that slow the absorption of carbohydrates (e.g. α-glucosidase inhibitors) and SGLT2 inhibitors (Chemistry to Clinics 3.17).

Chemistry to Clinics: 3.17: Sodium-glucose Linked Transporter 2 (SGLT2) and Diabetes Mellitus

In the kidneys, >90% of the filtered glucose is reabsorbed by SGLT2 in the proximal convoluted tubules and the rest by SGLT1 in the proximal straight tubules. Recently, a new drug called canagliflozin has been introduced in the market which inhibits SGLT2. Thus, majority of the filtered glucose fails to get reabsorbed and is eliminated in the urine. This helps to reduce blood glucose levels and is useful in the treatment of T2DM.

In some cases, a patient with T2DM may be treated with insulin, just like the patient with T1DM.

TESTS FOR DIABETES MELLITUS

Estimation of Blood Glucose

Normal Values

Normal value for glucose, by the methods other than Folin-Wu, varies between 60 and 90 mg/dl of whole blood or 70 and 100 mg/dl of serum or plasma, in adults. In neonates, blood glucose concentration varies between 30 and 60 mg/dl of serum/plasma, which is still lower in premature neonates. Blood glucose concentration increases with age by about 2–3 mg/dl, per decade.

Glucose concentration in the cerebrospinal fluid (CSF) is nearly 60–65% of the serum/plasma level.

Hypoglycemia

Hypoglycemia (plasma glucose concentration below 40 mg/dl) is a common and potentially dangerous complication of insulin treatment, particularly, in tightly controlled diabetics. Insulinoma (benign adenoma of pancreatic islets) can also cause hypoglycemia. Estimation of plasma insulin concentration, which is raised during fasting, confirms diagnosis.

Estimation of blood glucose may include analysis of the:

- Random sample for blood glucose
- Fasting sample for blood glucose
- Two-hour's postprandial sample for blood glucose

Besides, one can perform oral glucose tolerance test (OGTT).

Glucose Tolerance Test

Glucose tolerance test (GTT) determines the ability of an individual to tolerate an extra load of glucose.

Oral GTT is helpful in patients who have fasting blood glucose concentration in the upper normal limits, those with transient or sustained glycosuria without the symptoms of diabetes or those with family history of the disease, etc.

Procedure

- For a standard routine GTT fasting venous blood sample (after 12–16 hours of fast) is drawn, in a fluoride-oxalate bottle.
- Thereafter, 75 g of glucose (about 1 g/kg body weight) is given, in nearly 200–300 ml of water, to drink. Blood samples are again drawn after every 30 minutes, till 2 to 2½ hours.
- Urine specimens are also collected, simultaneously.
- Each sample is analyzed and glucose tolerance curve is plotted.

Interpretation of the test

- Fasting blood glucose, maximum value of glucose, rate at which it returns to the fasting value and glycosuria gives idea about the disease.
- For a **normal individual fasting blood glucose** value is within the normal limit. It is increased by more than twofold within 60 min and thereafter returns to normal after about two hours of the ingestion of glucose. Moreover, glycosuria is not observed in any of the sample (Fig. 3.45).

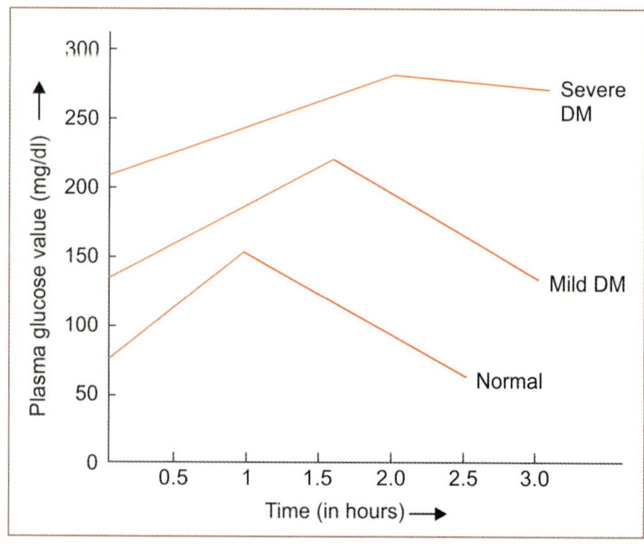

Fig. 3.45: Glucose tolerance curves

3

- Any deviation from the above is referred to as **abnormal glucose tolerance curve**. In a patient with diabetes mellitus fasting blood glucose level is above the normal and/or curve is raised as well as prolonged. This is also accompanied with glycosuria.
- In a patient of renal glycosuria, glucose tolerance curve is normal but there is glycosuria.

Fasting and postprandial blood glucose concentration

- Recently, International Committee of Diabetologists has recommended simplifying the glucose tolerance test to require only an overnight fasting measurement and 2 hours after a standard 75 g oral glucose load.
- An oral glucose tolerance test is normal if the fasting venous plasma glucose value is less than 100 mg/dl and the 2 hours value is below 140 mg/dl.
- A fasting value of 126 mg/dl or higher, or a 2-hour value of greater than 200 mg/dl is diagnostic of diabetes mellitus.
- Values between the upper limits of normal and those diagnostic of diabetes (fasting between 100 and 125 mg/dl and 2-hour value between 140 and

Hypoglycemia (plasma glucose concentration below 40 mg/dl) is a common and potentially dangerous complication of insulin treatment, particularly, in tightly controlled diabetes. Insulinoma (benign adenoma of pancreatic islets) can also cause hypoglycemia. Estimating plasma insulin concentration, which is raised during fasting, can make its diagnosis.

Besides the above, **glycated hemoglobin** (glycosylated hemoglobin or HbA1c) is ordered for monitoring type II diabetes, while it becomes essential to test for **insulin**, if a patient is on insulin therapy.

GLYCOGEN STORAGE DISEASES

This is a group of inherited disorders associated with glycogen metabolism where an abnormal type or quantity of glycogen is deposited in different tissues. According to the deficiency of the enzyme involved, there are several types of glycogen storage diseases. All these are autosomal recessive disorders except Her's disease which is autosomal dominant (Table 3.12).

LACTOSE INTOLERANCE

It is a condition resulting from a deficiency of intestinal **lactase** so that the individual is unable to digest the milk sugar. It is different from milk allergy that is due to an immune reaction to milk protein. Lactase deficiency results in the accumulation of undigested lactose which is osmotically active. Lactose moves to the colon where its bacterial fermentation generates

Table 3.12: Glycogen storage diseases

Type	Glycogen storage disease	Deficient enzyme	Features
I	von Gierke's disease	Glucose-6-phosphatase	Liver, renal and intestinal epithelial cells are loaded with glycogen. There also occurs hypoglycemia, lactic acidosis, ketosis, hyperlipemia and hyperuricemia.
II	Pompe's disease	Lysosomal acid maltase	Accumulation of glycogen in the lysosomes. It is fatal and may result in heart failure
III	Limit dextrinosis/Forbes' disease or Cori disease	Debranching enzyme	Accumulation of the branched polysaccharide in liver, muscle, heart and leukocytes
IV	Amylopectinosis or Andersen's disease	Branching enzyme	Accumulation of the polysaccharide having few branch points. Death may occur due to liver or cardiac failure within first year of life
V	McArdle's syndrome	Muscle phosphorylase	Muscle has abnormally high glycogen content. There is diminished exercise tolerance with little or no lactate in blood after exercise.
VI	Her's disease	Liver phosphorylase	High glycogen content in liver. There is also a tendency towards hypoglycemia
VII	Tarui disease	Phosphofructokinase	As in type V, but there is also a possibility of hemolytic anemia
VIII	—	Liver phosphorylase kinase	As in type VI

CO_2 and organic acids. The symptoms include abdominal cramps, diarrhea and flatulence.

It is very rare for an infant to be born with lactase deficiency. Lactase activity is highest immediately after birth and by adulthood only 5–10% of the initial activity remains. Only 30% of people retain enough lactase to digest lactose efficiently throughout adult life. Secondary lactase deficiency may result from damage to villi caused by drugs, prolonged diarrhea and malnutrition. Cheese is well tolerated since lactose gets removed with the whey during manufacturing.

The management strategy is to gradually decrease the intake of milk products, to take them with other foods and to spread their intake over the day. Further, medications containing lactose as filler must be avoided and adequate supplementation of riboflavin, calcium and vitamin D should be taken. **'Acidophilus milk'**, i.e. milk pre-treated with the bacteria *Lactobacillus acidophilus* is commercially available. The bacterial lactase cleaves lactose into glucose plus galactose, thus producing a sweet though lactose-free product.

Some Important Questions

1. Define carbohydrate. Give their classification.

2. What are polysaccharides? Classify them.

3. Outline the reactions of citric acid cycle. Give energetics of the cycle and explain the amphibolic role of this cycle.

4. Outline HMP shunt reactions. Discuss the significance of HMP pathway in the liver and erythrocytes.

5. Give outline of glycolytic reactions. What are the regulatory steps? What is the energy yield of this pathway?

6. Define glycogenolysis. Outline reactions of this pathway. How is it regulated?

7. What is glycogenesis? Give reactions of glycogenesis. How is it regulated?

8. Explain:

i. Why aerobic glycolysis releases more energy than anaerobic glycolysis?
ii. How glycolysis can be reversed?
iii. Anaplerotic reactions of TCA cycle and its energetics

9. Discuss briefly:

i. Metabolism of galactose
ii. Regulation of blood glucose
iii. Glycogenolysis
iv. Fructose metabolism

10. Write notes on:

i. Cellulose
ii. Inulin
iii. Homopolysaccharides
iv. Heteropolysaccharides
v. Hyaluronic acid
vi. Chondroitin sulfates
vii. Heparin
viii. Diabetes mellitus
ix. Galactosemia
x. Glycogenesis
xi. Glycated hemoglobin
xii. Artificial sweeteners
xiii. Energetics of TCA cycle
xiv. Gluconeogenesis
xv. Glycogen storage diseases

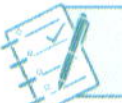

Multiple Choice Questions

1. An example of a nonreducing disaccharide is:

A. Maltose
B. Isomaltose
C. Lactose
D. Sucrose

2. The most notorious cariogenic sugar is:

A. Sucrose B. Glucose
C. Fructose D. Lactose

3. In the prophylaxis and treatment of deep vein thrombosis, low molecular weight derivatives of the following heteropolysaccharides are used:

A. Hyaluronic acid
B. Chondroitin sulphate
C. Heparan
D. Heparin

4. The following heteropolysaccharide is commercially available for injecting into synovial joints in patients suffering from advanced ostcoarthritis:

A. Hyaluronic acid
B. Chondroitin sulphate
C. Heparan
D. Heparin

5. Cornea and heart valves are rich in the following heteropolysaccharide(s):

A. Keratan sulphate
B. Chondroitin-4-sulphate and chondroitin-6-sulphate
C. Dermatan sulphate
D. Keratan sulphate and dermatan sulphate

6. Fluoroacetate inhibits:

A. Hexokinase
B. Pyruvate dehydrogenase
C. Aconitase
D. Lactate dehydrogenase

7. Essential fructosuria is due to a deficiency of:

A. Aldolase 'A'
B. Aldolase 'B'
C. Fructokinase
D. Phosphofructokinase 1

8. The following is called a glucose sensor in pancreatic α-cells:

A. Glucokinase
B. Insulin
C. Amylin
D. Glucose tolerance factor

9. Glycated hemoglobin levels in blood are an index of blood glucose control over the past:

A. 3 hours
B. 3 days
C. 3 months
D. 3 years

10. Anderson's disease is due to deficiency of:

A. Lysosomal acid maltase
B. Debranching enzyme
C. Branching enzyme
D. Muscle phosphorylase

CHAPTER 4

Chemistry and Metabolism of Lipids

Competency Achievement: The student should be able to:

BI4.1 Describe and discuss main classes of lipids (essential/nonessential fatty acids, cholesterol and hormonal steroids, triglycerides, major phospholipids and sphingolipids) relevant to human system and their major functions

BI4.2 Describe the processes involved in digestion and absorption of dietary lipids and also the key features of their metabolism

BI4.3 Explain the regulation of lipoprotein metabolism and associated disorders

BI4.4 Describe the structure and functions of lipoproteins, their functions, interrelations and relations with atherosclerosis

BI4.5 Interpret laboratory results of analytes associated with metabolism of lipids

BI4.6 Describe the therapeutic uses of prostaglandins and inhibitors of eicosanoid synthesis

BI4.7 Interpret laboratory results of analytes associated with metabolism of lipids

PY4.4 Describe the physiology of digestion and absorption of nutrients

IM2.3 Discuss and describe the lipid cycle and the role of dyslipidemia in the pathogenesis of atherosclerosis

IM2.12 Choose and interpret a lipid profile and identify the desirable lipid profile in the clinical context

Lipids (Greek *lipos*: Fat) are the heterogeneous group of largely hydrophobic organic molecules found in all cells. They are sparingly soluble in water but are soluble in organic solvents, such as acetone, ether, alcohol or chloroform. Lipids therefore, can be easily separated from other biological materials by their extraction into organic solvents.

CLASSIFICATION OF LIPIDS

Lipids are classified into three groups, i.e. simple lipids, compound lipids and derived lipids (Fig. 4.1).

Simple Lipids

Simple lipids are the esters of fatty acids with various types of alcohol, e.g. fats, oils and waxes.

Fats and oils are complex mixtures of triacylglycerols (triglycerides) whose fatty acid composition may vary with the source. Thus, 'lipids' and 'fats' are not synonymous; fats are just a type of simple lipids.

Fats and oils differ only in that **fats are solid while oils are liquid at room temperature.**

Fats are obtained from animal sources, have more saturated fatty acids and thus higher melting points.

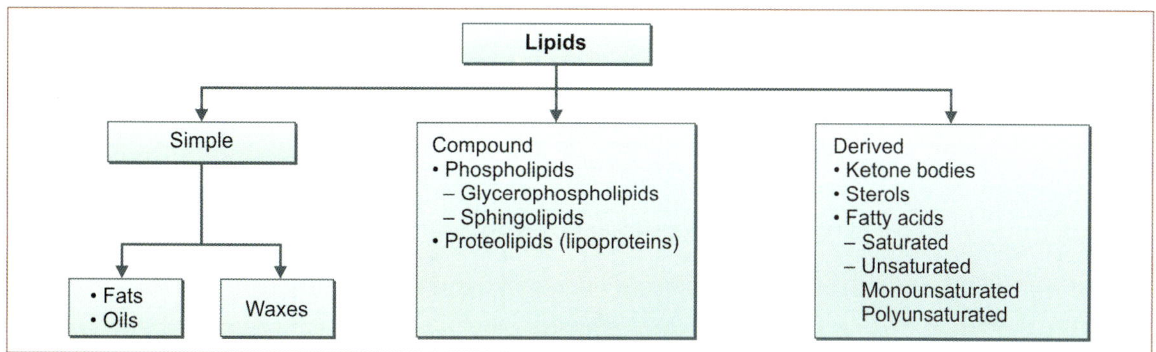

Fig. 4.1: Classification of lipids

Oils are abundant in plant seeds. These are usually rich in unsaturated fatty acids.

The esters of long chain fatty acids with high molecular weight monohydroxy aliphatic alcohols are called **waxes**. These are used in the manufacturing of various types of wax polish.

Compound Lipids

In addition to fatty acids and alcohol, certain lipids also contain some amphipathic group. These are thus called compound lipids, e.g. lipids conjugated with phosphate to form phospholipids.

Derived Lipids

These are derived from the hydrolysis of the simple lipids and the compound lipids, e.g. fatty acids, glycerol, etc.

Biological Significance of Lipids

1. Important dietary constituents of food; have high calorific value.
2. Enhance the palatability of food.
3. Dietary lipids are the source of lipid soluble vitamins and essential fatty acids.
4. Serve as energy stores.
5. Subcutaneous and perivisceral fat acts as a thermo-insulating material.
6. Lipids around the nerves, such as myelin sheath, act as electrical insulators.
7. Lipid bilayers together with proteins are important components of biological membranes.
8. Involved in various intra- and intercellular signaling events.

FATTY ACIDS

Fatty acids are the carboxylic acids with a long hydrocarbon chain. The hydrocarbon chain in turn may be **saturated** (no double bond) or **unsaturated** with one or more double bonds.

Most fatty acids in the body are esterified in triacylglycerols or phospholipids which act as storage or structural forms, or transport vehicles for fatty acids.

The major source of circulating free fatty acids is the adipose tissue which releases fatty acids after hydrolysis of its stored triacylglycerols. Although the plasma concentration of free fatty acids is low, they have a very rapid turnover and are an important source of energy for many tissues of the body. They have a limited solubility in water and are mainly bound to plasma albumin which has specific binding sites for free fatty acids.

Nomenclature of Fatty Acids

The nomenclature of fatty acids depends upon the name of the hydrocarbon chain with the same number of carbon atoms where the suffix '-oic' is substituted for the final 'e' in the name of the hydrocarbon. There are two systems of nomenclature:

Delta system: Various carbon atoms in a fatty acid are numbered, beginning with the **carboxyl carbon** (–COOH) as carbon atom number 1. The next carbon atom, to which the carboxyl carbon group is attached, is designated as α-carbon. Accordingly, carbon-3 (C_3) is the β-carbon and C4 is the γ-carbon. This system of numbering of the carbon atoms of a fatty acid is called delta (Δ) system of nomenclature of fatty acids.

Omega system: The carbon atoms in a fatty acid are counted beginning at the **methyl terminal** (CH_3-) end of the chain and the position where a double bond is first encountered. This carbon atom at the terminal CH_3-group is called omega (ω) carbon. Hence, this system of nomenclature of a fatty acid is called omega (ω) system (Fig. 4.2).

However, replacement of the symbol ω by the letter 'n' has been recommended as an n-numbering system.

Saturated and Unsaturated Fatty Acids

The hydrocarbon side chain in a fatty acid may be saturated or unsaturated. Accordingly, fatty acids may be divided into two groups, i.e. saturated fatty acids and unsaturated fatty acids.

Most of the naturally occurring fatty acids have even number of carbon atoms because they are synthesized

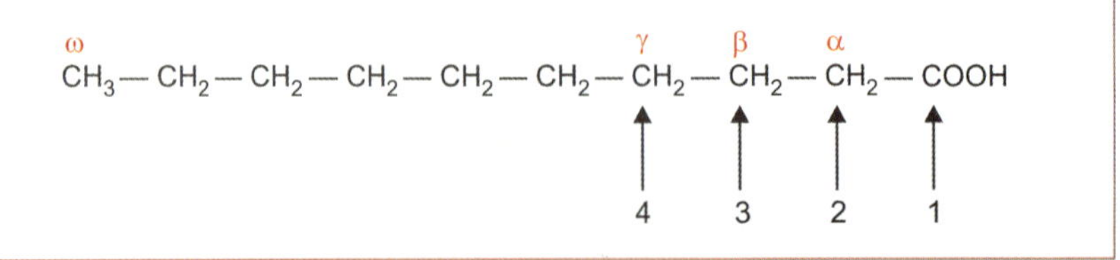

Fig. 4.2: Numbering of a fatty acid

4

from acetyl-CoA, i.e. by the combination of 2C units. They are divided into three groups, i.e. short chain (4–8C), medium chain (9–14C) and long chain fatty acids (15C or more). They have different physicochemical properties and are handled differently in the body. In higher plants and animals, the predominant fatty acids are those containing 16 or 18 carbon atoms, such as palmitic acid, oleic acid, linoleic acid and stearic acid.

Saturated fatty acids end in '-anoic', e.g. octadecanoic acid (stearic acid) is a fatty acid with 18 carbon atoms. Saturated fatty acids are highly flexible molecules and can assume a wide range of conformations because there is relatively free rotation around each of their C–C bonds. These are obtained from animal fats, e.g. butter fat. Saturated fatty acids of common biological significance are listed in Table 4.1.

Unsaturated fatty acids, i.e. those with one or more double bonds, end with '-enoic', e.g. octadecenoic acid (oleic acid), a fatty acid with 18 carbon atoms and a double bond. Widely used convention to name an unsaturated fatty acid is to indicate the number of carbon atoms, followed by the number of double bonds with their positions in the carbon chain, such as octadecenoic acid may be written as 18:1; 9, i.e. a fatty acid with 18 carbon atoms and one double bond present on C9, i.e. between C9 and C10 (Fig. 4.3).

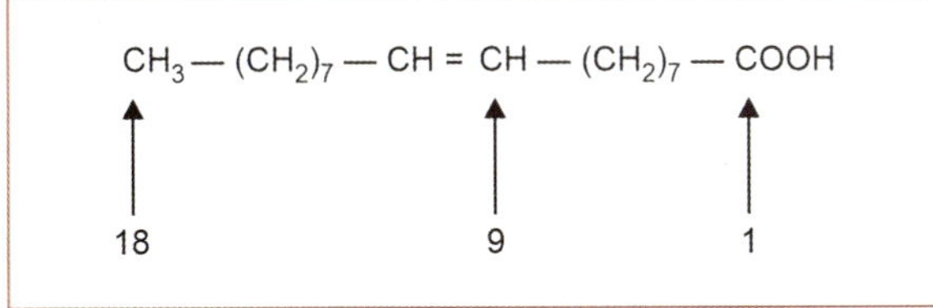

Fig. 4.3: Oleic acid or octadecenoic acid (18:1;9)

The location of double bond in linoleic acid can be indicated by the symbol Δ, followed by the number of carbon atom. Thus, linoleic acid, which has 18 carbons and two double bonds at C9 and C12, is written as 18:2;9,12.

According to the ω system, linoleic acid is designated as ω-6 fatty acid because the double bond (closest to the ω-end) is located six carbon atoms away from the ω-end (Fig. 4.4).

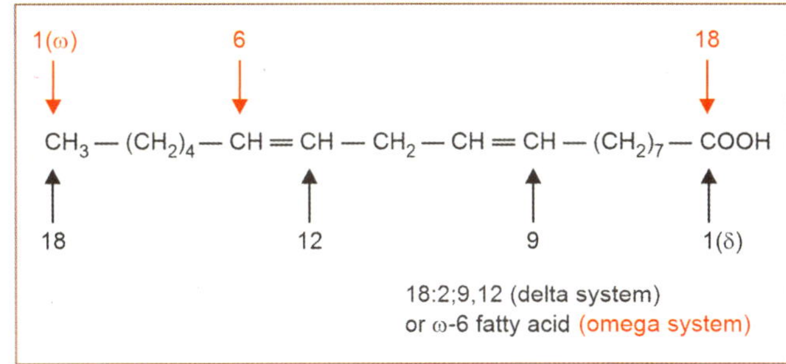

Fig. 4.4: Linoleic acid

Over half of the fatty acid residues of plant and animal lipids are unsaturated, i.e. they contain double bonds. The double bond of a monounsaturated fatty acid commonly occurs between C9 and C10, and is called a Δ9 double bond, e.g. oleic acid.

The double bonds may be *cis-* or *trans-* in their orientation. Naturally occurring fatty acids have predominantly *cis-* double bonds (Chemistry to Clinics 4.1).

Chemistry to Clinics 4.1: *Trans*-Fatty Acids

Majority of the unsaturated fatty acids occurring in nature are *cis*-fatty acids, i.e. the H-atoms next to the double bonds lie on the same side of the hydrocarbon chain. Only a few are *trans*-fatty acids, i.e. the H-atoms next to the double bonds lie on opposite sides of the hydrocarbon chain (Fig. 4.5).

Table 4.1: Saturated fatty acids

Fatty acids	No. of C-atoms	Formula	Sources
Acetic acid	2	CH_3–COOH	Carbohydrate fermentation
Butyric acid	4	CH_3–$(CH_2)_2$–COOH	Butter
Caproic acid	6	CH_3–$(CH_2)_4$–COOH	Butter and some plant fats
Caprylic acid	8	CH_3–$(CH_2)_6$–COOH	– do –
Capric acid	10	CH_3–$(CH_2)_8$–COOH	– do –
Lauric acid	12	CH_3–$(CH_2)_{10}$–COOH	Coconut oil
Myristic acid	14	CH_3–$(CH_2)_{12}$–COOH	– do –
Palmitic acid	16	CH_3–$(CH_2)_{14}$–COOH	Animal and plant fats
Stearic acid	18	CH_3–$(CH_2)_{16}$–COOH	– do –
Arachidic acid	20	CH_3–$(CH_2)_{18}$–COOH	Peanut oil

Fig. 4.5: *Cis-trans* isomerism in fatty acids: The steric geometry of unsaturated fatty acids can vary so that the acyl groups can be oriented on the same side or on opposite sides of the double bond. When both the acyl groups are on the same side of the double bond it is referred to as a *cis* bond, e.g. oleic acid (18:1). When the acyl groups are on opposite sides the bond is termed *trans* such as in elaidic acid, the *trans* isomer of oleic acid. The majority of naturally occurring unsaturated fatty acids exist in the *cis*-conformation. *Trans*-fatty acids occur in some foods and as byproducts of the process of hydrogenating saturated fatty acids to make them solids at room temperature, such as in partially hydrogenated vegetable oils

Milk fat and butter contain traces of *trans*-fatty acids. In the body, *trans*-fatty acids behave more like saturated fatty acids than like unsaturated fatty acids and are associated with cardiovascular disease.

Unsaturated fatty acids are chemically more reactive than the saturated fatty acids and are prone to alterations by processes such as lipid peroxidation. Unsaturated fatty acids pack together less efficiently than the saturated fatty acids. Unsaturated fatty acids also have reduced van der Waals interactions and low melting points; the melting point decreases with the degree of unsaturation. On the other hand, the fluidity of lipid increases with the degree of unsaturation.

Physical and Chemical Properties of Fatty Acids

- Generally, short chain fatty acids, i.e. those between 4C and 8C, are liquid while long chain fatty acids, i.e. those with >15 carbon atoms are solid at room temperature.
- Fatty acids present in various oils react with alkali and form salts. Salts of the various acids are used as soaps and emulsifying agents.
- Unsaturated fatty acids undergo reduction and are converted to saturated fats, such as hydrogenation of a vegetable oil results in the formation of ghee.
- Unsaturated fatty acids exhibit *cis-trans* isomerism, due to the presence of a double bond.
- Various fatty acids can be separated from a mixture by gas-liquid chromatography.

Polyunsaturated Fatty Acids

Fatty acids obtained from plant seeds usually contain two or more double bonds. These fatty acids are called polyunsaturated fatty acids (**PUFAs**). In PUFAs, double bonds generally occur after every three carbon atoms and always have a *cis*-configuration. The PUFAs are obtained mainly from plant oils, e.g. soya bean oil, sunflower oil, groundnut oil, etc.

Essential Fatty Acids

Though the body can introduce a double bond and prolong an aliphatic chain, some of the polyunsaturated fatty acids (PUFAs) cannot be synthesized in the body. Thus, they are to be essentially included in the diet and are called essential fatty acids. These include linoleic acid, linolenic acid and arachidonic acid (Figs 4.4, 4.6 and 4.7).

As linoleic acid can be converted to arachidonic acid in the body, hence, only two of these, i.e. **linoleic acid** and **linolenic acid** are truly essential in a human diet. Arachidonic acid, however, becomes essential, if there is insufficient amount of linoleic acid in the diet.

Deficiency of the essential fatty acids can lead to the development of a condition characterized by retarded growth, hair loss, dermatitis ('toad-skin' or phrenoderma) and poor wound healing (Fig. 4.8).

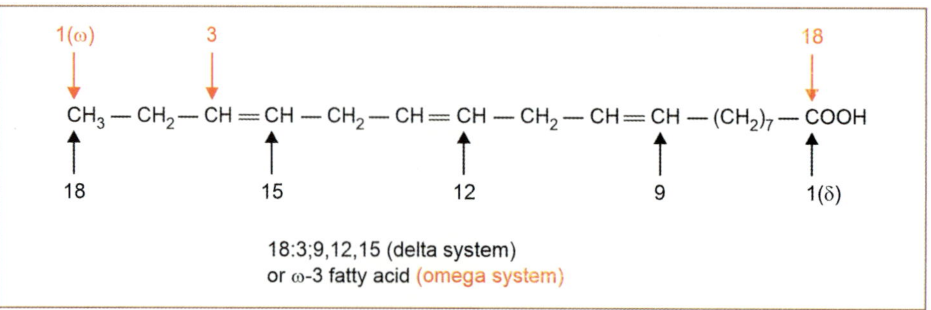

Fig. 4.6: Linolenic acid

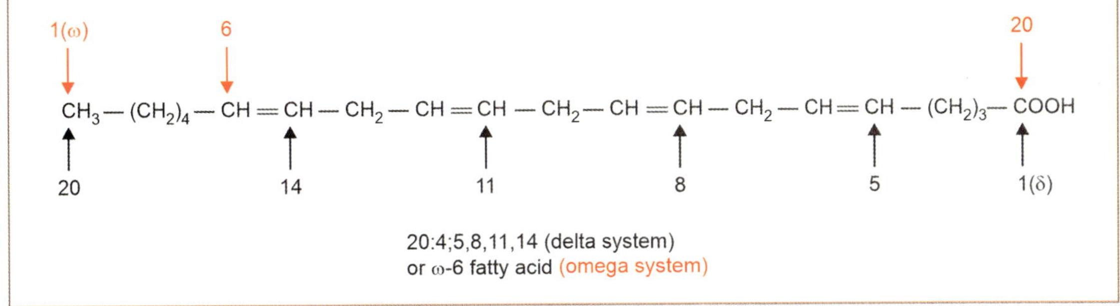

Fig. 4.7: Arachidonic acid

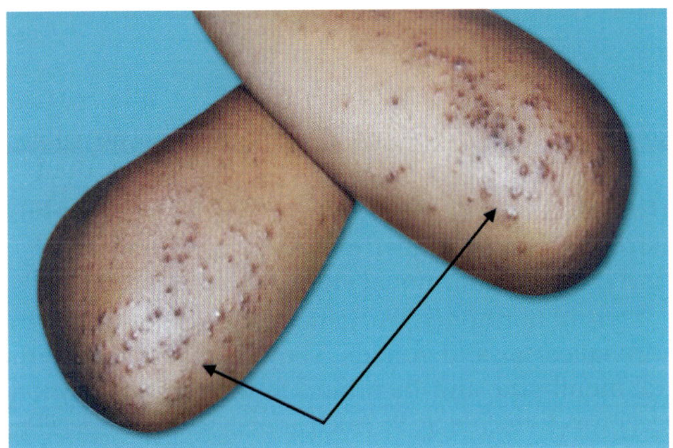

Fig. 4.8: Phrenoderma (or phrynoderma): A child with hard papules on the extensor surfaces (arrows) due to deficiency of essential fatty acids, resembling **'toad skin'**. However, sometimes, similar findings may be seen in vitamin A deficiency

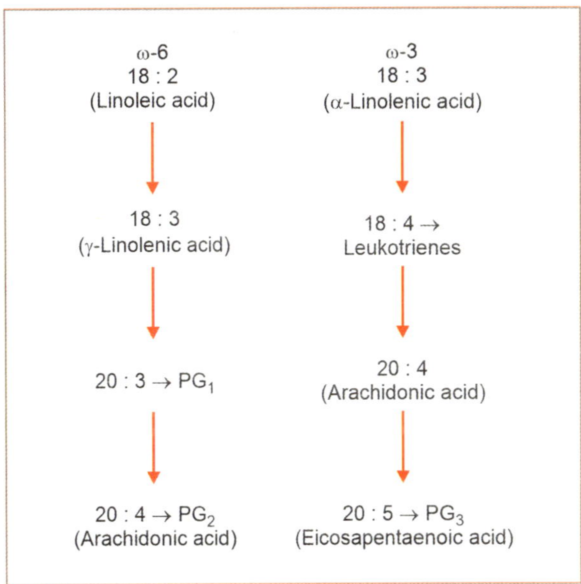

Fig. 4.9: Biological significance of essential fatty acids

Functions of Essential Fatty Acids

- They form an important constituent of the phospholipids.
- Essential fatty acids also help in lowering blood cholesterol level and help in its esterification in the liver.
- Arachidonic acid is also a precursor of eicosanoids such as prostaglandins, thromboxanes and leukotrienes.

Essential fatty acids are sometimes also classified by the position of the first double bond, numbered from the methyl (or ω) end of the fatty acid chain. Thus, linoleic acid is an example of an ω-6 and α-linolenic acid of an ω-3 fatty acid. Both types are essential and can be converted into many biologically important compounds (Fig. 4.9).

Arachidonic acid (20:4;5,8,11,14), an ω-6 fatty acid can be synthesized from linoleic acid. It is a precursor of the 2-series of prostaglandins and thromboxanes, and the 4-series of leukotrienes. The α-linolenic acid is converted in the body to eicosapentaenoic acid (20:5 ω-3), a precursor of the 3-series of prostaglandins and thromboxanes.

Biological Significance of PUFA

1. Necessary for normal growth and health.
2. Important constituents of all biological membranes.
3. Required for the esterification of cholesterol and thus help in its transport and metabolism.
4. Diet rich in ω-6 PUFA (principally linoleic acid) promotes a reduction in cholesterol level.
5. Diet rich in ω-3 PUFA promotes a reduction in plasma triacylglycerols.
6. Arachidonic acid is a precursor of eicosanoids.

CHOLESTEROL AND HORMONAL STEROIDS

Steroids are the derivatives of **cyclopentanoperhydrophenanthrene ring**, also called **steroid nucleus**, a component that consists of four fused, nonpolar rings labeled as A, B, C and D (Fig. 4.10).

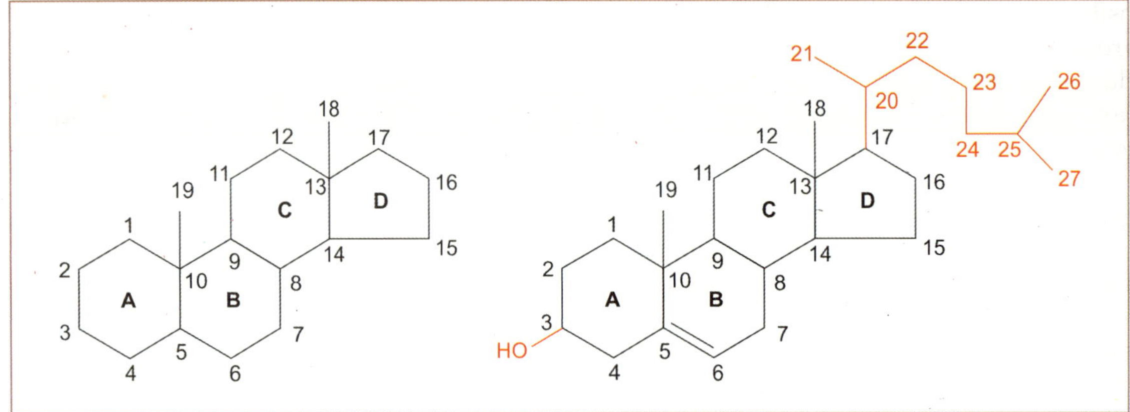

Fig. 4.10: Steroid nucleus (cyclopentanoperhydrophenanthrene ring) and cholesterol

CHOLESTEROL

Cholesterol is the most abundant steroid in animals. It has 27 carbon atoms, a hydroxyl group at C3, a double bond between C5 and C6, two methyl groups at C18 and C19, and a side chain at C17 (Fig. 4.10).

Because of the OH group (at C3), cholesterol is a steroid alcohol (sterol) and can be esterified to long chain fatty acids to form cholesteryl esters.

Functions of Cholesterol

1. The body of an adult contains about 1 g cholesterol/kg body weight. About 25% of it is in the membranes of the nervous system where it is a major component of the myelin sheath.
2. Cholesterol is a major component of all biological membranes where it exists as free/unesterified cholesterol.
3. It is a precursor of steroid hormones (glucocorticoids, mineralocorticoids, androgens and estrogens), vitamin D and bile acids.

Normal serum cholesterol level is 150–220 mg/dL although the desirable level in adults is <200 mg/dL. Eggs, meat and milk are the main dietary sources of cholesterol. It is also synthesized in the body by nearly all cells and the process is controlled by the intracellular cholesterol content. The amount synthesized each day is at least twice of that ingested in the average diet which is nearly 250–750 mg/day.

HORMONAL STEROIDS

Hormonal steroids are the steroids that act as hormones. They are a group of hormones which are **derived from cholesterol**. They are secreted by the adrenal cortex, testes and ovaries and during pregnancy by the placenta. On the basis of their receptors, steroid hormones have been classified into different groups as **glucocorticoids**, **mineralocorticoids**, **androgens**, **estrogens** and **progestins**. Besides, **vitamin D** is a closely related hormonal steroid (*see* Chapter 8).

Steroid hormones are, generally, synthesized in the adrenal cortex and gonads. They can pass through the cell membrane and then bind to the steroid hormone receptors (which may be nuclear or cytosolic depending on the steroid hormone) to bring about changes within the cell. They are transported through the bloodstream, bound to specific carrier proteins such as corticosteroid-binding globulin or sex hormone-bonding globulin. Further conversions and catabolism occurs in the liver, other peripheral tissues, and the target tissues.

Steroid hormones perform several functions, such as help control metabolism, inflammation, immune functions, electrolytes and water balance, development of sexual characteristics, and the ability to withstand illness and injury.

- **Glucocorticoids**, such as **cortisol**, control or influence many metabolic processes, including the formation of glucose (from amino acids) and fatty acids, and the deposition of glycogen in the liver. Glucocorticoids also help to maintain normal blood pressure, and have anti-inflammatory and immunosuppressive actions.
- **Mineralocorticoids**, such as **aldosterone**, help maintain the balance between water and electrolytes in the body, predominantly exerting their effects within the kidneys.
- **Androgens** are the male sex hormones. The principal androgen, **testosterone**, is produced, primarily, by the testes and in lesser amounts by the adrenal cortex and (in women) by the ovaries. They are, primarily,

responsible for the development and maintenance of reproductive function and stimulation of the secondary sex characteristics in the male. They also have an anabolic function in stimulating the production of skeletal muscle, bone and red blood cells.

- **Estrogens** are one of the two types of female sex hormones. They are secreted, mainly, by the ovaries and in smaller amounts by the adrenal glands and in men by the testes. The most potent of the estrogen is **estradiol**. Estrogens promote development of the primary and secondary female sex characteristics. They also stimulate linear growth and skeletal maturation. The ovarian production of estrogen plummets during menopause.
- **Progestins**, the most important of which is **progesterone**, are the other type of female sex hormones and are named for their role in maintaining pregnancy (progestation).

  Both, estrogens and progestins are secreted, cyclically, during menstruation. During the menstrual cycle, the corpus luteum produces progesterone, which renders the uterine lining receptive to the implantation of a fertilized ovum. The contraceptive quality of progesterone led to the development of structurally modified progestins and estrogens, the oral contraceptives, known as birth-control pills that are used by women to prevent unwanted pregnancy.

TRIGLYCERIDES

Triglycerides or neutral fats (also called triacylglycerols) are fatty acid tri-esters of glycerol (glycerin, a trihydric alcohol) and are simple lipids. Glycerol with one molecule of a fatty acid is called **monoacylglycerol**, with two molecules of fatty acids are called a **diacylglycerol** while with three fatty acid residues it is known as **triacylglycerol** (Fig. 4.11).

A molecule of triacylglycerol may contain three similar or dissimilar fatty acid residues which may be saturated and/or unsaturated. Triglycerides are named according to the presence of the fatty acid residues on the glycerol moiety, e.g. 1-palmitoyl-2-arachidonoyl-3-stearoylglycerol has palmitic acid at C1, arachidonic acid at C2 and stearic acid at C3 of glycerol. All natural fats and oils invariably are complex mixtures of triacylglycerols whose fatty acid composition varies with the source. Plant oils are usually rich in unsaturated fatty acids compared to animal fats. Generally, with the primary alcoholic groups, i.e. at the α positions (C1 and C3 of glycerol), there are saturated fatty acids while at C2 there is an unsaturated fatty acid.

$$\begin{array}{ll} CH_2-OH & \alpha_1\ CH_2-O-COR_1 \\ | & | \\ CH-OH & \beta\ CH-O-COR_2 \\ | & | \\ CH_2-OH & \alpha_2\ CH_2-O-COR_3 \\ \textbf{Glycerol} & \textbf{A triglyceride} \end{array}$$

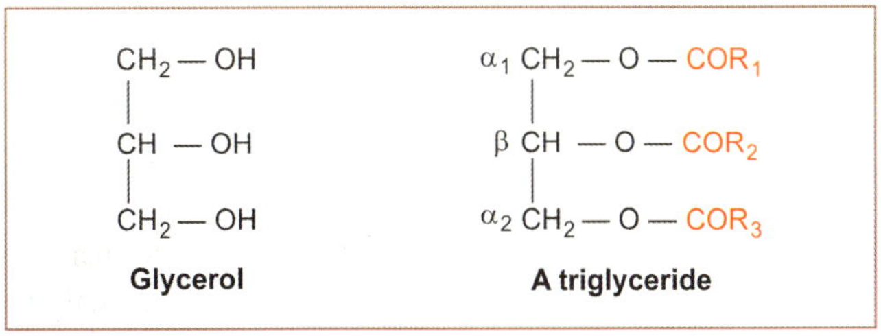

Fig. 4.11: Structure of glycerol and a triglyceride (triacylglycerol or neutral fat)

Dietary fat, which is an **important source of energy for the body**, mainly contains triacylglycerols. In the body also triacylglycerols are the store of energy. Fat is stored in the body in the form of triacylglycerols, mainly in the adipose tissue. Triacylglycerols are transported in the plasma either as chylomicrons (which are produced by the intestine for the transport of exogenous fat) or as very low density lipoprotein particles (which are produced in the liver for the transport of endogenous triglycerides).

Physical and Chemical Properties of Triacylglycerols

1. ***Energy reserve:*** Triacylglycerols are the major storage form of energy in the body. In animals, fat cells (adipocytes) are specialized for the synthesis and storage of triacylglycerols. The average fat content of normal human being is about 21% for man and 26% for woman. This allows them to survive for 2–3 months.
2. ***Hydrolysis:*** Triacylglycerols are hydrolysed by lipases to release free fatty acids and glycerol (Fig. 4.12).

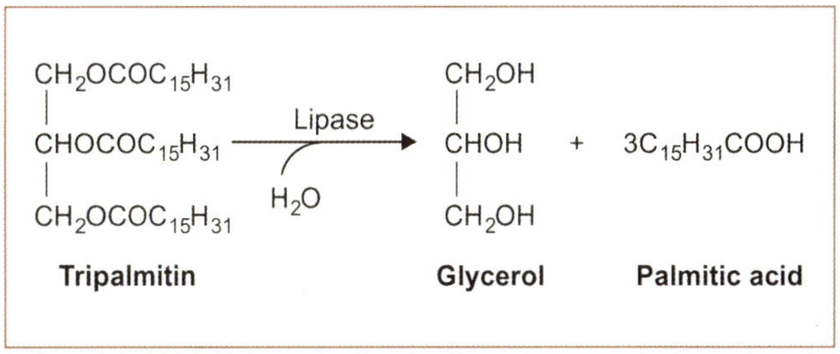

$$\begin{array}{l} CH_2OCOC_{15}H_{31} \\ | \\ CHOCOC_{15}H_{31} \\ | \\ CH_2OCOC_{15}H_{31} \\ \textbf{Tripalmitin} \end{array} \xrightarrow[H_2O]{\text{Lipase}} \begin{array}{l} CH_2OH \\ | \\ CHOH \\ | \\ CH_2OH \\ \textbf{Glycerol} \end{array} + \begin{array}{c} 3C_{15}H_{31}COOH \\ \textbf{Palmitic acid} \end{array}$$

Fig. 4.12: Hydrolysis of tripalmitin, a triglyceride

3. ***Rancidity:*** Naturally occurring fats, particularly from animal sources, develop unpleasant odor and taste, if stored under moist conditions. This is called rancidity. It is due to partial hydrolysis of triacylglycerols and the subsequent oxidation of the released fatty acids to aldehydes and ketones. Antioxidants, e.g. vitamin E can prevent atmospheric oxidation of fats and thus rancidity.

4. ***Iodine number:*** Unsaturated fatty acids, present in triacylglycerols can accept halogens, such as iodine at the double bond. This process is termed **halogenation**. It is a measure of the degree of unsaturation of a fat. Number of grams of iodine used for the iodination of 100 g of fat is referred to as iodine number. High iodine number indicates that more unsaturated fatty acids are present in a particular fat, thus suggestive of high degree of unsaturation.

PHOSPHOLIPIDS

Phospholipids are a heterogeneous group of compound lipids which contain one or more phosphoric acid and a polar group, which may be a nitrogenous base, an amino acid or a polyalcohol. In addition, they also contain long chain fatty acid residues. With cholesterol, phospholipids are the important constituents of the cell membrane. Classification of phospholipids is given in Table 4.2.

Table 4.2: Classification of phospholipids

Glycerophospholipids
• Phosphatidic acid • Lecithins (phosphatidylcholines) • Cephalins (phosphatidylethanolamine or phosphatidylserine) • Phosphatidylinositols • Plasmalogens
Sphingolipids
• Sphingomyelins • Cerebrosides (glycosphingolipids) • Gangliosides

GLYCEROPHOSPHOLIPIDS

Phospholipids which are derivatives of glycerol are called glycerophospholipids or phosphoglycerides. Glycerophospholipids are the major lipid components of the biological membrane. A glycerophospholipid consists of glycerol, two residues of fatty acids and a molecule of phosphoric acid. Phosphoric acid is attached at C3 of glycerol, forming glycerol-3-phosphate. The C1 and C2 positions of glycerol-3-phosphate are esterified with two fatty acids. A saturated fatty acid usually occurs at C1 (α_1-carbon) while a polyunsaturated fatty acid is commonly attached at C2 (β-carbon) of glycerol. Glycerophospholipids are thus amphiphilic molecules with nonpolar tails and polar heads.

1,2-Diacylglycerol

Some of the hydrolyzed products of glycerophospholipids, such as 1,2-diacylglycerol, serve as intra- and extracellular signaling molecules. 1,2-diacylglycerol is derived from membrane lipids by the action of phospholipase C. It is an intracellular signal molecule that activates protein kinase.

Phosphatidic Acid

The simplest glycerophospholipid is phosphatidic acid (Fig. 4.13).

Phosphatidic acid is produced by hydrolysis of the membrane lipids in blood platelets and injured cells, and stimulates cell growth as a part of the wound repair process. The phosphoryl group of phosphatidic acid may be linked to a nitrogenous compound such as ethanolamine, choline or serine, or to some other group like inositol thereby forming various glycerophospholipids, e.g. phosphatidylcholine (lecithin), phosphatidylethanolamine (cephalin), phosphatidylinositol, etc.

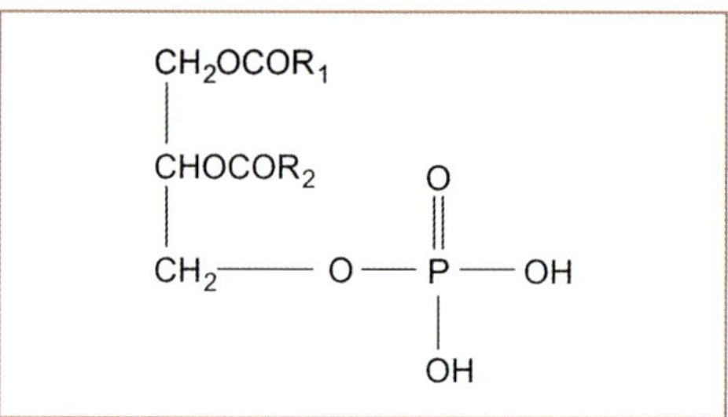

Fig. 4.13: Phosphatidic acid

Lecithins

Lecithins contain choline (a nitrogenous base) at C3 in a phosphatidic acid (Fig. 4.14).

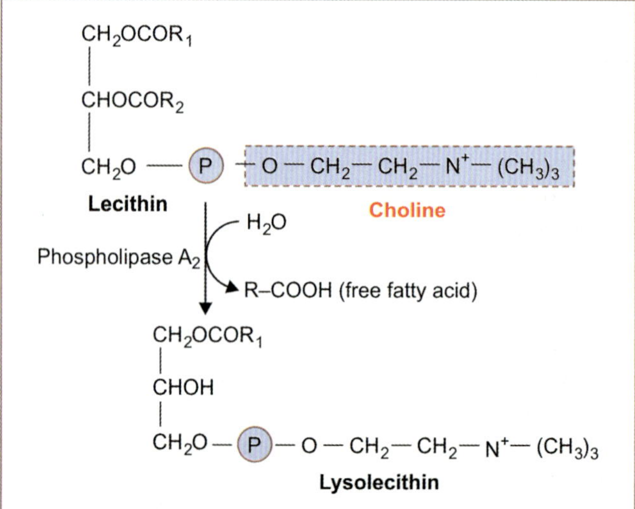

Fig. 4.14: Lecithins

Lecithins are surface active agents and help in emulsification of fat. These are widely distributed in brain, lungs, nerve cells, sperm and egg yolk.

Various hydrolytic enzymes, known as phospholipases, act at different sites in glycerophospholipids and hydrolyze them. This leads to the formation of various products, e.g. phospholipase A_2 hydrolytically removes a fatty acid residue from C2, leaving a lysophospholipid (Fig. 4.14; Chemistry to Clinics 4.2).

Chemistry to Clinics 4.2: Snake Venom

The venom of Indian cobra (*Naja naja*) is rich in phospholipase A_2. Entry of the venom into the circulation of a victim of cobra-bite results in extensive hydrolysis of fatty acids at position C2 of membrane glycerophospholipids. This alters the membrane integrity especially of RBC. Further, the released lysolecithin acts as detergent and disrupts the membrane leading to hemolysis. The liberation of hemoglobin into the circulation may be sufficiently high (exceeding the capacity of haptoglobin and hemopexin, the hemoglobin-binding plasma proteins) to block the renal tubules and cause acute renal failure.

Cephalins

Cephalins are glycerophospholipids where instead of choline present in lecithins, either ethanolamine or serine is attached as a nitrogenous base with the phosphoric acid residue. Cephalins are present in erythrocyte membrane, brain, etc.

Phosphatidylinositols

Phosphatidylinositols are glycerophospholipids containing phosphatidic acid bound to inositol instead of a nitrogenous base. These are found mainly in the brain.

Plasmalogens

Plasmalogens are glycerophospholipids in which C1 of glycerol is linked to an α, β-unsaturated fatty acid by an ether linkage in the *cis*-configuration, rather than to a saturated fatty acid through an ester linkage. Plasmalogens are present in cardiac and skeletal muscles, and in semen. Because of their large concentration in cardiac muscles these are also called cardiolipins.

SPHINGOLIPIDS

Sphingolipids do not contain glycerol but are derivatives of an unsaturated amino alcohol sphingosine which has 18 carbon atoms and a double bond with a *trans*-configuration. Most sphingolipids are sphingoglycolipids, i.e. their polar head groups consist of carbohydrate units.

N-Acyl derivatives of sphingosine (N-acyl sphingosines) are known as **ceramides**. The ceramides are parent compounds of most sphingolipids, e.g. sphingomyelins, cerebrosides and gangliosides.

Sphingomyelins

Sphingomyelins are ceramides with either phosphocholine or phosphoethanolamine. These are the most common sphingolipids and are also called sphingophospholipids. The membranous myelin sheath that surrounds and electrically insulates many nerve cell axons is particularly rich in sphingomyelins.

Sphingolipids, like glycerophospholipids, are a source of smaller lipids that have discrete signaling activity. Sphingomyelin as well as ceramide portions of the more complex sphingolipids, modulate activities of protein kinases and protein phosphatases that are involved in the regulation of cell growth and differentiation.

Lung Surfactant

Chemical nature: Pulmonary surfactant is a lipoprotein rich in phospholipid. The principal agent responsible for its surface tension reducing properties is dipalmitoyl phosphatidylcholine (DPPC), also called dipalmitoyl lecithin.

Biosynthesis: The alveolar epithelium consists of two cell types: Alveolar type I and type II cells. Alveolar type II cells, often referred to as type II pneumocytes, synthesize surfactant. Compared with type I cells, they are rich in mitochondria and are metabolically more active. Electron dense lamellar inclusion bodies are a distinguishing feature of the type II cell and are the storage sites for surfactant (Fig. 4.15).

Principle of Action

- The alveolar lining is coated with pulmonary surfactant which not only lowers surface tension at the gas-liquid interface but also changes surface tension with changes in alveolar diameter (Fig. 4.16).

  Therefore, pulmonary surfactant makes it possible for alveoli of different diameters that are connected in parallel to coexist and be stable at low lung volumes, by lowering surface tension proportionately more in the smaller alveoli.
- When the water and gas molecules are compressed during lung deflation, surfactant causes a decrease in surface tension. At low lung volume, when the

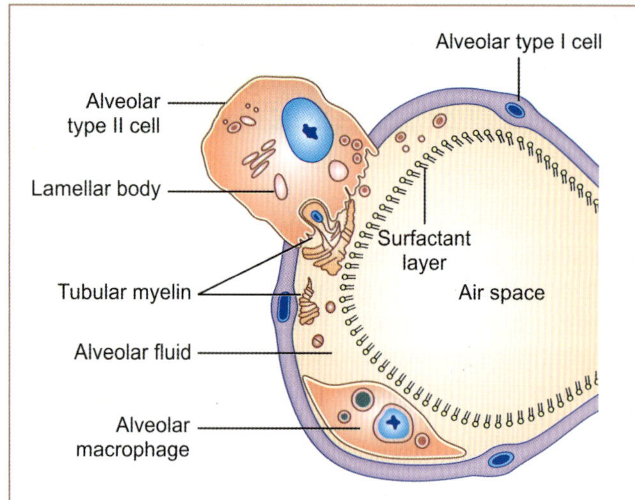

Fig. 4.15: Surfactant layer inside an alveolus. Alveolar type II cells synthesize surfactant and store it as lamellar bodies which are later exocytosed and complexed with proteins to form tubular myelin. Subsequently, the surfactant layer is formed

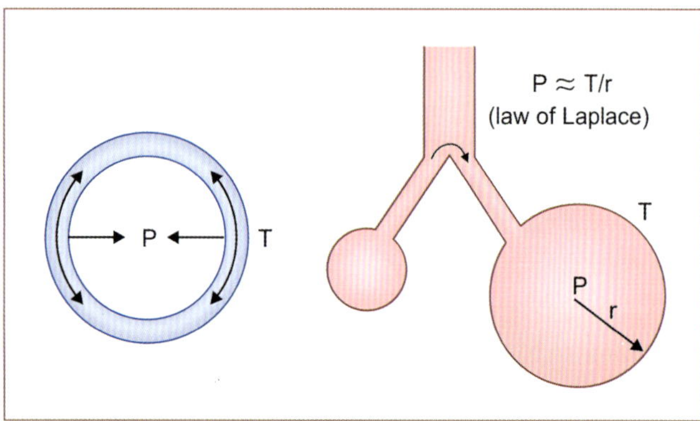

Fig. 4.16: The law of Laplace states that the pressure (P) inside a sphere is inversely proportional to the radius (r) at constant surface tension (T). Thus, if surface tensions are equal, during deflation (expiration), a small alveolus will experience a greater inward force than a large alveolus. If both alveoli are connected to the same airway, the small alveolus will be more likely to collapse, expelling its contents into the large alveolus. This is prevented by the **action of surfactant which lowers surface tension more in** the small alveolus

molecules are tightly compressed, some surfactant is squeezed out of the surface. On expansion (re-inflation), new surfactant is required to form a new film that is spread on the alveolar surface lining.

- In addition to lowering alveolar surface tension and promoting alveolar stability, surfactant helps to prevent edema in the lungs. The inwardly contracting force that tends to collapse alveoli also tends to lower interstitial pressure, which 'pulls' fluid from the capillaries. Pulmonary surfactant reduces this tendency by lowering surface forces.

4

The Lecithin:Sphingomyelin Ratio

The lecithin:sphingomyelin ratio (**L/S ratio**) in amniotic fluid is an index of fetal lung maturity. L/S ratio of more than 2 is indicative of fetal lung maturity.

Lung maturity: Because the lungs are among the last organs to develop, the synthesis of surfactant appears rather late in gestation. In humans, surfactant appears at about week 34 (a full-term pregnancy is 40 weeks). Failure of proper lung maturation during the perinatal period is still a major cause of death in newborns (Chemistry to Clinics 4.3).

Chemistry to Clinics 4.3: Infant Respiratory Distress Syndrome

Premature birth and certain hormonal disturbances (such as those seen in diabetic pregnancies) interfere with the normal control and timing of lung maturation. These infants have structurally intact but functionally immature lungs at birth which often leads to infant respiratory distress syndrome (IRDS), also called **hyaline membrane disease**. Breathing is extremely labored because surface tension is high, making it difficult to inflate the lungs. These infants develop pulmonary edema and atelectasis (alveolar collapse, Fig. 4.17).

On the other hand, surfactant deficiency in a mature lung may result in adult respiratory distress syndrome (Chemistry to Clinics 4.4).

Chemistry to Clinics 4.4: Adult Respiratory Distress Syndrome (ARDS)

It is the name given to diffuse lung injury of various causes which include trauma from chest injury (e.g. car accidents), long bone injury, and pelvic injury. Two other major causes include sepsis (presence of pathogen or toxin in the blood) and aspiration of gastric contents. The latter occurs with gastric reflux and usually occurs at night during sleep. Other causes include cardiopulmonary bypass, high altitude, smoke inhalation and exposure to irritant gases. Exposure to irritant gases was the cause of the widespread ARDS cases that occurred at the disaster in Bhopal, India. ARDS is characterized by decreased lung compliance, pulmonary edema, focal atelectasis and hypoxemia (low partial pressure of O_2 in the arterial blood), with an inflammatory reaction that leads to an infiltration of neutrophils into the lung.

They are at high risk until the lungs become mature enough to secrete surfactant. The syndrome can be diagnosed by obtaining amniotic fluid (amniocentesis) and calculating the lecithin: Sphingomyelin ratio (**L/S ratio**). L/S ratio of less than 2.0 is associated with a high risk of ARDS. The condition can be treated with exogenous surfactants and hydrocortisone injection during antenatal period (Fig. 4.18).

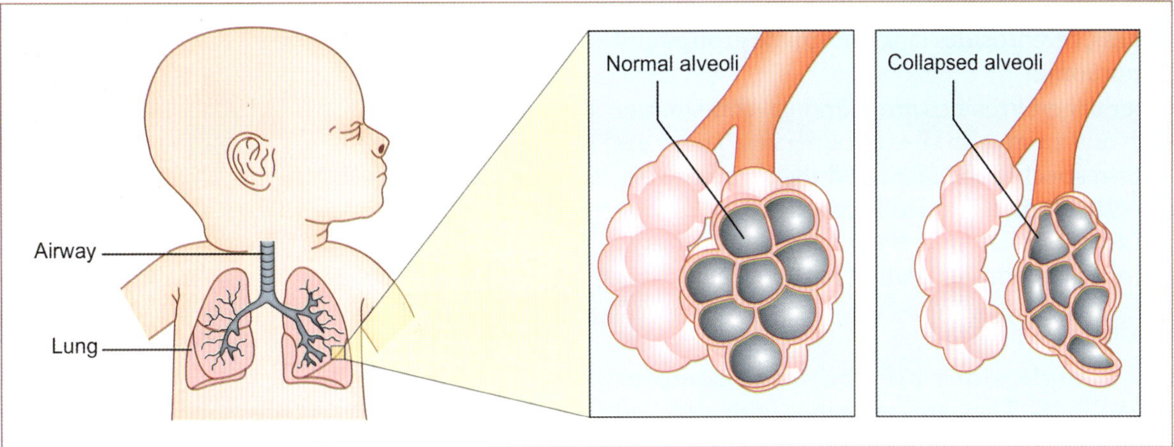

Fig. 4.17: Collapsed alveoli in infantile respiratory distress syndrome

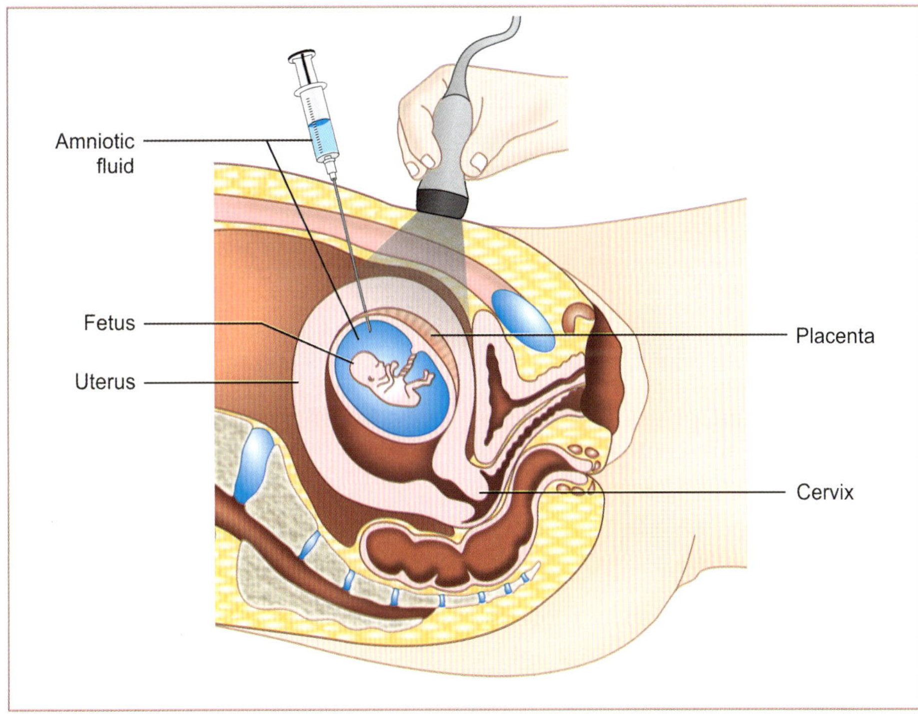

Fig. 4.18: Amniocentesis: The aspiration of amniotic fluid under ultrasound guidance. Lecithin:sphingomyelin ratio (L/S ratio) in the amniotic fluid is used for the evaluation of fetal lung maturity. Before 33–35 weeks of gestation, the ratio is nearly 1.0. At term, there is a marked increase in lecithin concentration and thus the L/S ratio increases to more than 5.0. In a premature low birth weight fetus, the ratio is <2.0. Such infants are likely to develop respiratory distress syndrome

Neutrophil aggregation is a key underlying mechanism of ARDS, causing capillary endothelial damage by releasing a number of toxic products. These include oxygen free radicals, proteolytic enzymes, arachidonic acid metabolites (leukotrienes, thromboxanes, prostaglandins), and platelet-activating factor. Collectively, these factors lead to a loss of surfactant and an increase in lung stiffness (i.e. decreased compliance). The condition warrants the use of mechanical ventilation and drugs to reduce neutrophil chemoattraction and aggregation in the pulmonary capillaries.

Cerebrosides

Cerebrosides are glycosphingolipids and contain a ceramide with a sugar residue (such as galactose or glucose), i.e. cerebrosides are ceramide monosaccharides. Most prevalent cerebrosides are galacto-

4

cerebrosides and glucocerebrosides. In contrast to phospholipids, cerebrosides lack phosphate groups and hence are nonionic.

A number of cerebrosides are found in white matter of the brain and in myelin sheath of nerves. These are named with respect to the fatty acid they contain, e.g. a galactosylceramide called cerebran contains cerebronic acid. Similarly, nervon has an unsaturated derivative of lignoceric acid called nervonic acid.

Gangliosides

Structure: Gangliosides are the most complex glycosphingolipids. They are ceramides with attached oligosaccharides that include hexosamines (glucosamine or galactosamine) and at least one molecule of N-acetylneuraminic acid (sialic acid). In other words, gangliosides are sialic acid containing ceramide oligosaccharides.s

Nomenclature: Numerous gangliosides are known and each one of them has different oligosaccharide head groups. These are designated as GM1, GM2, GM3, etc. (G refers to a ganglioside; M, D or T indicate mono-, di- or tri-sialic acid residues; the number with each subscript denotes the carbohydrate sequence that is attached to the ceramide).

Distribution: Gangliosides are primarily components of cell membrane surface and constitute a significant fraction of brain lipids. They are present in large amount in the ganglion cells of the central nervous system, particularly in the nerve endings.

Importance

1. Their complex carbohydrate head groups act as specific receptors for certain pituitary glycoprotein hormones that regulate a number of important physiological functions.
2. Gangliosides are receptors for certain bacterial protein toxins such as cholera toxin, tetanus toxin and certain viruses (Fig. 4.19).
3. Gangliosides are specific determinants of cell-recognition and thus have a role in growth and differentiation of tissues as well as in carcinogenesis.

DIGESTION AND ABSORPTION OF DIETARY LIPIDS

An adult human consumes nearly 50–100 g of lipids per day. Normally, triacylglycerols (triglycerides) constitute >90% of the dietary lipids with only a small amount of free fatty acids, phospholipids, cholesterol,

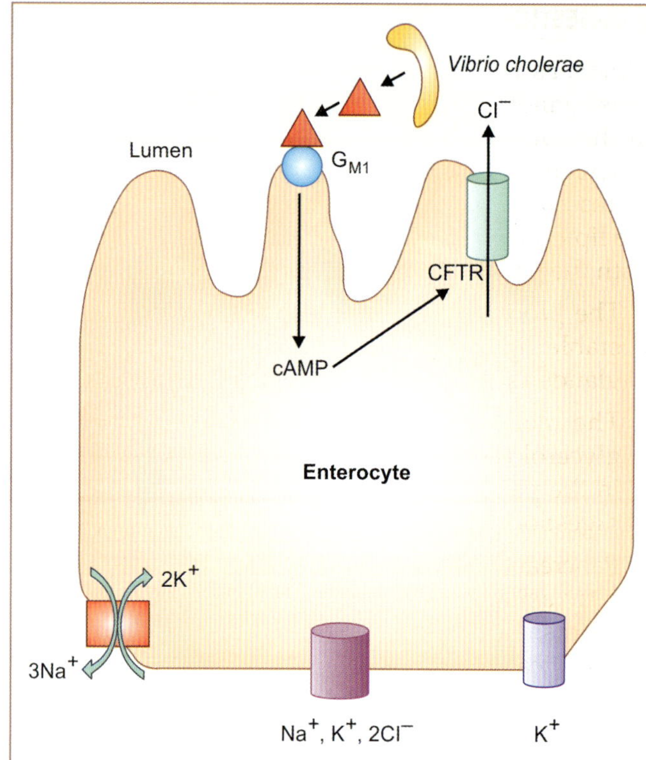

Fig. 4.19: Cholera toxin-induced diarrhea: The bacterium *Vibrio cholerae* secretes a toxin (red triangle) which binds to the ganglioside receptor G_{M1} (blue sphere) on the enterocyte luminal brush border membrane. Activation of adenylate cyclase forms cAMP which stimulates secretion of Cl^- through cystic fibrosis transmembrane regulator (**CFTR channels**), with associated sodium and water secretion. Cl^- and Na^+ reabsorption are also inhibited. The abundance of water and mucus in the stool gives the name rice watery diarrhea, causing severe dehydration. The various ion channels in the contraluminal membrane fail to compensate for the deficiency. The condition requires treatment with oral rehydration solution or, in an emergency, with intravenous fluids/electrolytes

vitamin A and their esters. Excess lipid consumption may result in turbid urine in some individuals (Chemistry to Clinics 4.5).

Chemistry to Clinics 4.5: Lipuria

Ingestion of large amounts of lipids may lead to a condition called alimentary lipuria (**adiposuria**). The urine of such individuals becomes opalescent, turbid or sometimes even milky. In rare instances, when its lipid content is very high, a peculiar creamy layer is also seen. Lipuria may also be observed in lipemia of diabetes mellitus, lipoid nephrosis, fractures of the long bones with injury to the bone marrow and in phosphorus poisoning.

DIGESTION OF DIETARY LIPIDS

Lipids, as we know, are poorly soluble in water and thus cannot be easily accessible to digestive enzymes in the aqueous phase. To facilitate the same, dietary triacylglycerols form emulsion droplets which, in turn, increases the interfacial area between the aqueous and the lipid phase. Digestion of dietary lipids takes place with the participation of several enzymes (Table 4.3).

- The process is initiated **in the stomach** by an acid stable lipase which is present in the sublingual glands as well as in the stomach.
- The main enzyme for the hydrolysis of triacylglycerol is the **pancreatic lipase (steapsin)** present in the pancreatic juice. Thus, the main site of lipid digestion is the **small intestine**.
- Pancreatic lipase is an α-lipase and prefers long chain fatty acids, i.e. fatty acids of more than 10 carbon atoms. It also requires a colipase. The enzyme specifically attacks ester linkages at 1- and 3-position of a triacylglycerol, leaving monoacylglycerol with a fatty acid at C2 of glycerol, i.e. a β-monoacylglycerol. The free fatty acids and β-monoacylglycerol are released at the surface of the lipid emulsion droplet and are incorporated into **micelles**.

  Micelles provide a major vehicle for moving lipids from the intestinal lumen to the cell surface where absorption occurs. Micelles also serve as a transport vehicle for cholesterol and lipid-soluble vitamins.
- In addition to lipase, pancreatic juice also contains a less specific lipid esterase which acts upon monoacylglycerols, cholesterol esters and esters of retinoic acid.
- Dietary phospholipids are hydrolyzed by specific phospholipases. Pancreatic juice is especially rich in proenzyme for phospholipase A_2 which is activated by trypsin. Phospholipase A_2 also requires bile acids for its activity.

Bile Acids

Bile acids are composed of 24 carbon atoms and are synthesized in the hepatocytes, directly from the cholesterol. **Primary bile acids**, i.e. cholic acid and chenodeoxycholic acid, are derivatives of cholanic acid. They contain two or three OH groups and have a side chain with a carboxyl group which is often conjugated via amide linkage either to glycine or to taurine and form glycocholic acid or taurocholic acid. Since the carboxyl group is ionized at pH 7.0, hence these are named as ***bile salts***. They can bind to cations and commonly exist as sodium glycocholate, sodium taurocholate, potassium glycocholate and potassium taurocholate.

Bile acids are secreted into bile canaliculi and carried to the gallbladder for storage and ultimately to the small intestine for excretion. With the removal of one OH group by microorganisms in the gut, the **primary bile acids**, i.e. cholic acid and chenodeoxycholic acid are converted to deoxycholic acid and lithocholic acid, respectively. These are called as **secondary bile acids**. Enterohepatic circulation carries bile acids from the intestine back to the liver.

Functions of Bile Acids

1 Cholesterol is excreted in the bile as free cholesterol and as bile acids.
2. Bile acids and phospholipids function to solubilize cholesterol in the bile and act as emulsifying agents (Fig. 4.20).
3. Bile acids are the biological detergents; they reversibly form aggregates, called micelles, without

Table 4.3: Digestion of dietary lipids

Enzyme	Site of action	Action of the enzyme
Lingual lipase (important in neonates)	Mouth	Triglycerides ⟶ Fatty acids, monoglycerides, glycerol
Lipase/colipase	Pancreas	Triglycerides ⟶ Fatty acids, monoglycerides, glycerol
Phospholipase A/B	Pancreas	Lecithin ⟶ Fatty acid, lysolecithin
Cholesterol esterase	Pancreas	Cholesterol ester ⟶ Cholesterol, fatty acid
Retinyl ester hydrolase	Pancreas	Retinyl ester ⟶ Retinol, fatty acid
Monoglyceride lipase	Small intestine	Monoglyceride ⟶ Glycerol, fatty acid
Lecithinase	Small intestine	Lecithin ⟶ Fatty acids, glycerol, phosphoric acid, choline

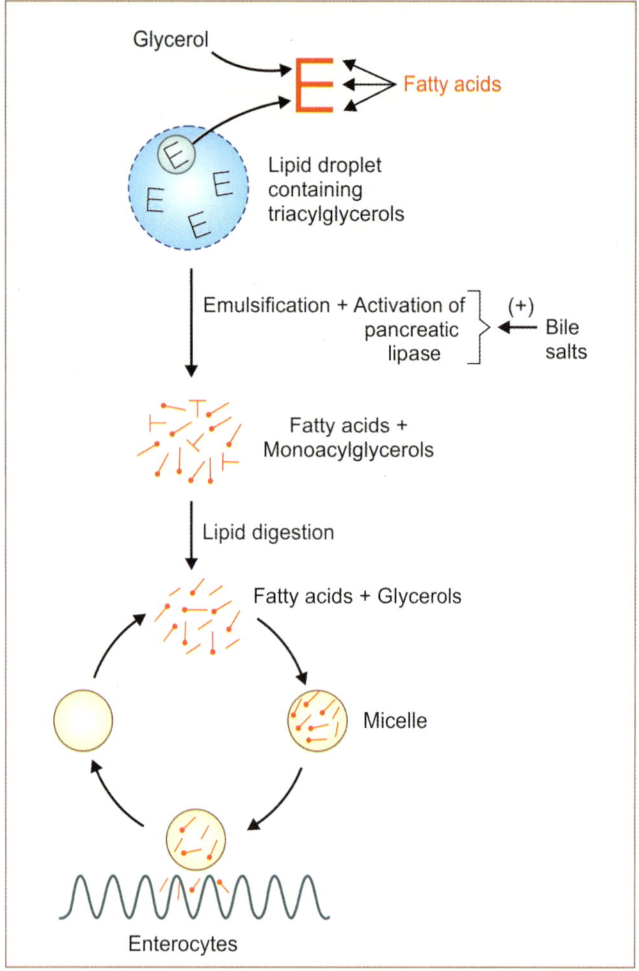

Fig. 4.20: Role of bile salts in emulsification, digestion and absorption of dietary lipids

which dietary lipids cannot be digested and absorbed (Chemistry to Clinics 4.6).

4. Bile acids also play a role in the activation of pancreatic lipase.
5. They also facilitate the absorption of lipid soluble vitamins from the intestine.

Chemistry to Clinics 4.6: Steatorrhea

Digestion and absorption of triacylglycerols is drastically reduced in the absence of bile acids. As a result, a bulk of the dietary lipids is excreted in the stool which becomes clay-colored. This condition is known as steatorrhea. Naturally, the absorption of lipid soluble vitamins is also compromised. The first vitamin whose deficiency becomes manifest clinically is that of vitamin K (increased bleeding tendency after minor cuts). Steatorrhea is commonly seen in obstructive jaundice (impaired flow of bile from the liver to the small intestine) and in advanced cases of hepatic jaundice (decreased hepatic synthesis of bile acids).

4

ABSORPTION OF DIETARY LIPIDS

- **Absorption of the products of lipid digestion**, primarily **free fatty acids** (≈70%) and **β-monoacylglycerols** (≈25%), occurs from micelles in the brush border of the enterocytes by passive diffusion. Within the enterocytes, the fate of the absorbed fatty acids depends on their chain length.
  - **Short** to **medium chain fatty acids** (4–12 C-atoms) as well as unsaturated fatty acids are absorbed more readily and without any modification. These fatty acids thus reach the liver directly via portal blood, for their utilization in the hepatic tissue.
  - On the other hand, **long chain fatty acids**, i.e. those with chain length of >12 C-atoms, bypass the liver. These fatty acids bind to a fatty acid binding protein in the cytoplasm and are transported to the endoplasmic reticulum where they are used for the resynthesis of triacylglycerols. Glycerol required for this purpose is obtained from the absorbed β-monoacylglycerols, and a small amount from glucose, via glycolysis.
- **Absorption of the hydrolyzed products of phospholipids**, i.e. fatty acids, glycerol, phosphoric acid and nitrogenous bases are absorbed along with the digestive products of triacylglycerols. Phospholipids are then resynthesized in the intestinal mucosa and form a part of the chylomicrons.
- **Cholesterol is absorbed** in the free form but is re-esterified in the intestinal mucosa. Cholesterol esters are also incorporated into the chylomicrons.

Formation of Chylomicrons

The resynthesized **triacylglycerols** form **fat globules** onto which phospholipids and some specific proteins, designated as apoproteins, are absorbed. Within the membrane bound vesicles, the complexes migrate through Golgi apparatus to the basolateral plasma membrane and released into the intercellular space. Since these fat globules are several microns in diameter and are released from the intestine as milky juice via lymph vessels called chyle, these fat globules are termed chylomicrons. Apolipoprotein B is essential for the release of chylomicrons from enterocytes into the lymphatics.

Thus, ***all dietary lipids***, i.e. triacylglycerols, phospholipids, free and esterified cholesterol along with the apoproteins (apolipoproteins) are incorporated into and released as chylomicrons (Fig. 4.21).

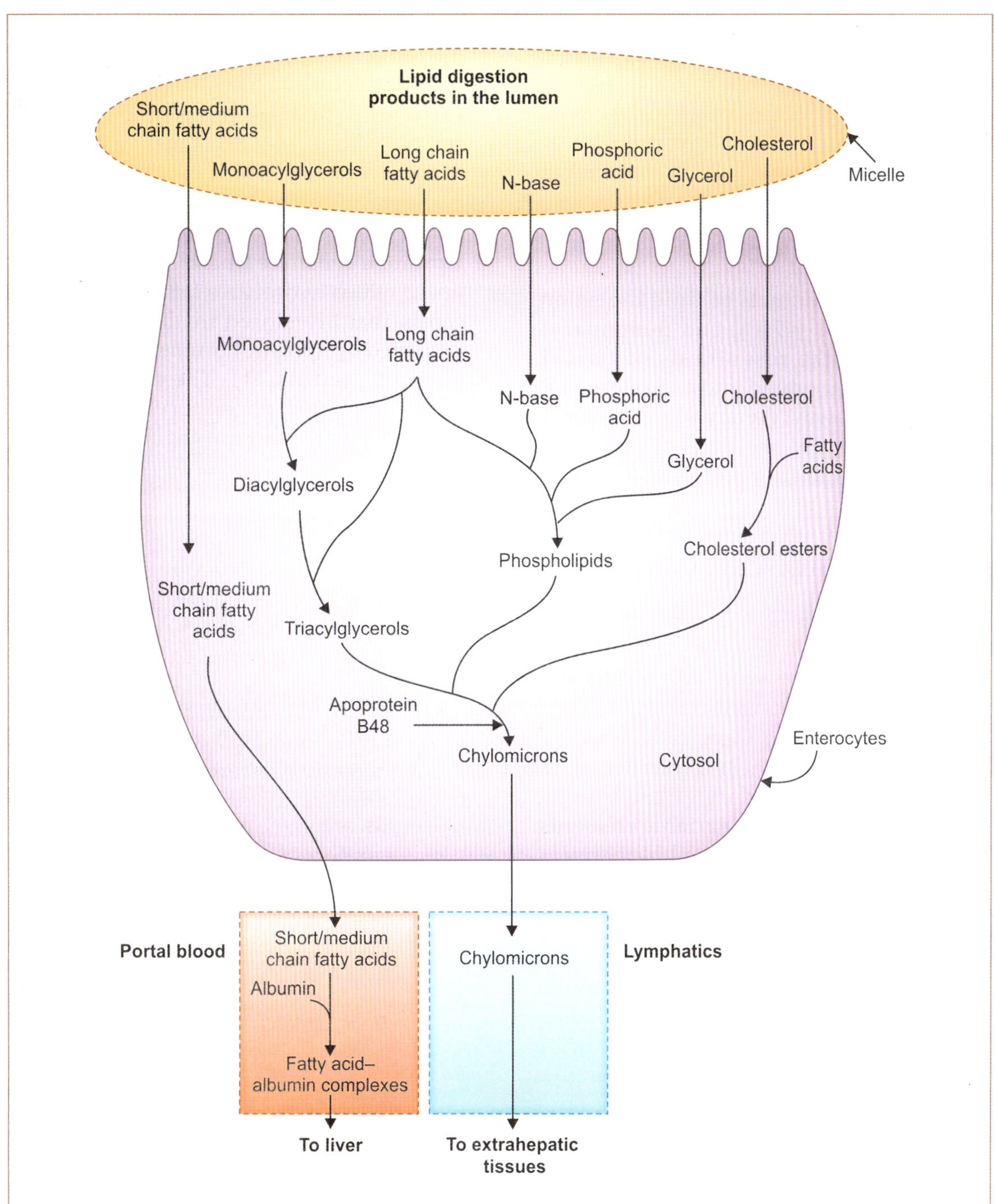

Fig. 4.21: Lipid absorption in the intestine

Via the thoracic duct, intestinal lymph vessels drain into the large veins and thus (through blood), dietary triacylglycerols finally reach the peripheral tissues (Chemistry to Clinics 4.7).

Cells of the adipose tissues and the muscles take up large amounts of these dietary lipids for either storage or metabolism, and bypass the liver from a lipid overload after a meal. Intestinal lipid absorption is

Chemistry to Clinics 4.7: Chyluria

An obstruction to the thoracic duct may result in milky appearance of the urine. This is due to the reason that lymph vessels of the urinary tract become distended and burst thereby allowing lymph to pass directly into the urine. Hence, this condition, i.e. the presence of chylomicrons in the urine, is called chyluria. It is common in endemic zones of lymphatic filariasis.

associated with a marked increase in lymph flow called the **lymphagogic effect of fat feeding**. This increase in lymph flow plays an important role in the transfer of lipoproteins from the intercellular spaces to the central lacteal. Apoprotein A–IV (Apo A–IV) secreted by the small intestine, may be an important factor contributing to anorexia after fat feeding.

METABOLISM OF DIETARY LIPIDS

As discussed above, **the products of lipid digestion**, primarily, **free fatty acids** (≈70%) and **β-monoacylglycerols**, are used for the **resynthesis of triacylglycerols**, which are incorporated into and **released as chylomicrons**. It is in this way, **dietary triacylglycerols reach peripheral tissues** and are either stored in the adipose tissue (for use at the time of necessity) or are oxidized in the liver and muscle.

METABOLISM OF TRIACYLGLYCEROLS IN ADIPOSE TISSUE

A major part of the dietary lipids is stored in the fat depots, called adipose tissue (**white adipose tissue**), which are utilized during prolonged starvation.

In a homeostatic situation, there is continuous synthesis and breakdown of triacylglycerols in the adipose tissue. As the levels of triacylglycerols in the fat depots vary, these are called the **variable elements**. On the other hand, other lipids, such as phospholipids, form an essential component of the cell and the membrane structure, since their levels do not alter during fasting these are called **constant elements**.

Brown adipose tissue: Besides white adipose tissue, newborns also have another type of adipose tissue called brown adipose tissue. It disappears during growth of the child. Brown adipose tissue has a **higher metabolic activity** and is capable of producing **large amount of heat**.

Catabolism of Triacylglycerols

The process of breakdown of triacylglycerols is called **lipolysis** and the key enzymes for the release of energy from these stores are called **lipases**.

There are two types of lipases involved in the hydrolysis of triacylglycerols:

- **Lipoprotein lipase:** This enzyme is located on the surface of the endothelial cells of capillaries and possibly of the adjoining tissues. Lipoprotein lipases remove fatty acids from 1 and/or 3 positions of triacylglycerols and/or diacylglycerols when they are present in lipoproteins (VLDL and chylomicrons). The enzyme requires apoprotein C-II for its activity. Insulin also activates the enzyme.

  Fatty acids that are released are either bound to serum albumin or are taken up by the tissues. Monoglycerides, which are produced, may either pass into the cells or are further hydrolyzed by the serum monoacylglycerol hydrolase.
- **Hormone sensitive lipase:** This is a distinct type of lipase which hydrolyzes fatty acids from triacylglycerols that are stored in the adipose tissue. It is regulated by lipolytic hormones such as epinephrine, glucagon and ACTH. These hormones stimulate cAMP-mediated phosphorylation of the inactive enzyme. Insulin and prostaglandins inhibit enzyme activity.

The Process of Lipolysis

The sequence of hydrolysis of fatty acids from 3 positions of glycerol depends upon the specificities of the particular lipase (Fig. 4.22).

Fatty acids and glycerol so produced are released into the circulating blood. Fatty acids are bound to serum albumin, transported to different tissues and are oxidized to CO_2 and H_2O with the liberation of large amount of energy. Glycerol returns to the liver where it is converted to dihydroxyacetone phosphate and enters the glycolytic pathway or is converted to glucose via gluconeogenesis.

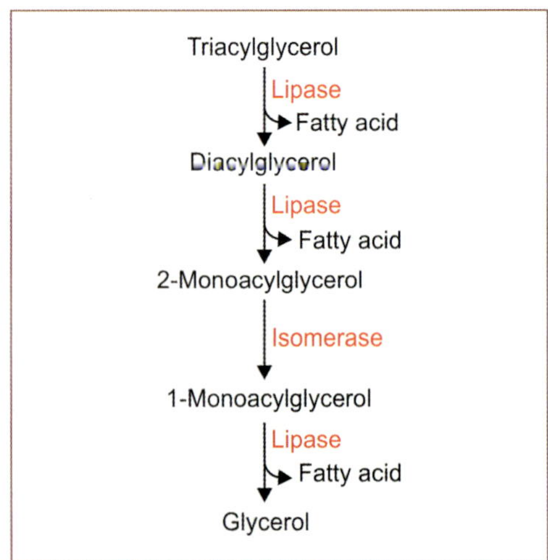

Fig. 4.22: Catabolism of a triacylglycerol

BIOSYNTHESIS OF TRIACYLGLYCEROLS

Triacylglycerols, as mentioned above, are the principle dietary lipids as well as lipids of the fat depot in the body. Excessive amounts of dietary carbohydrates are also stored as triacylglycerols in the adipose tissue. The process of biosynthesis of triacylglycerols is referred to as **lipogenesis**, which, though mainly, occurs in the liver and adipose tissue; lactating mammary glands, kidneys and epithelial cells of the intestinal mucosa are also active in this respect.

The Process of Lipogenesis

Lipogenesis involves activation of free fatty acids and α-glycerol phosphate (Fig. 4.23).

- **Synthesis of L-α-glycerol phosphate:** L-α-glycerol phosphate, required for the esterification of fatty acids, can be synthesized in two ways:
  1. In most of the tissues which contain glycerol kinase, glycerol is directly converted to L-α-glycerol phosphate.
  2. Alternatively, in muscle and adipose tissue which lack glycerol kinase, L-α-glycerol phosphate is formed by the reduction of dihydroxyacetone phosphate, an intermediate of glycolysis. The reaction is catalyzed by glycerol-3-phosphate dehydrogenase.
- **Activation of fatty acids:** Free fatty acids, in the presence of ATP and CoA, are activated to acyl-CoA, by thiokinase (fatty acyl-CoA synthetase).
- **Re-esterification of glycerol phosphate**

  After the synthesis of L-α-glycerol phosphate and the activation of fatty acids, triacylglycerols are synthesized by a process called re-esterification:
  1. A molecule of acyl-CoA combines with α-glycerol phosphate and forms 1-acylglycerol-3-phosphate (lysophosphatidic acid). The reaction is catalyzed by glycerol-3-phosphate acyltransferase.
  2. L-Acylglycerol-3-phosphate acyltransferase (lysophosphatidyl acyltransferase) converts 1-acylglycerol-3-phosphate to 1,2-diacylglycerol phosphate (phosphatidic acid), a common intermediate for the biosynthesis of both triacylglycerols as well as phospholipids.
  3. A phosphatase (phosphatidic acid phosphohydrolase) hydrolyzes phosphatidic acid and forms 1,2-diacylglycerol. In many tissues, especially in the intestinal mucosa, 1,2-diacylglycerol is also formed from 2-monoacylglycerols since monoacylglycerols are directly absorbed in the intestinal mucosa. The reaction involves the transfer of an acyl group by the enzyme monoacylglycerol acyltransferase.
  4. Diacylglycerol acyltransferase esterifies diacylglycerol and forms triacylglycerol.

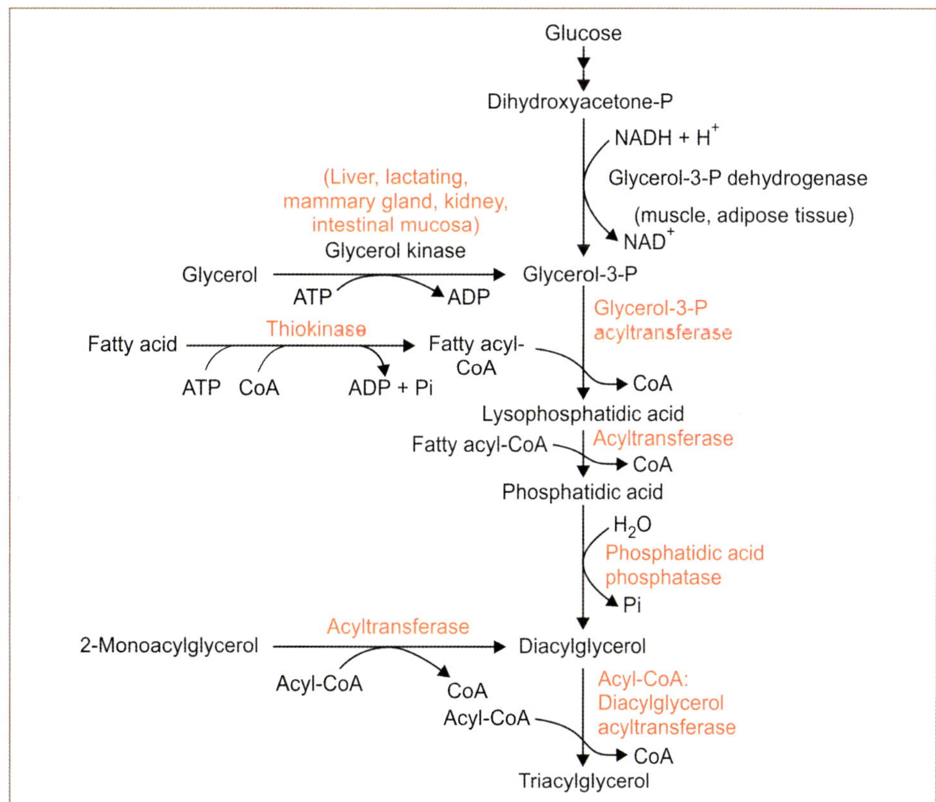

Fig. 4.23: Biosynthesis of a triacylglycerol

4

Generally, palmitic acid is mainly present in position 1 while oleic acid at positions 2 and 3 of a triacylglycerol in the human adipose tissue.

OXIDATION OF FATTY ACIDS

Fatty acids that arrive at the surface of the tissues are taken up by the cells and are used (oxidized) for the production of **energy**. Oxidation of fatty acids takes place, mainly, in the **mitochondria** where various enzymes for the oxidation of fatty acids are present, close to the enzymes of the electron transport chain. Besides, small amounts of some of the fatty acids are oxidized in the peroxisomes and endoplasmic reticulum.

THE PROCESS OF β-OXIDATION OF FATTY ACIDS IN MITOCHONDRIA

It is the most important mechanism for the oxidation of fatty acids that occurs in mitochondria. The process of β-oxidation of fatty acids was proposed by Knoop and requires CoA, FAD and NAD. Oxidation of a fatty acid occurs at the β-carbon atom (carbon atom number 2) and results in the **elimination of two terminal carbon atoms as acetyl-CoA**, leaving fatty acyl-CoA which has two carbons less than the original fatty acid (Fig. 4.24).

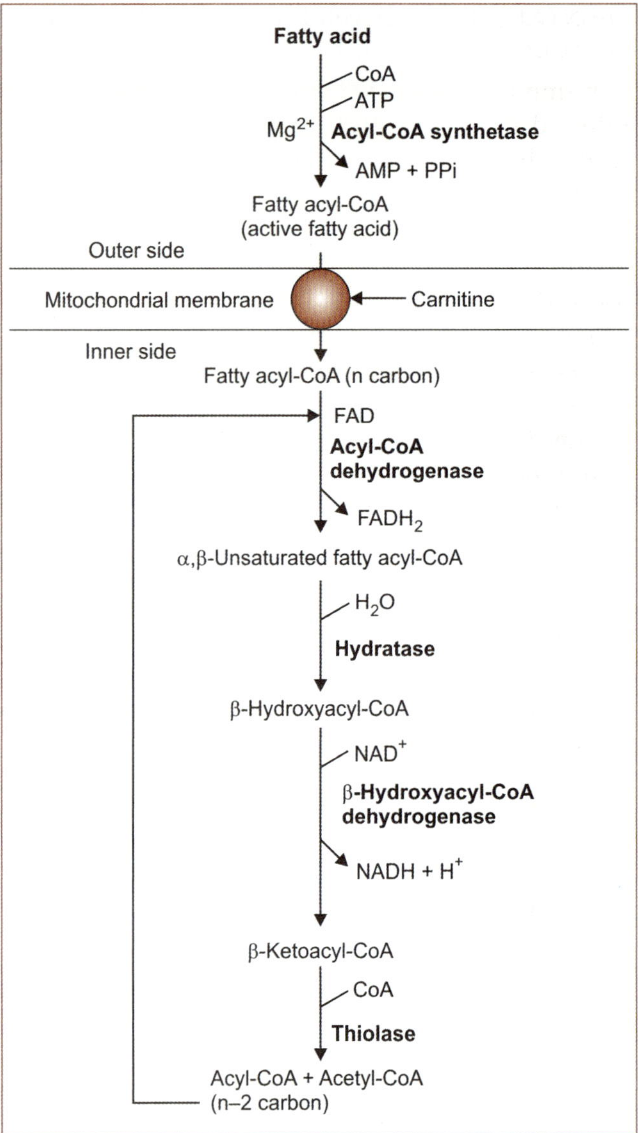

Fig. 4.24: The process of β-oxidation of fatty acids

It involves **activation of fatty acids** in cytoplasm, their **transport into mitochondria** and their **oxidation in the mitochondria**.

1. **Activation of fatty acids in cytoplasm:** The first step in the oxidation of a fatty acid is its **activation**. Fatty acid activation occurs in the cytoplasm, in the presence of ATP and is catalyzed by a thiokinase (acyl-CoA synthetase). Thiokinases are fatty acid activating enzymes found, both, inside as well as outside the mitochondria. Several thiokinases are known, each one of which is specific for a group of fatty acids. These include:
   - **Acetyl-CoA thiokinase:** This is found in the mitochondria and causes activation of acetic, propionic and butyric acids.
   - **Short chain fatty acyl-CoA thiokinases:** These are also found in the mitochondria and cause activation of fatty acids with 4–12 carbons.
   - **Long chain fatty acyl-CoA thiokinases:** These are found in the cytoplasm and cause activation of long chain saturated as well as unsaturated fatty acids.
2. **Transport of fatty acids from cytoplasm to mitochondria:** As mentioned above, short chain fatty acids can cross the inner mitochondrial membrane as such and are activated to their CoA derivatives directly within the mitochondria. On the other hand, activation of long chain fatty acids (>12C) occurs outside the mitochondria. Since the machinery for their oxidation is present within the mitochondria and the inner mitochondrial membrane is impermeable to CoA as well as to its derivatives, the long chain fatty acids are thus to be transported from the cytoplasm to the mitochondria. This takes place with the help of **carnitine** which acts as a carrier of acyl group across the membrane. The enzymes that transfer a fatty acyl group between CoA and carnitine are found on both sides of the inner mitochondrial membrane.

4

Role of Carnitine in the Transport of Long chain Fatty Acids: Carnitine Shuttle

Carnitine (4-trimethylamino-3-hydroxybutyrate) is widely distributed in all the tissues especially the muscles. It is synthesized from **lysine and methionine** in the liver and the kidney and then redistributed to other tissues. It is used as a carrier of acyl group (chain length 12C–18C) across the mitochondrial membrane (Fig. 4.25).

The outer mitochondrial membrane contains an enzyme, carnitine palmitoyltransferase I (CPT-I). The enzyme converts long-chain fatty acyl-CoA to acylcarnitine that exchanges across the inner mitochondrial membrane with free carnitine by a carnitine: acylcarnitine antiporter translocase. Finally, the fatty acyl group is transferred back to CoA by carnitine palmitoyltransferase II (CPT-II), which is located on the matrix side of the inner membrane. The entire mechanism is also called carnitine shuttle and several disorders are associated with it (Chemistry to Clinics 4.8).

Carnitine is also emerging as an important health supplement (Chemistry to Clinics 4.9).

Secondary carnitine deficiency: It is associated with inherited defects in β-oxidation pathway resulting in the accumulation of acyl-CoA and acylcarnitine. Acylcarnitine is excreted in the urine and further lowers carnitine levels in the body.

Chemistry to Clinics 4.8: Carnitine Deficiency Disorders

Primary carnitine deficiency: The entry of carnitine into the cell across the plasma membrane requires a sodium-dependent transporter encoded by the solute carrier family 22 member 5 (*SLC22A5*) gene. Mutations in *SLC22A5* result in autosomal recessive primary carnitine deficiency, which manifests with cardiac and skeletal symptoms because low levels of carnitine affect oxidation of long chain fatty acids. It requires lifelong oral L-carnitine supplementation.

Chemistry to Clinics 4.9: Carnitine Supplements

Intensive research on the role of carnitine supplements has shown partial benefit in the following conditions:

- Heart failure
- Peripheral vascular disease
- Muscle wasting (as in cancer patients)
- Hepatic encephalopathy
- Type 2 diabetes mellitus

Mutations in the carnitine palmitoyltransferase II (*CPT II*) gene: These give rise to partial loss of CPT II activity. Patients generally experience muscle weakness during prolonged exercise. Myoglobinuria, due to breakdown of muscle tissue, is frequently observed. Severe deficiency of the enzyme may be precipitated by prolonged period of fasting and leads to hypoketotic hypoglycemia, hyperammonemia, cardiac malfunctions, etc.

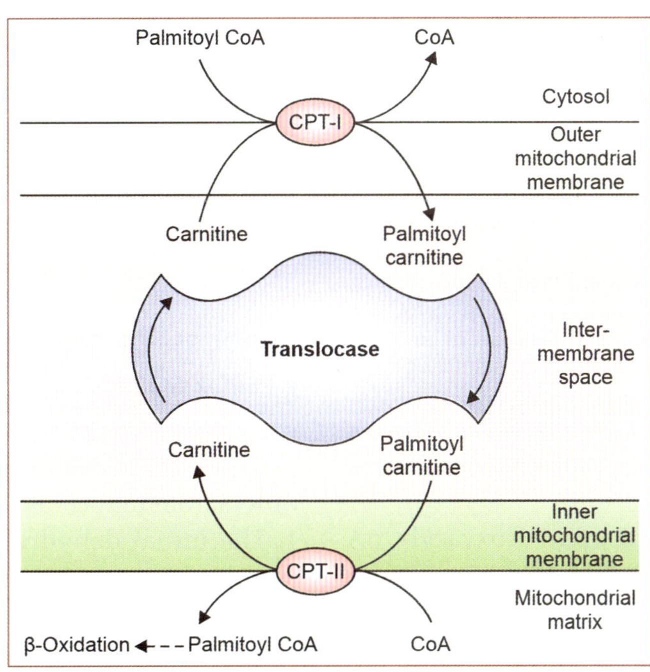

Fig. 4.25: Role of carnitine in transport of fatty acid from cytosol to mitochondria

4

3. **The process of β-oxidation in the mitochondria**

   Oxidation of fatty acids in mitochondria occurs in four different steps:

   i. After activation and entry of the fatty acid into the mitochondria, flavoprotein containing acyl-CoA dehydrogenase removes two hydrogen atoms from α- and β-positions of the fatty acyl-CoA. It forms enoyl-CoA with a *trans*-double bond between C2 and C3, i.e. an α, β-unsaturated fatty acyl-CoA.

   Mitochondria contain several acyl-CoA dehydrogenases with different chain length specificities. These are designated as short chain fatty acyl-CoA dehydrogenase, medium chain fatty acyl-CoA dehydrogenase and long chain fatty acyl-CoA dehydrogenase. There may be a genetic deficiency of any of the three enzymes with several common clinical features. These are collectively called acyl-CoA dehydrogenase deficiency diseases. Medium chain acyl-CoA dehydrogenase deficiency disease is called sudden infant death syndrome (Chemistry 15 Clinics 4.10).

Chemistry to Clinics 4.10: Sudden Infant Death Syndrome (Reye's Syndrome)

Acyl-CoA dehydrogenase deficiency diseases are a group of inherited autosomal recessive defects resulting in impairment of the process of β-oxidation of fatty acids. The most common amongst them is the medium chain fatty acyl-CoA dehydrogenase deficiency. This is also referred as sudden infant death syndrome (SIDS) or Reye's syndrome. Impairment in β-oxidation of medium chain fatty acids results in their accumulation in tissues, such as in the muscle. This, in turn, leads to their metabolism via ω-oxidation and transesterification to glycine and carnitine. Medium chain dicarboxylic acids as well as their glycine and carnitine esters may be detected in the urine of the affected individuals. Typical features include vomiting, lethargy and frequently coma, accompanied with hypoketotic hypoglycemia and dicarboxylic aciduria. Symptoms appear after more than 12 hours of fast and are more complicated on prolonged starvation, usually within first two years of life.

   ii. Enoyl-CoA hydratase adds a molecule of water at the double bond as a result of which α, β-unsaturated fatty acyl-CoA is converted to β-hydroxyacyl-CoA.

   iii. In the presence of NAD^+, β-hydroxyacyl-CoA dehydrogenase oxidizes β-hydroxyacyl-CoA to β-ketoacyl-CoA.

   iv. β-ketothiolase, in the presence of CoA, cleaves β-ketoacyl-CoA and yields acetyl-CoA and fatty acyl-CoA having two carbons less than the original fatty acyl-CoA. The enzyme is of clinical importance (Chemistry to Clinics 4.11).

Chemistry to Clinics 4.11: β-Ketothiolase

Heart muscles utilize free fatty acids as their primary fuel, via β-oxidation. In patients suffering from angina pectoris, parts of the heart muscles become ischemic. Under these conditions, one of the aims of treatment is to shift the metabolic fuel of heart muscles from fatty acids to glucose which also helps to reduce the accompanying acidosis. This is accomplished by administering trimetazidine, a drug which inhibits β-ketothiolase and thus stops β-oxidation, helping in a faster recovery from ischemia.

The newly formed fatty acyl-CoA again undergoes a similar set of reactions, starting with acyl-CoA dehydrogenase and is subsequently degraded to acetyl-CoA.

Regulation of β-oxidation: Availability of the substrates and the cofactors as well as the rate of removal of the product (acetyl-CoA) regulates the process of β-oxidation.

Energy production during β-oxidation: When palmitic acid (C_{15}, H_{31}, COOH) undergoes β-oxidation, it releases 8 molecules of acetyl-CoA in 7 rounds of the oxidative process. In each round of β-oxidation, one molecule of FADH2 and one molecule of NADH are produced. These, in turn, generate 1.5 and 2.5 ATP molecules, respectively. Thus, a total of 28 ATP are obtained during 7 rounds of the process. In addition, each molecule of acetyl-CoA when oxidized in the citric acid cycle, gives 10 ATP. Therefore, additionally 80 ATP are produced from 8 molecules of acetyl-CoA. A total of 108 ATP are hence generated from a molecule of palmitic acid.

As two high energy phosphate bonds are hydrolyzed from one molecule of ATP which is changed to AMP, a total of two ATP are used in the activation of a fatty acid. Therefore, there is a **net yield of 106 ATP when one molecule of palmitic acid (fatty acid with 16 carbons) is completely oxidized**.

PROCESS OF OXIDATION OF FATTY ACIDS IN PEROXISOMES

Besides β-oxidation, fatty acid oxidation also occurs in peroxisomes of the liver, kidney and other tissues. It differs from mitochondrial β-oxidation in two ways:

1. The initial dehydrogenation is carried out by a cyanide insensitive oxidase system. This results in the production of H_2O_2 which is detoxified by a catalase.
2. Specificity of the peroxisomal enzymes is for the long chain fatty acids. This, in turn, results in chain

shortening of the long chain fatty acids to the stage of octanoyl-CoA, i.e. up to 8C only.

THE PROCESS OF α-OXIDATION OF FATTY ACIDS IN ENDOPLASMIC RETICULUM

The process of α-oxidation of fatty acids in endoplasmic reticulum is an alternative pathway of fatty acid oxidation, where some of the fatty acids are oxidized in the liver and the brain. α-oxidation occurs at carbon-2 (α-carbon) instead of the carbon-3 (β-carbon) in β-oxidation.

In α-oxidation, there is a sequential removal of one carbon atom from the carboxyl end of a fatty acid which **neither forms CoA intermediates nor generates ATP** but is removed as CO_2. Reactions of α-oxidation are, particularly, important in the metabolism of methylated fatty acids, such as phytanic acid, a constituent of lipids in milk and other animal fats.

During the process of α-oxidation, a fatty acid is metabolized by α-hydroxylation followed by dehydrogenation and decarboxylation (Fig. 4.26).

Deficiency of the α-hydroxylating enzyme results in Refsum's disease (Chemistry to Clinics 4.12).

Chemistry to Clinics 4.12: Refsum's Disease

Genetic deficiency of the α-hydroxylating enzyme (a monooxygenase) of the α-oxidation system, results in the accumulation of large quantities of phytanic acid in tissues and plasma. This leads to a neurological disorder called Refsum's disease.

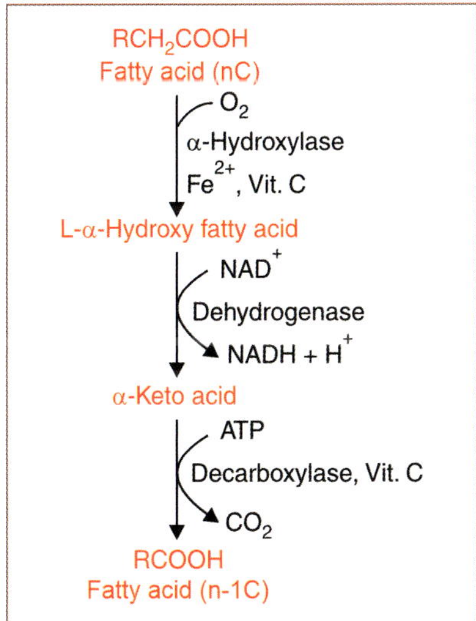

Fig. 4.26: Process of α-oxidation of a fatty acid

ω-OXIDATION OF FATTY ACIDS

This is another minor pathway, where oxidation of medium and long chain fatty acids may occur from **both the ends, simultaneously**. Firstly, the end methyl group ($-CH_3$) of the acyl chain, called the ω-carbon, is oxidized to a carboxylic group (–COOH) and forms a dicarboxylic acid. The reaction is catalyzed by ω-hydroxylase in the presence of **cytochrome P450**. The dicarboxylic acid thereafter undergoes β-oxidation from both the ends, in a chain reaction (Fig. 4.27).

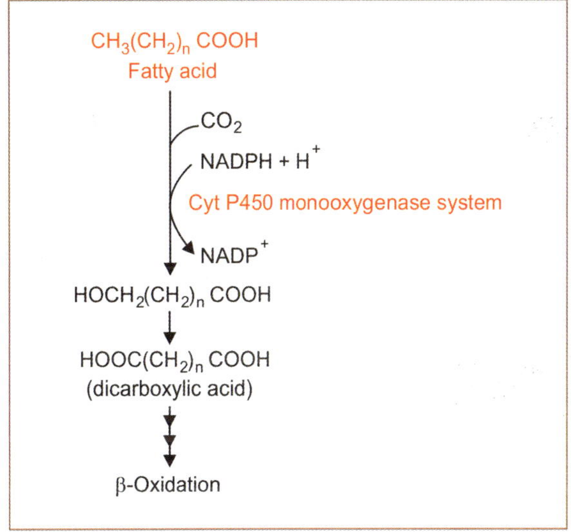

Fig. 4.27: ω-Oxidation of fatty acid

OXIDATION OF FATTY ACIDS WITH ODD NUMBER OF CARBON ATOMS

Fatty acids with odd number of carbon atoms are also oxidized by the process of β-oxidation which in turn removes 2 carbon atoms as acetyl-CoA in each round of the oxidative process. A molecule of **propionyl-CoA,** containing 3 carbon atoms, is formed as the final product (Fig. 4.28).

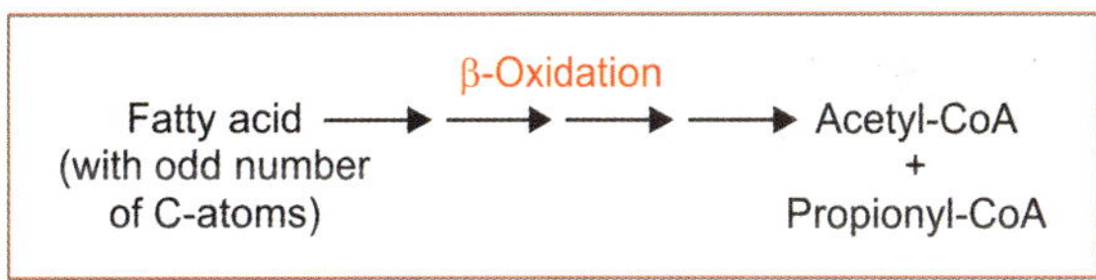

Fig. 4.28: Oxidation of fatty acid containing odd number of carbon atoms

Thereafter, propionyl-CoA undergoes carboxylation, molecular rearrangement and is converted to succinyl-CoA. This, in turn, forms an intermediate of the Krebs cycle (Fig. 4.29).

4

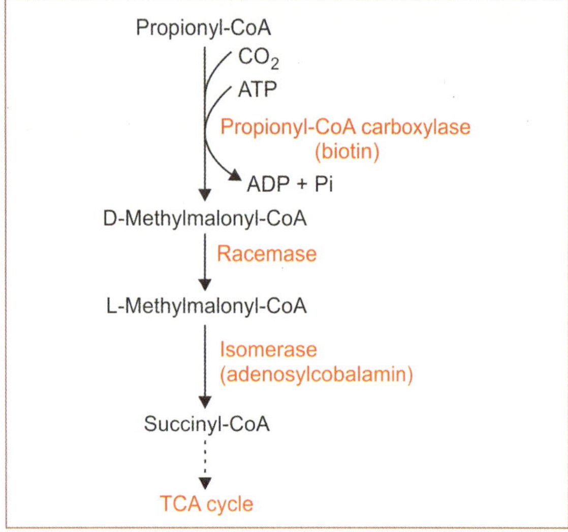

Fig. 4.29: Conversion of propionyl-CoA to succinyl-CoA

OXIDATION OF UNSATURATED FATTY ACIDS

Unsaturated fatty acids are also activated, transported across the inner mitochondrial membrane and undergo β-oxidation, similar to that of saturated fatty acids. But the double bonds of the naturally occurring unsaturated fatty acids are in the *cis*-configuration, whereas those produced during β-oxidation have the *trans*-configuration. Hence, **three additional enzymes** are required for the oxidation of unsaturated fatty acids (Fig. 4.30):

1. An unsaturated fatty acid, such as linoleic acid, when undergoes the process of β-oxidation, after three rounds, it results in the formation of enoyl-CoA. This, however, has a *cis*-configuration and cannot be further oxidized by enoyl-CoA hydratase since this enzyme acts only if the double bond has a *trans*-configuration. The shift of the double bond, from *cis*- to *trans*-configuration, is catalyzed by enoyl-CoA isomerase. The process of β-oxidation thereafter again continues.
2. During the second round of β-oxidation, the product which is formed has a double bond at even numbered carbon atom, i.e. dienoyl-CoA with Δ4 double bond which is reduced by NADPH-dependent dienoyl-CoA reductase and the product is converted to *trans*-3-enoyl-CoA.
3. *Trans*-3-enoyl-CoA is subsequently isomerized to *trans*-2-enoyl-CoA by 3, 2-enoyl-CoA isomerase.

Thereafter, the process of β-oxidation again continues resulting in complete oxidation of the unsaturated fatty acid.

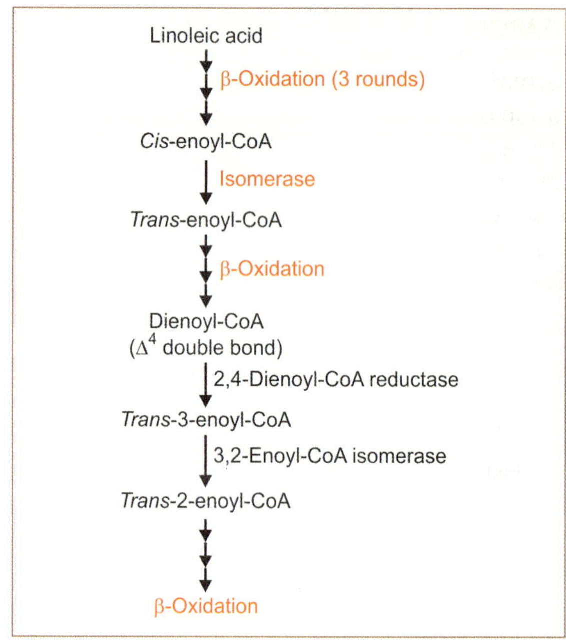

Fig. 4.30: Oxidation of an unsaturated fatty acid

Age pigments/lipofuscin: Auto-oxidation of lipids particularly that of PUFAs, result in the formation of hydroperoxides and dialdehydes, such as malondialdehyde (MDA) in the cell. These oxidized products of lipids and proteins accumulate in the cell in the form of a chemically heterogeneous pigmented substance called **lipofuscin** or **lipochrome.** Since lipofuscin, normally, accumulates in the cells of the older individuals and has been implicated in the aging process, it is also called **age pigments** or **'wear and tear' pigments** (Fig. 4.31).

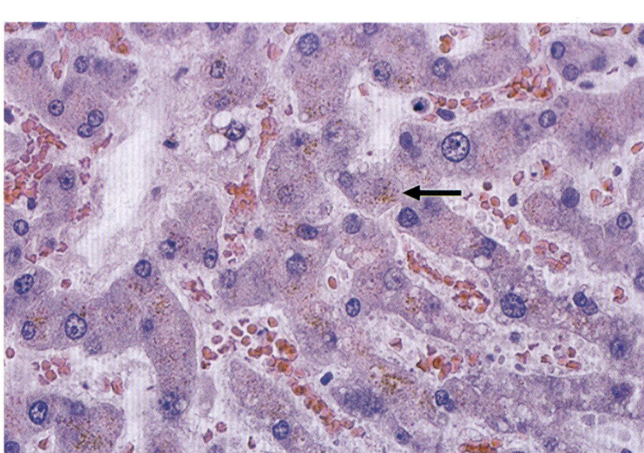

Fig. 4.31: Lipofuscin: The yellow-brown granular pigment (arrow), also called residual body or lipochrome or 'wear and tear' pigment, seen in the hepatocytes. It is the end result of autophagocytosis in which intracellular debris are sequestered and turned into lipofuscin in the cytoplasm

METABOLIC FATES OF ACETYL-CoA

In normal metabolic processes, as discussed above, oxidation of glucose (in glycolysis) as well as oxidation of fatty acids (via β-oxidation) produces acetyl-CoA, which is mainly used in the **Krebs cycle**. Besides, it is also used for the **synthesis of fatty acids** and **cholesterol**. A small quantity is converted to **ketone bodies** in the liver (Fig. 4.32).

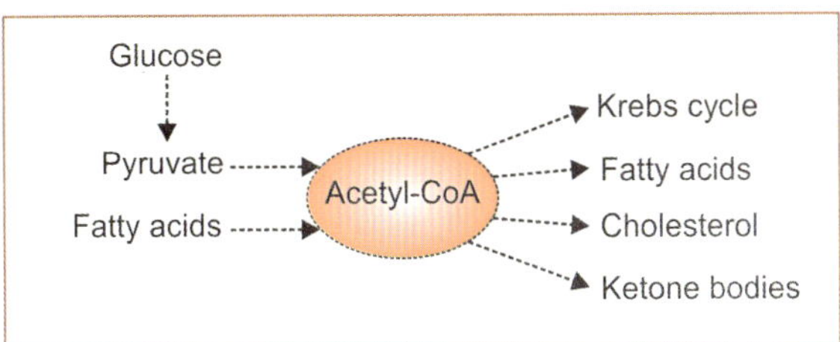

Fig. 4.32: Metabolic fates of acetyl-CoA

BIOSYNTHESIS OF FATTY ACIDS

Other than the availability of fatty acids from dietary lipids, the second major source of fatty acids in the body is their biosynthesis from small molecules (intermediates) which are obtained as a result of the metabolism of sugars, some amino acids and fatty acids. Mammals can synthesize a major portion of the saturated as well as monounsaturated fatty acids. Saturated straight chain 16C fatty acid, i.e. **palmitic acid, is first synthesized** and all the other fatty acids are formed by modifications of the palmitic acid.

DE NOVO SYNTHESIS OF A FATTY ACID

Acetyl-CoA is a direct source of all the carbon atoms for the biosynthesis of a fatty acid which mainly occurs in the liver, the mammary gland and the adipose tissue. Since the main enzymes for fatty acid synthesis, i.e. acetyl-CoA carboxylase and fatty acid synthetase are found, primarily, in the cytosol, synthesis occurs in the **cytoplasm** by the sequential addition of the two-carbon units to the activated carboxyl end of a growing chain. This process of the biosynthesis of fatty acid is called *de novo* synthesis (*de novo* = 'a new', i.e. starting 'from scratch').

Acetyl-CoA, as discussed earlier, is produced in the mitochondria from different sources, such as from pyruvate (obtained from carbohydrates via aerobic glycolysis) and glucogenic amino acids or directly from lipids (β-oxidation) and ketogenic amino acids. Since the mitochondrial membrane is impermeable to acetyl-CoA, a bypass mechanism moves it to the cytosol.

1. Transport of Acetyl-CoA into Cytosol

For its entry into the cytosol, acetyl-CoA first condenses with oxaloacetate and forms citrate. Citrate then enters the cytoplasm and is degraded to acetyl-CoA and oxaloacetate by ATP citrate lyase (Fig. 4.33).

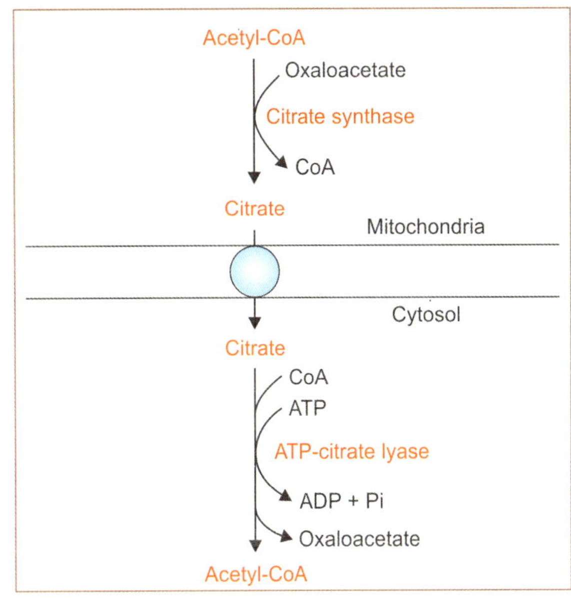

Fig. 4.33: Transport of acetyl-CoA from mitochondria to cytosol

2. Synthesis of Malonyl-CoA

In the cytoplasm, acetyl-CoA is first converted to malonyl-CoA by a biotin containing enzyme acetyl-CoA carboxylase, irreversibly. The reaction occurs in the presence of ATP and CO_2 (HCO_3^-). Formation of malonyl-CoA is a committed step in the synthesis of a fatty acid (Fig. 4.34; reaction 1).

Acetyl-CoA carboxylase regulates fatty acid synthesis by allosteric regulation, covalent modification, induction and repression. Acetyl-CoA carboxylase is controlled by cAMP-mediated phosphorylation-dephosphorylation. Phosphorylation of the enzyme is promoted by glucagon and inactivates the enzyme. High carbohydrate or fat free diet increases the rate of synthesis of the enzyme while fasting or high fat diet decreases its rate of synthesis.

3. Synthesis of Palmitic Acid

Biosynthesis of palmitic acid requires NADPH besides biotin and pantothenic acid. Various reactions are catalyzed by fatty acid synthase which is a multienzyme complex.

Fatty acid synthase complex: It is composed of **two identical subunits, each one of which is a multi-**

enzyme complex containing **6 enzymes** and an **acyl carrier protein (ACP)**. Six subunits of the multienzyme complex are designated as acetyl-CoA-ACP transacylase, malonyl-CoA-ACP transacylase, β-ketoacyl-ACP synthase (condensing enzyme), β-ketoacyl-ACP reductase, β-hydroxyacyl-ACP dehydratase, and enoyl-ACP reductase. The acyl carrier protein (ACP) contains pantothenic acid and has two –SH groups called the pantotheinyl –SH group and the cysteinyl –SH group.

The **reaction sequence for the synthesis of palmitic acid** is as follows (Fig. 4.34):

I. After the synthesis of malonyl-S-ACP, there occur the transfer of an acetyl-CoA onto the cysteinyl –SH group of ACP. The reaction is catalyzed by acetyl-CoA-ACP transacylase subunit of the fatty acid synthase complex and leads to formation of the acetyl-S-ACP.

II. At the same time, malonyl-CoA-ACP transacylase transfers malonyl-CoA onto the pantotheinyl –SH group of ACP and forms malonyl-S-ACP.

III. Next, the condensing enzyme (β-ketoacyl-ACP synthase) condenses acetyl-S-ACP with malonyl-S-ACP and forms acetoacetyl-S-ACP (β-ketoacyl-ACP).

IV. β-Ketoacyl-ACP reductase with NADPH + H^+ reduces acetoacetyl-S-ACP to form β-hydroxy-butyryl-S-ACP (-hydroxyacyl-S-ACP).

V. β-Hydroxyacyl-ACP dehydratase removes H_2O from β-hydroxyacyl-S-ACP and forms α-,β-transbutenoyl-ACP (crotonyl-S-ACP).

VI. α, β-Transbutenoyl-ACP is reduced by enoyl-ACP reductase, utilizing NADPH + H^+ and is converted to butyryl-S-ACP (acyl-ACP).

VII. In the next cycle of reactions, butyryl-S-ACP again condenses with a molecule of malonyl-CoA, chain elongation continues with the repeated rounds and finally palmitoyl-S-ACP is synthesized.

VIII. Thereafter, palmitoyl thioesterase removes ACP and yields palmitate. The reducing equivalents (NADPH + H^+) used in the biosynthesis of fatty acids are derived from pentose phosphate pathway.

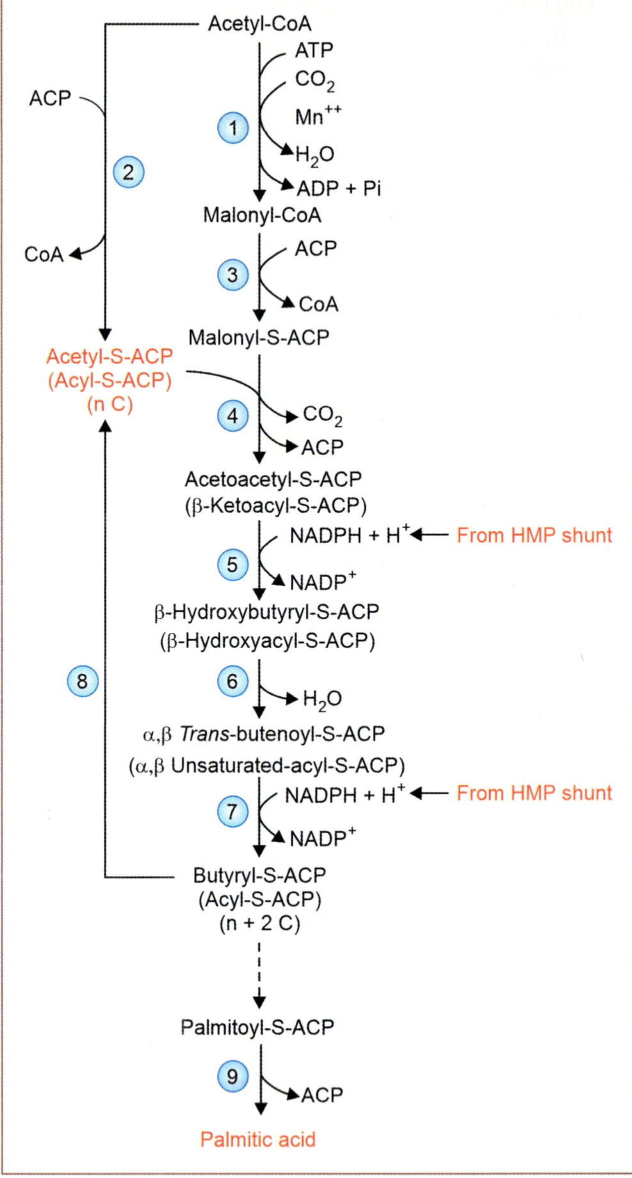

Fig. 4.34: *De novo* synthesis of palmitic acid: (1) Acetyl-CoA carboxylase, (2) Acetyl-CoA-ACP transacylase, (3) Malonyl-CoA-ACP transacylase, (4) Condensing enzyme (β-ketoacyl ACP synthase), (5) Reductase, (6) Dehydratase, (7) Reductase, (8) Further condensation and chain elongation, (9) Thioesterase

Advantages of FAS existing as multienzyme complex: Multienzyme complexes are called '**metabolons**' because they function as a discrete metabolic unit with distinct advantages:

i. The proximity of one enzyme to another minimizes the diffusion of the reaction intermediates thereby enhancing the overall reaction rate.

ii. The channeling of intermediates between successive enzymes reduces the opportunity for these intermediates to react with other molecules, thereby minimizing side reactions.

iii. The complex is more stable as compared to the constituent enzymes present in isolation.

iv. The individual enzymes are encoded by the same structural gene, hence all the enzyme constituents are coordinately expressed.

v. The multienzyme complexes are regulatory proteins so the reactions catalyzed by them are coordinately regulated.

4. Conversion of Palmitate to other Fatty Acids

As discussed above, the first fatty acid which is synthesized within the body is a saturated straight chain 16C fatty acid, called palmitic acid or palmitate. Palmitate is converted to various long chains unsaturated and hydroxy fatty acids by chain elongation, desaturation and hydroxylation.

Chain Elongation

Chain elongation of a fatty acid occurs either in the mitochondria or in the endoplasmic reticulum.

In mitochondria: Chain elongation in the mitochondria takes place by the successive additions of acetyl-CoA as two carbon units where both NADH as well as NADPH can serve as the reducing agent. The system operates by reversal of the pathway of β-oxidation with the exception that NADPH-linked enoyl-CoA reductase replaces FAD-linked acyl-CoA dehydrogenase. This process, primarily, results in the elongation of palmitate.

- Firstly, acyl-CoA condenses with acetyl-CoA and forms β-ketoacyl-CoA which utilizes NADH + H^+ and is reduced to β-hydroxyacyl-CoA.
- Removal of a molecule of water converts β-hydroxyacyl-CoA to α, β-unsaturated fatty acyl-CoA (enoyl-CoA).
- The latter is reduced to a higher member of the series (Fig. 4.35).

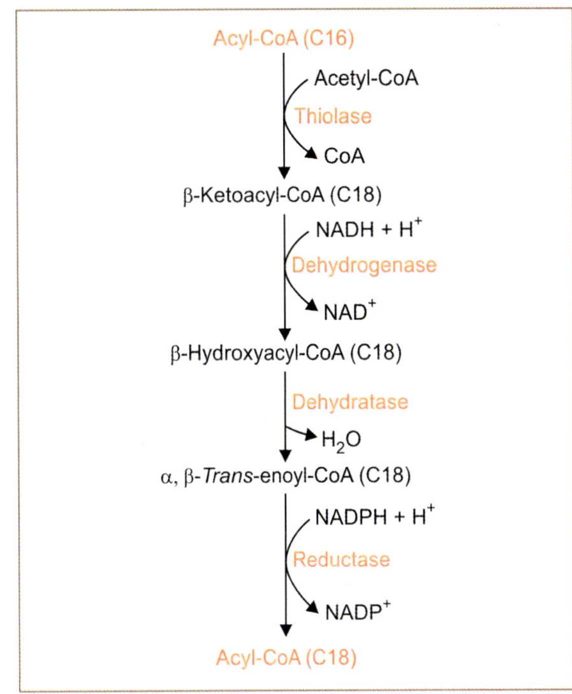

Fig. 4.35: Chain elongation of a fatty acid in the mitochondria

In endoplasmic reticulum: The process of chain elongation in the endoplasmic reticulum is similar to fatty acid biosynthesis (*de novo* synthesis) in the cytoplasm. It utilizes malonyl-CoA as the source of two carbon units but in the endoplasmic reticulum fatty acid is elongated as its CoA derivative rather than as ACP derivative as in fatty acid synthesis in the cytoplasm. In most of the tissues, chain elongation system in the endoplasmic reticulum converts palmitate to stearate. Brain, however, contains one or more additional elongation systems for the synthesis of long chain fatty acids (up to 24C), which are needed for the synthesis of complex lipids within the brain.

Desaturation

Desaturation of a fatty acid occurs in higher animals in the endoplasmic reticulum, by desaturases, also termed mixed function oxidases (Fig. 4.36).

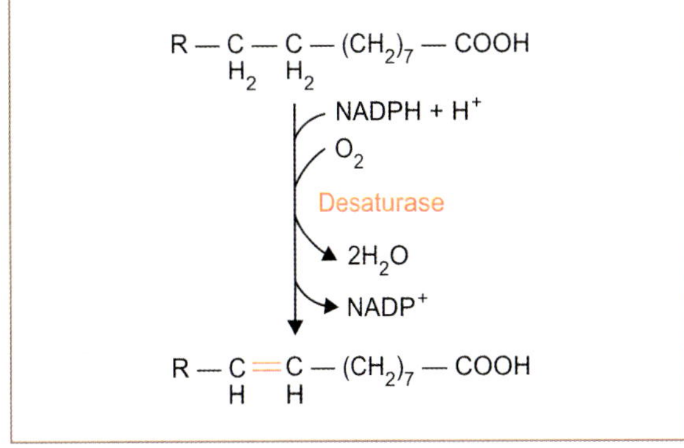

Fig. 4.36: Desaturation of a fatty acid in the endoplasmic reticulum

Desaturase is a multienzyme complex that has 3 components, i.e. a desaturase, cytochrome *b*5 and NADPH-cytochrome *b*5-reductase.

A committed step in the formation of an unsaturated fatty acid from palmitic acid or stearic acid is the introduction of the first double bond between C9 and C10 by stearoyl-CoA desaturase, to form palmitoleic acid or oleic acid, respectively. The activity of this enzyme and its synthesis are controlled by both dietary as well as hormonal mechanisms.

Increasing amounts of PUFA in the diet decreases the activity of this enzyme in the liver, whereas insulin, triiodothyronine and hydrocortisone induce the enzyme.

4

Once the initial double bonds have been introduced between carbons 9 and 10 by stearoyl-CoA desaturase, additional double bonds can be introduced beyond C4, C5 or C6.

Hydroxylation

Formation of α-hydroxy fatty acids in higher animals occurs in the mitochondria with the mixed function oxidase system which requires molecular oxygen and NADH or NADPH. Their synthesis is closely co-ordinated with the biosynthesis of sphingolipids that contain hydroxylated fatty acids in the nervous tissue.

Regulation of Fatty Acid Biosynthesis

- The conversion of acetyl-CoA to malonyl-CoA is a rate-limiting step in the biosynthesis of fatty acids. This reaction is catalyzed by **acetyl-CoA carboxylase** which is stimulated by citrate, isocitrate and α-ketoglutarate. Citrate allosterically activates acetyl-CoA carboxylase while long chain fatty acyl-CoA acts as an allosteric inhibitor for the same. Insulin also stimulates the activity of the enzyme, whereas glucagon inhibits it.
- **High carbohydrate diet** increases the production of acetyl-CoA which also increases the citrate pool. Citrate leaves the mitochondria and is cleaved by citrate lyase to produce acetyl-CoA. Citrate also stimulates acetyl-CoA carboxylase. Thus, high carbohydrate diet leads to increased synthesis of fatty acids.
- **Hormones** also regulate fatty acid biosynthesis. Insulin reduces cAMP levels, inhibits the activation of hormone sensitive lipase and favors lipogenesis. Glucagon, on the other hand, increases cAMP levels, activates hepatic lipase and inhibits fatty acid synthesis. Glucagon thus promotes the release of fatty acids from the adipose tissue (lipolysis) and opposes lipogenesis.
- **Fatty acid synthase** is the other key enzyme of palmitate biosynthesis. A high carbohydrate diet or a fat free diet stimulates fatty acid synthase activity by increasing enzyme synthesis. On the other hand, a high fat diet, fasting and glucagon decrease enzyme synthesis. Phosphorylated sugars, e.g. glucose-6-phosphate also cause allosteric activation of the enzyme.

4

LIPOPROTEINS

As discussed above, **lipids** are sparingly soluble in the aqueous solution. Hence, they are transported in blood **complexed with proteins** (called apolipoproteins or simply as **apoproteins**) as the hydrophilic complexes called **lipoproteins**.

STRUCTURE OF LIPOPROTEINS

These are globular micelle-like particles that consist of nonpolar core of triacylglycerols and cholesteryl esters surrounded by an amphiphilic coating of proteins, phospholipids and cholesterol with various **apoproteins (apolipoproteins)**.

Apolipoproteins

- Protein components of lipoproteins are known as apolipoproteins or apoproteins.
- Functions:
  1. Transport lipids (water insoluble by nature) in plasma in a water-miscible form.
  2. Serve as structural components of lipoproteins.
  3. Provide recognition sites for cell surface receptors.
  4. Serve as activators for enzymes involved in lipoprotein metabolism.
- Various apolipoproteins are divided into different classes from A to E, and at least nine are distributed in the lipoproteins, i.e. A1, A2, B48, B100, C1, C2, C3, D and E.
- All apoproteins except B100 are water-soluble. Apolipoprotein B100 (Apo B100) is one of the largest monomeric proteins known. It is synthesized by the liver and is present in LDL.

CLASSIFICATION OF LIPOPROTEINS

There are four major types of lipoproteins, which are designated as chylomicrons (CM), very low density lipoproteins (VLDL), low density lipoproteins (LDL) and high density lipoproteins (HDL; Table 4.4).

SEPARATION OF LIPOPROTEINS

According to their densities, various lipoproteins can be separated by ultracentrifugation (Fig. 4.37).

They can also be separated, according to their protein contents, by electrophoresis (Fig. 4.38).

METABOLISM AND FUNCTIONS OF LIPOPROTEINS

As mentioned above, there are four major types of lipoproteins that are designated as chylomicrons, very low density lipoproteins (VLDL), low density lipoproteins (LDL) and high density lipoproteins (HDL).

Table 4.4: Physical properties and chemical composition of human serum lipoproteins

	Chylomicrons	VLDL	LDL	HDL
Density (g/ml)	<1.006	<1.006	1.019–1.063	1.063–1.125
S_f	>400	20–400	0–12	3.6–9.0
Electrophoretic mobility	Origin	Pre-β	β	α
Protein concentration (%)	2–4	8–12	20–25	40–45
Free cholesterol (%)	1–3	5–10	7–10	5
Cholesterol esters (%)	2–4	10–15	35–40	12–18
Triacylglycerols (%)	85–90	50–65	6–10	4–6
Phospholipids (%)	8–10	16–20	20–24	25–30

VLDL rich or CM rich
IDL
LDL
HDL_2 rich/HDL_3 poor
HDL_2 poor/HDL_3 rich

Fig. 4.37: Separation of serum lipoproteins by ultracentrifugation

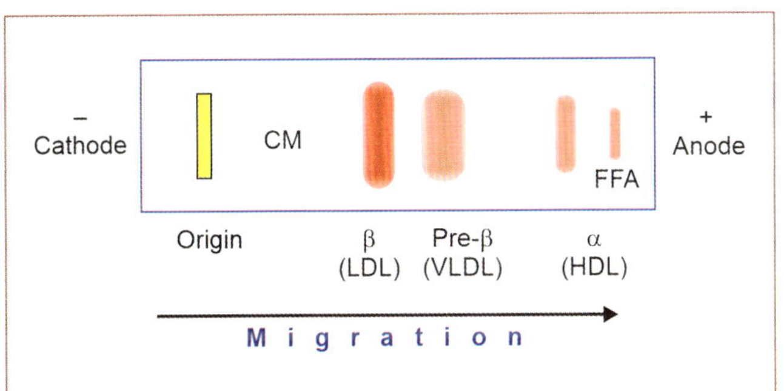

Fig. 4.38: Electrophoretogram of serum lipoproteins after 12 hours of fasting. For approximately 2-8 hours following a meal, there is an additional lipoprotein class (position indicated by blue arrow), called chylomicrons (CM), representing the transport of dietary lipids absorbed in the intestine. The small band to the right of HDL represents free fatty acid-albumin complex (FFA)

Chylomicrons

Chylomicrons are **triacylglycerol-rich particles** that are assembled in the **intestinal mucosal cells**. They carry **dietary/exogenous triacylglycerols** (the major lipids of chylomicrons), cholesterol and cholesteryl esters **to the peripheral (extrahepatic) tissues** where these lipids are subsequently metabolized (Fig. 4.39).

Intestinal mucosal cells release **nascent chylomicrons** which contain **Apo B48** that is synthesized in the intestine. These nascent chylomicron particles receive Apo E and Apo C from the circulating HDL. Apo C2, in turn, activates lipoprotein lipase and hydrolyzes triacylglycerols to monoacylglycerols, free fatty acids and glycerol. As a result, chylomicron particles decrease in size and increase in density. Thereafter, Apo C is returned back to HDL and the leftover particles are called **chylomicron remnants**.

Chylomicron remnants bind to Apo E receptors on the hepatocytes. These particles are then internalized and their lipids including cholesteryl esters can be either utilized or stored intracellularly. A small amount of the released fatty acids enters circulation and contributes directly to the plasma free fatty acid pool.

Very Low Density Lipoproteins

Very low density lipoproteins (VLDL), also called **pre-β-lipoproteins**, are composed of triacylglycerols like chylomicrons but their function is to transport these lipids (**endogenous triacylglycerol**) from the **liver to the peripheral tissues (extrahepatic tissues)**. VLDL are released from the liver as **nascent VLDL** particles, similar to the release of nascent chylomicrons from the intestinal mucosa. Nascent VLDL particles contain **Apo**

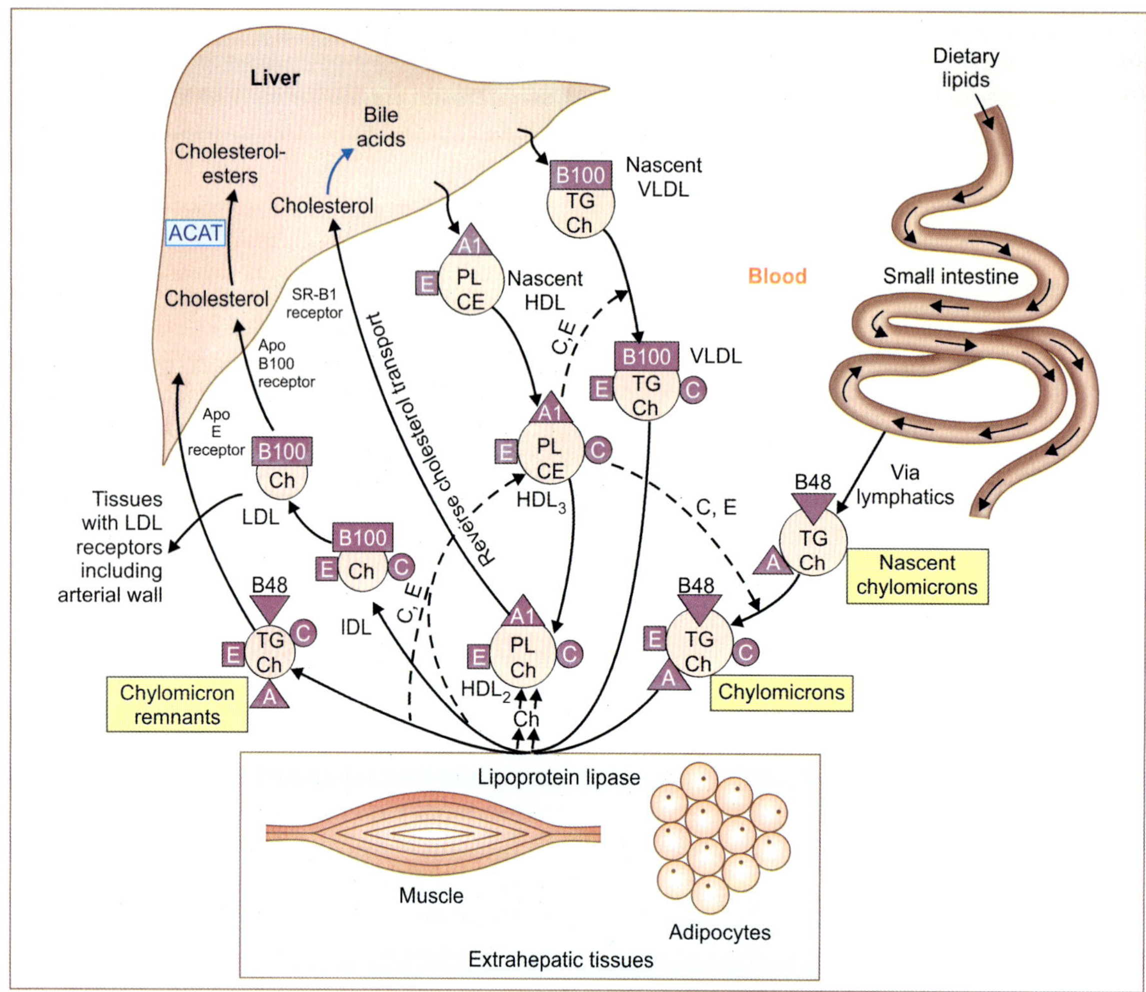

Fig. 4.39: Metabolism of lipoproteins

B100 and Apo A1. They, subsequently, acquire Apo C2 and Apo E from the circulating HDL and are converted to VLDL (Fig. 4.39).

During circulation, lipoprotein lipase hydrolyzes triacylglycerols and releases free fatty acids which are taken up by the peripheral tissues. Subsequently, Apo C and Apo E are transferred to HDL. In addition, cholesteryl esters are transferred from HDL to VLDL in exchange with the transfer of triacylglycerols and phospholipids from VLDL to HDL. As a result, their particle size is reduced and density is increased. VLDL particles are hence converted into **VLDL remnants** which are also designated as **intermediate density lipoproteins (IDL)**.

The **IDL particles are either removed by the liver or are further converted into circulating LDL particles**. During the process of this conversion (of IDL) to LDL, surface lipids and apoproteins, other than the molecule of Apo B100, are removed. Cholesteryl esters, which are synthesized in plasma as a result of the action of lecithin cholesterol acyltransferase (LCAT, discussed later) on HDL particles, are transferred from HDL to VLDL and IDL via cholesteryl ester transfer protein (CETP).

Low Density Lipoproteins

Low density lipoproteins (LDL) contain **high concentration of cholesterol and its esters**. They retain **Apo B100** and lose other apoproteins to HDL. The primary function of the LDL is to transport **cholesterol (initially released from the liver in VLDL) to the extrahepatic tissues**. For their metabolism, LDL particles bind to their receptors on the cell membrane.

LDL receptors are negatively charged glycoproteins that are clustered in pits on the cell membrane and recognize Apo B100 of the LDL. The intracellular side of the pit is coated with a protein called **clathrin**, which stabilizes the shape of the pit. The number of these receptors is regulated by the cholesterol content of the cell. The ability of a tissue to take up LDL depends upon the rate of transcapillary transport as well as the number of receptors. The liver and the adrenals which have a fenestrated epithelium as well as large number of receptors, may take up LDL rapidly while the muscle and the adipose tissue which lack such an epithelium and have a few LDL receptors, take up LDL slowly.

After binding, LDL particles are **internalized** by endocytosis, in the form of vesicles. These LDL vesicles rapidly lose the clathrin coat, fuse with other similar vesicles and form endosomes (large vesicles). The receptors are recycled, whereas LDL remnants, in the vesicles, are degraded and release cholesterol, fatty acids, phospholipids and amino acids (Fig. 4.39).

Free cholesterol can be used for membrane biosynthesis or for its conversion to steroid hormones and bile acids. Excess of the cholesterol is re-esterified by acylcholesterol acyltransferase (**ACAT**) and is stored as cholesteryl esters.

Nearly 70–80% of the LDL particles are removed via LDL receptors while the rest of them are removed by nonspecific endocytosis, via the scavenger pathway. The latter is also a receptor mediated process involving phagocytic cells, in the reticuloendothelial system.

There are two LDL subtypes that are clinically important (Chemistry to Clinics 4.13).

Chemistry to Clinics 4.13: LDL Subtypes

There are two LDL subtypes: Type A or large, **buoyant LDL** and type B or small, **dense LDL**. Both subtypes are found in the circulation although their relative proportion differs from person to person. Their size depends on genetic as well as nutritional factors. The small, dense LDL has greater ability to penetrate the tunica intima, is more prone to oxidation (forming pro-atherogenic oxidized LDL) and binds more strongly to proteoglycans in the extracellular matrix of the arterial wall. Thus, it is highly atherogenic. It is recommended that at the time of plasma LDL determinations, the concentrations of the specific subtypes should also be ascertained.

Lecithin–Cholesterol Acyltransferase (LCAT) and Reverse Cholesterol Transport (RCT)

HDL and the enzyme lecithin–cholesterol acyltransferase (LCAT) are important for the removal of cholesterol from the body. LCAT is a plasma enzyme produced mainly by the liver. The enzyme transfers a fatty acid from C2 position of lecithin to the 3-hydroxyl of cholesterol. The reaction is freely reversible and utilizes cholesterol which is present in HDL. Cholesterol esters so formed, diffuse into the core of the HDL particles where these are transported from tissues via plasma to the liver, the only organ capable of metabolizing and excreting cholesterol as bile acids. This mechanism, i.e. the action of LCAT on HDL is referred to as **reverse cholesterol transport (RCT)**. HDL thus provides a vehicle for the transport of cholesterol from peripheral tissues to the liver and **protects from atherosclerosis**.

LCAT versus ACAT: Although both the enzymes are involved in acyl group transfer, they differ with respect to their location, the esterifying unit, activator and function (Table 4.5).

High Density Lipoproteins

High density lipoprotein (HDL) particles are synthesized in the **liver** and secreted into the bloodstream by exocytosis, as **nascent HDL** particles. They are discoidal in shape and are composed of Apo A, Apo E, phospholipids and free cholesterol. Among the various lipoproteins, they contain **highest concentration of phospholipids**.

As discussed above, there also occur the transfer of Apo C to the nascent HDL from chylomicrons and VLDL. Nascent HDL particles are thus converted to **mature HDL** called **HDL_3**. From HDL_3, cholesteryl esters (produced by the action of LCAT) are shifted to VLDL and IDL. At the same time, HDL_3 also acquires free cholesterol from the cell membrane. These HDL_3 particles are thus converted to **HDL_2.** (Note: HDL_1 is a

Table 4.5: Difference between LCAT and ACAT

Parameter	LCAT	ACAT
Site of esterification	Intravascular, extracellular	Extravascular, intracellular (hepatocytes)
Esterifying unit	Polyunsaturated fatty acids	Monounsaturated fatty acids
Activator	Apo A1 in HDL	Unesterified cholesterol
Metabolic purpose	To esterify free cholesterol derived from peripheral tissues and transport it to the liver via HDL	To store excess cholesterol as esters so as to maintain low intracellular free cholesterol levels

4

very minor HDL fraction with higher phospholipid and lower Apo A1 content, detected in some patients of primary hyperlipoproteinemia or cholestasis). This is an important mechanism for the removal of excess cholesterol from the peripheral tissues and is called reverse transport of cholesterol transport (Fig. 4.39).

HDL thus performs several important functions

1. It is a circulating reservoir of Apo C2 which is transferred to chylomicrons and VLDL for the activation of lipoprotein lipase.
2. It removes free cholesterol from the extrahepatic tissues and esterifies it with the help of LCAT. HDL thus transports cholesterol from the extra-hepatic tissues to the liver.
3. It transfers cholesteryl esters to VLDL and LDL in exchange for triacylglycerols and phospholipids from these particles.
4. It also carries cholesteryl esters to the liver.

In the liver, HDL is taken-up via SR-B1 (scavenger receptor class B, type 1) receptors, degraded and releases cholesterol. Cholesterol, in turn, is either repacked within the lipoproteins or is converted into bile acids and secreted into the bile for its removal from the body. Thus, HDL protects an individual against atherosclerosis.

Good cholesterol versus bad cholesterol: The risk of developing atherosclerosis is directly related to the plasma concentration of LDL cholesterol but inversely related to HDL cholesterol. Therefore, **LDL cholesterol** is called the **'bad cholesterol'** while **HDL cholesterol** is referred to as the **'good cholesterol'**, although chemically there is only one cholesterol.

DISORDERS OF LIPOPROTEIN METABOLISM

HYPERLIPOPROTEINEMIAS

Increased rate of synthesis or reduced clearance of lipoproteins from the bloodstream may result in a group of disorders referred to as hyperlipidemias or hyperlipoproteinemias (Table 4.6).

Usually, they are detected by measuring plasma triacylglycerols and cholesterol, and are classified accordingly as follows:

Type I hyperlipoproteinemia: This condition is also called **hyperchylomicronemia or familial fat-induced hyperlipemia**. This is due to the accumulation of chylomicrons. These patients have very high levels of triacylglycerols in their plasma (over 1000 mg/dl) with a proportionally smaller increase in cholesterol. On electrophoresis, chylomicrons remain at the origin. Type I hyperlipoproteinemia may be due to **three different types** of genetic abnormalities:

Table 4.6: Classification of hyperlipoproteinemias

Type	↑ Lipoproteins
Primary	
I Exogenous hypertriglyceridemia	Chylomicrons
IIa Hypercholesterolemia	LDL
IIb Combined hyperlipidemia	LDL + VLDL
III Remnant hyperlipidemia `	Remnant VLDL
IV Endogenous hyperlipidemia	VLDL
V Mixed hyperlipidemia	VLDL + Chylomicrons
Secondary	
Type IV pattern: Diabetes mellitus, alcoholism, von Gierke's disease, lipodystrophies, acromegaly, oral contraceptives, uremia, hypothyroidism, high carbohydrate diet	VLDL

- **Familial lipoprotein lipase deficiency:** It is usually present in infancy or childhood. There are recurrent episodes of abdominal pain due to attacks of acute pancreatitis which are triggered by very high plasma levels of triacylglycerols (Chemistry to Clinics 4.14).

Chemistry to Clinics 4.14: Hypertriglyceridemia and Acute Pancreatitis

Chylomicrons are usually formed 1–3 hours postprandially and cleared within 8 hours. However, in hypertriglyceridemia, chylomicrons are almost always present thereby increasing the viscosity of blood. Further, these particles are very large and may obstruct pancreatic capillaries leading to local ischemia and acidemia followed by cell necrosis and apoptosis. This local damage exposes triglycerides to pancreatic lipases. Triglycerides are hydrolyzed to free fatty acids which form self-aggregating micelles with detergent properties, damaging capillaries, platelets and pancreatic tissue. Cytotoxic injury, release of inflammatory mediators and free radicals, eventually manifests as acute pancreatitis.

Patients may also have skin lesions called **eruptive xanthomata** which appear on buttocks, back, knees and elbows. These lesions contain a lot of triacylglycerols due to the deposition of chylomicrons. Serum has a lipemic appearance and after an overnight refrigeration at 4°C, chylomicrons rise to the surface (Fig. 4.40).

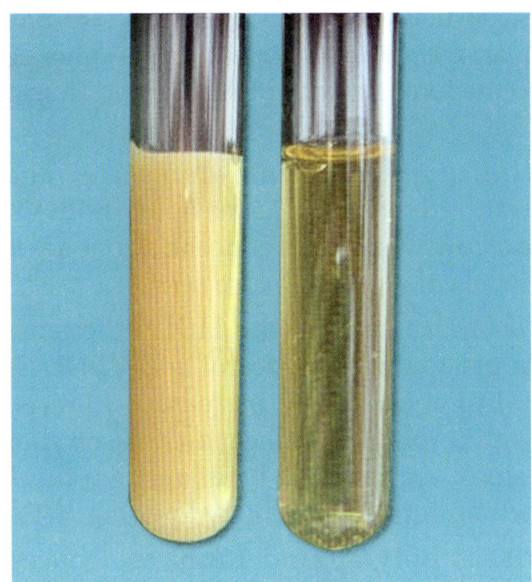

Fig. 4.40: Serum of a patient with triglyceride-related acute pancreatitis. Left: Lipemic serum before treatment with insulin and heparin. Right: Clear serum after 5 days of therapy

Its diagnosis can be confirmed by measuring lipoprotein lipase activity in the plasma after a bolus injection of heparin.

- **Familial Apo C2 deficiency:** It is a rare condition, which is inherited as an autosomal recessive disorder. It is due to the deficiency of Apo C2 which is essential for the activation of lipoprotein lipase. Hence, there is impaired removal of both chylomicrons and VLDL from the plasma. This, in turn, results in the lipoprotein pattern which may be of type I or type V.
- **Familial lipoprotein lipase inhibitor:** It is an autosomal dominant condition of the type I hyperlipoproteinemia. The patient has low post-heparin plasma lipolytic activity but high levels of lipoprotein lipase in the adipose tissue. Plasma of the affected individuals contains a nondialyzable, heat stable inhibitor of lipoprotein lipase. Occasionally, subjects with type I phenotype may also show a type V pattern, due to the accumulation of VLDL in their plasma. This is common if they ingest a high carbohydrate diet.

Type II hyperlipoproteinemia: It may be further subclassified as:

- **Type IIa hyperlipoproteinemia:** It is also called **familial hypercholesterolemia or familial hyperbetalipoproteinemia**. There is high cholesterol in fasting plasma without increase in triacylglycerols. Electrophoretic pattern also shows an increase in β-lipoproteins. It may be a primary disorder due to some genetic abnormality or a secondary lipoprotein disorder.

  Primary type IIa hyperlipoproteinemia also called familial type IIa hyperlipoproteinemia may be seen in heterozygotes or homozygotes. Heterozygous familial type IIa hyperlipoproteinemia is an autosomal dominant inherited disease, usually from many different genetic mutations, affecting the gene for LDL, for Apo B and Apo E receptors. Mutations for LDL receptor gene can cause four different types of disorders:
  - The most common type is mutant allele where no receptors are synthesized.
  - The second common type of disorder is the one where receptors are synthesized but are transported slowly from the endoplasmic reticulum to the Golgi apparatus.
  - Receptors are processed and reach the cell surface but fail to bind LDL.
  - Receptors reach the surface and bind LDL but fail to cluster in the coated-pits, and cannot be internalized.

  The heterozygotes have very high levels of plasma cholesterol and LDL.

  Homozygous familial type IIa hyperliporoteinemia is generally seen in children who present with planar or tuberous xanthomata since birth. Yellowish plaques or lumps occur on buttocks, knees, elbows and hands. Cardiovascular disease may develop before the age of 10 years.

  Plasma LDL is several times higher than normal. Some of these patients may also show moderate elevation of triacylglycerols.

  Secondary type IIa hyperlipoproteinemia results in hypercholesterolemia which can be caused by several common disorders unrelated to familial conditions, such as Cushing's syndrome, hypothyroidism, anorexia nervosa, nephrotic syndrome, primary liver cell carcinoma or diabetes mellitus.
- **Type IIb hyperlipoproteinemia:** It is called **familial combined hyperlipidemia or multiple lipoprotein-type hyperlipidemia**. There is an increase in total plasma cholesterol and triacylglycerols. On electrophoresis, there is an increase in the intensity of both β- and pre-β-bands, due to increased production of VLDL and LDL. Composition of the individual lipoproteins is normal. Obesity, high serum uric acid levels and glucose intolerance are common in patients with this pattern.

Type III hyperlipoproteinemia: It is also called **dysbetalipoproteinemia or remnant hyperlipoproteinemia or broad, floating beta disease or familial type III hyperlipoproteinemia**. There is a moderate

4

hypercholesterolemia while hypertriacylglyceridemia is relatively uncommon. This is associated with the presence of chylomicron remnants and IDL in plasma. The disease rarely manifests itself before early adult life in males or before the menopause in females. Fasting serum or plasma is often turbid. The characteristic finding on electrophoresis is a broad β-band but on ultracentrifugation these particles are isolated in the VLDL region.

Type IV hyperlipoproteinemia: This condition is also called **hyper-pre-beta-hyperlipoproteinemia or endogenous hyperlipidemia or diet-induced hypertriglyceridemia or familial type IV hyperlipoproteinemia**. These patients have a marked elevation of plasma triacylglycerols in VLDL. In some families, there is excessive VLDL secretion while in others the removal rate of VLDL from plasma is reduced. Fasting serum or plasma is turbid. On electrophoresis, there is a marked pre-β-band with normal β and a normal or reduced α-band.

A **secondary type IV pattern** is quite common (Table 4.7).

Type V hyperlipoproteinemia: It is also called **mixed hyperlipidemia**, since large amounts of, both, chylomicrons and VLDL are seen in the fasting plasma. It is occasionally seen in patients whose characteristic pattern is like type I (due to lipoprotein lipase deficiency) but rarely of type IV. Whole blood may be lipemic. Plasma is white and turbid. The electrophoretic pattern is characterized by raised chylomicrons and VLDL levels.

HYPOLIPOPROTEINEMIAS

- ***Abetalipoproteinemia***: Fat malabsorption is present from birth. In neonates, there is poor appetite, vomiting, diarrhea and failure to thrive. All plasma lipids, particularly triacylglycerols, are reduced to less than 50% of the normal levels. This is mainly due to the total absence of Apo B, and thus of VLDL and LDL.
- ***Familial hypobetalipoproteinemia***: There is a moderate reduction of plasma lipids. Both VLDL and LDL are low while HDL concentrations are variable. Low levels of Apo B are also seen.
- ***Tangier disease***: It is the HDL deficiency state, where plasma triacylglycerol and VLDL levels are normal or moderately increased. LDL is rich in triacylglycerols. Total plasma cholesterol and LDL cholesterol are reduced by about two-thirds while HDL cholesterol is extremely low (Fig. 4.41).

  Apo A1 is only around 1% of the concentration normally found in plasma and Apo A2 is only about 5–8% of the normal. Besides Apo A1 and Apo A2, there is also a moderate reduction in all the other apoproteins.

Table 4.7: Causes of secondary type IV hyperlipoproteinemia
• Diabetes mellitus
• Alcoholism
• Hypothyroidism
• von Gierke's disease
• Lipodystrophies
• Acromegaly
• ↑use of oral contraceptives
• Uremia
• High carbohydrate diet

ATHEROSCLEROSIS

Atherosclerosis (arteriosclerosis) is a disease of arterial wall. It is characterized by the accumulation of **cholesterol** and its esters of lipoproteins containing Apo B100 in cells which are derived from monocyte-macrophage that line smooth muscle cells. This, in turn, results in the formation of **atherosclerotic plaque, which narrows the blood vessels** and serves as the site of thrombus formation (Fig. 4.42).

High calorie diet, or diet rich in saturated fat and cholesterol, hypercholesterolemia, sedentary lifestyle, stress and strain, obesity, hypertension and smoking are important contributory factors, favorable in the development of atherosclerosis.

Risk of developing the disease is directly related to the concentration of the LDL-cholesterol in plasma. It is also inversely related to the plasma concentration of HDL-cholesterol. Therefore, **LDL-cholesterol is called bad cholesterol** while **HDL-cholesterol** is referred to as **good cholesterol**. Diseases with prolonged elevated level of LDL, VLDL, IDL or chylomicron remnants in blood, like diabetes mellitus, hypothyroidism, lipid nephrosis, etc. are associated with severe atherosclerosis. Lipoprotein(a) or Lp(a) is considered to be an independent risk factor. It contains apo(a) which is similar to plasminogen in structure. It competes with plasminogen for conversion to plasmin which degrades fibrin in the blood clots. This apo(a) is different from Apo A of HDL.

Indians are genetically predisposed and are at an increased risk of developing atherosclerosis at an early

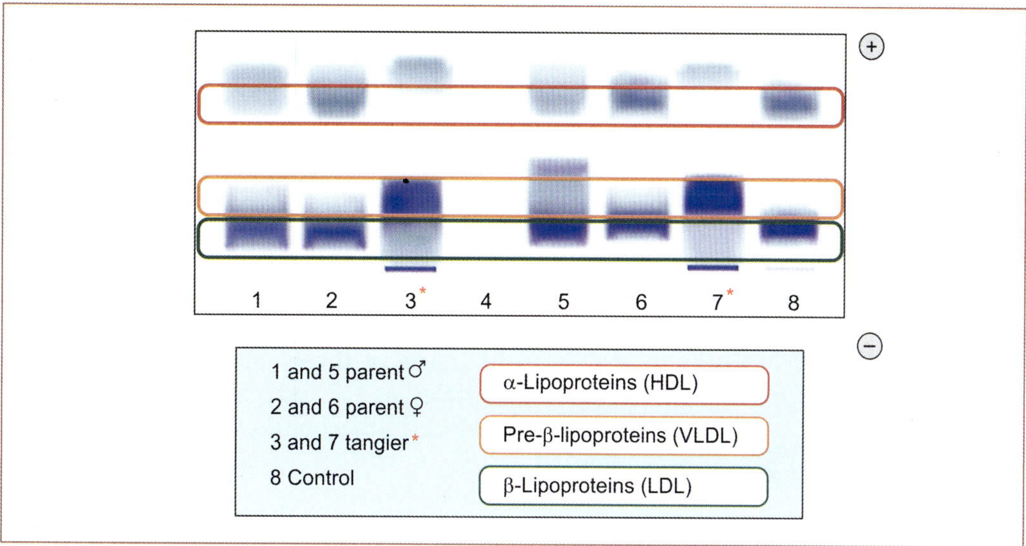

Fig. 4.41: Tangier disease. Two-dimensional lipoprotein electrophoresis: Patient sample (*columns 3 and 7) shows the **absence of α-band (red zone) indicating the absence of HDL**. Columns 1 and 5 show the father's sample; columns 2 and 6 show the mother's sample; and column 8, the control sample. The orange zone shows pre-β-lipoproteins; green zone, β-lipoproteins

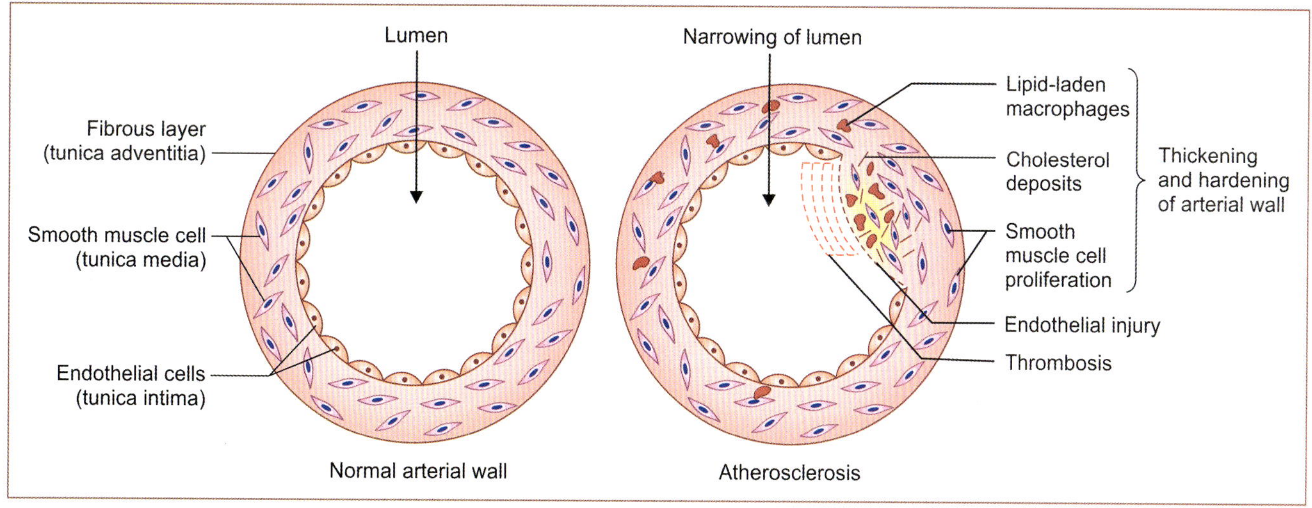

Fig. 4.42: Atherosclerosis

age, hence sometimes known as premature atherosclerosis. About 40% Indians have higher levels of Lp(a).

Drugs like **cholestyramine** bind bile salts and promote their excretion in stool. This, in turn, **increases the rate of bile salt synthesis** and LDL uptake by the liver. **Lovastatin**, the drug that is used in the treatment of **hyperlipidemia**, is an **inhibitor of the enzyme HMG-CoA reductase**. Hence, it decreases endogenous synthesis of cholesterol and stimulates LDL uptake (via LDL receptors) by the tissues. Sitosterol decreases intestinal cholesterol absorption. Clofibrate decrease the hepatic endogenous cholesterol secretion by inhibiting VLDL secretion. Nicotinic acid reduces lipolysis thereby decreasing acetyl-CoA, the precursor of cholesterol.

Dietary Recommen.dations

- Reduce the total amount of fat. Not more than 30% of total energy intake should come from fat.
- Reduce the use of animal fat. Not more than one-third of the total fat (less than 10% calories/day) should come from saturated fat, with the remainder from unsaturated fat.
- Reduce the intake of cholesterol. Dietary cholesterol should be less than 300 mg/day.
- Trans-fatty acid intake should limit to less than 1% calories/day.
- Increase omega-3 fatty acid intake from dietary or supplementary fish oil.

- Eat five or more servings of fruits and vegetables/day.
- Reduce salt intake.

Other Lifestyle Interventions

In addition to dietary advice, other lifestyle interventions include:

- Promotion of physical activity, e.g. adults should perform at least 30 minutes of moderate activity (brisk walking), at least 5 days per week. Maintaining ideal body weight emphasizes activity.
- Limit sedentary activities and give up smoking.

LIPID PROFILE

Serum lipids and lipoprotein fractions are, generally, measured after 12 hours of fasting, to allow complete clearing of chylomicrons. Serum may appear hazy when serum triglycerides exceed 200 mg/dl. Chylomicrons can be easily detected because they form a white supernatant after refrigeration.

The following parameters are included under a serum **lipid profile** or **lipidogram**:

- **Total cholesterol** (which is a sum of cholesterol distributed in LDL, VLDL and HDL): 150–220 mg/dl (desirable 140–200 mg/dl)
- **LDL-cholesterol:** 60–160 mg/dl
- **VLDL-cholesterol:** <32 mg/dl
- **HDL-cholesterol:** 30–60 mg/dl
- **Triglycerides:** 50–160 mg/dl

  According to **Friedwald's formula**, VLDL-cholesterol is given by triglycerides/5, provided triglycerides are <400 mg/dl. Thus, LDL-cholesterol can be calculated as follows:

  LDL-cholesterol = Total cholesterol – [HDL-cholesterol + Triglycerides/5]
- **Cardiac risk ratio** = Total-cholesterol: HDL-cholesterol. A ratio >5 indicates an increased cardiovascular risk.

Special investigations may be performed in some cases and include plasma troponin, myoglobin, homocysteine, lipoprotein(a) Creactive protein, etc. (Chemistry to Clinics 12.14).

EICOSANOIDS AND PROSTAGLANDINS

EICOSANOIDS

4

Eicosanoids (Greek *eicosa*: Twenty) are physiologically and pharmacologically active compounds such as prostanoids (prostaglandins, prostacyclins and thromboxanes), and the leukotrienes. Eicosanoids are derived from 20C containing polyunsaturated fatty acids (20C PUFA), also called eicosapolyenoic fatty acids, such as arachidonic acid. Three different eicosapolyenoic fatty acids, i.e. eicosatrienoic acid (20C:3), eicosatetraenoic acid (20C:4 or arachidonic acid), and eicosapentaenoic acid (20C:5) with 3, 4 and 5 double bonds, respectively, can be synthesized in the body from linoleic acid (Fig. 4.43).

Three different eicosapolyenoic acids act as precursors of three separate series of eicosanoids designated as 1, 2 and 3 (i.e. the compounds containing 3, 4 and 5 double bonds, respectively, such as PG_1, PG_2 and PG_3 series of prostaglandins). Variations in the substituent groups attached to the cyclic ring present in the eicosanoids further give rise to different types of compounds in each series. For example, the E type of prostaglandin (such as PGE_2) has a keto group in position 9 while the F type (such as PGF_1) has a hydroxyl group.

The Cyclooxygenase and Lipoxygenase Pathways

Eicosapolyenoic acids such as arachidonic acid follow one of the two metabolic pathways—the cyclooxygenase (COX) pathway or the lipoxygenase (LOX) pathway, producing different series of products. Cyclooxygenase pathway of eicosapolyenoic acid metabolism results in cyclization at the center of the 20 carbon chain. This results in the formation of a cyclopentane ring containing endoperoxides called PGG_2 which acts as precursors for the synthesis of

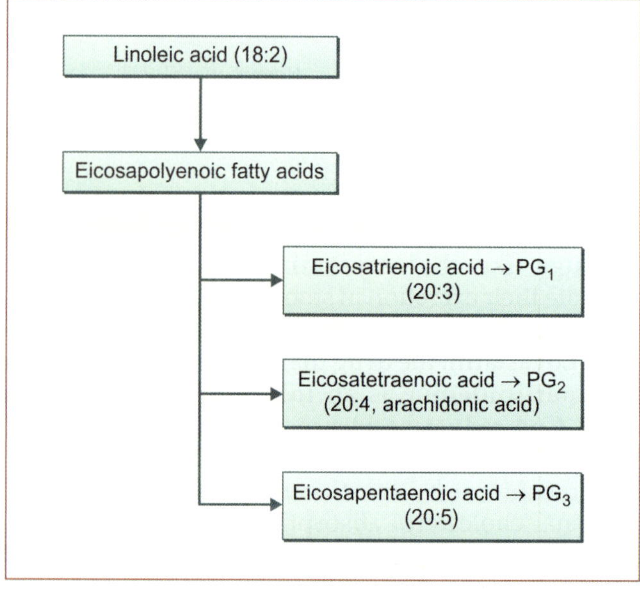

Fig. 4.43: Conversion of linoleic acid to eicosanoids (eicosapolyenoic fatty acids)

prostaglandins, prostacyclins and thromboxanes. On the other hand, lipoxygenase pathway leads to the formation of leukotrienes (Fig. 4.44).

The specific products, so formed, are tissue dependent. For example, the endothelial cells predominantly synthesize prostacyclins, whereas platelets produce thromboxanes. Eicosanoids act at very low concentrations and are important for the regulation of blood pressure, blood coagulation, vascular tone, inflammatory response, immune response, reproduction, gastric HCl secretion, maintaining the patency of fetal ductus arteriosus, smooth muscle contraction, etc.

Isoenzymes of cyclooxygenase (COX): Prostaglandin endoperoxide synthase (PGH_2 synthase) or cyclooxygenase (COX) catalyzes two steps in succession, i.e. oxidation of arachidonate to PGG_2 and the latter to PGH_2. The enzyme has two isoforms. COX-1 is responsible for the normal production of prostaglandins. COX-2 is induced by cytokines, mitogens and endotoxins during inflammation (Chemistry to Clinics 4.15).

Chemistry to Clinics 4.15: Anti-inflammatory Drugs and Prostaglandin Synthesis

There are two broad categories of anti-inflammatory drugs:

- The **nonsteroidal anti-inflammatory drugs** (NSAIDs) such as aspirin irreversibly acetylate Ser530 of both COX-1 and COX-2. Others, such as indomethacin and ibuprofen, inhibit COX-1/COX-2 by other mechanisms and thus block the conversion of eicosanoic acids, e.g. arachidonic acid to cyclic endoperoxides thereby inhibiting the biosynthesis of various prostaglandins. These drugs are nonspecific COX inhibitors. Recently, specific COX-2 inhibitors have been developed that selectively suppress the role of eicosanoids during inflammation only. Such inhibitors, called 'coxibs' (e.g. celecoxib and etoricoxib), also produce less gastric and renal side effects.
- The **steroidal anti-inflammatory drugs** like hydrocortisone, prednisone and betamethasone, on the other hand, block the entire eicosanoid biosynthetic pathway by inhibiting phospholipase A_2 activity so as to interfere with the mobilization of arachidonic acid, an essential substrate for the subsequent reactions. Thus, steroids are more potent anti-inflammatory drugs than NSAIDs.

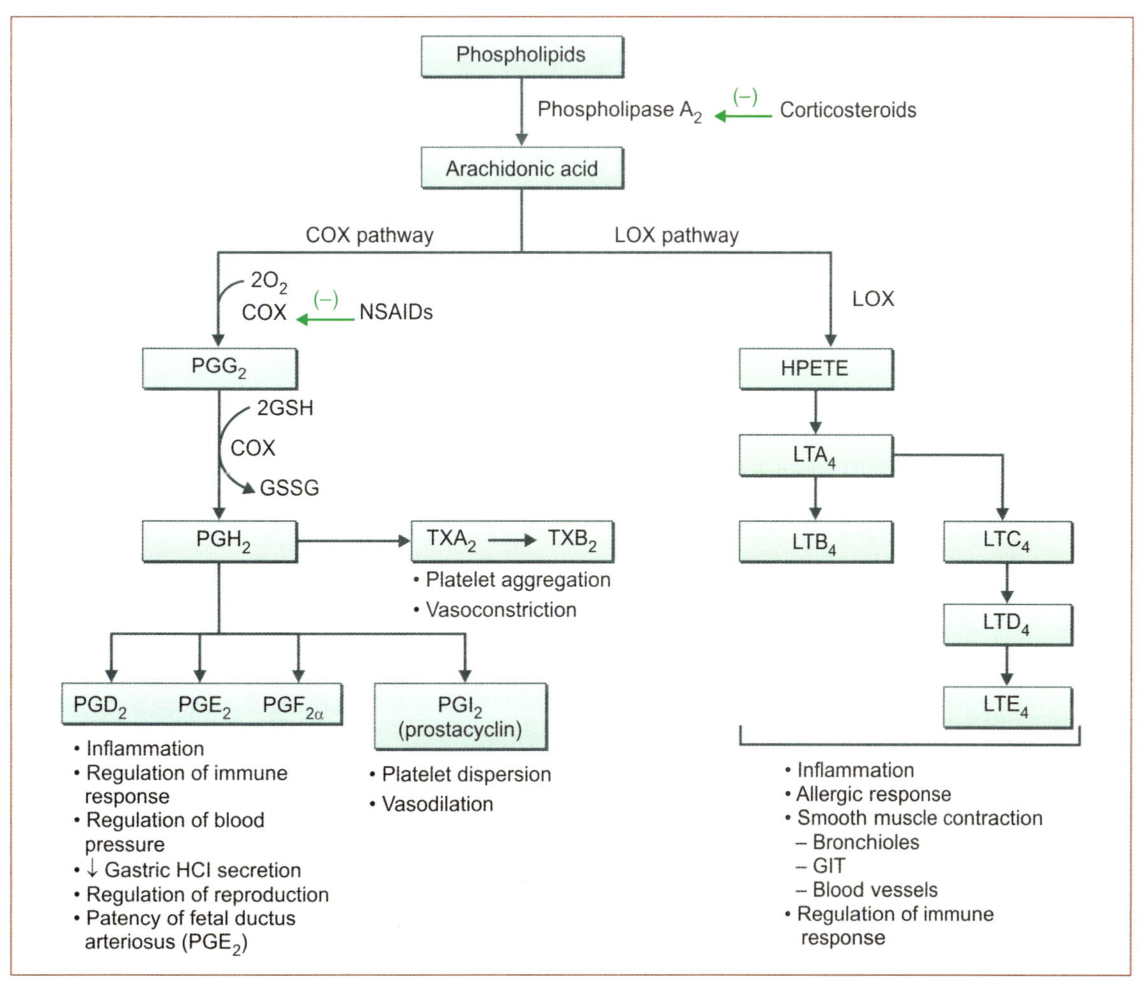

Fig. 4.44: Metabolism of arachidonic acid (COX pathway and LOX pathway)

4

PROSTAGLANDINS

Prostaglandins are 20 carbon containing fatty acid derivatives having one or more unsaturated bonds, several hydroxyl groups, sometimes a keto group and a cyclopentane ring. Prostaglandins are so named because of their initial isolation from the prostate gland secretion. They are now known to be produced and released by nearly all mammalian cells except red blood cells. Prostaglandins act as local hormones and have a very short half-life. Soon after their release, they are rapidly taken up by the cells where they exert very short-lived effects and are rapidly catabolized.

There are three major classes of primary prostaglandins, i.e. the A, E and F series. All are related to the hypothetical parent compound, prostanoic acid (Fig. 4.45).

Fig. 4.45: Prostanoic acid

Prostaglandins can be distinguished on the basis of functional groups around the cyclopentane ring, i.e. the E series contains a β-hydroxyketone, the F series are 1,3-diols, and those in the A series are α, β-unsaturated ketones. The subscript numerals 1, 2 and 3 refer to the number of double bonds in the side chain.

Prostacyclins

Prostacyclins (PGI_2) are derived from eicosapolyenoic acids such as arachidonic acid in the vascular endothelium. These have a powerful vasodilatory action especially on the coronary arteries. These are also responsible for inhibiting platelet aggregation.

Thromboxanes

The term 'thromboxane' is derived from the fact that these compounds have thrombus-forming potential. They are highly active metabolites of PGG_2 and PGH_2 type prostaglandin endoperoxides whose cyclopentane ring is replaced by a six-membered oxygen containing ring called oxane ring (Fig. 4.46).

The substituent groups attached to different positions of the ring give rise to different types in each series of thromboxanes, i.e. A, B, etc.

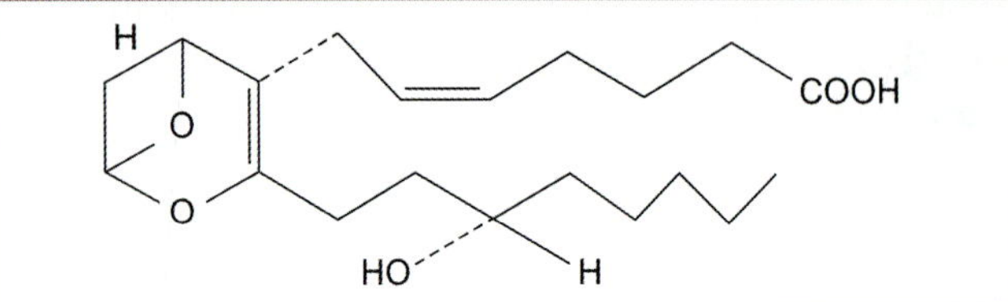

Fig. 4.46: Thromboxane A_2 (TXA_2)

The TXA_2 is the main prostaglandin endoperoxide formed in platelets. It causes release of serotonin and Ca^{2+} from platelet granules. It produces vasoconstriction and increase blood pressure besides contraction of arterial smooth muscle and platelet aggregation.

Leukotrienes

Leukotrienes are a family of conjugated trienes formed from eicosapolyenoic fatty acids by the lipoxygenase pathway. Twenty carbon polyunsaturated fatty acids, such as arachidonic acid, are first converted to their hydroperoxyeicosatetraenoic acids (HPETE) and serve as precursors of different types of leukotrienes. Leukotrienes do not have a ring in their structure but have three conjugated double bonds (Fig. 4.47).

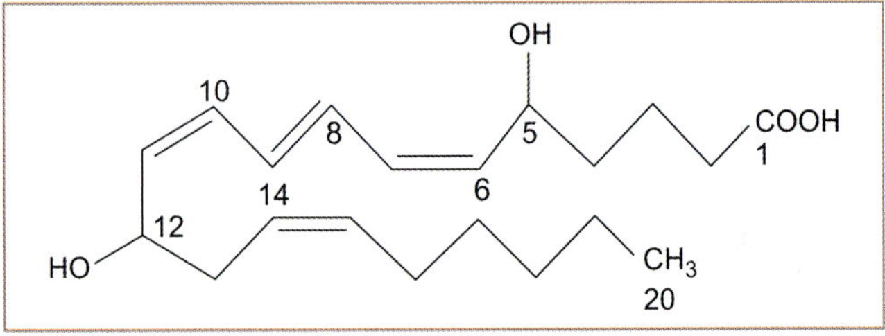

Fig. 4.47: Leukotrienes B_4 (LTB_4)

Leukotrienes are synthesized in leukocytes, mast cells and macrophages in response to immunologic and noninflammatory stimuli. They stimulate mucus secretion and cause constriction of the bronchial smooth muscles (Chemistry to Clinics 4.16).

Chemistry to Clinics 4.16: Leukotrienes and Bronchial Asthma

Elevated levels of leukotrienes (LT) are associated with various inflammatory and hypersensitivity disorders, such as bronchial asthma. Specifically, a combination of LTC4, D4 and E4, previously known as the 'slow reacting substance of anaphylaxis or SRSA', is notorious to produce bronchospasm. Drugs blocking the leukotriene receptors are currently being used in the treatment of bronchial asthma. Further, it is useful to bear in mind that aspirin and other NSAIDs suppress the cyclooxygenase pathway and thereby divert the eicosanoid pathway towards the synthesis of leukotrienes. This can precipitate an asthmatic attack in aspirin sensitive individuals.

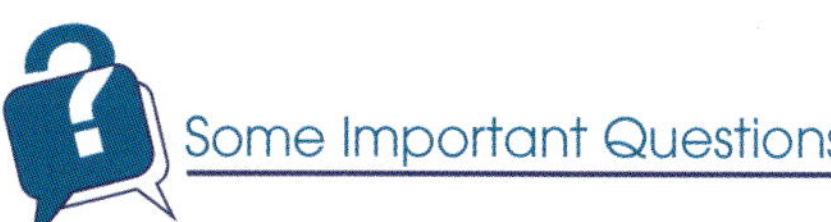

Some Important Questions

1. What are lipids? Classify them. Give biological significance of lipids.

2. What are phospholipids? Describe various types of phospholipids with example.

3. What are fatty acids? Classify them. Write biological significance of polyunsaturated fatty acids.

4. Outline β-oxidation of fatty acids. How much energy is produced when one molecule of palmitic acid is completely metabolized to acetyl-CoA?

5. Outline *de novo* synthesis of fatty acids. What is the source of reducing equivalents? How does *de novo* fatty acid synthesis differ from the microsomal and the mitochondrial fatty acid synthesis?

6. What are triacylglycerols? How triacylglycerols are synthesized in the adipose tissue?

7. Discuss:

i. Hyperlipoproteinemias
ii. Tangier disease
iii. Abetalipoproteinemia

8. Describe briefly:

i. Chemistry and functions of prostaglandins.
ii. Classification of lipids with suitable examples
iii. Leukotrienes
iv. Lipoproteins and their functions
v. Lung surfactants
vi. Sphingolipids
vii. Chemistry and functions of cholesterol
viii. Cerebrosides
ix. Lipoproteins
x. Apolipoproteins
xi. Role of carnitine in fatty acid metabolism
xii. Oxidation of fatty acids with odd number of carbon atoms

9. Write notes on:

i. Triacylglycerols
ii. Iodine number
iii. PUFA
iv. Thromboxanes
v. Essential fatty acids
vi. Eicosanoids
vii. Lecithins
viii. Respiratory distress syndrome
ix. L/S ratio
x. Cardiolipins
xi. Ketone bodies
xii. PUFA
xiii. β-Oxidation
xiv. Atherosclerosis
xv. Lipuria
xvi. Digestion and absorption of dietary lipids
xvii. Carnitine deficiency disorders
xviii. α-Oxidation of a fatty acid
xix. Steatorrhea
xx. Refsum's disease
xxi. Chyluria
xxii. Lipofuscin
xxiii. Sudden infant death syndrome
xxiv. Metabolic fates of acetyl-CoA
xxv. LCAT
xxvi. Catabolism of triacylglycerols
xxvii. Hormone sensitive lipase
xxviii. Lung surfactant
xxix. Lipoproteins
xxx. Bile acids

4

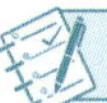

Multiple Choice Questions

1. The following are associated with an increased risk of cardiovascular disease:

A. Diet rich in saturated fatty acids
B. Diet rich in *trans*-fatty acids
C. Increased plasma oxidized LDL
D. All of the above

2. Phrenoderma results from a dietary deficiency of:

A. Essential amino acids
B. Essential fatty acids
C. Phytanic acid
D. Propionic acid

3. N-acyl sphingosine is:

A. Ceramide
B. Choline
C. Cephalin
D. Cardiolipin

4. Infantile respiratory distress syndrome is most likely with an amniotic fluid L/S ratio:

A. <2
B. 3
C. 4
D. >5

5. Phosphate groups are absent in:

A. Cerebrosides
B. Lecithin
C. Cephalin
D. Plasmalogen

6. The commonest deficiency in Reye's syndrome is of:

A. Short chain acyl-CoA dehydrogenase
B. Medium chain acyl-CoA dehydrogenase
C. Long chain acyl-CoA dehydrogenase
D. None of the above

7. Hormone sensitive lipase is stimulated by the following *except*:

A. ACTH
B. Insulin
C. Glucagon
D. Epinephrine

8. Very low density lipoproteins (VLDL) transport triacylglycerols from:

A. Liver to small intestine only
B. Small intestine to liver
C. Small intestine to extrahepatic tissues
D. Liver to extrahepatic tissues

9. The following is not a risk factor for atherosclerosis:

A. Increased plasma homocysteine
B. Increased plasma lipoprotein(a)
C. Increased plasma LDL-cholesterol
D. Increased plasma HDL-cholesterol

10. Tangier's disease is characterized by deficiency of circulating:

A. LDL
B. VLDL
C. Chylomicrons
D. HDL

CHAPTER 5

Chemistry and Metabolism of Proteins

Competency Achievement: **The student should be able to:**

BI5.1 Describe and discuss structural organization of proteins
BI5.2 Describe and discuss functions of proteins and structure–function relationships in relevant areas, e.g. hemoglobin and selected hemoglobinopathies
BI5.3 Describe the digestion and absorption of dietary proteins
BI5.4 Describe common disorders associated with protein metabolism
BI5.5 Interpret laboratory results of analytes associated with metabolism of proteins
PY2.2 Discuss the origin, forms, variations and functions of plasma proteins
PY4.4 Describe the physiology of digestion and absorption of nutrients

Proteins (Greek *proteios*, primary) are polymers of amino acids linked through peptide bonds in a specific sequence dictated by the corresponding DNA sequence. They are a class of macromolecules containing nitrogen. All proteins are composed of 20 different amino acids.

The commonly occurring amino acids are α-amino acids because they have a primary amino group ($-NH_2$) and a carboxylic group ($-COOH$) as substituents on the α-carbon atom. The general structure of an amino acid is represented in Fig. 5.1.

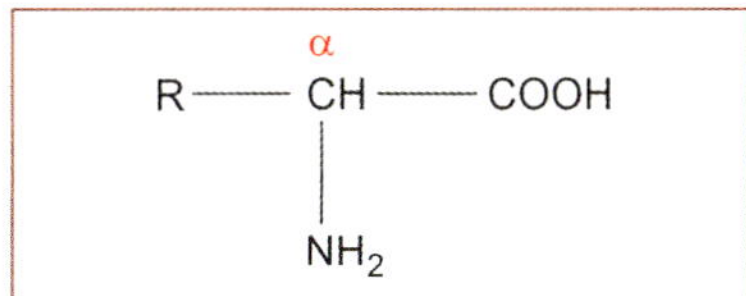

Fig. 5.1: General structure of an amino acid

Classification of Amino Acids

Amino acids may be classified either based on their side chains or according to their nutritional requirements.

Depending upon the presence of their side chain (the R group attached to the α-carbon atom), amino acids are classified into different groups, as follows (Table 5.1)

Neutral Amino Acids

These amino acids are neutral in reaction and have one amino ($-NH_2$) and one carboxylic ($-COOH$) group. These are also called monoamino monocarboxylic acids. According to the presence of the R group, neutral amino acids are further subdivided into two categories, i.e. the aliphatic amino acids and the aromatic amino acids.

Aliphatic Amino Acids

i. **Simple aliphatic amino acids:** Such as glycine and alanine. Glycine has the smallest possible side chain, i.e. a hydrogen atom (–H) as the R group. Alanine has a methyl group ($-CH_3$) in its side chain (Fig. 5.2).

ii. **Branched-chain amino acids:** These amino acids have an aliphatic hydrocarbon side chain which has a branch in its structure, i.e. some group is attached to one of the carbon atoms of the aliphatic side chain. There are 3 amino acids which are labeled as branched-chain amino acids. These are valine, leucine and isoleucine (Fig. 5.3).

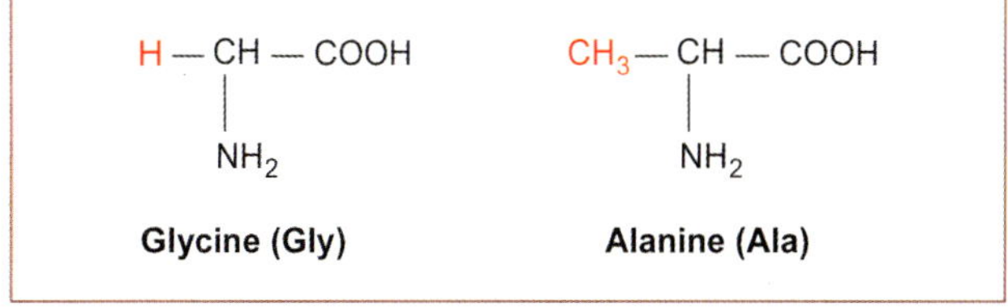

Fig. 5.2: Simple aliphatic amino acids

Table 5.1: Classification of amino acids

Amino acid	Abbreviation*
NEUTRAL AMINO ACIDS	
Simple Amino Acids	
Glycine	Gly
Alanine	Ala
Branched-Chain Amino Acids	
Valine	Val
Leucine	Leu
Isoleucine	Ile
Hydroxy Amino Acids	
Serine	Ser
Threonine	Thr
Aromatic Amino Acids	
Phenylalanine	Phe
Tyrosine	Tyr
Tryptophan	Trp
Sulfur-containing Amino Acids	
Cysteine	Cys
Methionine	Met
ACIDIC AMINO ACIDS	
Aspartic acid	Asp
Glutamic acid	Glu
Amides of the Acidic Amino Acids	
Asparagine	Asn
Glutamine	Gln
BASIC AMINO ACIDS	
Lysine	Lys
Arginine	Arg
Histidine	His
IMINO ACID	
Proline	Pro

*Three letters abbreviation is widely used. This, generally, includes first three letters of an amino acid.

iii. **Hydroxy amino acids:** There are 2 amino acids which have a hydroxyl (–OH) group in their aliphatic side chain. These are serine and threonine (Fig. 5.4).

iv. **Sulfur** (also spelt as 'sulphur') **containing amino acids:** Some amino acids, in addition to C, H, O and

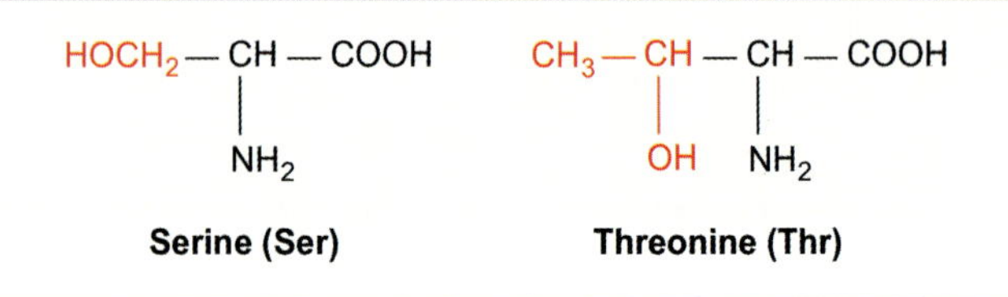

Fig. 5.4: Hydroxy amino acids

N, also contain sulfur (S) as a part of its aliphatic side chain. These are cysteine and methionine.

Cysteine has a free thiol group (–SH) which can form a disulfide bond (–S–S–) with another cysteine residue. Through the oxidation of the two thiol groups, it can form another amino acid called cystine or dicysteine. Certain oxidative processes can convert two molecules of cysteine to cystine, in a protein, in the body.

Methionine does not contain a free –SH group. Instead, it has a thiol linkage as CH3–S– in its side chain (Fig. 5.5).

Aromatic Amino Acids

These amino acids have an aromatic ring which is neutral in reaction. There are three amino acids which are grouped as aromatic amino acids. These are phenylalanine (alanine with a phenyl group), tyrosine (4-hydroxyphenylalanine) and tryptophan (alanine attached to an indole ring), as shown in Fig. 5.6.

Acidic Amino Acids and their Amides

These amino acids are acidic in reaction since they have one amino group but more than one (generally two) carboxylate groups. These amino acids are also called as monoamino dicarboxylic acids. There are two amino acids which are acidic in nature. These are aspartic acid and glutamic acid. Besides, there are two other amino acids which are not actually acidic in nature but are derived from the acidic amino acids. These are thus the amides of the acidic amino acids (Fig. 5.7).

The amide of aspartic acid is called asparagine. It is required in cell multiplication. The amide of glutamic acid is called glutamine. Its formation within the body

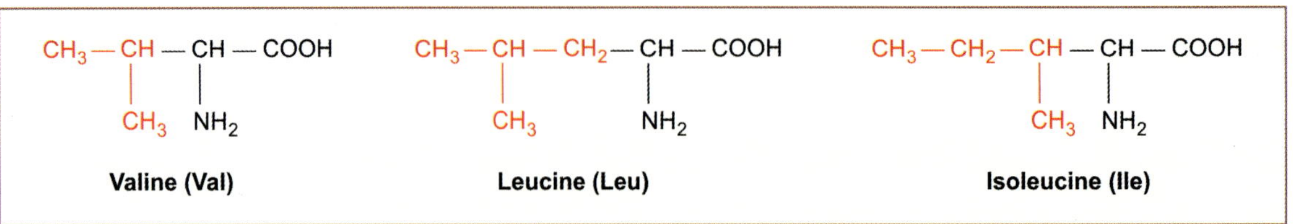

Fig. 5.3: Branched-chain amino acids

$HS—CH_2—CH(NH_2)—COOH$

Cysteine (Cys)

$HOOC—CH(NH_2)—CH_2—S—S—H_2C—HC(NH_2)—COOH$

Cystine (Cys – Cys)

$CH_3—S—CH_2—CH_2—CH(NH_2)—COOH$

Methionine (Met)

Fig. 5.5: Sulfur-containing amino acids

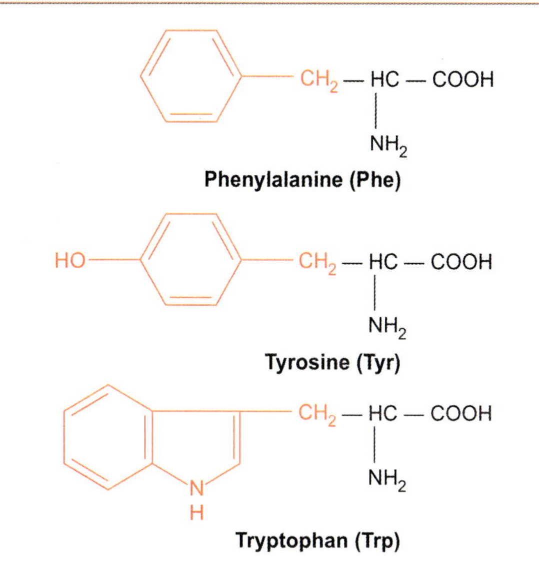

Fig. 5.6: Aromatic amino acids

helps to remove ammonia from the brain. Glutamine is also needed in many biosynthetic reactions.

Basic Amino Acids

These amino acids are basic in reaction and have one carboxylic group but either >1 amino group in the aliphatic side chain or a heterocyclic ring which is basic in reaction. These are lysine, arginine and histidine:

- Lysine has two $–NH_2$ groups.
- Arginine has a guanidino group in the aliphatic chain.
- Histidine has a heterocyclic imidazole ring (Fig. 5.8).

Imino Acids

In addition to the above amino acids which are found in most proteins, collagen is rich in proline, which is an imino acid. Proline does not contain a primary α-amino group ($–NH_2$) but has a secondary imino group (–NH–) in a heterocyclic ring (pyrrolidine ring). In collagen, proline is converted to its 4-hydroxy derivative

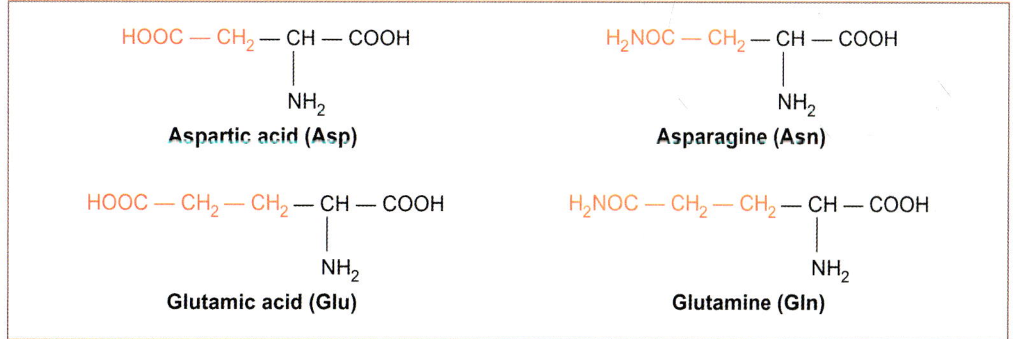

Fig. 5.7: Acidic amino acids and their amides

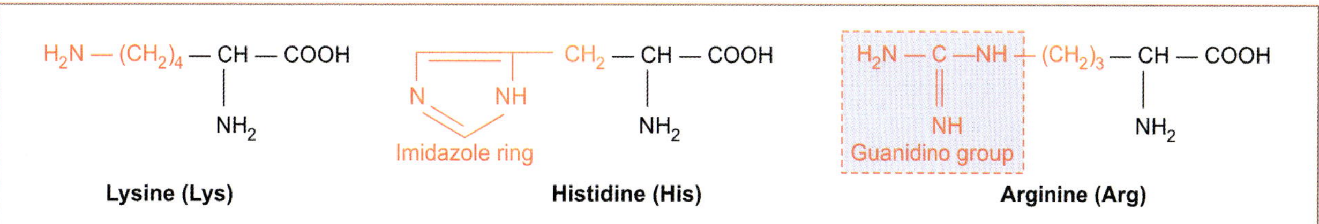

Fig. 5.8: Basic amino acids

called 4-hydroxyproline. Though proline has a secondary imino group, for the uniformity of classification, it is also referred as an α-amino acid (Fig. 5.9).

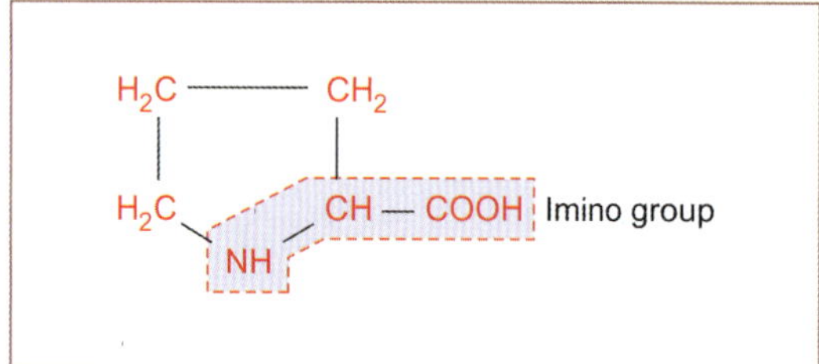

Fig. 5.9: Proline (Pro), an imino acid

Depending upon the nutritional requirement, amino acids are divided into three groups, as essential amino acids, semi-essential amino acids and non-essential amino acids (Table 5.2).

Among the various amino acids found in proteins, all cannot be synthesized in the body. Those which cannot be synthesized are essentially required in the diet and are called indispensible or **essential amino acids**. There are eight amino acids which are essential for an adult human being. These are methionine, threonine, tryptophan, valine, isoleucine, leucine, phenylalanine and lysine.

Arginine and histidine, though are not essential for normal adult human beings but their synthesis is not sufficient during growth, pregnancy and lactation or during high-grade fever and chronic infections when their requirements are increased. Under these conditions arginine and histidine also become essential. These two amino acids are thus called **semi-essential amino acids** or conditionally essential amino acids.

The remaining amino acids are **nonessential** and can be synthesized in the human body.

Table 5.2: Classification of amino acids according to their dietary requirement

Essential	Semi-essential	Nonessential
• Methionine	• Arginine	• Glycine
• Threonine	• Histidine	• Alanine
• Tryptophan		• Serine
• Valine		• Cysteine
• Isoleucine		• Tyrosine
• Leucine		• Aspartate
• Phenylalanine		• Glutamate
• Lysine		• Asparagine
		• Glutamine
		• Proline

A protein which has the right quantity of each essential amino acid required for growth and maintenance has **high biological value** (nutritionally superior), e.g. milk proteins and egg albumin. On the other hand, a protein with **poor biological value** (nutritionally inferior) has a limited supply of one or more essential amino acids, e.g. proteins from cereals and pulses. Besides the contents of essential amino acids, biological value of a protein is also influenced by digestibility of the protein.

Amino Acids form Peptide Bonds

- The most important property of amino acids is the formation of a peptide bond (–CO–NH) where an α-carboxylic group from one amino acid reacts with the α-amino group of the other amino acid.
- It is a condensation reaction resulting in a covalent (amide) linkage with the elimination of a molecule of water (Fig. 5.10).

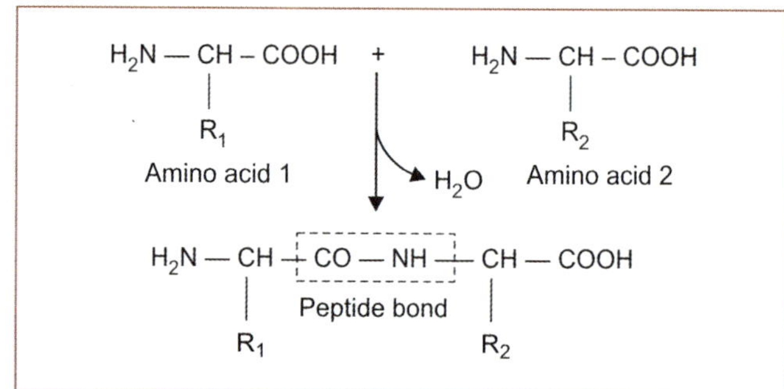

Fig. 5.10: Formation of a peptide bond

- It is planar, rigid with partial double bond character and no freedom of rotation.
- The –C=O and –NH groups are *trans*, polar and participate in H-bonding.
- It is the backbone of a polypeptide which is formed when several amino acids are linked together through peptide linkages (Fig. 5.11).

H_2N — AA_1 — AA_2 — AA_3 .... AA_{n-1} — AA_n — COOH

N-terminal end C-terminal end

Fig. 5.11: A polypeptide

- The C_α–C and N–C_α bonds are single bonds allowing adequate rotational freedom and hence the folding of the polypeptide.

PROTEINS, POLYPEPTIDES, OLIGOPEPTIDES AND PEPTIDES

Each protein has a free α-amino group (from the first amino acid) represented on the left hand side of the protein chain. It is called an **amino terminal or N-terminal end**. A protein also has free α-carboxylic group (from the last amino acid), which is present on the right hand side of the chain and is called the **carboxy terminal or C-terminal end**.

The term '**polypeptide**' is used when the number of amino acids is 51–100, e.g. insulin (51 amino acids). **Peptides** contain ≤50 amino acids and those which contain ≤20 amino acids are called **oligopeptides**. A **dipeptide** and a **tripeptide** contain two and three amino acids respectively. Some physiologically important peptides are listed in Table 5.3.

CLASSIFICATION OF PROTEINS

Several criteria are used to classify proteins (Fig. 5.12).

1. **Depending upon the physical and chemical properties:** Depending upon the physical and chemical properties, proteins are divided into three

Table 5.3: Physiologically important peptides

Peptide	Source	Importance
Glutathione (tripeptide = 3 amino acids; γ-glutamylcysteinylglycine)	All cells especially RBCs	Detoxification of peroxides
Thyrotropin releasing hormone (TRH; tripeptide = 3 amino acids)	Hypothalamus	Release of thyrotropin (thyroid stimulating hormone—TSH) from anterior pituitary
Angiotensin II (octapeptide = 8 amino acids)	Plasma angiotensin I	Vasoconstrictor, maintains blood pressure
Oxytocin (nonapeptide = 9 amino acids)	Posterior pituitary	Parturition; milk ejection
Antidiuretic hormone (ADH, nonapeptide = 9 amino acids)	Posterior pituitary	Water reabsorption from distal nephrons
Substance P (undecapeptide = 11 amino acids)	Sensory nerve terminals	Pain perception

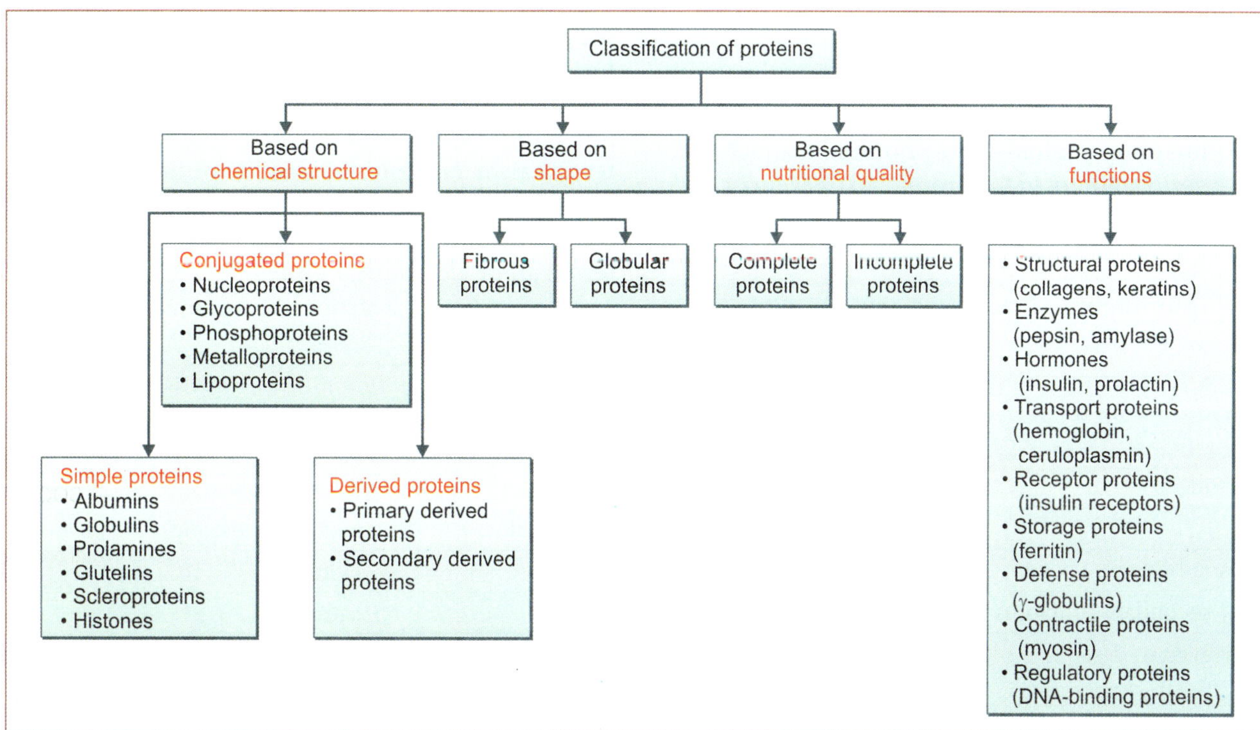

Fig. 5.12: Classification of proteins based on several criteria

5

categories, i.e. simple proteins, conjugated proteins and derived proteins.

- **Simple proteins:** Based on their solubility, simple proteins are further subdivided into different groups, as follows:
  - **Albumins:** Present in serum, milk and eggs. These are soluble in water as well as in a neutral salt solution.
  - **Globulins:** Also present in serum, milk and eggs. These are, however, sparingly soluble in water but are soluble in dilute neutral salt solutions.
  - **Prolamines:** Gliadin of wheat and zein of maize are the examples. These are insoluble in water but are soluble in 60–80% alcohol.
  - **Glutelins:** Soluble in dilute acids and alkalis, e.g. gluten in wheat and oryzenin in rice.
  - **Scleroproteins:** Highly insoluble proteins present in supporting tissues, such as bones and cartilages. These are also present in the protective tissues like skin, hair, nail and horn.
  - **Histones:** Rich in basic amino acids and are soluble in water, e.g. nucleohistones.
- **Conjugated proteins:** These are simple proteins which are conjugated with a nonprotein molecule, called a **prosthetic group. For example:**
  - **Nucleoproteins**—histones conjugated with nucleic acids
  - **Glycoproteins**—proteins in combination with carbohydrates,
  - **Phosphoproteins**—phosphoric acid attached to a serine moiety of the protein, like casein of milk
  - **Metalloproteins**—metal containing proteins, such as ceruloplasmin, a cuproprotein
  - **Lipoproteins**—lipid associated proteins.
- **Derived proteins:** These are the derivatives of simple proteins, such as denatured and coagulated proteins. These are classified as:
  - **Primary derived proteins—**those which are produced due to the cleavage of the peptide bonds
  - **Secondary derived proteins** such as proteoses and peptones.

2. **Depending on their overall morphology/shape**
   Depending on their overall morphology/shape proteins are classified as **fibrous** or **globular** proteins, based on their axial ratio, i.e. length/width ratio (Table 5.4).
3. **From the nutritional perspective:** From the nutritional perspective, proteins are categorized into complete and incomplete proteins.
   - **Complete proteins** such as milk casein and egg albumin contain all the essential amino acids.
   - **Incomplete proteins:** Cereal proteins, collagens and gelatin (obtained by denaturation of collagens) lack one or more essential amino acids and are called **incomplete proteins**.

STRUCTURAL ORGANIZATION OF PROTEINS

Proteins are made up of a long chain of amino acids. Even with a limited number of amino acid monomers, there are only 20 amino acids commonly seen in the human body, they can be arranged in a vast number of ways to alter the three-dimensional structure and function of the protein. Each protein has a free α-amino group (from the first amino acid), represented on the left hand side of the protein chain, called **amino-terminal or N-terminal end**. A protein also has free α-carboxylic group (from the last amino acid), present on the right hand side of the chain, called **carboxy-terminal or C-terminal end**.

There are 4 levels of structural organization of proteins:

Table 5.4: Fibrous versus globular proteins

Parameter	Fibrous proteins	Globular proteins
Axial ratio	>10	<10, usually <5
Shape	Rod-like, elongated and cylindrical	Nearly spheroidal
Water solubility	Lower	Higher
Regular secondary structures	Predominant	Variable
Biological role	Structural: Protective, connective, supportive	Functional: Catalysts, transporters, metabolic regulators
Examples	Collagen, α-keratin, tropomyosin	Hemoglobin, myoglobin, triose phosphate isomerase

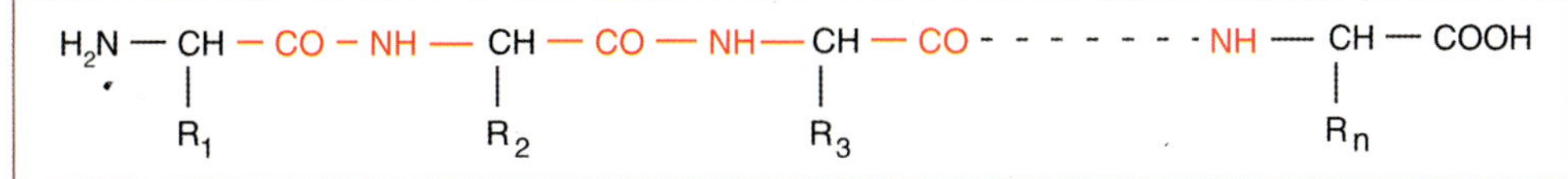

Fig. 5.13: Primary structure of a protein

PRIMARY STRUCTURE OF PROTEIN

The simple sequencing of the protein is known as its primary structure. It refers to the order and sequence of covalently linked amino acid residues in a polypeptide chain (Fig. 5.13).

Some proteins are synthesized as single polypeptides that are later cleaved into two or more chains, such as insulin. Such molecules may also have intra-chain as well as inter-chain disulfide linkages.

SECONDARY STRUCTURE OF PROTEIN

The secondary protein structure depends on the local interactions between parts of a protein chain, which can affect the folding and three-dimensional shape of the protein.

Various forces which stabilize protein conformation include hydrogen bonds, hydrophobic interactions, electrostatic interactions and van der Waals forces.

There can also be a several functional groups such as alcohols, carboxamines, carboxylic acids, thioesters, thiols and other basic groups linked to each protein. These functional groups also affect the folding of the proteins and, hence, its function in the body.

There are two main types of structures that characterize the secondary level of protein structure. These are referred to as α helix and β-pleated sheet structure:

- **α-Helix Structure**

  Since α-helix is the lowest energy and most stable conformation for a polypeptide chain, it forms spontaneously. A coil or helix is formed by twisting the backbone of a polypeptide chain. As a result of its folding, hydrogen bonds may be formed between –CO (of residue 'n') and –NH (of residue 'n + 4') groups within the same polypeptide chain (Fig. 5.14). Hydrogen bonds and van der Waals forces stabilize α-helices. α-Helices may be amphipathic. While commonly on the surface of proteins, α helices may also be wholly or partially buried in the interior of the protein. Proteins such as, hemoglobin, myoglobin, myosin, tropomyosin, fibrin and α-keratin are rich in α-helices.

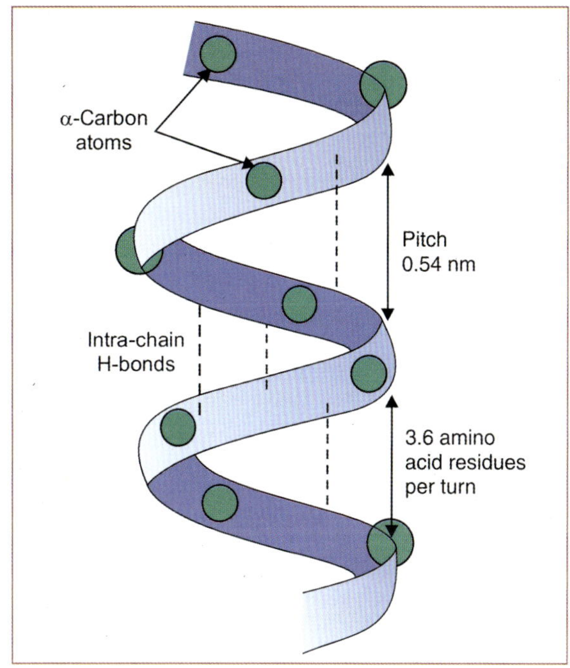

Fig. 5.14: Right-handed α-helix structure

- **β-pleated Sheet Structure**

  The N-H groups in the backbone of one strand form hydrogen bonds with C=O groups in the backbone of a fully extended strand next to it.

  It is the second regular structure that was described after α-helix.

  It is stretched-out with a rippled or pleated appearance when viewed from edge/side, hence called pleated sheet-like structure. β-pleated sheet orientation is formed due to stretching of the helices of the polypeptide chains, as a result of formation of hydrogen bonds between –CO and –NH groups of the neighboring strands of the polypeptide rather than within one strand (as in an α-helix). Therefore, it has inter-chain linkages (Fig. 5.15).

  β-Pleated sheets may be parallel or antiparallel depending upon the direction of adjacent polypeptide chains. Almost all β-pleated sheet strands are twisted in a right-handed sense. Proteins, such as ribonuclease A, carbonic anhydrase, flavodoxin, silk fibroin and wool are rich in β-pleated sheets.

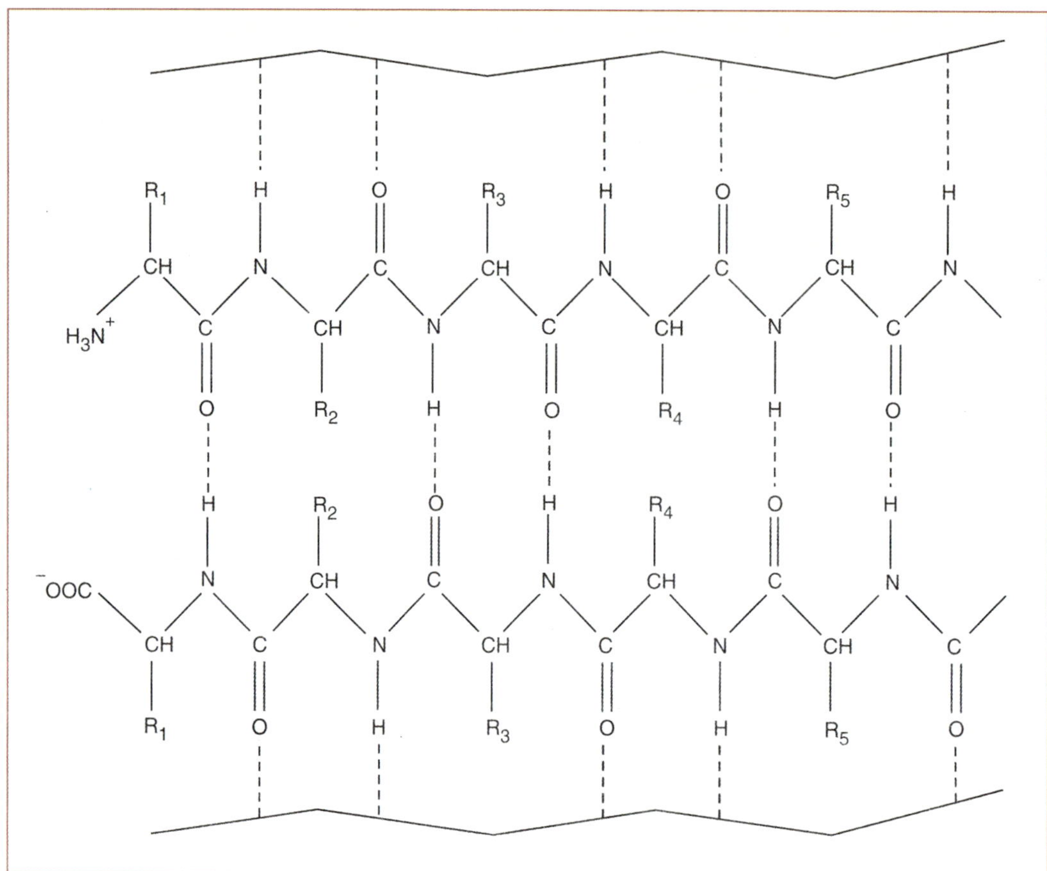

Fig. 5.15: β-Pleated sheet structure

Supersecondary structures: Certain combinations of secondary structure are also observed in different folded protein structures. They are referred to as **structural motifs**. These longer pattern lengths of secondary structure may include multiple structural motifs and when commonly observed in more than one protein are referred to as **supersecondary structures**. These include helix-turn-helix, leucine-zipper, zinc-finger (found in DNA binding proteins), etc.

TERTIARY STRUCTURE OF PROTEIN

The tertiary structure of proteins refers to the overall three-dimensional shape, after the secondary interactions. These include the influence of polar, nonpolar, acidic, and basic R groups that exist on the protein.

Tertiary structure involves the intra-molecular folding of the polypeptide chain into a compact three-dimensional structure with a specific shape (Fig. 5.16).

Tertiary structure is maintained by electrostatic linkages, hydrogen bonds, disulfide bridges, van der Waals forces and hydrophobic interactions. Hydrophobic interactions are the major forces in maintaining the unique tertiary structure of a protein.

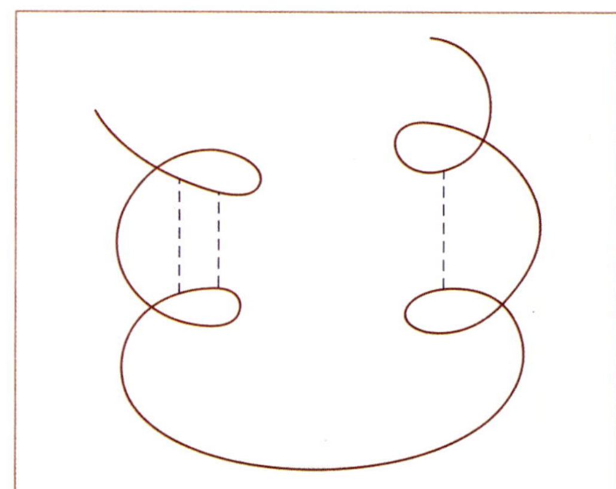

Fig. 5.16: Tertiary level of protein structure

Protein Folding

Correct and timely folding is an important phenomenon critical to the biological function of a protein. Its salient features are:

- ***Formation of secondary structure***: Initially, the secondary structures (α-helices and/or β-pleated sheets) are formed which associate and pack close together. The peptide segments between the secondary structures are short and direct, without any complicated twist or turn.

- ***Stabilization*:** The most stable structure is preferred which is characterized by:
  i. Large number of intra-molecular H-bonds.
  ii. Reduced exposed surface area accessible to solvents.
  iii. Buried hydrophobic core and hydrophilic surface, driven by hydrophobic interactions.
- ***Chaperones*:** The folding process may be assisted by other proteins called molecular chaperones, e.g. hsp60 (known as chaperonins), hsp70 and hsp90. The 'hsp' refers to 'heat-shock proteins' (originally observed in cells given brief exposure to high temperature, nearly 42°C) and the numbers are their Mr in kD. The chaperones help in:
  i. Appropriate burial of hydrophobic core, otherwise adjacent proteins may aggregate.
  ii. Moving proteins to their cellular destinations.
  iii. Rescuing and refolding of mature proteins that become partly unfolded.
- ***Abnormal or delayed folding*:** It is associated with diseases such as Alzheimer's disease, Creutzfeldt-Jakob disease, hereditary emphysema and cystic fibrosis (Chemistry to Clinics 5.1).

Chemistry to Clinics 5.1: Disorders of Protein Folding

It has been observed that many diseases result from an abnormal or delayed folding of a protein. Interestingly, the primary structure of the protein may be normal or altered, i.e. mutated. Important examples include:

- **Alzheimer's disease:** Misfolded β-amyloid peptide accumulates as plaques in the brain (Fig. 5.17).
- **Creutzfeldt-Jakob disease:** Normal cellular prion protein (PrPC) is replaced by protease-resistant prion protein (PrPSC) in the brain. Prion refers to '**pr**ote**i**nace**o**us i**n**fectious particles'.
- **Hereditary emphysema (called Z-variant):** Correct but slow folding of mutated α_1-antitrypsin in the lungs. Unopposed action of neutrophil elastase degrades the lung elastin.
- **Cystic fibrosis:** Mutant CFTR (**C**ystic **F**ibrosis **T**ransmembrane **R**egulator, a membrane Cl^- channel protein in the exocrine glands) fails to dissociate from chaperones and thus cannot reach its destination, i.e. cell membrane.

QUATERNARY STRUCTURE OF PROTEIN

The quaternary protein structure refers to the orientation and arrangement of subunits in proteins with multi-subunits. This is only relevant for proteins with multiple polypeptide chains. Proteins fold up into specific shapes according to the sequence of amino acids in the polymer, and the protein function is directly related to the resulting 3D structure.

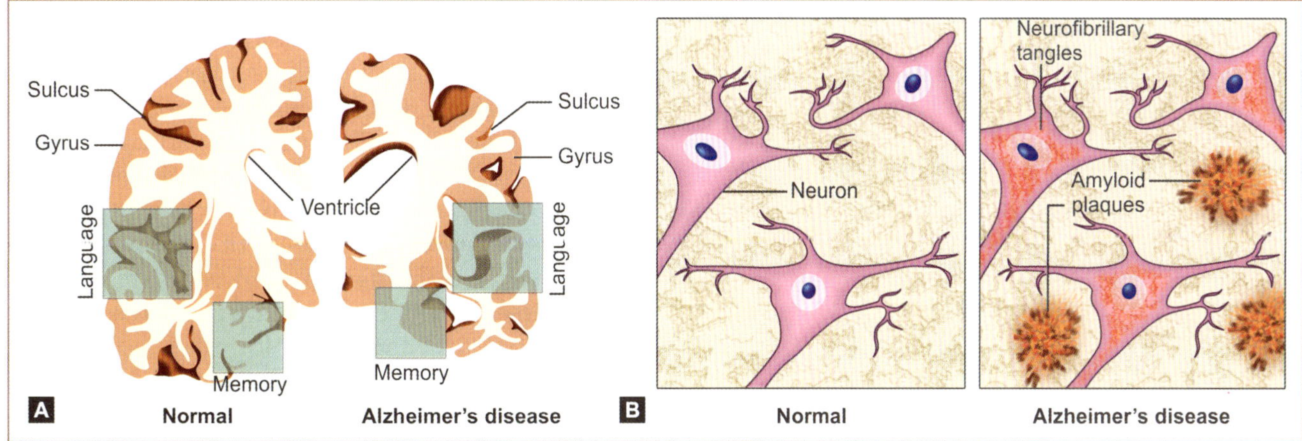

Fig. 5.17: Alzheimer's disease (AD). (A) Cut section of brain showing shrinkage of gyri and widening of sulci, particularly involving the memory and language areas of the brain, explaining the symptoms of AD. (B) **Hallmarks of AD:** β-Amyloid plaques and neurofibrillary tangles. β-Amyloid is a protein fragment cleaved from an amyloid precursor protein. In a healthy brain, these protein fragments are broken down and eliminated. In AD, the fragments accumulate to form insoluble plaques between the neurons. Neurofibrillary tangles are insoluble twisted fibers found inside the neurons, consisting primarily of a protein called tau (normal components of microtubules). The microtubule helps transport nutrients and other important substances from one part of the neuron to another. In AD, the tau protein is abnormal and the microtubule structures collapse. Both β-amyloid plaques and neurofibrillary tangles contribute to the neuronal loss in AD

Proteins may also interact with each other or other macromolecules in the body to create complex assemblies. In these assemblies, proteins can develop functions that were not possible in the standalone protein, such as carrying out DNA replication and the transmission of cell signals.

The nature of proteins is also highly variable. For example, some are quite rigid, whereas others are somewhat flexible. These characteristics also fit the function of the protein. For example, more rigid proteins may play a role in the structure of the cytoskeleton or connective tissues. On the other hand, those with some flexibility may act as hinges, springs, or levers to assist in the function of other proteins.

Proteins with more than one subunit are also called **oligomers** while their individual units are called **protomers** which may or may not be identical (Figs 5.18 and 5.19).

The structure of protein sets the foundation for its interaction with other molecules in the body and, therefore, determines its function.

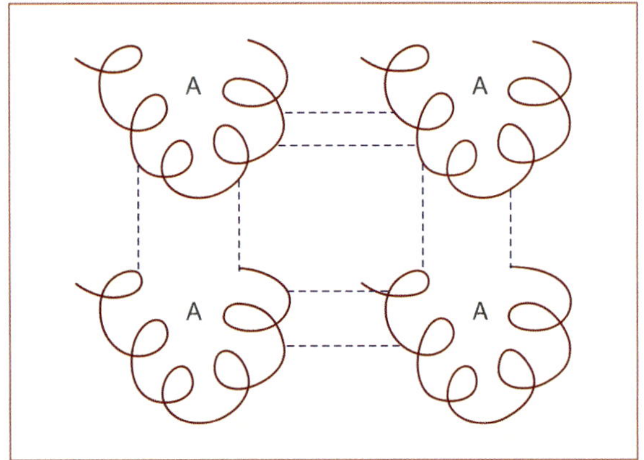

Fig. 5.18: Quaternary level of protein structure with four identical protomers = A_4

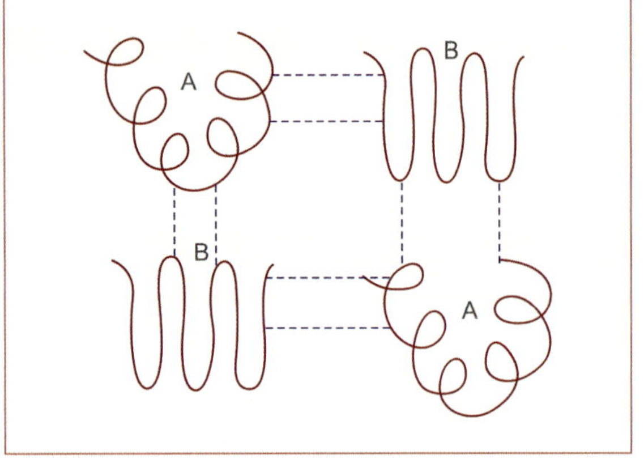

Fig. 5.19: Quaternary level of protein structure with two pairs of different protomers = A_2B_2

FUNCTIONS OF PROTEINS

Proteins play an important role in many crucial biological processes and functions. They are very versatile and have many different functions in the body (Table 5.5).

Table 5.5: Biological importance of proteins

Biological importance	Examples of proteins
As structural proteins	Collagen, keratins, etc.
As enzymes	Pepsin, amylase, etc.
As hormones	Insulin
As transporters	Hemoglobin
As receptors	Hormone receptors
As storage molecules	Ferritin
In immune response	γ-Globulins

- **Act as catalysts:** Some of the proteins, such as pepsin, catalyze biological reactions and act as enzymes.
- **Transport other molecules:** Several proteins serve as a carrier for the transport of a substance, within the body. For example, **hemoglobin is important** for the transport of oxygen, **ceruloplasmin** transports copper, etc.
- **Store other molecules:** Some of the proteins bind to a substance for its storage in different tissues in the body, e.g. **ferritin** stores Fe^{3+}.
- **Provide immune protection:** Some proteins, such as **γ-globulin**, act as antibodies and provide immunity.
- **Provide shape and structure:** Some of the proteins, e.g. **collagens** (found in bone and cartilage), **keratins** (found in hair and nail), etc., form an essential part of the particular structure within the body.
- **Generate movement:** Some of the proteins act as hormones, e.g. **insulin**, and regulate metabolic processes within the cell. Others, such as **hormone receptors**, act as receptors for other molecules and play an important role in signal transduction.
- **Transmit nerve impulses.**
- **Control cell growth and differentiation.**

STRUCTURE–FUNCTION RELATIONSHIPS

The extent to which the structure of proteins has an impact on their function is shown by the effect of changes in the structure of a protein. Any change to a protein at any structural level, including slight changes in the folding and shape of the protein, may render it nonfunctional.

Proteins are the most versatile macromolecules in living systems and serve crucial functions in essentially all biological processes. They function as catalysts, transport and store other molecules such as oxygen, provide mechanical support and immune protection, generate movement, they transmit nerve impulses, and they control growth and differentiation. Several key properties enable proteins to participate in such a wide range of functions:

1. **Proteins are linear polymers built of monomer units called amino acids:** The construction of a vast array of macromolecules from a limited number of monomer building blocks is a recurring theme in biochemistry. The function of a protein is directly dependent on its three-dimensional structure. Remarkably, proteins, spontaneously, fold up into three-dimensional structures that are determined by the sequence of amino acids in the protein polymer. Thus, proteins are the embodiment of the transition from the one-dimensional world of sequences to the three-dimensional world of molecules capable of diverse activities.
2. **Proteins contain a wide range of functional groups:** These functional groups include alcohols, thiols, thioethers, carboxylic acids, carboxamides and a variety of basic groups. When combined in various sequences, this array of functional groups accounts for the broad spectrum of protein function. For instance, the chemical reactivity associated with these groups is essential to the function of enzymes, the proteins that catalyze specific chemical reactions in biological systems.
3. **Poteins interact with one another, and with other biological macromolecules to form complex assemblies:** The proteins within these assemblies can act synergistically to generate capabilities not afforded by the individual component proteins. These assemblies include macromolecular machines that carry out the accurate replication of DNA, the transmission of signals within cells, and many other essential processes.
4. **Some proteins are quite rigid, whereas others display limited flexibility:** Rigid units can function as structural elements in the cytoskeleton (the internal scaffolding within cells) or in connective tissue. Parts of proteins with limited flexibility may act as hinges, springs and levers that are crucial to protein function, to the assembly of proteins with one another and with other molecules into complex units, and to the transmission of information within and between cells.

HEMOGLOBIN AND HEMOGLOBINOPATHIES

Hemoglobin is a metalloprotein that has hem and globin chains. It has a **quaternary structure**, i.e. it is a tetramer having four protein subunits (globin chains). **Normal adult hemoglobin** (**HbA1**) has two alpha and two beta chains, i.e. its subunit composition is as $\alpha_2\beta_2$. Any change in its subunit composition alters its type (structure) and functions.

For example

- **Minor adult hemoglobin:** It consists of two alpha and two delta chains, i.e. as $\alpha_2\delta_2$. It is referred to as **HbA$_2$**. It has a reduced efficiency to transport oxygen and comprises **only about 2.5%** of the normal adult hemoglobin.
- **Embryonic hemoglobin:** It contains two zeta chains along with either two epsilon ($\zeta_2\Upsilon_2$) or two gamma chains ($\zeta_2\varepsilon_2$), which are referred to as **Hb Gower 1** and **Hb Portland**, respectively. It is present in the embryonic stage, i.e. in the **first month after conception**.
- **Fetal hemoglobin:** It contains two alpha chains along with two gamma chains ($\alpha_2\Upsilon_2$). It is designated as HbF and predominates in blood of the human fetus. After birth, fetal hemoglobin is rapidly replaced with the adult hemoglobin (HbA1), whose synthesis, actually, starts in the late fetal life. HbF comprises only about 0.5% of the total hemoglobin in adults.

HEMOGLOBINOPATHIES

Hemoglobinopathies refer to a group of disorders, which are characterized by **structurally and/or functionally abnormal hemoglobin**, due to a **genetic** or **acquired** defect in **heme** or **globin**.

These include

- **Methemoglobin:** Methemoglobin (**Met-Hb**) is nonfunctional hemoglobin which has **Fe^{3+}, instead of Fe^{2+}** present in normal hemoglobin. Normally, Met-Hb levels are <1%. Elevated level of Met-Hb may be **congenital** (either due to the deficiency of Met-Hb reductase or due to mutated hemoglobin, i.e. HbM) or **acquired** due to exposure to certain drugs/chemicals. This, in turn, **reduces the ability of RBC to release oxygen to tissues**, **hypoxia** and **cyanosis** (bluish color of the skin).
- **Sickle cell hemoglobin:** Hemoglobin S **(HbS)** is a **variant of** normal adult hemoglobin (**HbA1**), where a substitution occurs in the sixth position of the β-globin chain. In HbA1 this position is occupied by

glutamic acid (Glu), whereas **in HbS, Glu is substituted by** valine **(Val)**. The molecular basis for this is a **point mutation**. HbS gets **polymerized** and **precipitate within RBCs**, particularly in the deoxygenated state. This, in turn, makes RBCs assume a **sickle shape**, instead of the normal biconcave shape. As a result of it, such distorted **RBCs** lose their deformability, resulting in **higher rate of hemolysis**. This type of hemolytic anemia is designated as **sickle cell anemia**.

- **Thalassemias:** Thalassemias are a family of related **genetic disorders**, which arise due to **deletion of one or more globin-like genes**, in either globin gene clusters or due to a defect in transcription and/or processing of mRNA of the globin gene. If there is a reduced synthesis, or total lack of synthesis, of the α-globin mRNA, the disease is classified as **α-thalassemia**. On the other hand, if β-globin mRNA level is affected, it is called **β-thalassemia**. When the child inherits the defective gene(s) from one parent, symptoms are usually minor and the condition is called **thalassemia minor**. On the other hand, if inheritance of the defective gene(s) is from both the parents, it results in a symptomatic disease requiring treatment and is called **thalassemia major**. Thalassemias are associated with **mild to moderate anemia** with different degrees of severity, **requiring repeated blood transfusions**.

DIGESTION AND ABSORPTION OF DIETARY PROTEINS

Digestion of Dietary Proteins

Digestion of dietary proteins begins with the hydrolysis of the peptide bonds, which link successive amino acid residues together, in a polypeptide chain. The process is known as **proteolysis** and the enzymes responsible for hydrolysis of the peptide linkages are called **proteases (peptidases)**. Endoproteases, i.e. those acting on peptide linkages other than the N- or C-terminal peptide bonds, are called **endopeptidases (proteinases)**, whereas exoproteases, i.e. those acting on the N- or the C-terminal peptide bonds are called **exopeptidases**.

Proteolytic digestion of the dietary proteins takes place in the gastrointestinal tract and is carried out by proteases secreted by the stomach, the pancreas and the small intestine:

- Digestion of proteins starts ***in the stomach*** by the action of a proteolytic enzyme **pepsin**, at pH of the gastric juice (1.5–2.5). Pepsin is secreted by chief cells of the gastric mucosa in the form of a zymogen (proenzyme) called **pepsinogen A** which is activated by hydrogen ions of the gastric juice (HCl) and later on autocatalytically by the pepsin itself (Fig. 5.20).

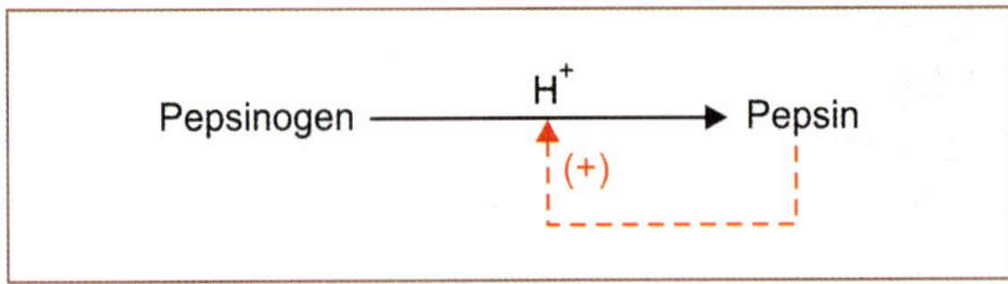

Fig. 5.20: Activation of pepsinogen

Pepsin preferentially hydrolyzes peptide linkages towards the amino group of either an aromatic amino acid (phenylalanine and tyrosine) or a dicarboxylic acid (aspartate or glutamate; Fig. 5.21).

In infants, another enzyme rennin hydrolyzes milk protein casein.

- Proteolytic products of pepsin pass on to the ***small intestine*** where they are attacked by proteases that are secreted by the pancreas, i.e. trypsin, chymotrypsin and carboxypeptidases.
  - **Trypsin** is secreted in the zymogen form as **trypsinogen,** which is converted to trypsin by another enzyme called enterokinase (enteropeptidase) that acts as an activator of trypsinogen and is secreted by the intestinal mucosa (Fig. 5.22).

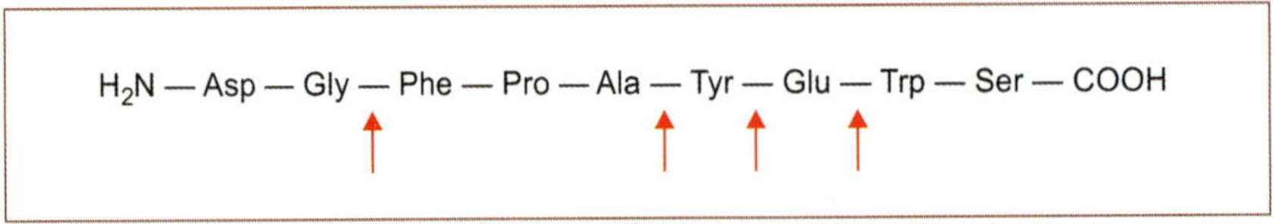

Fig. 5.21: Sites of action of pepsin

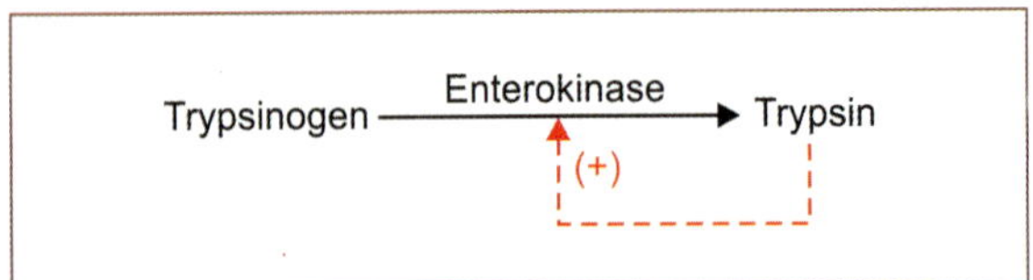

Fig. 5.22: Activation of trypsinogen

5

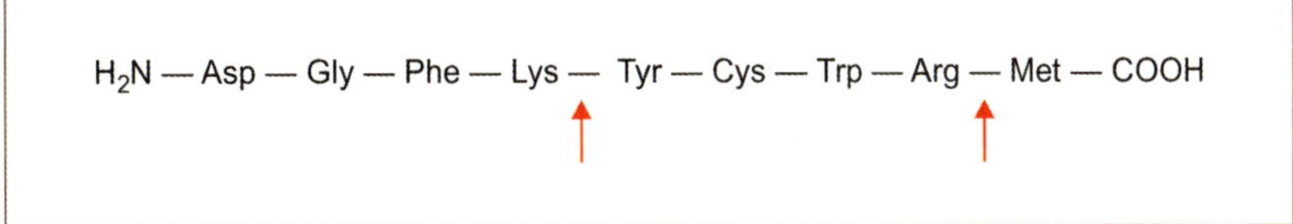

Fig. 5.23: Sites of action of trypsin

Once trypsin is formed, it acts on trypsinogen and converts it to trypsin, autocatalytically. Trypsin is most effective on a partially digested protein and hydrolyzes peptide linkages formed by carboxylate group contributed by a basic amino acid, i.e. arginine or lysine (Fig. 5.23).

- **Chymotrypsin** is also synthesized and secreted as a zymogen designated as **chymotrypsinogen**. It is activated by trypsin (Fig. 5.24).

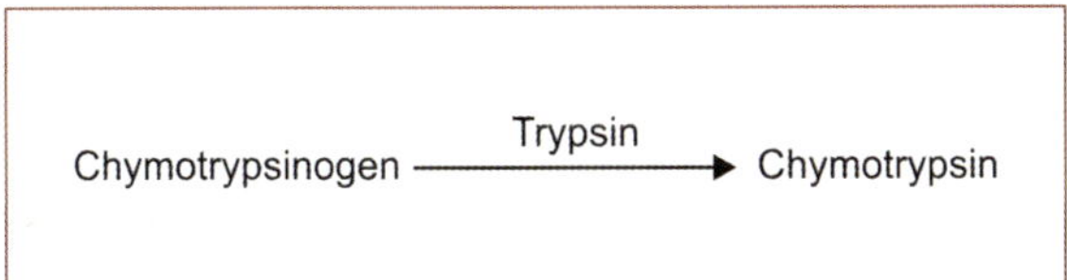

Fig. 5.24: Activation of chymotrypsin

Trypsin, preferentially, cleaves peptide bonds involving the carboxyl group contributed by the aromatic amino acids as well as those of leucine, methionine, asparagine and histidine (Fig. 5.25).

- Pancreatic juice also contains collagenase and elastase which specifically act on collagen and elastin, respectively.
- In addition to the above endopeptidases, two exopeptidases are also secreted by the pancreatic juice in the zymogen forms. These are procarboxypeptidase A and procarboxypeptidase B. These zymogens are also activated by trypsin (Fig. 5.26).

  Both of these enzymes attack peptide linkages specifically those having a free carboxyl group. **Carboxypeptidase A** hydrolyzes the C-terminal amino acid in peptides particularly of those where the terminal amino acid is an aromatic or aliphatic amino acid while **carboxypeptidase B** hydrolyzes the terminal peptide bond of the basic amino acids (arginine and lysine).

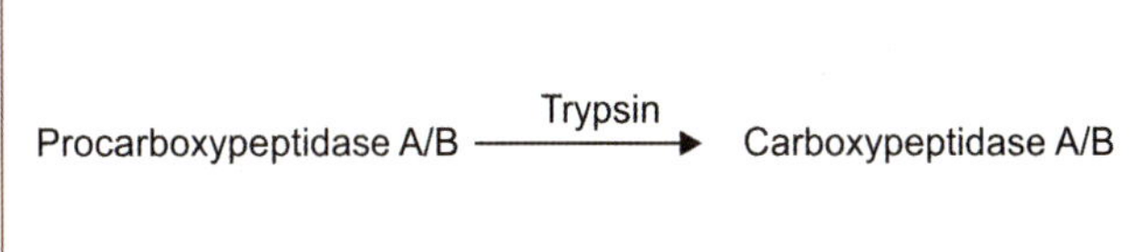

Fig. 5.26: Activation of procarboxypeptidase A and B

- The digestion of proteins thereafter is completed by the action of **aminopeptidases** and **dipeptidases** which are secreted by mucosa of the small intestine.

Absorption of Amino Acids

The end products of digestion of proteins are amino acids which are absorbed from the small intestine into the portal blood. Amino acid content of the portal blood rises only temporarily during digestion of proteins, indicating that absorption mechanisms are so efficient that amino acids are absorbed immediately after they are formed from digestion of proteins.

Absorption of L-amino acids is a Na^+-dependent active transport and requires ATP and specific transport proteins. Pyridoxal phosphate (vitamin B_6) is also required for the absorption of amino acids.

- Both an L-amino acid and the Na^+ attach to the carrier protein which is present on the mucosal surface of the microvillous membrane and form L-amino acid-carrier protein-Na^+ complex.
- The complex passes into the inner surface of the membrane and dissociates to liberate free amino acid and Na^+.
- Carrier protein returns to the brush border while the amino acid, through portal blood, enters the liver. On the other hand, Na^+ is actively pumped out of the cell membrane by the Na^+/K^+ pump. At the same time, ATP is hydrolyzed by ATPase, to release energy required for this process.

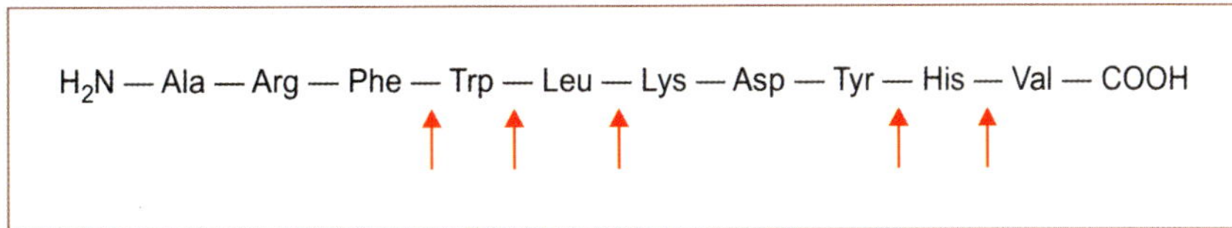

Fig. 5.25: Sites of action of chymotrypsin

At least seven different brush-border specific transport systems have been identified for the uptake of different classes of L-amino acids and the dipeptides in the luminal membrane. These include:

1. A carrier for neutral amino acids with short or polar side chains, such as for Ala, Ser and Thr;
2. A carrier for neutral amino acids with an aromatic or hydrophobic side chain, such as for Phe, Tyr, Met, Val, Leu and Ile;
3. A specific carrier for imino acids, i.e. for Pro and hydroxyproline (HO-Pro);
4. A separate carrier for Lys, Arg and Cystine (Cys-Cys);
5. A carrier for acidic amino acids, i.e. for Asp and Glu;
6. A separate carrier for β-amino acids, e.g. for β-Ala and taurine; and
7. A separate carrier for dipeptides, e.g. peptide 1 (Pep-1), glycylsarcosine, etc. The dipeptides are absorbed through the intestinal cells where they are hydrolyzed by dipeptidases to the constituent amino acids.

Besides, the small intestine of the fetus and the neonate can absorb intact proteins by endocytosis (pinocytosis).

Glutathione also participates in the active transport of L-amino acids in some of the tissues such as in the small intestine, kidneys and liver. The process is called group translocation (Fig. 1.18; *see* Chapter 1).

Absorption of amino acids may be affected in specific transport disorders or other diseases involving the small intestine or the immune system (Chemistry to Clinics 5.2 and 5.3).

Chemistry to Clinics 5.2: Genetic Disorders of Amino Acid Transport Carriers

- **Hartnup's disease:** It is a genetic lesion in epithelial amino acid transport named after the family in which the disease was first recognized. The transport and absorption of neutral amino acids including that of tryptophan is decreased in epithelial cells of the small intestine and proximal tubules of the kidney. The intestinal defect results in malabsorption of free amino acids from the diet. The inability to reabsorb amino acids by the kidney manifests in the excretion of neutral amino acids including that of tryptophan and other indole derivatives in the urine resulting in **neutral amino aciduria**. Symptoms of the disease are mainly those due to essential amino acid and nicotinamide deficiencies. Due to tryptophan deficiency there are **pellagra-like features**, such as dermatitis, diarrhea and dementia. Women are more susceptible to pellagra since kynurenine hydroxylase (an enzyme of the tryptophan-niacin pathway) is inhibited by estrogen.
- **Cystinuria:** It involves the carrier for sulfur-containing amino acids (e.g. cystine) and the basic amino acids (e.g. lysine and arginine). Because the apical membrane of enterocytes also possess a peptide transport system that is unaffected in these disorders, treatment with supplemental dipeptides containing the specific amino acids is possible. However, the treatment fails if the renal transporter is also involved as in the case of cystinuria.

Chemistry to Clinics 5.3: Celiac Disease

It is also called **celiac sprue** or **gluten-sensitive enteropathy**, a common disease caused by the sensitivity of the small intestine to gluten, the protein presents in cereal grains such as wheat, barley, rye and oats. Wheat gluten proteins consist of two major fractions: The gliadins (monomeric) and the glutenins (polymeric). Tissue transglutaminase (tTG, an enzyme present in many tissues including small intestine) is the autoantigen in celiac disease since anti-tTG antibodies (IgA and IgG) are found in the sera of these patients. Besides, anti-gliadin antibodies are also found. Upon exposure to gliadins, tTG modifies the proteins which then bind to specific HLA molecules in the intestine to trigger an inflammatory reaction.

It is important to note that celiac disease is different from '**wheat allergy**' characterized by an exaggerated mast cell-mediated IgE response to wheat proteins.

The disorder can result in the malabsorption of all nutrients as a result of the shortening or total loss of intestinal villi, which reduces the mucosal enzymes for nutrient digestion and the mucosal surface for absorption. The elimination of dietary gluten is a standard treatment for these patients. Occasionally, the symptoms are improved with glucocorticoid therapy because of the immunosuppressive and anti-inflammatory actions of these hormones. tTG is a potential target for therapeutic intervention.

PLASMA PROTEINS

Plasma contains over 300 proteins. Albumin, globulins and fibrinogen are the major plasma proteins, all of which are synthesized in the liver (except γ-globulins). Others include apolipoproteins (present in lipoproteins), protein hormones (such as insulin, prolactin etc.), enzymes and coagulation proteins.

Total plasma protein concentration varies from 6.3–8.0 g/dl out of which albumin constitutes 3.7–5.3 g/dl while globulins constitute 1.8–3.7 g/dl. The range for the various globulin fractions are—α_1 plus α_2 = 0.4–1.4 g/dl, β = 0.5–1.3 g/dl and γ = 0.6–1.5 g/dl.

ALBUMIN

Albumin performs several functions:
- Maintenance of **plasma colloidal osmotic pressure** and hence the regulation of blood volume.
- **Transport** of various molecules such as long chain fatty acids, unconjugated bilirubin, steroids, Cu^{2+} and drugs like salicylates, barbiturates, penicillin, sulfonamides and warfarin.
- As plasma **antioxidant** because of the presence of sulfhydryl (–SH) groups.
- **As protein reserve** in case of nutritional depletion.

GLOBULINS

The α and β globulins transport various molecules such as hormones, copper, iron, etc. (Table 5.6).

γ-globulins constitute the defense proteins that combat antigenic challenge.

Table 5.6: Transport proteins and their ligands

Protein	Ligand
Albumin	Cu^{2+}, Fe^{3+}, bilirubin, free fatty acids, steroids, heme
Ceruloplasmin	Copper
Transferrin, ferritin, hemosiderin	Iron
Haptoglobin, hemopexin	Free hemoglobin
Thyroid binding globulin	Thyroid hormones
Cortisol binding globulin	Cortisol
Sex hormone binding globulin	Androgens, estrogens

Clinical Uses of Plasma Proteins

- **Treatment of hypoalbuminemia:** A 20 40% colloidal solution of human albumin is administered by intravenous infusion to treat patients suffering from gross hypoalbuminemia and massive edema.
- **Diagnosis of pulmonary embolism:** Radiolabeled albumin is used in the screening of pulmonary embolism (the movement of a blood clot or other plug from the systemic veins through the right heart and into the pulmonary circulation, where it lodges in one or more branches of the pulmonary artery). It involves the injection of aggregates of human serum albumin labeled with a radionuclide into a peripheral vein. These albumin aggregates travel through the right side of the heart, enter the pulmonary vasculature and lodge in small pulmonary vessels. Only those lung areas receiving blood flow will manifest an uptake of the tracer; the nonperfused region will not show any uptake of the tagged albumin. The aggregates fragment and are removed from the lungs in about a day.
- **Passive immunization:** Sera rich in γ-globulins (hyperimmune sera) are used to confer artificial passive immunity in certain cases, e.g. administration of anti-tetanus serum (ATS) in tetanus.

Plasma Protein Disorders

Hypoalbuminemia

It refers to low plasma albumin and may arise due to a number of reasons such as:
- Protein malnutrition, e.g. kwashiorkor and marasmus.
- Malabsorption, e.g. inflammatory bowel disease and following bowel resection.
- Impaired synthesis in chronic liver disease, e.g. cirrhosis.
- Excessive losses in urine (nephrotic syndrome) or stool (protein losing enteropathy) or through skin (severe burns).
- Leakage and trapping in extravascular sites known as 'third space fluid losses, e.g. ascitis (accumulation in peritoneal cavity and pleural effusion (accumulation in pleural cavity).
- Increased catabolism (major surgery or trauma, sepsis, malignancy and following repeated radiation therapy).
- Overhydration (artifact causes), e.g. pregnancy or dilution of sample due to taking a blood sample from a site close to an intravenous infusion.

Analbuminemia

Analbuminemia refers to a condition in which plasma albumin is almost completely absent (<100 mg/dl). There may be compensatory increase in plasma globulins concentrations.

Hyperglobulinemia

Increase in globulins occurs most commonly in:
- Advanced liver disease, e.g. cirrhosis.
- Chronic diseases which may be infectious (tuberculosis, viral hepatitis) or non-infectious (rheumatoid arthritis).
- Multiple myeloma.

Liver disease, chronic infection or an autoimmune disease such as rheumatoid arthritis give rise to sustained stimulation of B lymphocytes and hence an increased production of γ-globulins, which is revealed as a broad/diffuse band on serum protein electrophoresis (Fig. 5.27C and H).

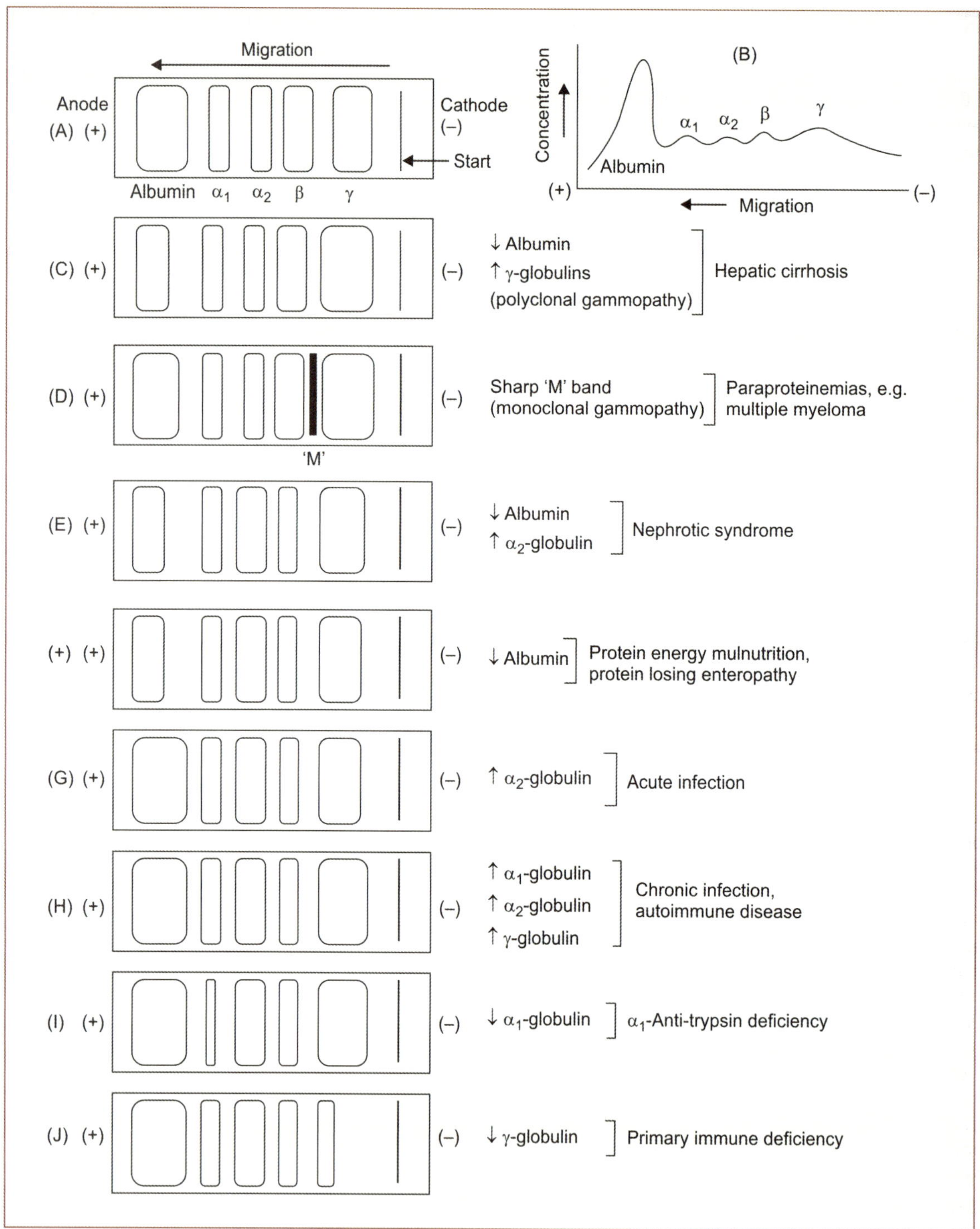

Fig. 5.27: Plasma proteins pattern on electrophoresis in some of the diseases. (A: Electrophoresis bands in normal serum; B: Bands on densitometer; C: Pattern in hepatic cirrhosis; D = Multiple myeloma; E: Nephrotic syndrome; F: Protein energy malnutrition (PEM); G: Acute infection; H: Autoimmune disease; I: α_1-Anti-trypsin deficiency; J: Primary immune deficiency

5

Paraproteinemia

Discrete immunoglobulin bands visible on serum protein electrophoresis are known as **paraproteins** or monoclonal components. They are observed in multiple myeloma and lymphoid tumors. They are due to overproduction of a single immunoglobulin class or immunoglobulin fragment by a single class (clone) of B cells (Chemistry to Clinics 5.4).

Chemistry to Clinics 5.4: Multiple Myeloma and Bence Jones Proteins

Normally, B lymphocytes mature into plasma cells which are responsible for the production of immunoglobulins/antibodies. **Multiple myeloma** is a disease characterized by malignant proliferation of B lymphocyte precursors generating excessive plasma cells, which overproduce complete IgG or IgA immunoglobulins and the amount is proportional to the tumor mass. Plasma protein electrophoresis reveals a characteristic, intense and narrow **'M' band** with the γ-globulin (Fig. 5.27D).

In some patients, dimers of immunoglobulin light chains (either κ or λ) are found in the urine. These are called **Bence Jones proteins** and they show a characteristic differential heat solubility—gradual heating of the urine sample kept in a water bath results in precipitates between 40°C and 50°C, disappearing at nearly 90°C. On cooling, the precipitates reappear at nearly 70°C.

ALBUMIN/GLOBULIN RATIO

Albumin:globulin ratio (A/G ratio) refers to the ratio of the serum concentration of albumin to the serum concentration of globulins. Normal serum A/G ratio is 1.2–2.0:1, which may be altered in a number of conditions (Chemistry to Clinics 5.5).

Chemistry to Clinics 5.5: A/G Ratio

- An increase in total plasma proteins occurs in dehydration due to prolonged diarrhea, vomiting and diabetes insipidus. Because of hemoconcentration, both albumin and globulins are increased proportionately so that A/G ratio remains unaltered.
- A decrease in total plasma proteins is generally due to hypoalbuminemia as seen in liver cirrhosis, nephrotic syndrome, kwashiorkor, etc. It may be accompanied by either no increase in globulins or an increase in globulins that is proportionately less than the fall in albumin, resulting in a reversal of A/G ratio. It is clinically manifested as edema involving the feet, pre-tibial area, pre-sacral area, periorbital area, etc. (Fig. 5.28).
  If not timely diagnosed and treated, it leads to generalized edema known as **anasarca**.
- Reversal of A/G ratio due to increased γ-globulins is observed in gammopathies such as multiple myeloma.

ACUTE-PHASE PROTEINS

The liver has the capacity to enhance or reduce the synthesis of various proteins in response to diseases. These are called acute-phase proteins or acute-phase reactants (Chemistry to Clinics 5.6).

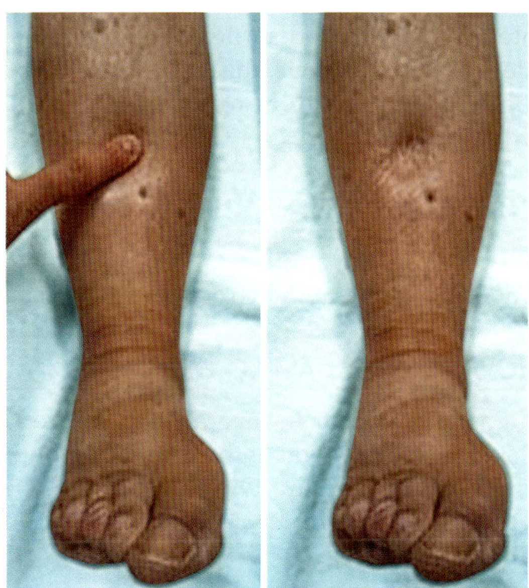

Fig. 5.28: Pitting edema of the lower extremity: The depression persists for sometime after the finger is removed

Chemistry to Clinics 5.6: Acute-phase Proteins

The liver responds to inflammation by increasing the synthesis of some plasma proteins and decreasing the synthesis of others. These proteins are called 'positive acute-phase proteins' or 'negative acute-phase proteins' respectively and the overall response is called the **acute-phase response**. Common examples include:

Positive acute-phase proteins: C-reactive protein (so named because it was first identified as a substance in the serum of patients with acute inflammation that reacted with the C-polysaccharide of Pneumococcus), fibrinogen, α_1-antitrypsin, β_2-macroglobulin, ferritin, ceruloplasmin, etc.

Negative acute-phase proteins: Albumin, transferrin, transthyretin, transcortin, retinol-binding protein, etc.

COMMON DISORDERS ASSOCIATED WITH PROTEIN METABOLISM

Inborn errors of protein metabolism include inherited biochemical disorders in which specific enzyme defects interfere with the normal metabolism of exogenous (dietary) or endogenous protein, a key constituent of most foods we eat, including meat, beans, milk products and grains. Infants with protein metabolism disorders cannot drink human milk because it also contains proteins and amino acids that cannot be metabolized. Since, they are unable to metabolize certain amino acids and require specialized formulas without the offending amino acid, allowing the baby to receive essential nutrients for growth.

Protein metabolism disorders include **metabolic disorders of the urea cycle** (the end product of protein metabolism or **disorders of the metabolism of individual amino acids**.

METABOLISM OF AMINO ACIDS

First step in the metabolism of amino acids is the removal of the alpha-amino group as ammonia.

REMOVAL OF THE α-AMINO GROUP

Although it may occur in several tissues, liver is the major site for the removal of the α-amino group from an amino acid. There are two major routes for the removal of α-amino group, i.e. **transamination** and **deamination**.

Transamination

- Transamination is a process of transfer of the α-amino group from an amino acid to a keto acid, forming **a new amino acid and a keto acid** (Fig. 5.29).

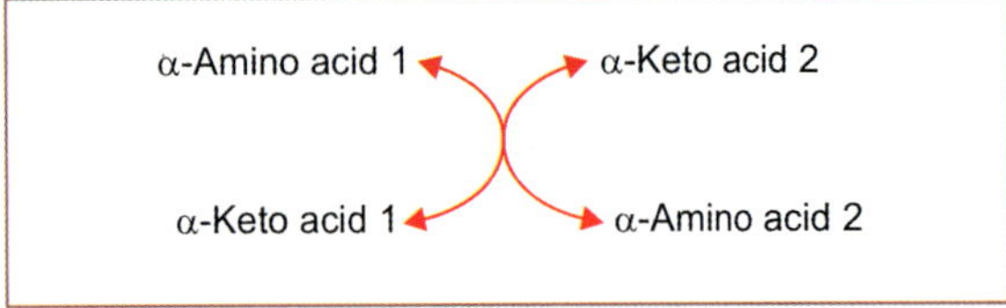

Fig. 5.29: The process of transamination of an amino acid

Enzymes which catalyze this reversible set of reactions are called **transaminases or amino-transferases**.

- It is the **commonest reaction** involving free amino acids. **Threonine** and **lysine** (and **proline**, an imino acid), however, **do not participate** in this reaction.
- An obligate amino acid and α-keto acid pair in all these reactions is that of glutamate and α-ketoglutarate. Although liver contains several transaminases (except for threonine, lysine and proline), most important of these are glutamate pyruvate transaminase (**GPT**) also called alanine aminotransferase (**ALT**), and glutamate oxalo-acetate transaminase (**GOT**) which is also known as aspartate aminotransferase (**AST**).
- Transaminases require **vitamin B_6 (pyridoxal-5-phosphate)** as a **coenzyme** (Fig. 5.30).

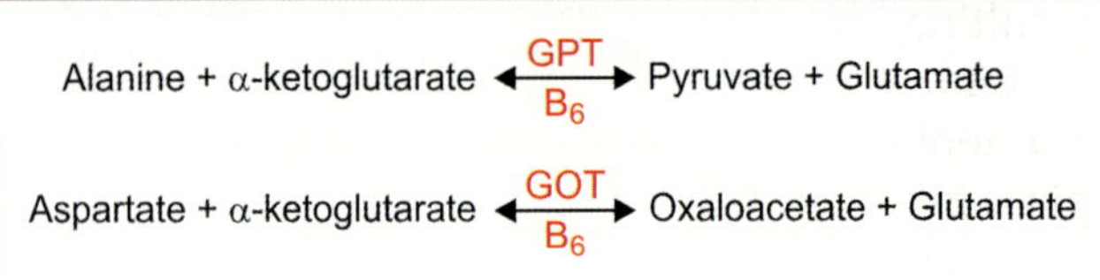

Fig. 5.30: Reactions catalyzed by two important transaminases, GPT (ALT) and GOT (AST)

- An amino acid first reacts with the coenzyme pyridoxal-5-phosphate (PLP) and forms a Schiff's base. The coenzyme is protonated and is subsequently hydrolyzed to release α-keto acid of the corresponding amino acid while retaining the α-amino group ($-NH_2$). The coenzyme thus gets aminated and is converted to pyridoxamine-5-phosphate. Thereafter, another α-keto acid (generally α-ketoglutarate) combines with the coenzyme bound amino group. This, in turn, releases the amino acid (mostly as glutamate) and regenerates the coenzyme (Fig. 5.31).

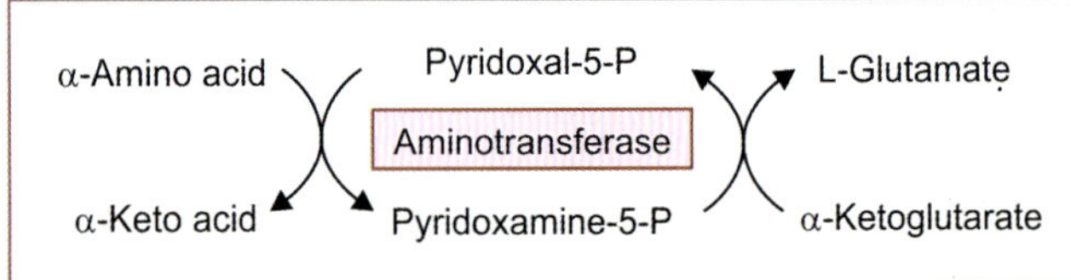

Fig. 5.31: Role of pyridoxal-5-phosphate in transamination

Importance of Transamination

1. **Nonessential amino acids can be synthesized** from α-keto acid precursors via transfer of an amino group from another amino acid by various transaminases.
2. Transamination followed by oxidative deamination (= **transdeamination**) ultimately releases the amino acid nitrogen as ammonia, to be detoxified in the urea cycle.
3. Transaminases have clinical importance (Chemistry to Clinics 5.7).

> **Chemistry to Clinics 5.7: Diagnostic Significance of Transaminases**
>
> Both the enzymes, i.e. GOT and GPT are of diagnostic significance. They are present in large amounts in the cardiac muscle and the liver, respectively. Although serum levels of both the enzymes are raised in heart as well as liver diseases, serum levels of GOT (**SGOT** levels) are markedly raised in myocardial infarction while **SGPT** levels are more increased in liver disorders, such as in viral hepatitis and toxic liver necrosis.

Deamination

- As discussed above, transamination involves only the transfer of α-amino group from an amino acid to α-keto acid and as such there is no net loss of the amino group, deamination is the actual process resulting in the removal of the α-amino group from an amino acid which is released in the form of ammonia. Though the process of deamination takes place in several tissues, the **liver** and the **kidney** are the main organs responsible for deamination of amino acids.

Deamination may take place as a result of removal of electrons which requires oxygen (**oxidative deamination**) or without the transfer of electrons (**nonoxidative deamination**).

- **Oxidative deamination:** The liver and the kidney contain several enzymes which catalyze deamination of amino acids, such as L-amino acid oxidases, D-amino acid oxidases, and glutamate dehydrogenase, etc.
  - **Amino acid oxidases**
    - **L-amino acid oxidases** catalyze o1xidation of L-amino acids. An α-keto acid and ammonia are released as the final products. The enzyme has FMN as a prosthetic group (Fig. 5.32).
    - **Glutamate dehydrogenase:** Glutamate mostly acts as a common intermediate between free ammonia and amino group of majority of the amino acids. Glutamate is produced via α-ketoglutarate by incorporating ammonia, as the amino group of nitrogen by the enzyme glutamate dehydrogenase. At the same time, this enzyme is also important in the production of ammonia from amino acids when these are catabolized for energy or are used as substrate for gluconeogenesis.

      Glutamate dehydrogenase thus catalyzes a reversible set of reactions where NADPH is used as a coenzyme in the synthetic reaction while NAD^+ is used in the liberation of ammonia, in the degradative reaction.

      Glutamate dehydrogenase is allosterically regulated by purine nucleotides. Its activity is increased by ADP and GDP in the direction of glutamate degradation when there is a need for the oxidation of amino acids for energy. On the other hand, ATP and GTP are allosteric activators in the direction of glutamate synthesis (Fig. 5.34).

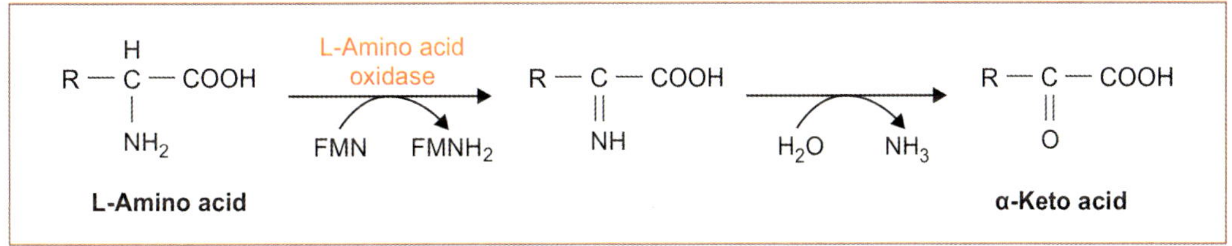

Fig. 5.32: Reaction catalyzed by L-amino acid oxidase

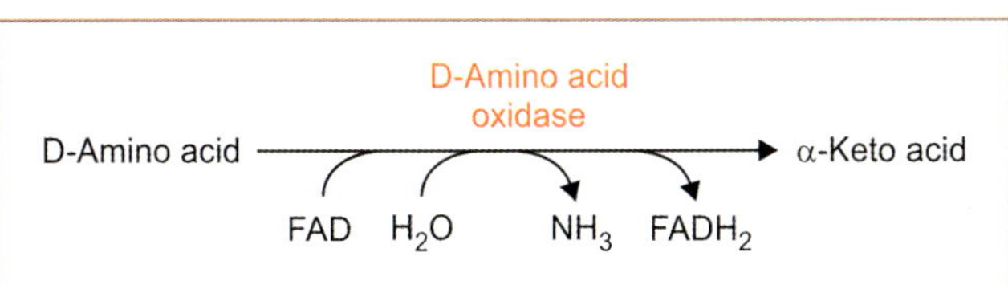

Fig. 5.33: Reaction catalyzed by D-amino acid oxidase

- Tissues also contain FAD-linked **D-amino acid oxidase** which catalyzes the oxidation of D-amino acids, derived from the intestinal bacteria, and of glycine (Fig. 5.33).

- **Nonoxidative deamination:** Deamination of some of the amino acids such as **serine, cysteine and histidine** is catalyzed by dehydratase, desulfhydrase and histidase, respectively. These enzymes require pyridoxal-5-phosphate as a coenzyme and cause dehydration of the amino acid, spontaneously, followed by (non-oxidative) deamination ultimately resulting in the removal of NH_3 (Fig. 5.35).

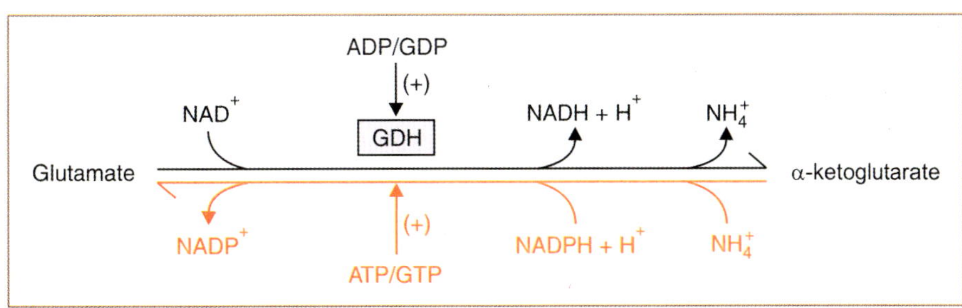

Fig. 5.34: Reactions catalyzed by glutamate dehydrogenase

5

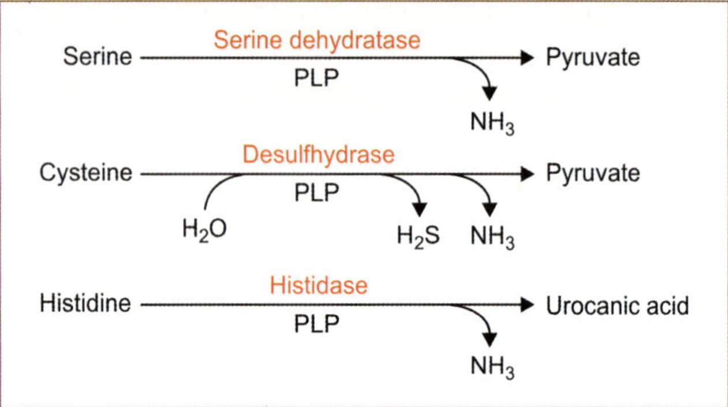

Fig. 5.35: Non-oxidative deamination of amino acids

DETOXIFICATION AND DISPOSAL OF AMMONIA

Ammonia, a highly toxic molecule, is detoxified and disposed-off by two processes:

- **First line of defense:** Ammonia, a highly toxic molecule, is trapped by glutamate to form glutamine, especially in the brain. This is catalyzed by **glutamine synthetase** (Fig. 5.36).

  Further, glutamine is an important form for the transport of ammonia to the kidney where glutaminase hydrolyzes amide group of glutamine to glutamic acid and ammonia. The amide group of glutamine is also important as a nitrogen donor for purine bases, amino group of cytosine and amide group of asparagine.

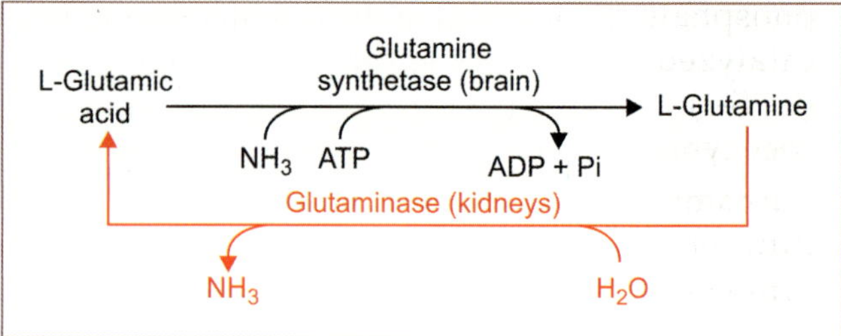

Fig. 5.36: Formation and disposal of glutamine

- **Second line of defense:** The **urea cycle** is a process by which ammonia is converted to urea, a less toxic and a soluble excretory waste product, in the liver, by the process referred to as urea cycle (Fig. 5.37).

UREA CYCLE

As mentioned above, urea is a major analyte of protein metabolism, which is synthesized by the process referred to as urea cycle.

1. In the first step, ammonia is activated by ATP and combines with carbon dioxide to form carbamoyl

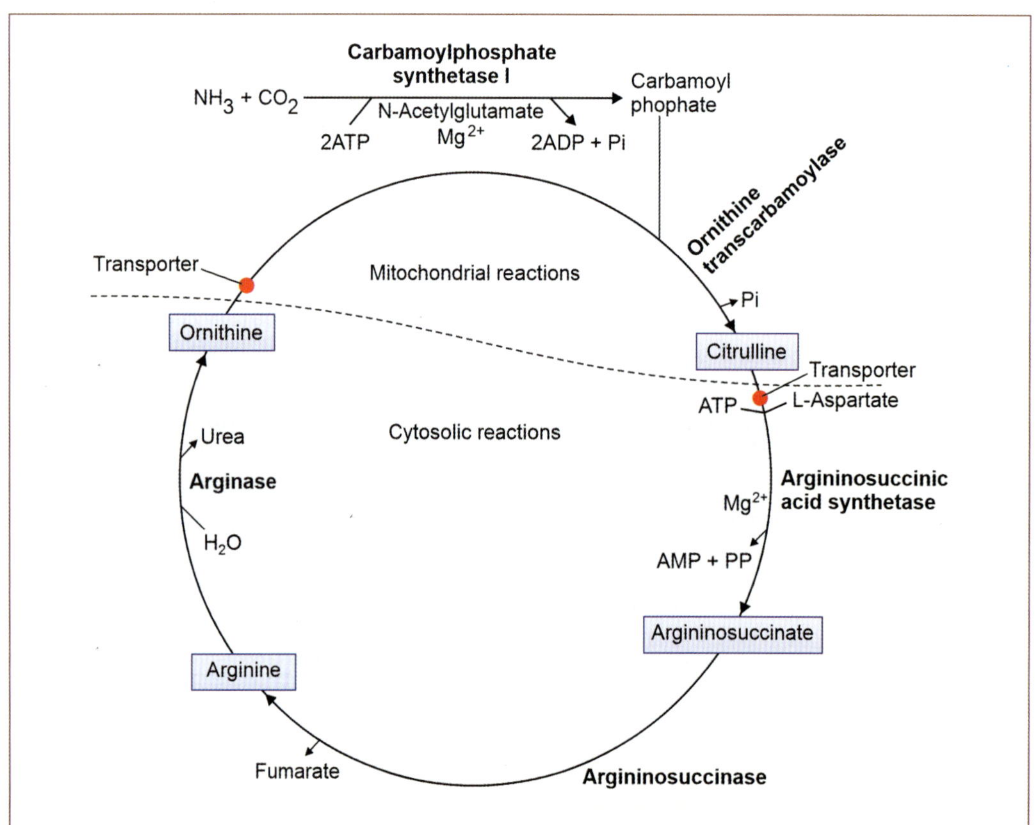

Fig. 5.37: Urea cycle

5

phosphate, in the mitochondria. The reaction is catalyzed by carbamoyl phosphate synthetase I (CPS-I) and requires N-acetyl glutamate as a coenzyme.

Carbamoyl phosphate synthetases: There are two different enzymes called carbamoyl phosphate synthetase I (CPS-I) and CPS-II (Table 5.7).

Table 5.7: Differences between CPS-I and CPS-II

	CPS-I	CPS-II
Location	Mitochondria	Cytosol
Nitrogen donor	NH_3	Glutamine
Metabolic pathway	Urea cycle	Pyrimidine biosynthesis
Allosteric regulator	N-Acetyl-glutamate (Activator)	CTP (Inhibitor)

2. Ornithine transcarbamoylase transfers the carbamoyl group from carbamoyl phosphate to ornithine and produces citrulline, in the mitochondrial matrix. Citrulline is transported from the mitochondria to the cytosol where other reactions of the urea cycle occur.
3. In the presence of argininosuccinic acid synthetase and ATP, citrulline combines with L-aspartate and forms argininosuccinic acid (argininosuccinate).
4. Subsequently, argininosuccinase hydrolyzes argininosuccinic acid to liberate arginine and fumaric acid. Carbons from aspartate are released as fumarate and enter the mitochondria where it is metabolized to oxaloacetate, by the tricarboxylic acid cycle. Hence, urea cycle is coupled with the Krebs cycle, as **Krebs bicycle**, both of which were discovered by Krebs and coworkers.
5. In the last step, arginine is hydrolyzed by arginase to regenerate ornithine and forms urea.
   Ornithine is transported to the mitochondria and re-enters the cycle.

Importance of Urea Cycle

1. Urea cycle is the mechanism for **nitrogen excretion** in humans and other primates. The two nitrogen atoms in each urea molecule are derived from two different sources, i.e. one from free NH_3 and the other from the amino group of aspartate. As human beings cannot metabolize urea, it is transported to the kidney for filtration and excretion (Fig. 5.38).
2. A small amount of urea may enter the **small intestine** where it is cleaved by bacteria. The NH_3 so formed is diffused into the circulation and used by the liver.
3. Fumarate is the link between urea cycle and Krebs cycle (**Krebs bicycle**).
4. Synthesis of **arginine**, a semiessential amino acid.
5. Disorders of urea cycle result in hyperammonemias.
6. Ornithine is regenerated which helps in the synthesis of polyamines.

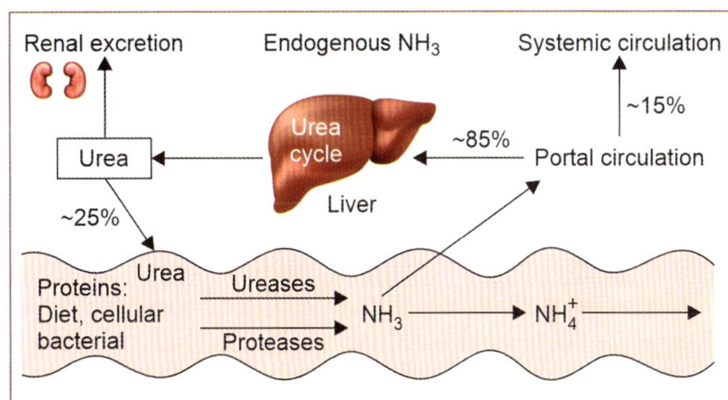

Fig. 5.38: Metabolic fate of urea

Regulation of Urea Synthesis

- Carbamoyl phosphate synthetase is absolutely dependent on N-acetylglutamate which acts as an allosteric activator for the enzyme. N-acetylglutamate is synthesized when acetyl-CoA combines with glutamate. The reaction is catalyzed by N-acetylglutamate synthase and requires arginine.
- Induction of the urea cycle enzymes occurs when delivery of ammonia or amino acids to the liver increases. Thus, a high protein diet as well as starvation, which results in catabolism of protein, cause induction of the enzymes of urea cycle.
- Compartmentalization of the cycle between the mitochondria and the cytosol.
- Presence of an ornithine-citrulline antiporter in the mitochondrial membrane ensures adequate exchange of the two compounds.

METABOLIC DISORDERS OF THE UREA CYCLE

As urea cycle is the major pathway for the elimination of **ammonia** from the body, which is a very **toxic** substance, metabolic disorders that may arise from abnormal function of the enzymes of urea synthesis are therefore potentially fatal and may cause coma when ammonia concentration becomes very high (Chemistry to Clinics 5.8).

5

Chemistry to Clinics 5.8: Hyperammonemias and Ammonia Toxicity

Increased NH_3 in the brain is toxic for two reasons:

- First, the glutamate dehydrogenase reaction is favored in the direction of glutamate synthesis thereby depleting α-ketoglutarate, an intermediate of Krebs cycle. This results in slowing of the Krebs cycle and reduced ATP synthesis. Lack of ATP not only compromises neuronal functions but also slows the glutamine synthetase reaction that converts glutamate to glutamine by trapping NH_3 (Fig. 5.34).
- Second, increased glutamate synthesis promotes the synthesis of γ-aminobutyric acid (GABA), an inhibitory neurotransmitter that can cause CNS depression. It should be noted that a similar clinical picture is observed in acquired liver diseases where the liver fails to detoxify ammonia, e.g. liver cirrhosis.

Inborn errors of all the enzymes of urea cycle have been reported and are shown in Table 5.8.

Urea cycle disorders occur when any defect, or total absence, of any of the enzymes, or the cofactors, used in the urea cycle results in the accumulation of ammonia in the blood. As discussed above, the urea cycle converts waste nitrogen into urea and excretes it from the kidneys. Since there are no alternate pathways to clear the ammonia, dysfunction of the urea cycle results in neurologic damages. Hyperammonemia is a biochemical manifestation of all these disorders. Treatment includes restriction of dietary protein to the amount tolerated without causing hyperammonemia and to prevent excessive body protein catabolism. Essential amino acids should be replaced with the corresponding α-keto acids, which in turn will reduce nitrogen disposal without causing deficiency of essential amino acids. Also, maximum calories should be provided in the form of glucose and lipids to reduce protein catabolism. Metabolic disorders of urea cycle include:

- **Hyperammonemia Type I**
  - This is a familial disorder, which occurs due to deficiency of the enzyme carbamoylphosphate synthetase.
  - It produces the symptoms of ammonia toxicity.
- **Hyperammonemia Type II**
  - Patients suffer from a deficiency of ornithine transcarbamoylase.
  - There is enhanced synthesis of glutamine by the glutamine synthetase reaction and tissue level of ammonia is increased.
  - The clinical finding is an elevation of glutamine in the blood, cerebrospinal fluid and urine.
  - The mothers show hyperammonemia and intolerance to high protein diet.
- **Citrullinemia**
  - It is due to complete absence of argininosuccinate synthetase activity.
  - Large quantities of citrulline are excreted in the urine, and plasma and CSF citrulline levels are elevated.
  - Citrulline and arginosuccinate act as alternative carriers of waste nitrogen, since they contain nitrogen used for urea synthesis.
  - Arginine feeding accelerates citrulline excretion in these patients.
  - Benzoate feeding diverts ammonium nitrogen to hippuric acid via glycine.
  - The form of citrullinemia called classic citrullinemia, usually, appears in the first few days after birth. If untreated, a baby with classic citrullinemia can die within the first week of life.
  - Health problems caused by citrullinemia can include brain damage, intellectual and developmental disabilities, liver problems and coma.

Table 5.8: Inborn errors of urea cycle

Deficient enzyme	Metabolic disorder	Product accumulates	Clinical features
Carbamoyl phosphate synthetase I	Hyperammonemia type I	Ammonia	Severe hyperammonaemia, mental retardation and developmental delay
Ornithine transcarbamoylase	Hyperammonemia type II	Ammonia	Channelling of carbamoyl-phosphate to pyrimidine biosynthesis and orotic aciduria
Argininosuccinic acid synthetase	Citrullinemia	Citrulline	Citrullinuria (breast milk is to be avoided)
Argininosuccinase	Argininosuccinic aciduria	Argininosuccinate	Metabolic acidosis, friable brittle tufted hair, trichorrhexis nodosa
Arginase	Hyperargininemia	Arginine accumulates in CSF and blood	cystinuria and lysinuria

- **Arginosuccinic aciduria**
  - Arginosuccinic aciduria (**argininosuccinic academia)** is caused due to the absence of arginosuccinase activity. This enzyme is also absent from brain, liver, kidney and erythrocytes of patients with this disease.
  - The disease is characterized by the increased level of arginosuccinic acid in blood, CSF and urine.
  - It is frequently associated with the occurrence of tufted hair.
  - The disease always appears by age 2 and, generally, terminates fatally early in life.
  - It needs measurement of erythrocyte arginosuccinase activity for confirmative diagnosis.
  - Arginine and benzoate feedings accelerate nitrogen excretion in these patients.
- **Hyperargininemia**
  - Low erythrocyte level of arginase causes this disease.
  - The urinary amino acid pattern resembles that of lysine cystinuria.
  - A low protein diet results in the lowering of plasma ammonia and abolishes urinary lysine cystinuria.

Acquired hyperammonemia (Hepatic coma)

It is also called hepatic encephalopathy which occurs due to hepatic failure and leads to hepatic coma and death. Patient has altered sensorium, convulsions, ascites, jaundice, hepatomegaly, cerebral edema, spider navi, etc.

Treatment

- Lactulose laxative which results in sterilization of gut.
- Treat the underlying cause of hepatic failure.
- Finally liver transplantation.

Neonatal hyperammonemia is also a medical emergency which requires rapid lowering of NH_3. Exchange transfusion is required. Hemodialysis or peritoneal dialysis also has a role.

BIOSYNTHESIS OF CREATININE

Creatinine is the **anhydride** form of creatine, which is synthesized from **glycine, arginine and methionine** (Fig. 5.39).

1. Firstly, guanidino group of arginine is transferred to glycine, to form guanidoacetic acid. The reaction is catalyzed by arginine-glycine transamidinase in the **kidney**.
2. Guanidoacetate methyltransferase transfers a methyl group from S-adenosylmethionine forming creatine. This reaction occurs in the **liver**.
3. Creatine enters the blood and transported to **muscles** where a high energy phosphate group is transferred from ATP and **creatine phosphate** is formed, catalyzed by creatine kinase (CK), reversibly (Chemistry to Clinics 5.9).

> **Chemistry to Clinics 5.9: Creatine Deficiency**
>
> Recently, creatine deficiency disorders have been identified due to deficiency of arginine glycine transamidinase or guanidoacetate methyltransferase or mutated *SLC6A8*. Due to the importance of creatine phosphate in muscles and brain, the disease is characterized by muscular weakness and neurological impairment. The therapeutic benefit of creatine supplementation is being explored.

Significance of Creatine Phosphate

1. Creatine phosphate is the form in which high energy phosphate is stored in the muscles. It is a **phosphagen**. During exercise, ATP is used as a source of energy and is converted to ADP. During resting conditions, creatine phosphate is utilized to phosphorylate this ADP while creatine is released as creatinine. The reaction is called Lohmann reaction and is catalyzed by creatine kinase. It is a reversible reaction which can also lead to the synthesis of creatine phosphate from creatine and ATP.
2. Only traces of creatine are normally present in the urine. Large quantities may be excreted in muscular dystrophies, during starvation and pregnancy.

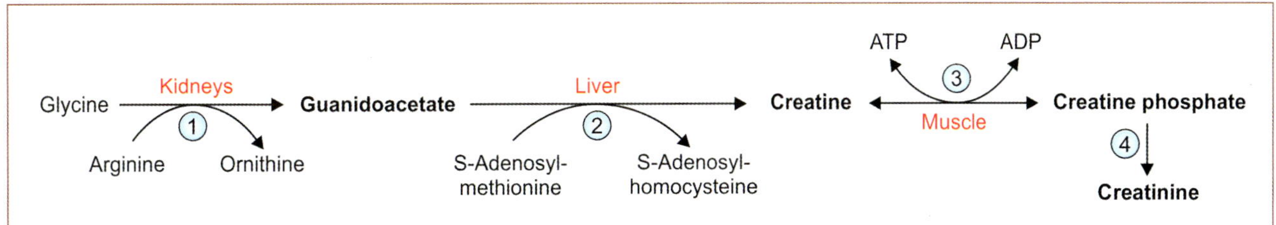

Fig. 5.39: Creatine metabolism: (1) Transaminidase; (2) Methyltransferase; (3) Creatine phosphokinase; (4) Nonenzymatic

5

Creatinine

Creatinine is formed in the muscle from creatine or creatine phosphate by a nonenzymatic reaction, irreversibly (Fig. 5.39).

Creatinine is one of the major **nonprotein nitrogenous** excretory products after urea. Nearly 1.0–1.5 g of creatinine is excreted in the urine in 24 hours. Its total excretion is independent of the amount of dietary protein but is related to **muscle mass.** Serum creatinine as well as the amount of the creatinine excreted by an individual remains constant from day-to-day, and by calculating creatinine clearance one can **determine the renal function in terms of glomerular filtration rate.**

DISORDERS OF THE METABOLISM OF INDIVIDUAL AMINO ACIDS

Disorders of the metabolism of individual amino acids are characterized by the inability of the body to metabolize a particular amino acid. Accumulation of the amino acid or any of its metabolite can be toxic.

HYPERGLYCINEMIA

- Hyperglycinemia (nonketotic hyperglycinemia) is due to the **deficiency of the enzyme glycine cleavage complex**, which degrades glycine to ammonia and carbon dioxide (Fig. 5.40).
- It is characterized by hyperglycinemia, a major inhibitory neurotransmitter, which, in turn, results in severe mental retardation.

PRIMARY HYPEROXALURIA

- This is an inherited disorder characterized by increased urinary excretion of oxalate (not related to dietary intake of oxalate) due to the **deficiency of the enzyme glycine transaminase**.
- Glycine is oxidatively deaminated by the enzyme glycine oxidase and forms glyoxylate. Glyoxylate can be transaminated back to glycine, by glycine transaminase. Due to deficiency of glycine transaminase, glyoxylate gets oxidized to oxalate (Fig. 5.41).
- Excessive production of oxalate (due to glycine transaminase deficiency) together with impairment of glycine oxidation (to formate) is the cause of hyperoxaluria.
- Oxalate forms calcium oxalate, high excretion of which leads to renal calculi (Fig. 5.42).
- The clinical features exhibit progressive bilateral calcium oxalate urolithiasis, nephrocalcinosis and recurrent infection of the urinary tract.
- Death occurs in childhood, or in early adult life, from renal failure or hypertension.

PHENYLKETONURIA

- Phenylketonuria (PKU) is an inherited disorder due to the **absence of the enzyme phenylalanine hydroxylase**, which converts phenylalanine to tyrosine in the presence of molecular oxygen and tetrahydrobiopterin (BH_4). In this process, BH_4 is converted to dihydrobiopterin (BH_2) and requires NADPH-dependent reductase for its regeneration (Fig. 5.43).
- Autosomal recessive deficiency of hepatic phenylalanine hydroxylase is referred to as **type I phenylketonuria (classical phenylketonuria)**. Deficiency of dihydrobiopterin reductase is referred to as **type II phenylketonuria**.
- Excess of phenylalanine, which cannot be converted to tyrosine, gets catabolized by the alternative pathway, where phenylalanine is transaminated to phenylpyruvic acid. Phenylpyruvate is subsequently reduced to phenyllactate as well as is decarboxylated to phenylacetate.
- Due to increased urinary excretion of phenylpyruvic acid (a phenylketone), the disease is called phenylketonuria.
- Increased level of the three phenylketoacids in the blood causes mental retardation and convulsions among infants and children.
- Besides, severe neurological symptoms and very low IQ, there is also light color of the skin and the eyes. This is due to underpigmentation, a result of tyrosine (and hence melanin) deficiency.

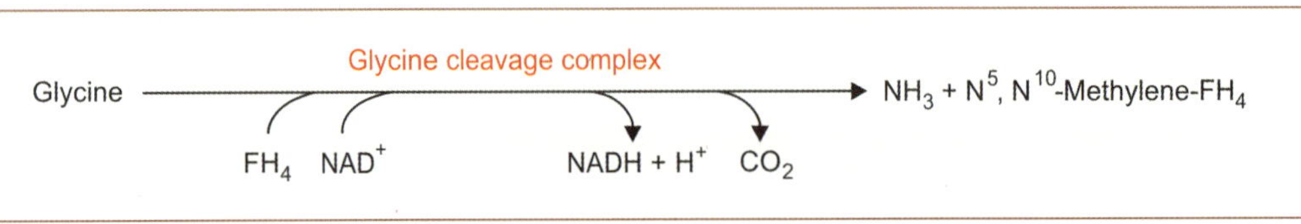

Fig. 5.40: Degradation of glycine

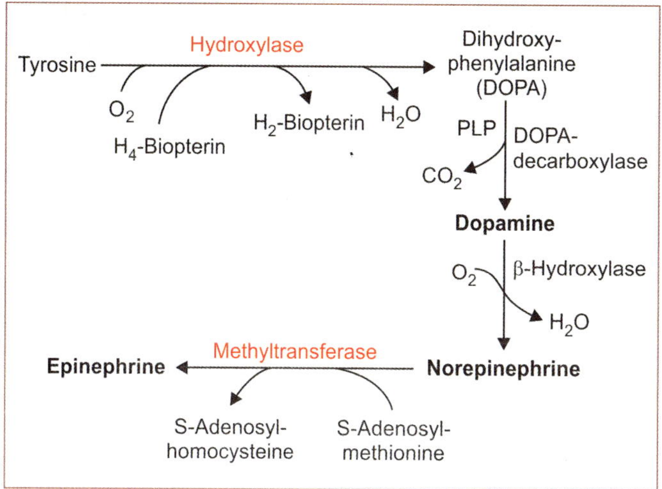

Fig. 5.41: Synthesis of catecholamines from tyrosine

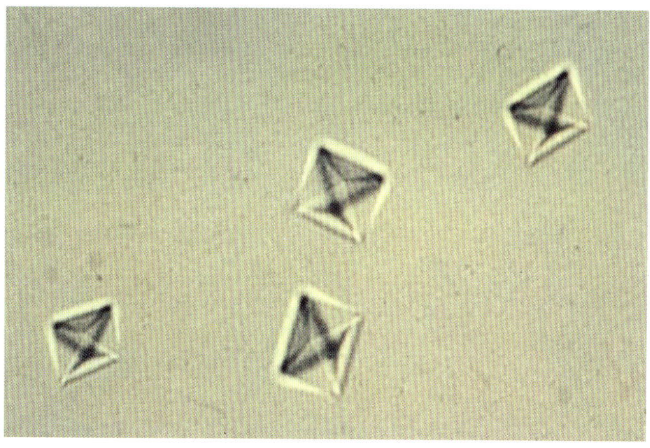

Fig. 5.42: Calcium oxalate crystals: Square shape with a characteristic 'X' mark. Calcium oxalate stones are the most prevalent renal stones

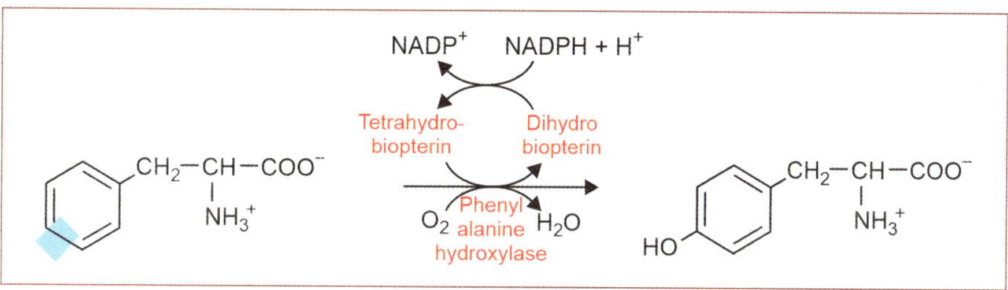

Fig. 5.43: Conversion of phenylalanine to tyrosine

- Patients with phenylketonuria tend to have a deficiency of serotonin. This may be connected with the defect of myelin synthesis.
- Ds k/a phenylketonuria. Phenylactate in sweat and urine imparts mousy body odour.
- Screening test for phenylketonuria can be done by addition of $FeCl_3$ to the urine which imparts blue green colour.
- Second is Guthrie test. Addition of blood sample of a PKU patient leads to growth of Bacillus subtilis which requires phenylalanine as an essential growth factor.
- Plasma phenylalanine level of >20 md/dL is the confirmatory test for PKU.
- The accumulation of phenylalanine also impairs melanin synthesis and children with this defect tend to have fair skin and fair hair.
- Early diagnosis (shortly after birth) and extreme restriction of phenylalanine intake is effective in preventing this disorder. Hence, such infants should be given **low phenylalanine diet**. Under these conditions **tyrosine becomes dietary essential**.

TYROSINEMIAS

Tyrosinemias is a group of autosomal recessive disorders due to **defects in tyrosine metabolism, in the liver**, which, in turn, lead to accumulation and excretion of tyrosine and its metabolites.

Catabolism of tyrosine in the liver occurs as follows:

- It starts with the transamination of tyrosine to *p*-hydroxyphenylpyruvate by the enzyme tyrosine aminotransferase (tyrosine transaminase).
- In the next step, a copper-containing enzyme complex, *p*-hydroxyphenylpyruvate oxidase converts *p*-hydroxyphenylpyruvate to homogentisic acid. The enzyme requires ascorbic acid and catalyzes decarboxylation, oxidation and migration of the carbon side chain, and hydroxylation of the substrate.
- Thereafter, an iron-containing enzyme homogentisic acid oxidase, oxidizes homogentisic acid.
- Subsequent reactions, catalyzed by maleylaceto-acetate isomerase (which requires glutathione for its activity) and fumarylacetoacetate hydrolase, lead to formation of the end products of tyrosine catabolism, i.e. fumarate and acetoacetate (Fig. 5.44).

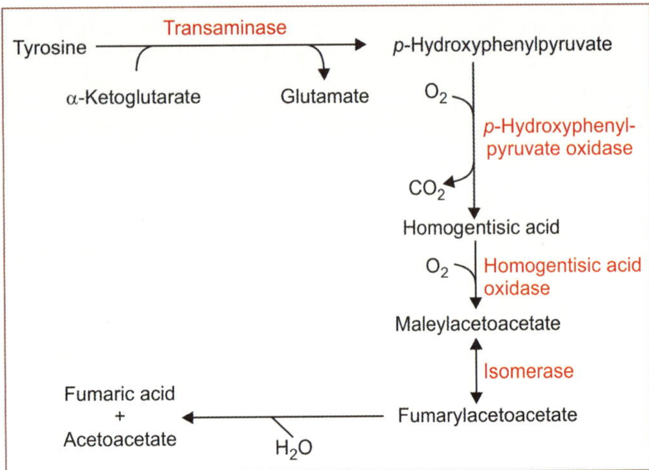

Fig. 5.44: Degradation of tyrosine in the liver

Tyrosinemias include

- **Type I tyrosinemia**
  - It is also called **hepatorenal tyrosinemia** and is caused by the **deficiency of the enzyme fumaryl-acetoacetate hydrolase**.
  - Fumarylacetoacetate and its precursor (maleyl-acetoacetate) get accumulated, both, of which are alkylating agents, and can lead to DNA alkylation and carcinogenesis.
  - It is a more serious type of the disease and involves liver failure, renal tubular dysfunction, rickets and polyneuropathy.
- **Type II tyrosinemia**
  - It is also called **oculocutaneous tyrosinemia** and is caused by the **deficiency of the enzyme tyrosine transaminase**.
  - It results in eye and skin lesions, and mental retardation.
- **Neonatal tyrosinemia**
  - It occurs in newborns, due to transient **deficiency of the enzyme *p*-hydroyphenylpyruvic acid oxidase**.
  - Tyrosine, *p*-hydroxyphenylpyruvic acid, *p*-hydroxyphenyllactic acid and *p*-hydroxyphenyl-acetic acid appear in the urine.
  - The condition lasts for a few weeks. Administration of ascorbic acid and reduction of protein intake brings about the normal condition.
- **Hereditary tyrosinemia**
  - It is due to the **inherited deficiency of *p*-hydroxyphenylpyruvic acid oxidase.**
  - This disorder is similar to neonatal tyrosinemia, but the amount of *p*-hydroxyphenyllactic acid in the urine is greater.
  - This disorder is not controlled by the administration of ascorbic acid.
  - Liver failure and death can occur six months after birth and the infant has a characteristic odor.
  - Other patients develop the clinical findings, including hepatosplenomegaly, nodular cirrhosis of the liver, abnormalities of tyrosine and methionine metabolism, multiple defects in renal tubular reabsorption, rickets, hyperphosphaturia, proteinuria and amino aciduria.
  - Diet containing low in tyrosine and phenylalanine improves renal function and also retards degenerative liver changes.

TYROSINOSIS

- This syndrome is due to the **absence of** either **hepatic *p*-hydroxyphenylpyruvate hydroxylase** or **tyrosine transaminase activity**.
- The patient excretes large quantities of tyrosine in the urine.
- Diet rich in tyrosine causes the excretion of other *p*-hydroxyphenyl acids, including 3,4-dihydroxyphenylalanine (DOPA) and *p*-hydroxyphenyllactic acid.

ALKAPTONURIA

- This condition is due to the **lack of homogentisic acid oxidase**.
- It is characterized by the excretion of homogentisic acid (dihydroxyphenylacetic acid) in the urine, where several grams of homogentisic acid may be excreted daily.
- Oxidation of homogenitisate by polyphenol oxidase forming benzoquinone acetate, which polymerizes to form black coloured alkapton bodies.
- The most common clinical manifestation is the dark urine due to the oxidation of homogentisic acid in air (Fig. 5.45).
- This condition is present at birth and persists throughout life.
- In later life, accumulation of dark pigment in cartilages and tendons gives rise to the condition known as **ochronosis**, which is accompanied by arthritic changes.

ALBINISM

- This condition appears in the total **absence of tyrosinase inside the melanocytes** in the skin, which is specific for the biosynthesis of melanin in melanocytes.

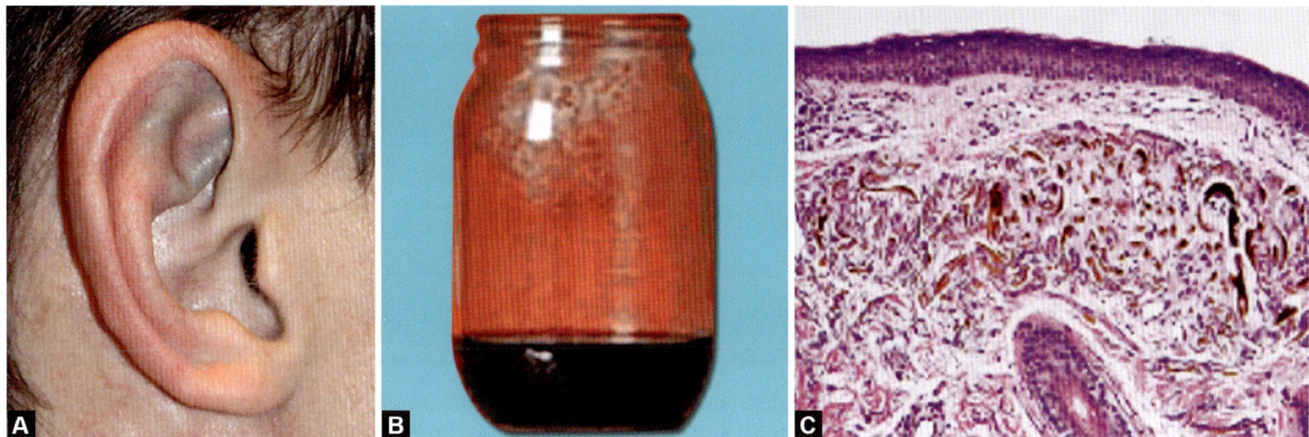

Fig. 5.45: Alkaptonuria: (A) Slate-blue discoloration of the antihelix of the ear; (B) Darkening of the urine on standing; (C) Ochronosis: Histopathology of the skin, showing sharply defined yellow-brown banana-shaped deposits within elastic fibers in the superficial dermis and scattered pigment-laden macrophages in the papillary dermis

- Besides its degradation in the liver, tyrosine also acts as a precursor of various compounds in different tissues. In the melanocytes, tyrosine is used for the synthesis of melanin, a brown-black pigment found in the skin, hair and retina (Fig. 5.46).
- **Synthesis of melanin** occurs as follows:
  - Firstly, by the enzyme tyrosinase (a copper-containing protein), tyrosine is first converted to DOPA and then to dopaquinone.
  - Subsequently, dopaquinone forms melanin.
- Deficiency of tyrosinase in melanocytes, in turn, affects the synthesis of melanin in the skin, eyes and hair, which leads to the appearance of white depigmented patches on the skin and iris (Fig. 5.47).
- Lack of melanin in the skin makes albinos more sensitive to sunlight and increases the risk of skin cancer. The diagnostic advice is for the prevention of exposure of sunlight.
- Lack of pigment in the eyes may also contribute to photophobia.

Parkinsonism

Dopamine deficiency due to degeneration of certain parts of brain mainly of substantia nigra is associated with Parkinson's disease. Commonly seen in elderly and is associated with muscular rigidity, mask-like face, lost body steps, lethargy, involuntary movements, etc. Treatment is administration of L-dopa.

Catecholamines and thyroxine are derived from tyrosine. Catecholamines are the amine derivatives of dihydroxylated phenyl ring and constitute dopamine, epinephrine and norepinephrine. There is tissue specificity in catcholamin formation. medulla synthesise epinephine and Adernal norepinephrine. Dophamine in sulstantia nigra and coeruleus of brain.

Vanillylmandelic acid (VMA) is produced from catabolism of catecholamines. Its normal level is 2–6 mg/24 hours. It is increased in pheochromocytoma and neuroblastoma.

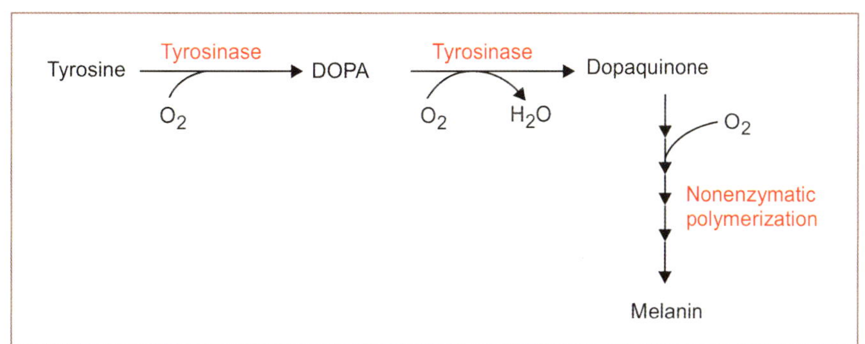

Fig. 5.46: Synthesis of melanin

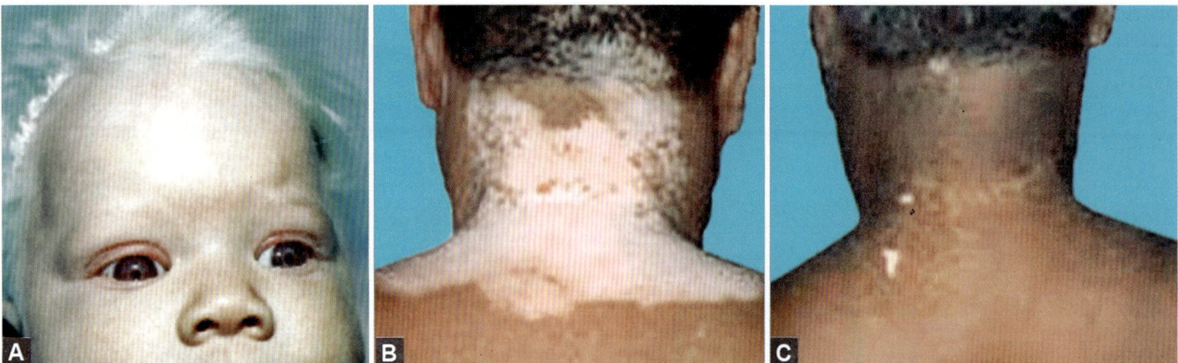

Fig. 5.47: (A) **Oculocutaneous albinism.** Hypomelanotic skin, white hair, and pink irides resulting from the **dysfunction of tyrosinase** in the melanocytes of these tissues and the subsequent lack of melanin synthesis; (B) **Vitiligo.** Hypopigmentation due to **lack of melanocytes** in the affected skin; (C) Same patient as in (B), improving **after UVB** (the B range of ultraviolet radiation) **phototherapy**

Hartnup's Disease

It is an inherited disorder of tryptophan metabolism. Autosomal recessive in character. There is impaired transport of tryptophan and neutral amino acids in intestinal mucosa, renal tubular ephithelial cells and brain clinical features include mental retardation, intermittent cerebellar ataxia and other neurological symptoms pellagra, etc.

Diagnosis is based on increased excretion of indole compounds that are derived from tryptophan, in use. It is also known as blue diaper syndrome.

MAPLE SYRUP URINE DISEASE

- This syndrome is characterized by the absence of the enzyme, **branched-chain α-keto acid dehydrogenase complex**, which is required for the oxidative decarboxylation of the keto acids that are derived from the branched-chain amino acids.
- Branched-chain amino acids include valine, leucine and isoleucine. These are oxidized in the liver and muscles. Although these three amino acids produce different end products, the first three steps in their catabolism, i.e. transamination, formation of CoA thioesters and their oxidation (Fig. 5.48).
- **Catabolism of branched-chain amino acids** include:
  1. **Transamination:** The first step in the oxidation of BCAA is the removal of α-amino group by transamination, forming the corresponding α-keto acids.
  2. **Oxidative decarboxylation:** Dehydrogenation of the branched-chain α-keto acid is carried out by

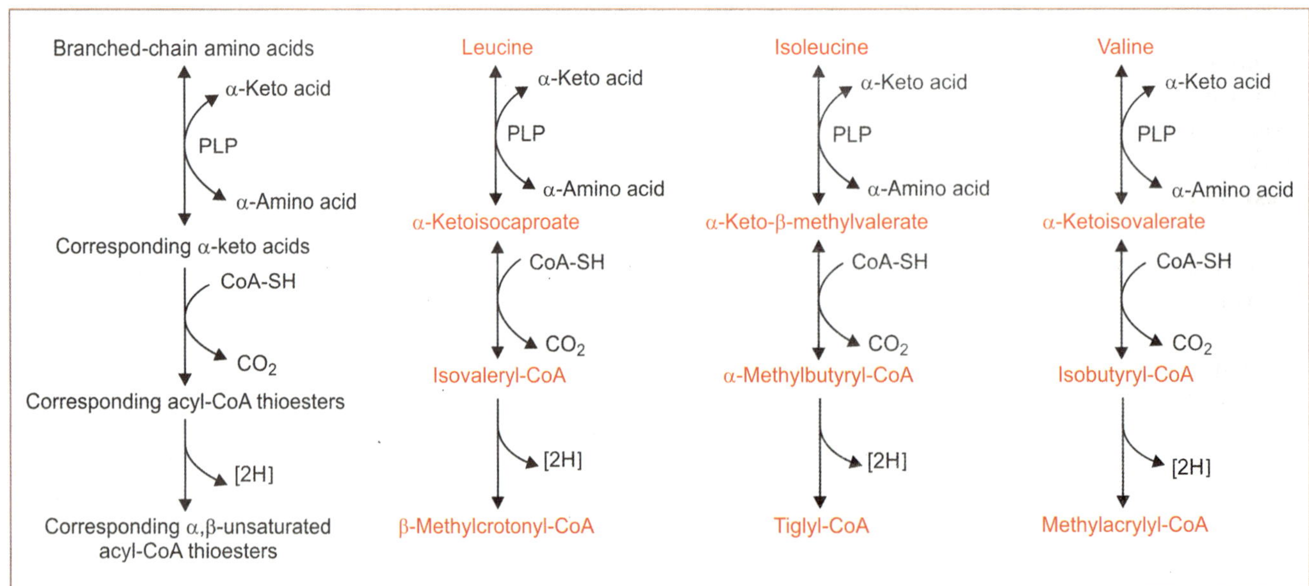

Fig. 5.48: Outline of metabolism of branched-chain amino acids

5

a branched-chain α-keto acid dehydrogenase complex. It results in the loss of a carboxylic group, forming CoA thioester of the corresponding BCAA. These are called branched-chain acyl-CoA thioesters, and are one carbon shorter than the original BCAA.

3. **Dehydrogenation:** In the next step, branched-chain acyl-CoA thioesters are oxidized to yield the corresponding α, β-unsaturated branched-chain acyl-CoA thioesters. Carbon skeleton of each of the branched-chain amino acid now follows a unique pathway to the amphibolic end products which determine that valine is glucogenic, leucine is ketogenic while isoleucine is both, i.e. ketogenic as well as glucogenic.

- As a result of the absence of the enzyme **branched-chain α-keto acid dehydrogenase complex**, branched-chain keto acids are accumulated in the blood and excreted in urine. The urinary excretion of these keto acids produces an odor like that of maple syrup or burnt sugar.
- This familial disorder is recognized by central nervous system manifestations of convulsions and attacks of flaccidity and apnea.
- The patients may be well treated with amino acid mixtures low in three branched-chain amino acids.
- The infant is difficult to feed and may vomit. The patient suffers from a significant degree of lethargy.
- Death may occur by the end of the first year of life without treatment.

CYSTINOSIS

- Cystinosis, also referred to as cystine storage disease, is a rare lysosomal disorder due to the impaired conversion of cystine to cysteine in the involved tissues as a result of the **deficiency of the enzyme cystine reductase** (Fig. 5.49).
- This disorder may also be characterized by **defective carrier-mediated transport of cystine**, resulting in cystine crystals.
- These cystine crystals are accumulated in liver, spleen, bone marrow, peripheral leukocytes, lymph nodes, kidney and cornea. These crystals are, particularly, accumulated in reticuloendothelial system.

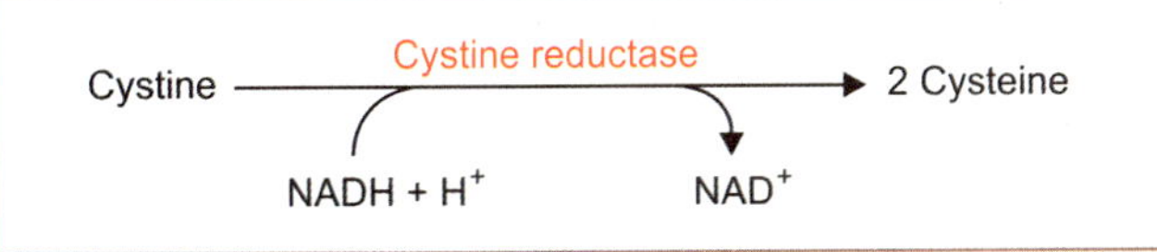

Fig. 5.49: Formation of cysteine from cystine

- Cystinosis is, usually, accompanied by aminoaciduria, glycosuria, polyuria, chronic acidosis leading to uremia and death.
- The renal functions are seriously impaired for which patients die in the young stage from acute failure.
- In adults, cystine gets deposited in cornea. Cystine crystals can be detected easily in cornea by slit lamp microscopy and confirmed by chemical determination of cystine crystals of peripheral leukocytes or cultured fibroblasts.

HOMOCYSTINURIA

- Homocystinuria is a **disorder of methionine metabolism**, leading to abnormal accumulation of, both, homocystine and methionine in blood and urine.
- **Methionine has various metabolic fates**
  1. **Formation of active methionine:** The first step, in the metabolism of methionine, is catalyzed by adenosyltransferase, which converts methionine to **S-adenosylmethionine (SAM)** or active methionine (Fig. 5.50).

     Active methionine acts as a methyl carrier and helps in the synthesis of several methylated products. The methylation reactions are catalyzed by the specific methyltransferases which transfer a methyl group from SAM to an acceptor molecule. This is important in the formation of methylated products of biological significance (Table 5.9).
  2. **Synthesis of homocysteine**: After the removal of its active methyl group by a methyltransferase, S-adenosylmethionine is converted to S-adenosylhomocysteine. Subsequently, adenosylhomocysteine hydrolase cleaves the adenosyl moiety (a molecule of adenosine) and forms homocysteine (which has one carbon more than cysteine; Fig. 5.51).
  3. **Metabolism of homocysteine:** Homocysteine can be utilized in different ways:
     i. **Methylation pathway:** It results in the **resynthesis of methionine**. When cells need to resynthesize methionine, **homocysteine methyltransferase** (methionine synthase) transfers a methyl group from N^5-methyltetrahydrofolate (N^5-methyl-FH_4) to cobalamin, forming methylcobalamin, which reconverts homocysteine to methionine (Fig. 5.51).

5

Table 5.9: S-Adenosyl methionine (SAM) as a methyl group donor

Methyl group acceptor	Methylated product	Biological importance
Ethanolamine	Choline	Choline-containing phospholipids
Guanidoacetate	Creatine	Creatine phosphate, a high-energy reservoir
N-Acetyl serotonin	Melatonin	Neurotransmitter
Norepinephrine	Epinephrine	Catecholamine
Epinephrine	Metanephrine	Metabolite of epinephrine
Lysine residues in some proteins	Trimethyl lysine	Precursor of carnitine which shuttles activated fatty acids from cytosol to mitochondria
DNA, RNA, proteins	Methylated nucleic acids and proteins	Regulation of gene expression

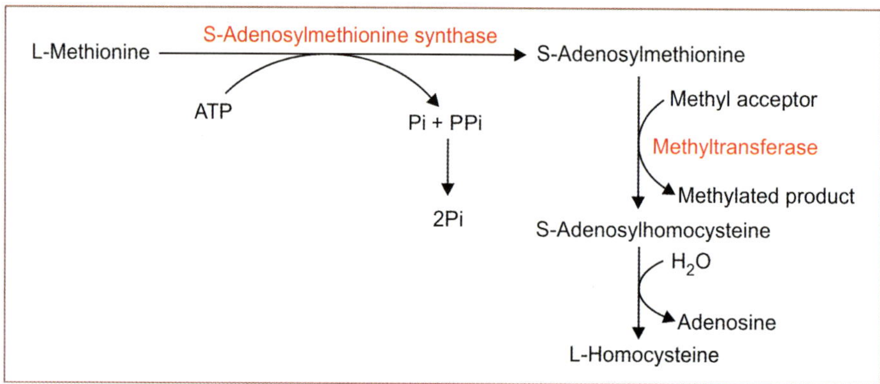

Fig. 5.50: Synthesis of S-adenosylmethionine and its role in transmethylation

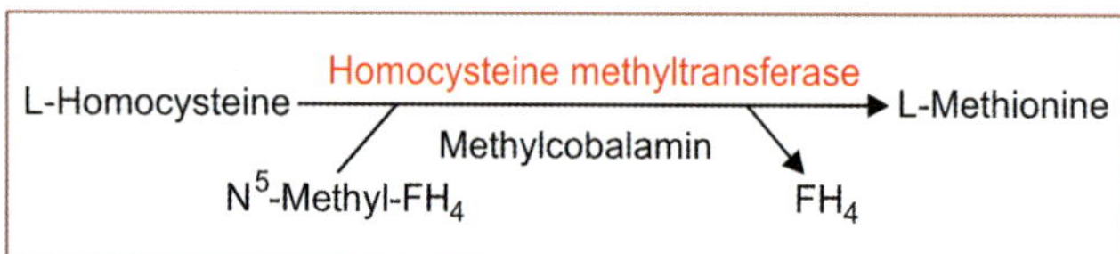

Fig. 5.51: Conversion of homocysteine to methionine

ii. **Trans-sulfuration pathway:** It results in the **synthesis of cysteine**. In this process, homocysteine is coupled with serine and forms cystathionine. This reaction is catalyzed by **cystathionine synthase** and requires pyridoxal-phosphate as a coenzyme. Thereafter, cystathionine is cleaved, by the splitting enzyme cystathione lyase (cystathionase), and forms cysteine and α-ketobutyrate (Fig. 5.52).

- Homocystinuria includes a group of autosomal recessively inherited defects either in the trans-sulfuration pathway or methylation pathway. There are four types of homocystinurias:
  - **Type I homocystinuria:** It is due to **deficiency of the enzyme cystathionine synthase** and results in osteoporosis, thrombosis, dislocation of lens and mental retardation.
  - **Type II homocystinuria:** It is due to **deficiency of the enzyme N^5,N^{10}-methylenetetrahydrofolate reductase** and can be corrected by vitamin B_6.
  - **Type III homocystinuria:** It is due to **deficiency of N^5-methyltetrahydrofolate:homocysteine transmethylase**, resulting in lack of methylcobalamin.
  - **Type IV homocystinuria:** It is due to **defect in intestinal absorption of cobalamin**, leading to defect in methylation cycle.
- If untreated, homocystinuria can cause problems with the blood, bones, eyes, heart and pancreas.

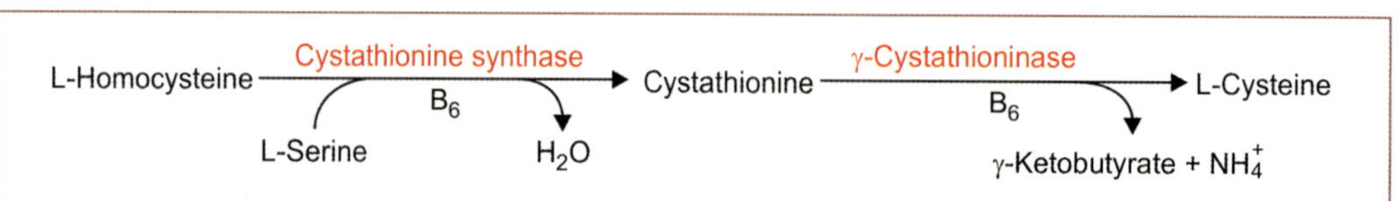

Fig. 5.52: Conversion of homocysteine to cysteine

5

- Babies with homocystinuria may look healthy at birth, but symptoms, usually, appear within the first year of life.
- The clinical findings of this disease are the occurrence of thrombosis, osteoporosis, dislocated lenses in the eyes and frequently mental retardation.
- A low methionine and a high cystine diet effectively prevent this condition if treated earlier.

HISTIDINEMIA

- It is an inherited disorder of histidine metabolism, **due to the insufficient activity of liver histidase,** which impairs the conversion of histidine to urocanic acid (Fig. 5.53).
- The amounts of histidine in the blood and urine are increased. There is also increased excretion of imidazole pyruvic acid.
- Development of speech in this condition is retarded. Mental development is also retarded.
- These histidinemic patients are treated well with a diet containing protein hydrolysate free from histidine, instead of intact protein.

ANALYTES ASSOCIATED WITH METABOLISM OF PROTEINS

As discussed above, degradation of proteins results in the release of **amino acids**, which are absorbed in the liver and are catabolized with the removal of ammonia. Ammonia is removed from the body as **urea**, which forms a **major analyte of protein metabolism**. Some of the amino acids are also used in the synthesis of **creatinine**. Thus, **urea** and **creatinine** are the two main analytes, which are associated with the metabolism of proteins.

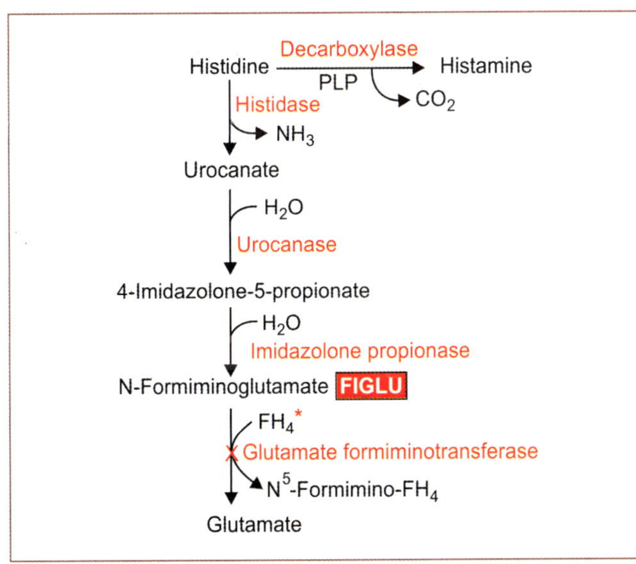

Fig. 5.53: Metabolism of histidine. *Site of block in folate deficiency

UREA

Urea is a major nitrogenous metabolic end product of protein catabolism in man, accounting for more than 75% of the nonprotein nitrogen, which is eventually excreted. Urea is freely filtered by the glomeruli. In a normal kidney, 40–70% urea moves passively out of the renal tubule into the interstitium.

Blood urea: Blood urea level, in a normal individual, may vary between 15 and 45 mg/dl. In patients with untreated chronic renal failure blood urea level may be increased to 100–150 mg/dl.

Measurement of blood urea is widely used as a test of renal function. However, a number of non-renal factors influence blood urea concentration. For example, urea production, and consequently blood urea concentration, is increased on a high protein diet, in protein catabolic states, gastrointestinal hemorrhage and treatment with cortisol in some cases of chronic liver disease and with decreased perfusion of the kidney. Blood urea also depends upon the state of hydration of the patient.

Urine urea: An adult excretes, nearly, 25–30 g of urea under normal conditions, in 24 hours. Urea excretion is increased on high protein diet or in protein catabolic states, such as fever. On low protein diet urea excretion is reduced. Decrease in urea excretion can also be observed in disorders associated with impaired liver function, such as cirrhosis, as well as in a kidney disease, such as nephritis.

Alterations in blood urea level

- **Increase in blood urea level:** Increased blood urea level, above normal, is termed **azotemia**. When this is associated with clinical symptoms, it is called **uremia**. **High blood urea** concentration may be due to several reasons, which may be subdivided into pre-renal, renal and post-renal:

  1. **Pre-renal**
     - Increased production by the liver, such as on a high protein diet.
     - Increased breakdown of tissue proteins, e.g. in protein catabolic states (high grade fever, trauma, major surgery, or starvation) and some toxic states.

- Dehydration, leading to low perfusion of kidneys and, therefore, decreased filtration of urea, e.g. in cases of:
  - Burn
  - Diarrhea
  - Vomiting
  - Severe hemorrhage
  - Diabetic ketoacidosis.

2. **Renal**
   - Glomerulonephritis, acute and chronic
   - Chronic renal failure
   - Chronic pyelonephritis
   - Poisoning, affecting kidneys
   - Nephrotoxic drugs, e.g. gentamicin, cephaloridine, sulfonamide, etc.
   - Diabetic and gouty nephropathy.
3. **Post-renal**
   - Stone, anywhere in the urinary tract
   - Malignancy
   - Stricture of the urinary tract
   - Prostate hypertrophy in the elderly

- **Decrease in blood urea level**

  Low blood urea concentration may be observed in situations such as reduced synthesis, e.g. on a low protein diet or in an acute liver disease. Blood urea level may also fall as a result of water retention.

Note: Estimation of plasma urea concentration, however, is a less valuable test of renal function than plasma creatinine concentration. This is due to the reason that nearly 50% of the urea, filtered at the glomerulus, is passively reabsorbed through the tubules and this fraction increases if urine flow rate increases, such as in dehydration. Plasma urea concentration is also affected by dietary protein intake.

CREATININE

Another important analyte associated with protein metabolism is creatinine.

Serum creatinine: Normal serum creatinine concentration varies between 0.8 and 1.5 mg/dl.

Determination of serum creatinine gives a useful indication of the degree of renal failure, because:

1. Plasma creatinine concentration, normally, remains fairly constant throughout adult life.
2. It correlates well with GFR in patients with a renal disease.
3. Sequential plasma creatinine concentration measurements enable the progress of a renal disease, to be followed with better precision.

Urine creatinine: Its daily excretion is related to muscle mass and does not vary greatly from day-to-day. Hence, its level in the blood remains fairly constant. Moreover, creatinine is freely filtered at the glomerulus. Although it is not reabsorbed to any great extent by renal tubules but a small amount of it is secreted. Its secretion is increased with the increasing level of plasma creatinine.

Creatinine content of urine is increased in conditions associated with increased muscular activity. A decrease in creatinine excretion may be observed in disorders, which are associated with muscular weakness as well as in a kidney disease.

Alterations in Serum Creatinine Concentration

- **Increase in serum creatinine**

  An increase in serum creatinine, due to fall in GFR is observed when:

  1. There is decreased renal perfusion, e.g. reduced blood pressure, fluid deprivation or renal arterial stenosis.
  2. There is a loss of functional nephrons, e.g. in acute and chronic glomerulonephritis
  3. Pressure is increased on the tubular side of the nephron, e.g. in urinary tract obstruction due to prostate enlargement.

  Besides

  4. High meat intake can cause temporary rise in plasma creatinine level.
  5. Transient small increase in plasma creatinine level may occur after vigorous exercise.
  6. Some drugs, e.g. salicylates, cimetidine, etc. reduce tubular secretion of creatinine, hence, exhibit elevated plasma creatinine concentration.
  7. High concentration of certain compounds, such as acetoacetate or cephalosporin antibiotic, exhibit analytical interference and result in its overestimation.

- **Decrease in serum creatinine**

  1. Decrease in serum creatinine concentration is found in subjects with a small total muscle mass. Thus, a lower value is found in children. Values are also, on average, normally lower in women than in men.
  2. Abnormally low values may be found in wasting diseases (reduced muscle bulk) and starvation, and in patients on steroid therapy, due to their protein catabolic effect.
  3. Plasma creatinine concentration is also usually low in pregnancy.

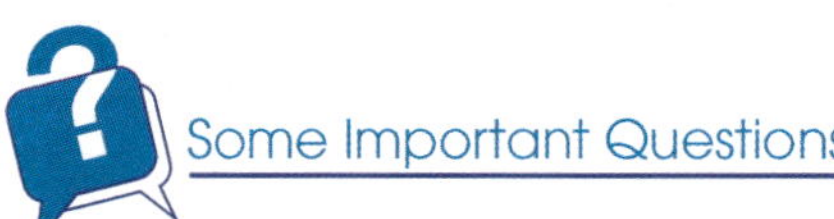

Some Important Questions

1. What are amino acids? Based on the ionic charge classify amino acids.

2. What are proteins? Based on their solubility classify proteins.

3. Outline urea cycle. What is the site of urea synthesis? What is the need for urea synthesis in the body?

4. Describe various processes of the removal of ammonia from amino acids.

5. How is ammonia detoxified in our body? Outline the reactions involved in this process.

6. Describe digestion and absorption of proteins.

7. Discuss briefly:

i. α-Helix
ii. β-Pleated sheets
iii. Quaternary structure of proteins
iv. Biosynthesis of creatine
v. Transamination and its importance
vi. Hyperhomocysteinemia

8. Write notes on:

i. Neutral amino acids
ii. Branched-chain amino acids
iii. Aromatic amino acids
iv. Acidic amino acids
v. Basic amino acids
vi. Essential amino acids
vii. Functions of plasma albumin
viii. Functions of plasma globulins
ix. A/G ratio
x. Hypoalbuminemia
xi. Hyperglobulinemia
xii. Bence Jones protein
xiii. Edema
xiv. Acute-phase proteins
xv. Alkaptonuria
xvi. Maple syrup urine disease
xvii. Phenyl-ketonuria
xviii. Hartnup's disease
xix. Deamination
xx. Hyperammonemias
xxi. Glucose alanine cycle
xxii. Primary hyperoxaluria

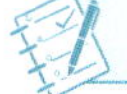

Multiple Choice Questions

1. The normal plasma albumin/globulin (A/G) ratio is:

A. 1.2 : 1 B. 2.2 : 1
C. 1 : 1.2 D. 1 : 2.2

2. Hyperglobulinemia may occur in:

A. Tuberculosis
B. Rheumatoid arthritis
C. Hepatic cirrhosis
D. All of the above

3. The following is a purely glucogenic amino acid:

A. Isoleucine B. Leucine
C. Tyrosine D. Methionine

4. In each urea molecule, the two nitrogen atoms are derived from:

A. One from ammonia, one from aspartate
B. One from ammonia, one from arginine
C. Both from ammonia
D. Both from glutamine

5. Deficiency of glycine cleavage complex leads to the following *except:*

A. Hyperglycinemia
B. Mental retardation
C. Ketosis
D. Death during infancy

6. Parkinson's disease is characterized by decreased neuronal synthesis of:

A. Acetylcholine
B. Dopamine
C. DOPA
D. Serotonin

7. Hepatorenal tyrosinemia is due to a deficiency of:

A. Tyrosine aminotransferase
B. Homogentisate oxidase
C. Tyrosinase
D. Fumarylacetoacetate hydrolase

8. In maple syrup urine disease, the typical odor of urine is due to:

A. Branched-chain amino acids
B. Branched-chain keto acids
C. Branched-chain amino acid acyl-CoA
D. Unsaturated branched-chain acyl-CoA

9. Daily urinary creatinine excretion is:

A. 0.1–0.5 g
B. 0.5–1.0 g
C. 1.0–1.5 g
D. 1.5–2.0 g

10. Rapid neuronal death during stroke is due to increased flux of the following ions through NMDA receptors:

A. Na^+
B. K^+
C. Ca^{2+}
D. Mg^{2+}

5

CHAPTER

6

Metabolism and Homeostasis

Competency Achievement: The student should be able to:

BI6.1 Discuss the metabolic processes that take place in specific organs in the body in the fed and fasting states

Metabolism is the sum of all chemical changes in the body. It consists of the sum of anabolism (synthesis) and catabolism (degradation) with the release of energy, and achieving a fairly constant internal environment referred to as homeostasis, the state of steady internal, physical and chemical conditions maintained by the living systems. The central theme of metabolism is to **extract energy from food, store excess of the energy for future needs**, and **to maintain tissue proteins** for performing various vital functions.

Homeostasis means the maintenance of internally stable conditions, in spite of changes in the person's environment. Homeostasis is often maintained by metabolic mechanisms. It is the condition of optimal functioning for the organism and includes many variables. For example, blood sugar concentration is kept **within certain preset limits**, referred to as **homeostatic range (reference range)**. When the **levels become higher** or **lower than the reference range**, it is referred to as **hyperglycemia** or **hypoglycemia**, respectively. A well-known example of a **homeostatic failure** is **type 1 diabetes mellitus**, where blood sugar regulation is unable to function, because the beta cells of the pancreatic islets are destroyed and cannot produce the necessary insulin. This, in turn, results in a rise in blood sugar level causing **hyperglycemia**.

METABOLIC PROCESSES THAT TAKE PLACE IN SPECIFIC ORGANS IN THE FED AND FASTING STATES

The homeostatic range of blood sugar is regulated within fairly narrow limits, despite changes in the environment, diet or level of physical activity. In humans, the primary **sensors** for this are the **beta cells of the islets of pancreas**, which secrete insulin.

- **In the fed state** there is an **increase in blood sugar concentration**, which in turn, stimulates the beta cells to **secrete insulin** into the blood and, simultaneously, **inhibits** the **alpha cells from secreting glucagon.**
- **In the fasting state** there is a **fall in blood glucose concentration**, which causes insulin secretion to be stopped, and glucagon to be secreted from the alpha cells into the blood. This, in turn, inhibits the uptake of glucose from the blood by the insulin sensitive cells.

  This combination, i.e. **high blood insulin** and **low glucagon levels**, act on the effector tissues, chief of which are the **liver**, **fat cells** (adipocytes) and **muscle cells**.

THE LIVER

Liver occupies a central position and maintains circulating levels of all the fuels for their oxidation by the other tissues, mainly brain and muscle. One of the important functions of the liver is to maintain blood glucose homeostasis. After a carbohydrate rich meal, i.e. in the postabsorptive state, when blood glucose concentration is high, liver takes up glucose from circulation and converts it to glucose-6-phosphate, which is used through various routes, depending upon the need of the body.

Metabolic processes that take place in the liver in the fed state

In the fed state, when blood glucose concentration is high, the **liver is inhibited from producing glucose.**

- The liver **converts glucose into glycogen** and **triglycerides**.
- The **glycogen is stored in the liver**, whereas the **triglycerides are secreted into the blood as VLDL** particles (very low density lipoprotein).
- VLDL particles are taken up **by the adipose tissue** and stored there **as triacylglycerols (fat)**
- **Amino acids**, which are absorbed **from the gut**, are taken up by the muscle and stored there as **proteins** (Fig. 6.1).

Metabolic processes that take place in the liver in the fasting state

In the fasting state, a **fall in blood glucose** concentration causes **insulin secretion to be stopped** and **glucagon to be secreted** from the alpha cells into the blood. This, in turn, **inhibits the uptake of glucose** from the blood by the liver, fat cells and muscle.

- The liver is strongly stimulated to **release glucose from glycogen**, through **glycogenolysis.**
- The glucose **synthesis** is also stimulated **from non-carbohydrate sources**, such as **glucogenic amino acids** (received by the liver as a result of proteolysis of tissue proteins, mainly the muscle) and **glycerol** (obtained from adipose tissue, as a result of hydrolysis of triacylglycerols), **by the process of gluconeogenesis**.
- The **glucose**, thus produced, is **released into the blood**, thereby correcting hypoglycemia and is also **transported to the brain** for its use there.
- A fall in the circulating concentration of insulin also results in the **release of free fatty acids** (from triacylglycerols) **from the adipose tissue**. These are **taken up by the liver and muscle**.
- Peripheral **muscles** and **liver** consume, progressively, less glucose and **switch-over to fatty acids** as the main **source of energy**.

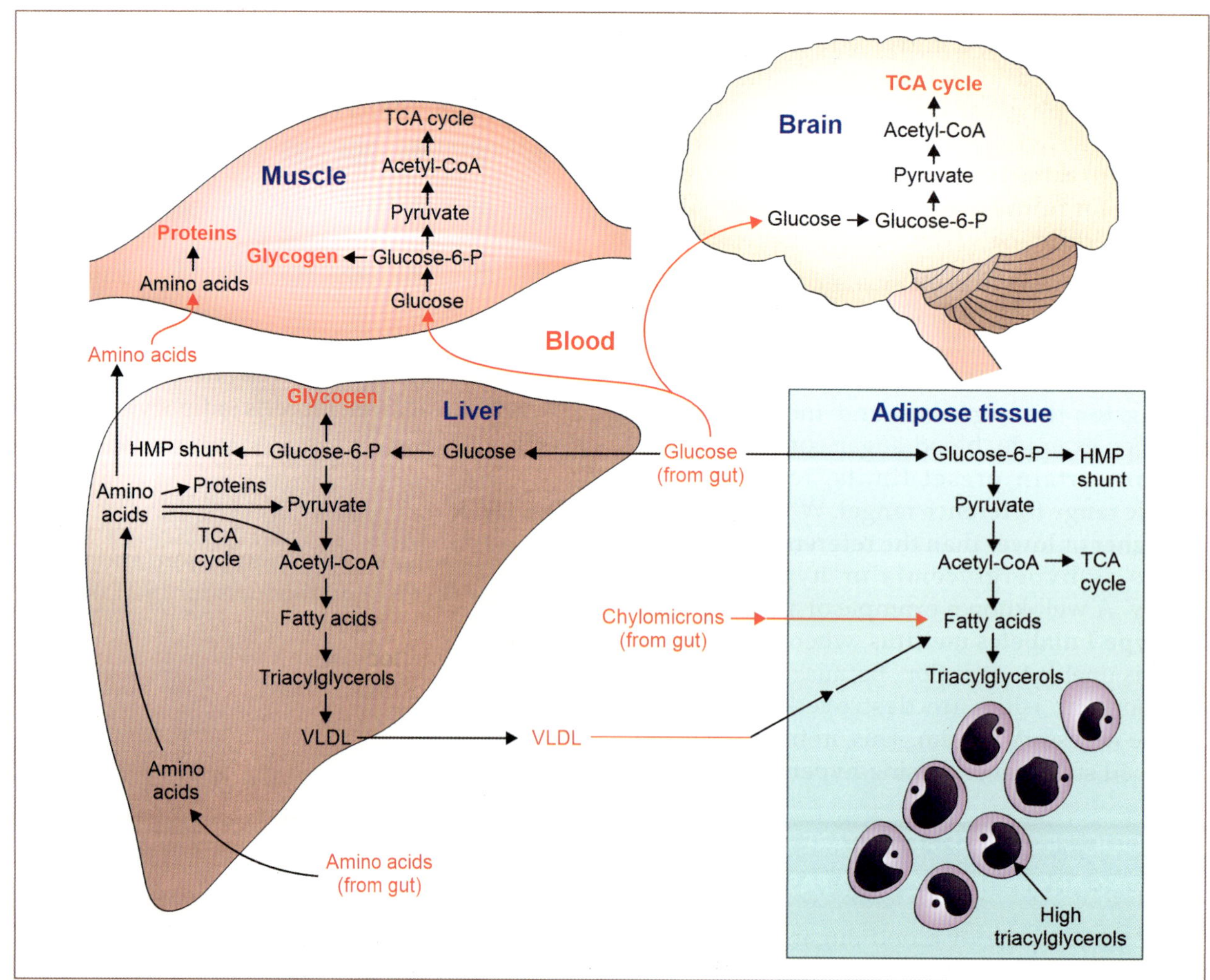

Fig. 6.1: Metabolic processes that take place in the specific organs in the fed state

6

- This, in turn, promotes β-oxidation of fatty acids, increases the production of acetyl-CoA and **stimulates ketogenesis**. As a result of it, plasma concentration of ketone bodies is increased.
- **Ketone bodies** are **released into the blood** are **used by** many tissues, including **muscle** and **brain** (Fig. 6.2).

THE ADIPOSE TISSUE

The adipose tissue, also known as **fat cells**, is a loose connective tissue composed, mostly, of **adipocytes** that are specialized in **storing energy, as triacylglycerols** (fat).

There are two types of adipose tissue, known as **white adipose tissue** (which stores energy) and **brown adipose tissue** (which generates body heat).

White adipose tissue is widely distributed throughout the body but is most prominent under the skin, and in the abdominal cavity and skeletal muscle. The main role of the white adipose tissue is to store energy (in the form of triacylglycerols) and release fatty acids, when needed.

Metabolic processes that take place in the adipose tissue in the fed state

- Adipocytes **take up glucose through GLUT4** (the special glucose transporters, whose number in the cell wall is increased as a direct effect of insulin acting on these cells).
- The **glucose** that enters the fat cells, in this manner, **is converted into triglycerides** (via the same metabolic pathways as used by the liver), which are **stored there**, together with the VLDL-derived triglycerides (from the liver) as well as in chylomicrons from the gut (Fig. 6.1).

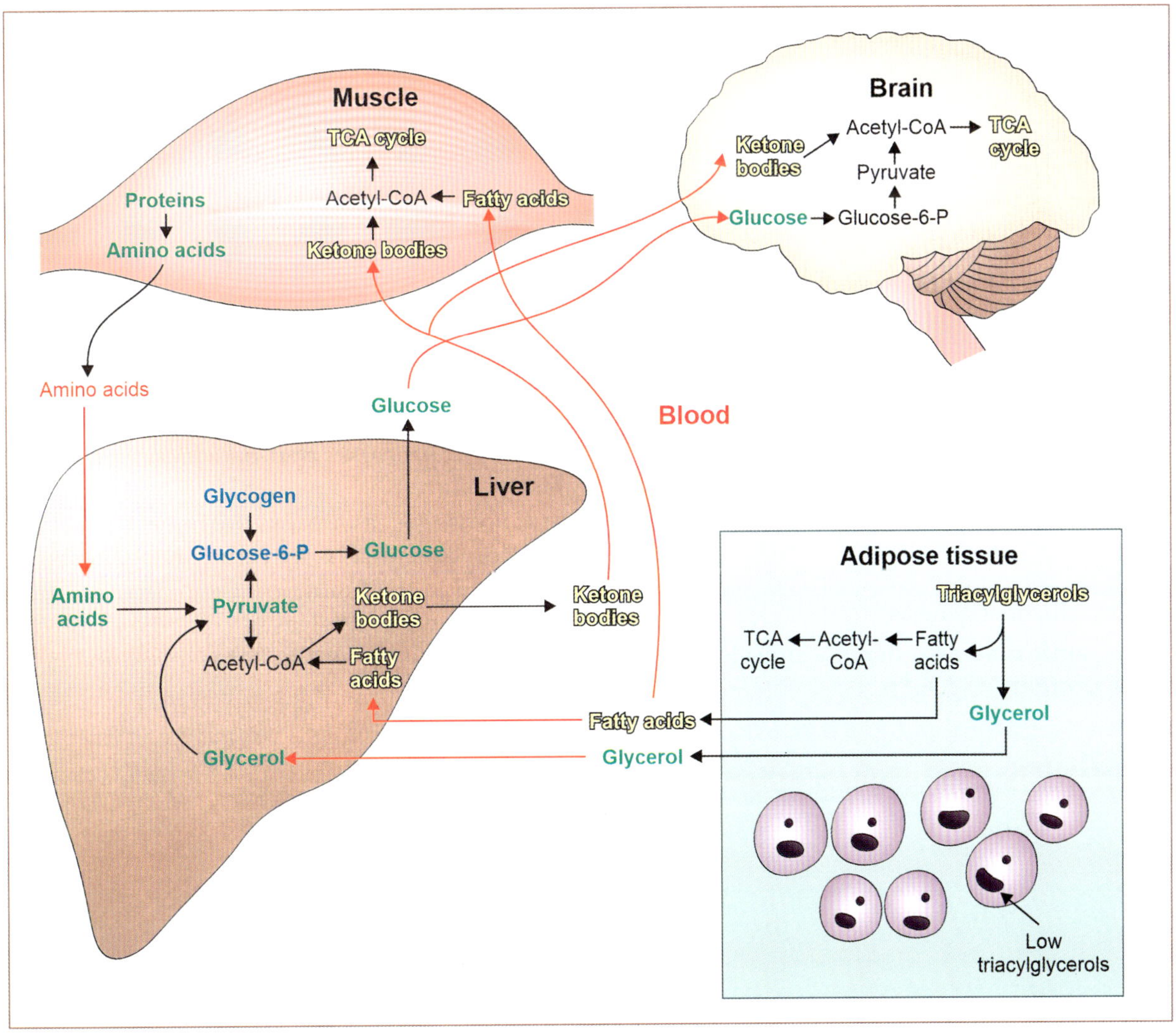

Fig. 6.2: Metabolic processes that take place in the specific organs in the fasting state

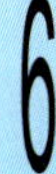

Metabolic processes that take place in the adipose tissue in the fasting state

- A fall in the circulating concentration of insulin **promotes lipolysis in the adipose tissue** and **releases free fatty acids**, and **glycerol** (from triacylglycerols), **which enter liver**.
- **Fatty acids** also **enter muscle** and are consumed there as the main source of energy (Fig. 6.2).

THE MUSCLE

The muscle cell, also known as **myocyte**, is the type of cell found in muscle tissue. Myocytes develop from **myoblasts** to form muscles in a process known as myogenesis. There are two specialized forms of **myocytes** with distinct properties, **cardiac** and **smooth muscle cells**. On the other hand, **skeletal muscles** are formed by morphological units referred to as **muscle fibers**.

- **Cardiomyocytes** are the cells that form the chambers of the heart, and have a single central nucleus.
- **Skeletal muscle** fibers help support and move the body.
- **Smooth muscle cells** control involuntary movements, such as the peristalsis contractions in the esophagus and stomach.

Metabolic processes that take place in muscles in the fed state

- Skeletal muscle, similar to live, **takes up glucose**, through insulin-sensitive GLUT4, and **converts it to glycogen**, which is stored there. The **glycogen stored in the muscle remains in the muscle**, and is **only broken down during exercise**, to glucose-6-phosphate and thence, to pyruvate (to be used in the citric acid cycle) and lactate (which is returned to the blood, taken up by the liver and converted to glucose by gluconeogenesis).
- Via liver, **amino acids** enter the muscle and are **stored as proteins** (Fig. 6.1).

Metabolic processes that take place in muscles in the fasting state

- **Free fatty acids** (released from triacylglycerols) are taken up by the muscle and **are used** as the **source of energy**.
- **Ketone bodies, released from liver into the blood**, are also **used by muscle** as a source of energy.
- **Proteins are degraded** and the **amino acids are transported to the liver**, where they are used for the **synthesis of glucose**, **by** the process of **gluconeogenesis** (Fig. 6.2).

THE BRAIN

The brain, particularly, the **hypothalamus**, plays a key role in the homeostatic regulation of energy and glucose metabolism. It modulates various aspects of metabolism, such as food intake, energy expenditure, insulin secretion, hepatic glucose production and glucose/fatty acid metabolism in the adipose tissue and the skeletal muscle. The brain also integrates metabolic signals from peripheral tissues (such as the liver, pancreas, adipose tissue, gut and muscle) and modulates various processes that consume energy (such as locomotor activity, fatty acid oxidation in the skeletal muscle, and thermogenesis).

Metabolic processes that take place in the brain in the fed state

Glucose is the primary fuel of the brain under normal conditions and that it requires a steady supply of glucose from the blood.

Metabolic processes that take place in the brain in the fasting state

- **Glucose**, released **from the liver** (formed **as a result of glycogenolysis** and **gluconeogenesis**), is **transported to the brain**, for use in there.
- **Ketone bodies, released from liver into the blood**, are also **used by** the brain as a source of energy (Fig. 6.2).

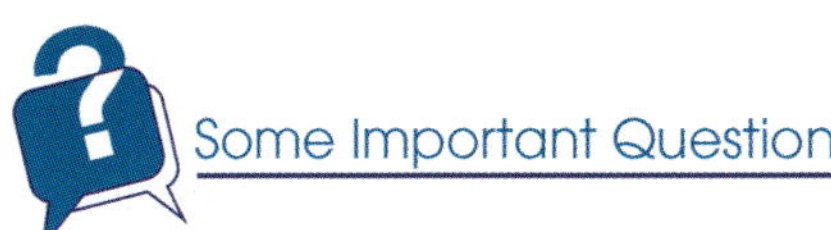

Some Important Questions

1. **Discuss the metabolic processes that take place in specific organs in the body in the fed and fasting states.**
2. **Write notes on:**
   i. Metabolic processes that take place in the liver in the fed state
   ii. Metabolic processes that take place in the liver in the fasting state

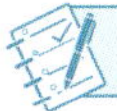

Multiple Choice Questions

1. **In a healthy 70 kg man, the fat content in adipose tissue is:**
   A. 5 kg B. 15 kg
   C. 25 kg D. 35 kg
2. **The preferred fuel for adipose tissue is:**
   A. Glucose B. Fatty acids
   C. Amino acids D. Ketone bodies
3. **The preferred fuel for exercising skeletal muscle is:**
   A. Glucose B. Fatty acids
   C. Amino acids D. Ketone bodies
4. **During exercise, the following is released from muscles into the circulation:**
   A. Glucose
   B. Ketone bodies
   C. Lactate
   D. Glycerol
5. **During starvation, the following is released from muscles into the circulation:**
   A. Glucose
   B. Ketone bodies
   C. Glycerol
   D. Branched-chain amino acids

CHAPTER 7

Chemistry and Metabolism of Nucleotides

Competency Achievement: **The student should be able to:**

BI6.2 Describe and discuss the metabolic processes in which nucleotides are involved
BI6.3 Describe the common disorders associated with nucleotide metabolism
BI6.4 Discuss the laboratory results of analytes associated with gout and Lesch-Nyhan syndrome

A **nucleotide** has 3 components, i.e. a pentose sugar, a nitrogenous base and phosphoric acid.

PENTOSE SUGARS

The presence of a pentose sugar defines the type of the nucleotide (such as nucleotide or deoxynucleotide) and nucleic acid (i.e. deoxyribonucleic acid or DNA, and ribonucleic acid or RNA). A nucleotide contains ribose sugar while a deoxynucleotide contains deoxyribose sugar.

- **Ribose** has three –OH groups at carbon numbers 1, 2 and 3 of the pentose molecule.
- **Deoxyribose**, on the other hand, does not contain an oxygen atom at the second carbon and thus has only two –OH groups, i.e. at carbon atoms, 1 and 3. Deoxyribose, thus, is also called 2-deoxyribose (Fig. 7.1).

  The sugar molecule is linked to a nitrogenous base on one side (through carbon atom one, i.e. C1) and to phosphoric acid on the other side (through carbon atom five, i.e. C5).

  To differentiate between the carbon atoms of a sugar molecule from the carbon atoms of the nitrogenous base, in the nomenclature of a nucleotide, the position of the carbon atom of the sugar moiety is represented by a sign called **prime (′)**. These are, thus, written as C1′ or C5′, etc. On the other hand, the carbon and the nitrogen atoms of the nitrogenous bases are written without the prime sign, such as N1 or C2, etc.

Ribose 2-Deoxyribose

Fig. 7.1: Sugars present in nucleic acids

NITROGENOUS BASES

Nitrogenous bases found in various nucleotides are either the derivatives of a purine ring or of a pyrimidine ring.

- A **Purine ring** is a nine-membered ring containing 5 carbon and 4 nitrogen atoms, whereas a **pyrimidine ring** is a six-membered ring which has 4 carbon and 2 nitrogen atoms (Fig. 7.2).

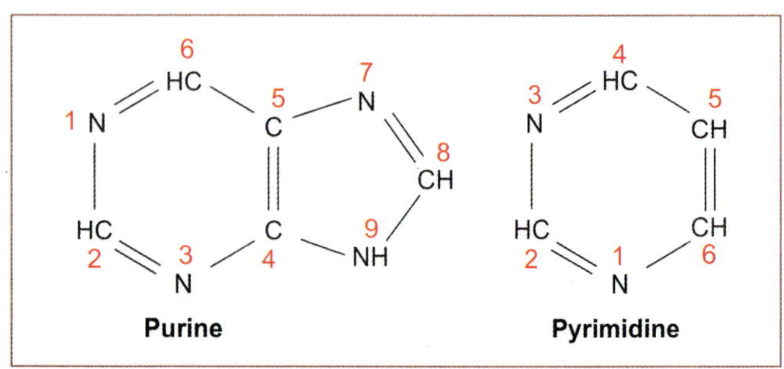

Fig. 7.2: Purine and pyrimidine rings

Various nitrogenous bases are formed with the appropriate substitutions on the parent heterocyclic ring, and are accordingly called the derivatives of purines and pyrimidines.

- **Purines:** There are two types of purine bases present in nucleic acids, viz. **adenine** (6-aminopurine) and **guanine** (2-amino-6-oxypurine).
- **Pyrimidines:** The pyrimidine bases, found in nucleic acids, are designated as **cytosine** (2-oxy-4-amino-pyrimidine), **uracil** (2,4-dioxypyrimidine) and **thymine** (2, 4-dioxy-5-methylpyrimidine, also called 5-methyluracil; Fig. 7.3).

Out of these three pyrimidines, only two are repeatedly found in a nucleic acid. Usually, cytosine and uracil are found in RNA while cytosine and thymine are found in DNA.

Unusual Nitrogenous Bases

- Besides the four nitrogenous bases (2 purines and 2 pyrimidines), which are commonly found in nucleic acids, there also occur some unusual nitrogenous bases in nucleic acids of certain bacteria and viruses. These are called minor bases, e.g. **5-methylcytosine, 5-hydroxymethylcytosine, pseudo-uracil** (where structural positions of N1 and C5 in the uracil molecule are interchanged), **N6-methy-ladenine, N7-methylguanine**, etc. (Fig. 7.4).

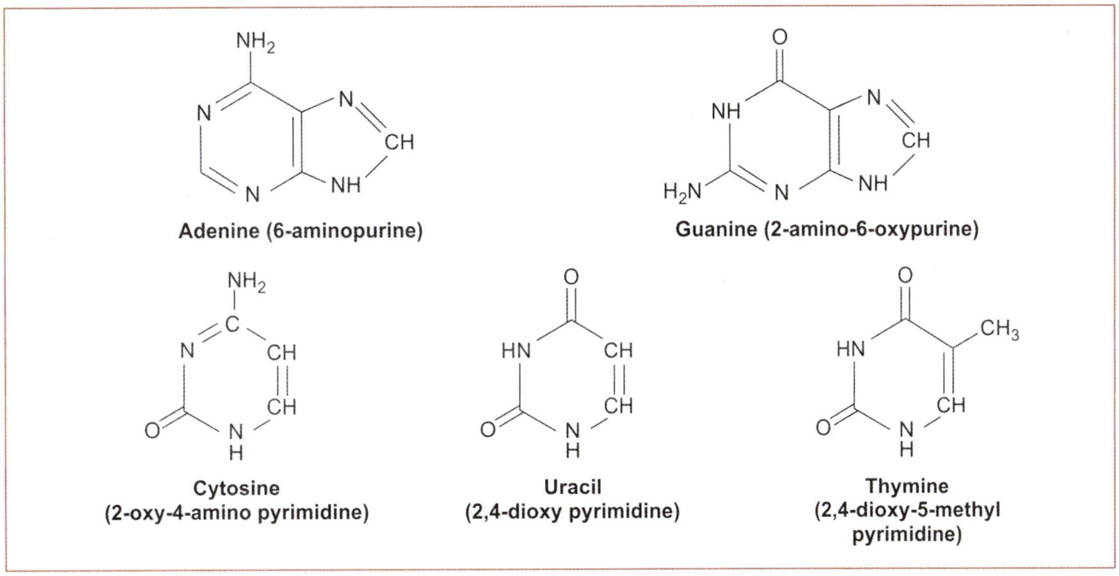

Adenine (6-aminopurine)

Guanine (2-amino-6-oxypurine)

Cytosine (2-oxy-4-amino pyrimidine)

Uracil (2,4-dioxy pyrimidine)

Thymine (2,4-dioxy-5-methyl pyrimidine)

Fig. 7.3: Nitrogenous bases found in nucleic acids

5-Methylcytosine

5-Hydroxymethylcytosine

Dihydrouracil

N^6-Methyladenine

N^7-Methylguanine

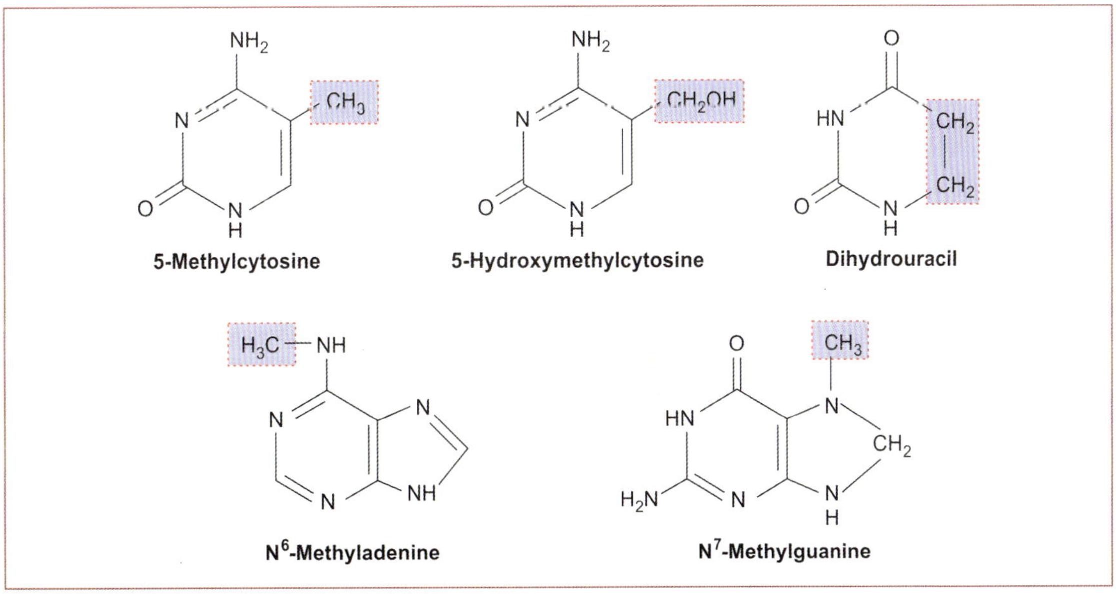

Fig. 7.4: Some unusual nitrogenous bases found in nucleic acids

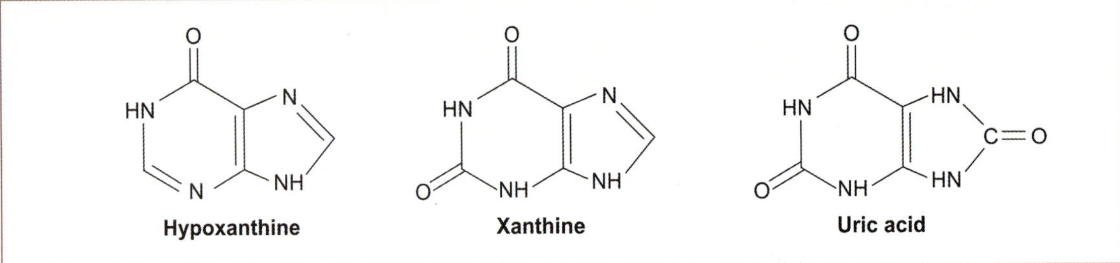

Fig. 7.5: Some purine bases of metabolic significance

- There are also some other purine derivatives which are of biological significance. These are either found as intermediates in purine biosynthesis, e.g. **hypoxanthine** and **xanthine**, or as the end product of their catabolism, such as **uric acid** (Fig. 7.5).

NUCLEOSIDES

A nucleoside has two components, i.e. it consists of a **nitrogenous base** and a molecule of **sugar**. In a nucleoside, a pentose sugar (ribose or deoxyribose) is linked to a nitrogenous base by an N-glycosidic linkage. The first carbon atom of the sugar moiety (C1) is linked either with the N1 of a pyrimidine or with N9 of a purine.

Base – N – (1/9)–C′ – **Sugar**

- **Ribonucleosides**
  - The nucleosides of ribose are called ribonucleosides. Ribonucleosides of adenine, guanine, cytosine and uracil are designated as **adenosine**, **guanosine**, **cytidine** and **uridine**, respectively (Fig. 7.6).

Adenosine has attained considerable clinical importance (Chemistry to Clinics 7.1).

Chemistry to Clinics 7.1: Significance of Adenosine

- Adenosine is a local hormone, known as an **autacoid**. During exercise, contracting muscles release adenosine which causes local vasodilation, thereby enhancing the supply of nutrients including oxygen to the muscles.
- Adenosine participates in sleep regulation. Prolonged wakefulness increases the extracellular adenosine levels in the brain which induce sleepiness by binding to specific adenosine receptors. Interestingly, this interaction is blocked by caffeine, explaining the tendency of coffee to promote wakefulness.
- Intravenous administration of adenosine is employed in the emergency treatment of supraventricular tachycardia characterized by uncontrolled rapid heartbeats (Fig. 7.7).

Deoxyribonucleosides

- Nucleosides of deoxyribose are designated as deoxyribonucleosides. Various deoxyribonucleosides are written with a prefix d-(deoxy). Thus,

Fig. 7.6: Ribonucleosides

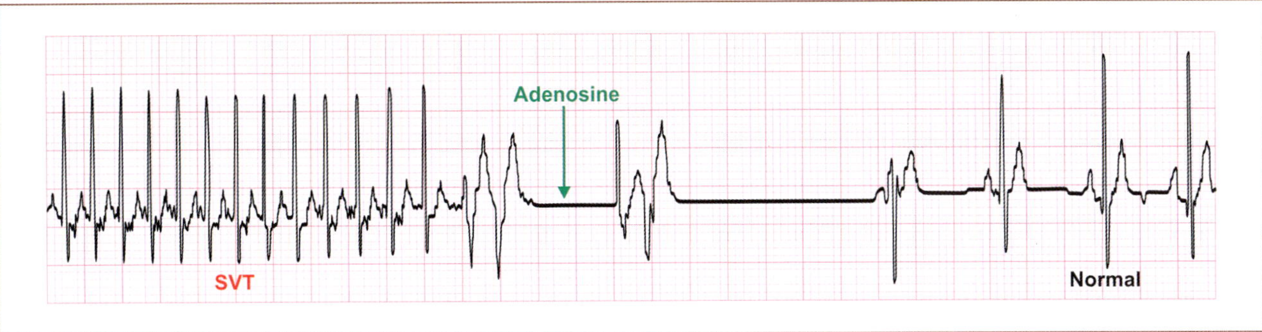

Fig. 7.7: ECG showing supraventricular tachycardia (SVT: Abnormally rapid heart rate which may be life-threatening) being normalized by intravenous **adenosine**

deoxyadenosine, deoxyguanosine, deoxycytidine and **deoxythymidine** are the nucleosides of deoxyribose with adenine, guanine, cytosine, and thymine respectively. Since thymine is usually found in DNA where it is linked to a deoxyribose only, its nucleoside is commonly designated as thymidine and not deoxythymidine (Fig. 7.8).

NUCLEOTIDES

In a nucleotide, the **sugar** molecule (ribose or deoxyribose) is linked both to a **nitrogenous base** on one side and to **phosphoric acid** on the other side. As in a nucleoside, C1 of the sugar molecule is linked to a nitrogenous base either through N1 of a pyrimidine or N9 of a purine. The sugar is also linked to phosphoric acid. Although any hydroxyl group (–OH) of the sugar can get esterified with phosphoric acid, more commonly C5 of the sugar is linked to a phosphate moiety.

Base – N – (1/9) –C1′ – **Sugar** – 5′ – **Phosphate**

During hydrolysis of a nucleic acid, the phosphate moiety may get attached even onto the –OH group at C3′, forming deoxyribonucleoside-3′-monophosphate (dN-3′-MP). The N refers to a nucleoside of any nitrogenous base.

In a ribose, since the –OH group is also present at C2′, in addition to N-3′-MP (nucleoside-3′-monophosphate) and N-5′-MP, N-2′-MP is also obtained during hydrolysis of an RNA molecule.

Ribonucleotides

- A nucleotide containing a ribose sugar is called ribonucleotide. Four ribonucleotides obtained on hydrolysis of RNA are designated as adenosine monophosphate or adenylate (**AMP**), guanylate (**GMP**), cytidylate (**CMP**) and uridylate (**UMP**; Fig. 7.9).

Deoxyribonucleotides

- The corresponding deoxyribonucleotides obtained on hydrolysis of a DNA molecule are designated as **dAMP, dGMP, dCMP** and **TMP**, respectively. Some of the deoxyribonucleotides are shown in Fig. 7.10.
- Various nitrogenous bases, nucleosides and nucleotides found in nucleic acids are shown in Table 7.1.

Fig. 7.8: Deoxyribonucleosides

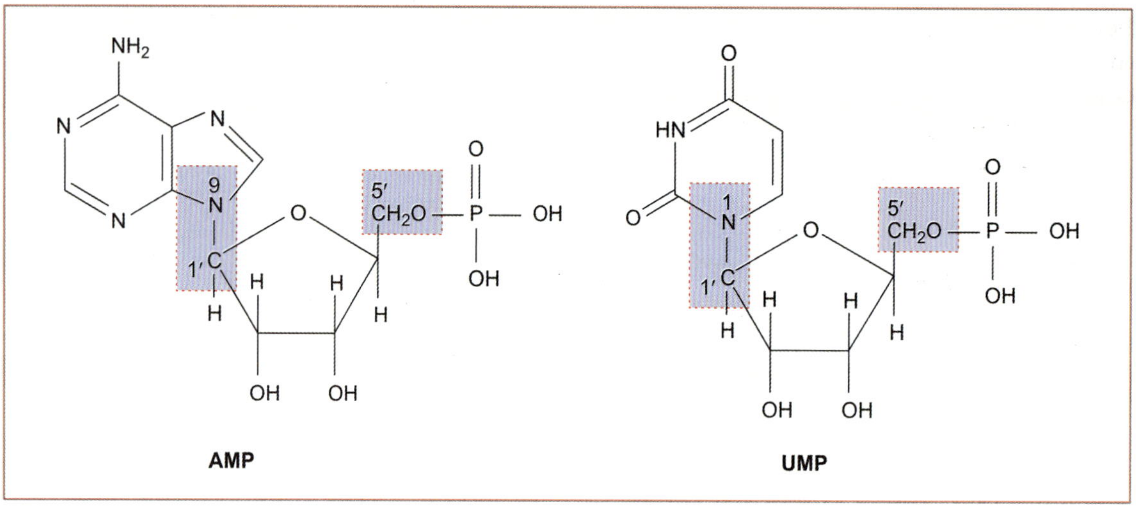

Fig. 7.9: Ribonucleotides

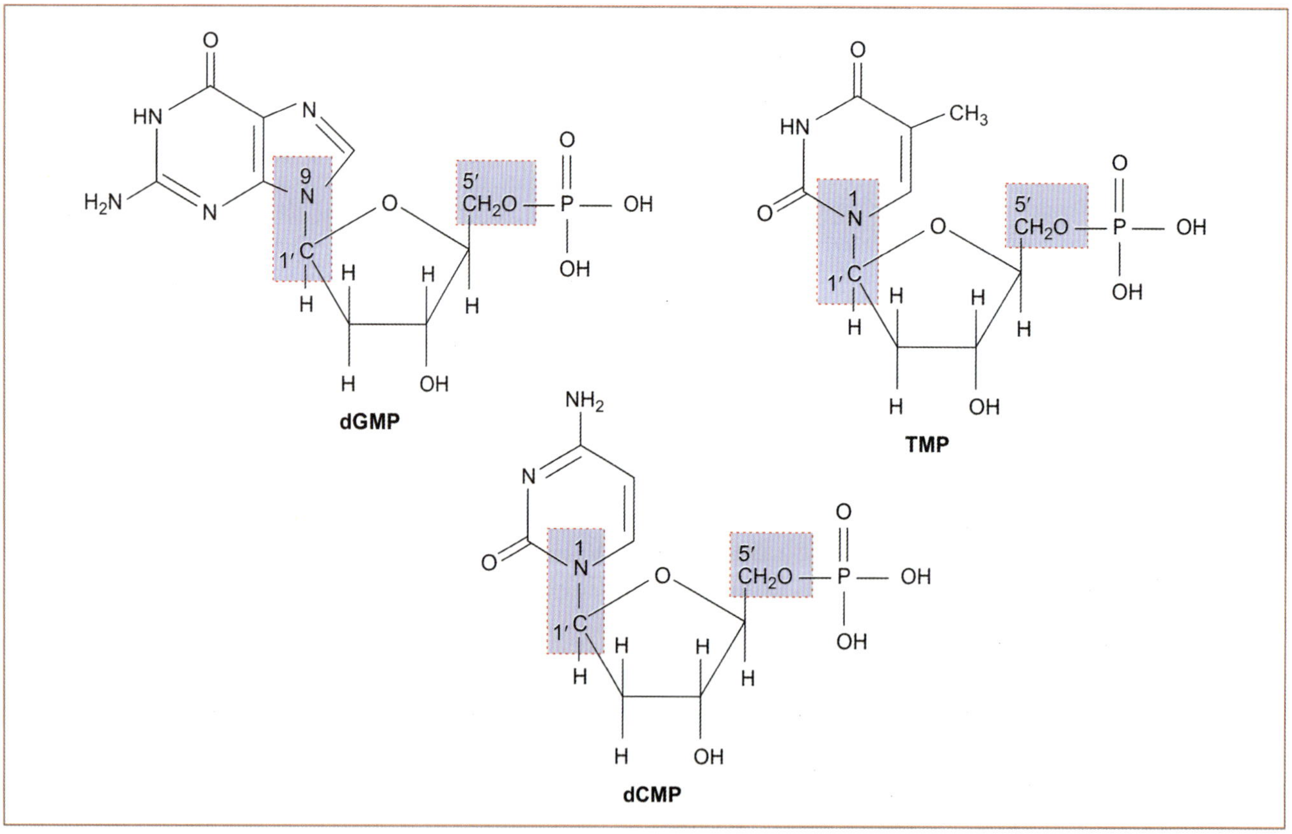

Fig. 7.10: Deoxyribonucleotides

7

Nucleotide Derivatives of Biological Significance

Besides the nucleotides of adenine, guanine, cytosine, uracil or thymine which are the hydrolyzed products of nucleic acids, there also occur di- and triphosphate derivatives of various nucleosides, e.g. ADP, ATP, GTP, CTP, UTP, etc. (Fig. 7.11).

Pharmacologically Active Purine/Pyrimidine Analogs

Any alteration either in the purine or pyrimidine ring, or in the sugar moiety, results in the production of various pharmacologically active compounds. When they get incorporated into the nucleic acid, they show toxic effects.

Some of them are inhibitory to several enzymes in DNA replication, inhibit DNA synthesis, and thus, are of therapeutic significance (Chemistry to Clinics 7.2).

Some analogs of sugar moiety, such as arabinosylcytosine (cytosine with arabinose instead of cytidine which contains cytosine and ribose) are also used in cancer chemotherapy (Fig. 7.12).

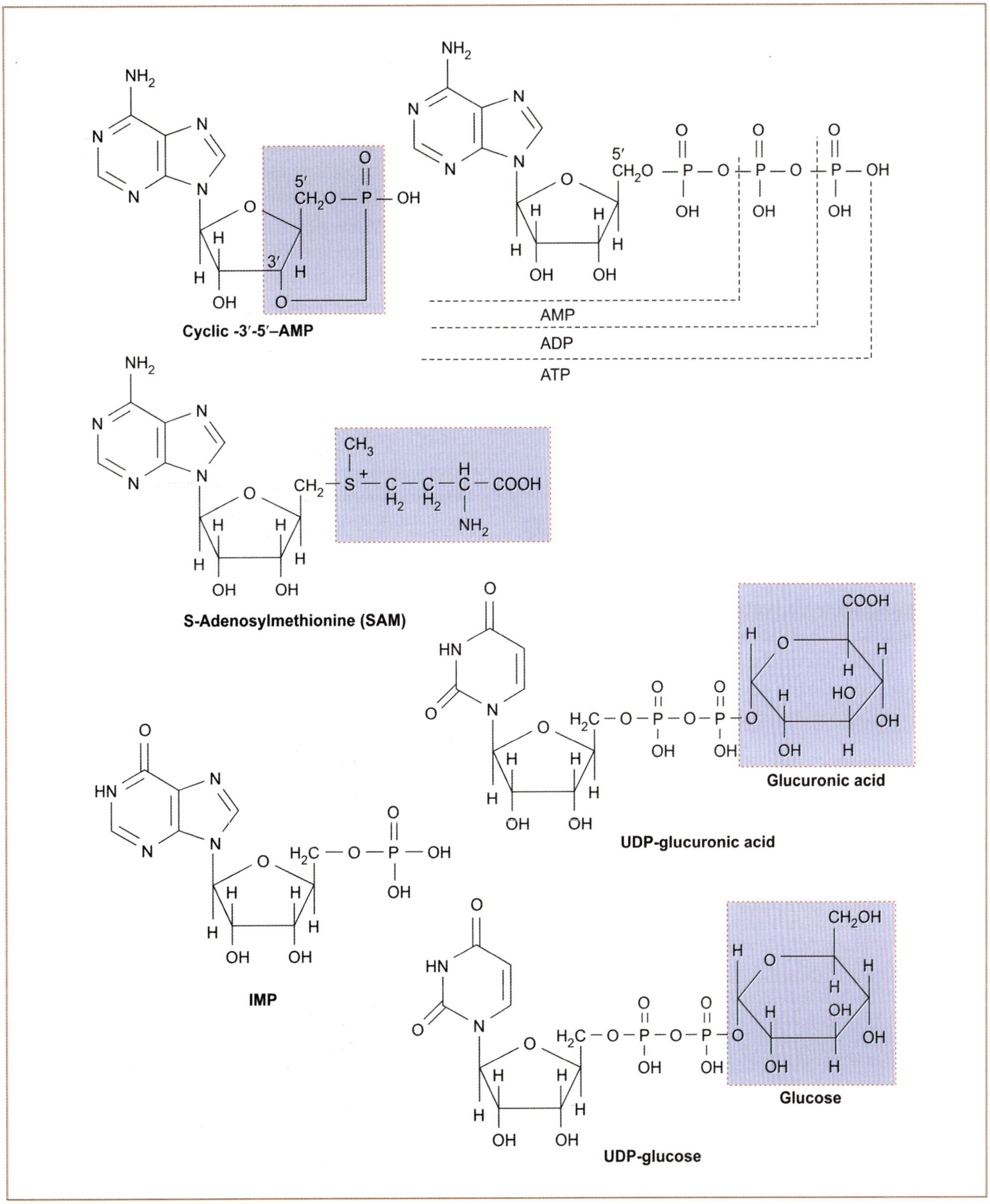

Cyclic -3′-5′–AMP

AMP

ADP

ATP

S-Adenosylmethionine (SAM)

Glucuronic acid

UDP-glucuronic acid

IMP

Glucose

UDP-glucose

Fig. 7.11: Some nucleotide derivatives of biological significance

Table 7.1: Different nitrogenous bases, nucleosides and nucleotides found in nucleic acids

Nitrogenous base	Nucleoside (base + sugar)	Nucleotide (base + sugar + P)
RNA		
Adenine	Adenosine	AMP
Guanine	Guanosine	GMP
Cytosine	Cytidine	CMP
Uracil	Uridine	UMP
DNA		
Adenine	Deoxyadenosine	dAMP
Guanine	Deoxyguanosine	dGMP
Cytosine	Deoxycytidine	dCMP
Thymine	Thymidine	TMP

Chemistry to Clinics 7.2: Purine/Pyrimidine analogs used as Drugs

Some of the synthetic analogs, such as 5-fluorouracil (a derivative of pyrimidine with the analogous heterocyclic ring), 6-thioguanine and 6-mercaptopurine (sulfur substituted analogs of purine) are used as anticancer drugs. Allopurinol (4-hydroxy-pyrazolopyrimidine, an analog of purine) is an inhibitor of xanthine oxidase and is used in the treatment of hyperuricemia.

METABOLIC PROCESSES IN WHICH NUCLEOTIDES ARE INVOLVED

Nucleotides and their derivatives play important role in several metabolic processes:

- **Synthesis of nucleic acids: Ribonucleotides** (AMP, GMP, CMP and UMP) and **deoxyribonucleotides** (dAMP, dGMP, dCMP and TMP) are the **monomeric units of nucleic acids**. These are obtained on hydrolysis of RNA and DNA, respectively. At the same time **ribonucleotide triphosphates** (ATP, GTP, CTP and UTP) and **deoxyribonucleotide triphosphates** (dATP, dGTP, dCTP and TTP) are used in the **synthesis of RNA** and **DNA**, respectively.
- **As energy currency of cell:** Nucleotide triphosphate, e.g. **ATP** is **the energy currency of cell.**
- **As metabolic precursors:** Some of the nucleotide triphosphates are used as metabolic precursors, e.g. **GTP for tetrahydrobiopterin synthesis**.
- **Act as allosteric effectors:** Some of the nucleotides **act as allosteric effectors**. For example, hexokinase is allosterically activated by ADP but inhibited by ATP.
- **Act as second messenger: Cyclic nucleotides act as physiological mediators**, e.g. cAMP acts as second messenger for epinephrine.
- **Components of coenzymes:** Some of the **nucleotide derivatives act as components of coenzymes**, e.g. NAD, FAD, etc.
- **Activated metabolic intermediates:** Some **nucleotide derivatives act as activated metabolic intermediates**, e.g. S-adenosylmethionine (SAM).
- **Used in the interconversion of monosaccharides:** Some of the nucleotide derivatives, such as UDP-glucose and UDP-galactose are used in the **interconversion of monosaccharides**.
- **Used as a carrier of monosaccharide unit:** Some of the nucleotide derivatives, such as UDP-glucose and

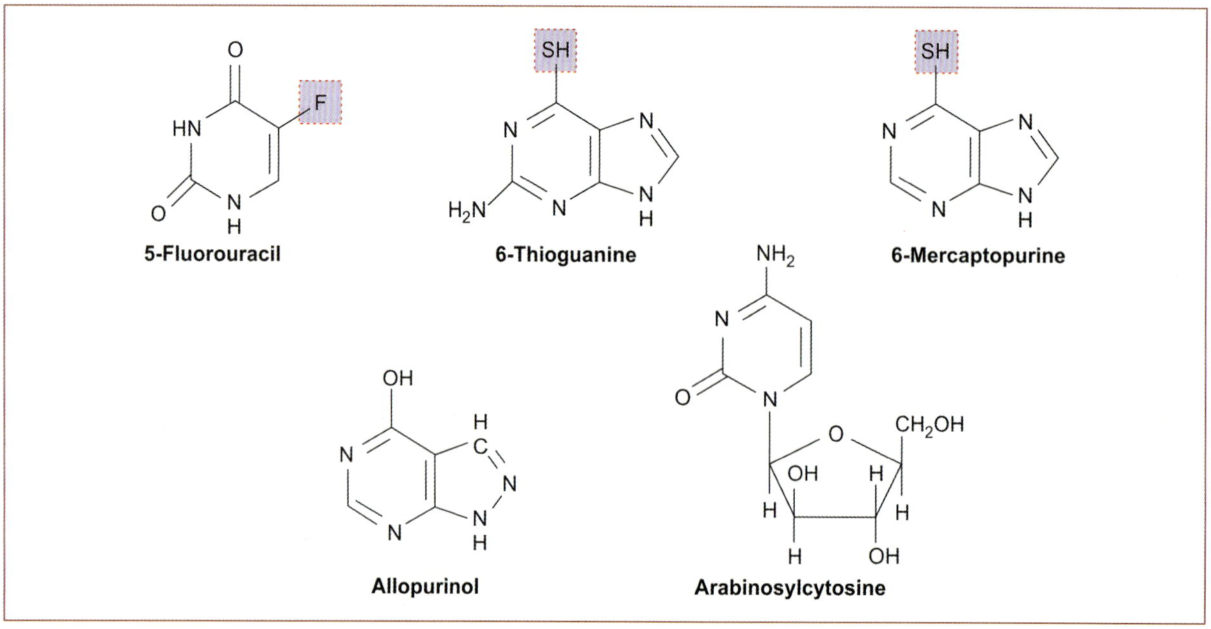

Fig. 7.12: Some pharmacologically active pyrimidines/purine analogs

UDP-galactose are also **used in glycogenesis** and **lactose synthesis**.

- **Used in conjugation reactions:** Some of the nucleotide derivatives are also used in **conjugation reactions**, e.g. UDP-glucuronic acid, for the conjugation of bilirubin.
- **Used as anticancer drugs:** Some of the **synthetic analogs**, such as 5-fluorouracil, are used **as anticancer drugs**.
- **Used in the treatment of hyperuricemia: Allopurinol** (an analog of purine) acts as an inhibitor of xanthine oxidase and is used in the **treatment of hyperuricemia**.

COMMON DISORDERS ASSOCIATED WITH NUCLEOTIDE METABOLISM

All cells can synthesize nucleotides, either by the biosynthetic process, called ***de novo*** synthesis, or from the degradation products of nucleic acids, i.e. free bases and nucleosides, by the process called **salvage pathway**.

METABOLISM OF PURINE NUCLEOTIDES

Synthesis of Purine Nucleotides

De novo Synthesis of Purine Nucleotides

The process of synthesis of complex end product(s) in a metabolic pathway from simple precursor molecules is called *de novo* synthesis (*de novo* = 'anew', i.e. starting 'from scratch'). A purine ring is synthesized, as a part of the nucleotide inosine-monophosphate (IMP), by utilizing three amino acids (aspartate, glutamine and glycine) as carbon and nitrogen donors, besides respiratory CO_2 (HCO_3–) and two 1C moieties (transferred via tetrahydrofolate, FH_4) as the carbon sources.

Accordingly, the N1 of a purine ring is derived from the amino group ($-NH_2$) of aspartate, C2 and C8 from N^{10}-formyltetrahydrofolate (N^{10}-formyl-FH_4), N3 and N9 from amide nitrogen ($-CONH_2$) of glutamine, C6 from CO_2 (HCO_3^-), and C4, C5 and N7 from glycine (Fig. 7.13).

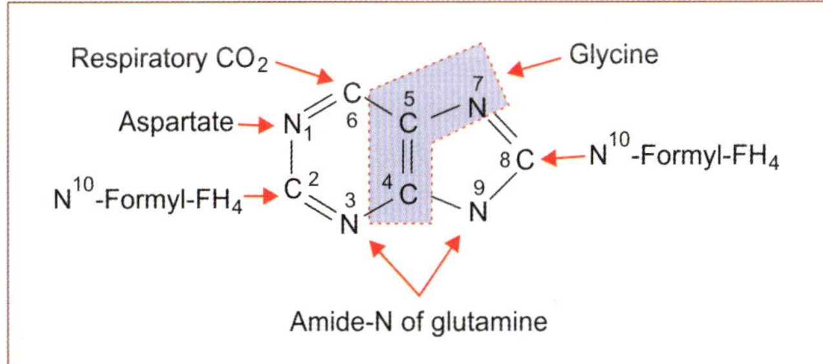

Fig. 7.13: Sources of carbon and nitrogen atoms in a purine ring

Synthesis of IMP

The starting material for the synthesis of a purine ring (IMP) is phosphoribosyl pyrophosphate (PRPP). PRPP is synthesized by the addition of pyrophosphate from ATP, onto ribose-5-phosphate (produced in the HMP shunt). This reaction is catalyzed by phosphoribosyl pyrophosphate synthetase (PRPP synthetase), also called ribose phosphate pyrophosphokinase, which is inhibited by, both, ADP as well as GDP (Fig. 7.14).

PRPP is used as a starting material, not only for the synthesis of purines but also for pyrimidines. PRPP is also used in the utilization of purine and pyrimidine bases by the salvage pathway.

1. The first step in IMP synthesis is the formation of 5'-phospho-ribosylamine. The reaction is catalyzed by an amido-transferase (glutamine PRPP amido-transferase), also called phosphoribosylamine synthetase. Pyrophosphate group is replaced by the amide nitrogen of glutamine. This, in turn, results in the acquisition of N9 of the purine ring and is a committed step. The rate of the reaction is controlled by intracellular concentrations of both the substrates, i.e. glutamine as well as PRPP.
2. In the next step, glycine gets conjugated with the amino group of phosphoribosylamine and forms 5-phosphoribosylglycinamide. The reaction is catalyzed by phosphoribosylglycinamide synthetase.
3. In the next reaction, N^{10}-formyl-FH_4 donates a formyl group and results in the formation of 5-phosphoribosylformylglycinamide. The reaction is catalyzed by formyltransferase or transformylase (phosphoribosylglycinamide transformylase).
4. Thereafter, through a series of reactions, **IMP** is synthesized as the **first purine nucleotide**.

Various enzymes involved in the synthesis of a purine nucleotide are found in the **cytosol** of a cell whereas energy, to drive some of these reactions, is obtained from the hydrolysis of ATP. During this process 6 moles of ATP are utilized per mole of IMP synthesized. This implies that the ***de novo*** synthesis of purines is **costly** in terms of the energy investment.

Synthesis of AMP and GMP

IMP serves as a common precursor for the synthesis of AMP as well as GMP (Fig. 7.15).

- **Synthesis of AMP:** IMP reacts with aspartate and is changed to adenylosuccinate (AMPS). The reaction is catalyzed by adenylosuccinate synthetase. Thereafter, adenylosuccinase (adenylosuccinate lyase) removes fumarate and forms AMP. Adeny-

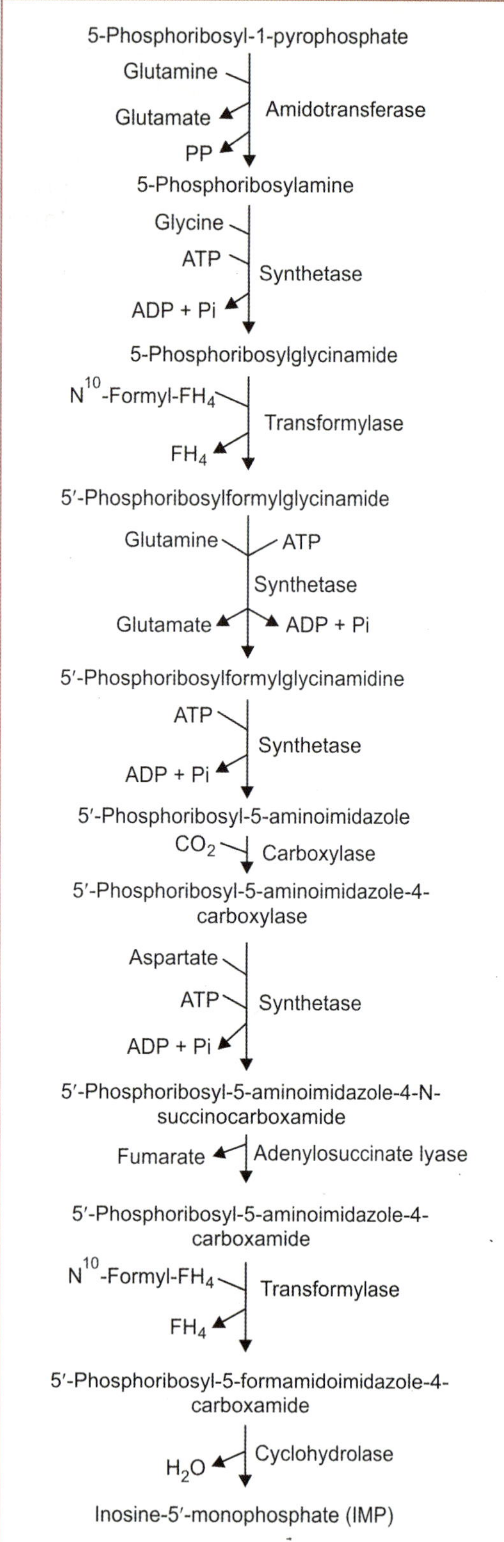

Fig. 7.14: Synthesis of IMP

losuccinate synthetase is a rate-limiting enzyme with AMP acting as a competitive inhibitor. GTP is used as a source of energy.

- **Synthesis of GMP:** IMP is converted to xanthosine monophosphate (XMP) by IMP dehydrogenase. Thereafter, GMP synthetase converts XMP to GMP. IMP dehydrogenase is a rate-limiting enzyme. It is regulated by GMP which acts as a competitive inhibitor for the enzyme.

  Formation of GMP from IMP requires ATP as a source of energy.

Regulation of biosynthesis of purine nucleotides: Biosynthesis of IMP is regulated at the first step of the pathway by the availability of ribose-5-phosphate and hence PRPP.

- The reaction catalyzed by **amidotransferase is a committed step**, i.e. the site of metabolic regulation. The enzyme glutamine: PRPP amidotransferase is regulated, allosterically, by the end products of the pathway, i.e. by IMP, GMP and AMP which serve as negative effectors. On the other hand, PRPP is a positive effector for the enzyme.
- Biosynthesis of AMP and GMP from IMP is also regulated. Both, AMP and GMP are competitive inhibitors of IMP in their own synthesis. From IMP to GMP, **IMP dehydrogenase is the rate limiting enzyme**. It is regulated by GMP which acts as a competitive inhibitor. Adenylosuccinate synthetase is a rate limiting enzyme in the conversion of IMP to AMP where AMP acts as a competitive inhibitor.
- The rate of GMP synthesis increases with the concentration of ATP while that of the AMP increases with the concentration of GTP (Fig. 7.16).

Salvage Pathway for Purine Nucleotides Synthesis

In mammals, **free purine bases**, i.e. hypoxanthine, guanine and adenine as well as their nucleosides can also be converted to the corresponding nucleotides in the salvage pathway.

The conversion of free base to the respective nucleotide requires phosphoribosyl transferase and PRPP as a source of ribose-5-phosphate. For the salvage, adenine mainly arises from the synthesis of polyamines, i.e. from 5'-methylthioadenosine. On the other hand, hypoxanthine and guanine arise from the degradation of purine nucleotides.

- **Adenine** is converted to AMP by adenine phosphoribosyltransferase (APRTase), whereas both **hypoxanthine** and **guanine** are converted to IMP

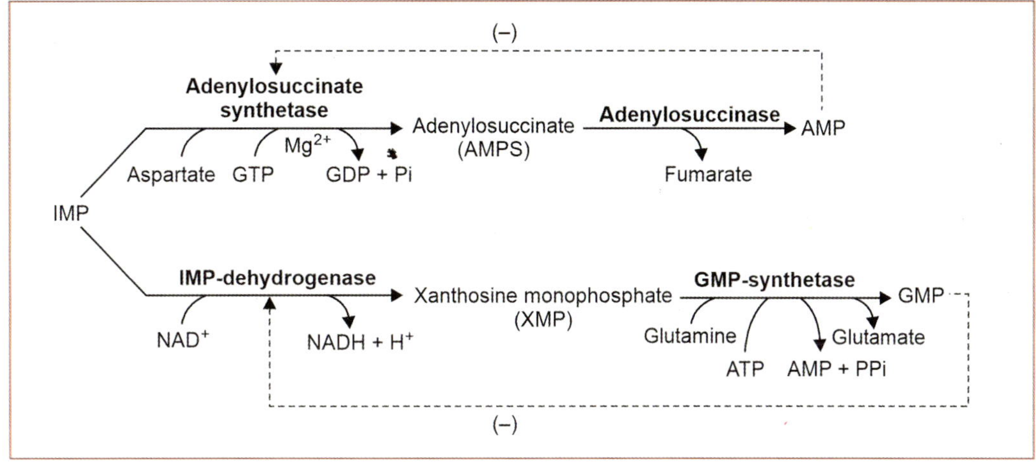

Fig. 7.15: Conversion of IMP to AMP and GMP

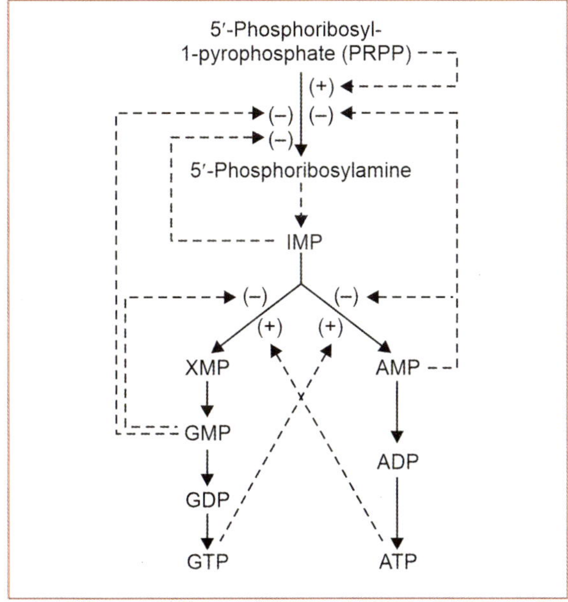

Fig. 7.16: Regulation of the synthesis of purine nucleotides

and GMP respectively, by the same enzyme, i.e. hypoxanthine–guanine phosphoribosyltransferase (HGPRTase; Figs 7.17 and 7.18).

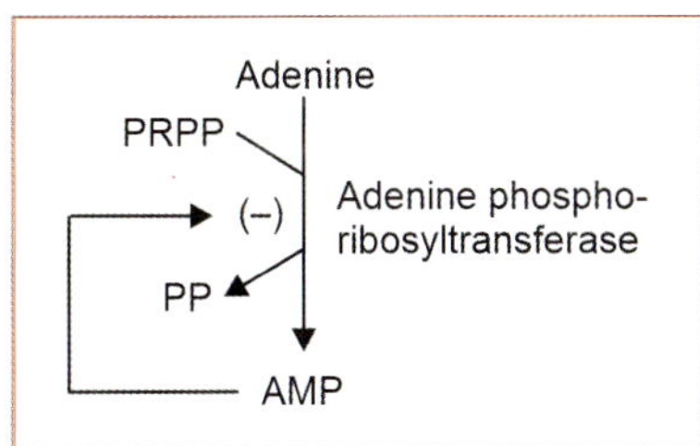

Fig. 7.17: Conversion of adenine to AMP by APRTase

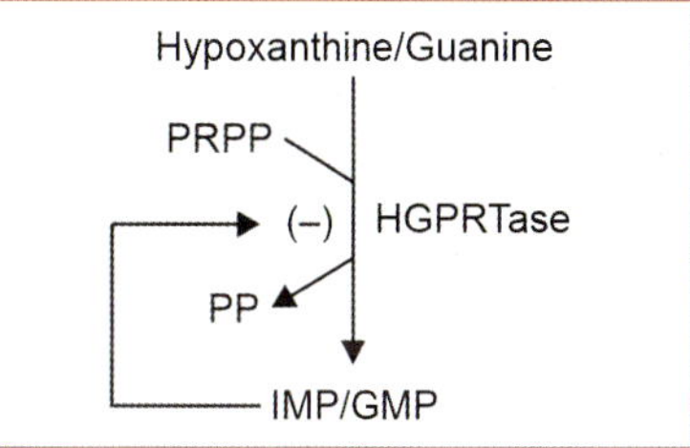

Fig. 7.18: Conversion of hypoxanthine/guanine to IMP/GMP by HGPRTase

Both the phosphoribosyltransferase reactions are regulated by their end products. Whereas AMP is a competitive inhibitor of APRTase, IMP and GMP competitively inhibit HGPRTase activity.

Lack of HGPRTase activity results in a condition designated as **Lesch-Nyhan syndrome** (Chemistry to Clinics 7.3).

- **Nucleosides** can be salvaged by the respective nucleoside kinases. For example, adenosine is salvaged by adenosine kinase, a 5′-phosphotransferase, that utilizes ATP as the phosphate donor (Fig. 7.19).

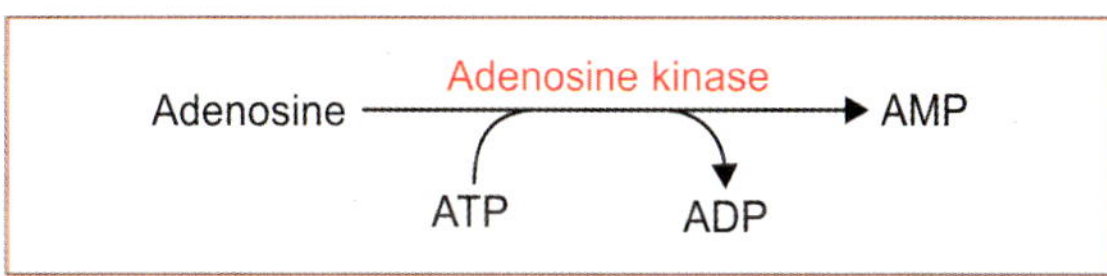

Fig. 7.19: Conversion of adenosine to AMP by adenosine kinase

Significance of Salvage Pathway

1. The ***de novo*** purine synthesis is energetically expensive. Salvage reactions **conserve energy**.

Chemistry to Clinics 7.3: Lesch-Nyhan Syndrome

Inability of the body to salvage hypoxanthine and guanine due to the complete **deficiency of HGPRTase**, leads to a condition called Lesch-Nyhan syndrome (partial deficiency causes Kelley-Seegmiller syndrome). Since the gene for HGPRTase is located on the X chromosome, this disease is limited to males only.

Features

1. In this condition, hypoxanthine and guanine are not salvaged. This, in turn, results in increased intracellular pool of PRPP and decreases IMP and GMP concentrations, thereby promoting *de novo* synthesis of purine nucleotides. This leads to excessive production of uric acid, hyperuricemia and gout.
2. Guanosine is an important modulator of glutamatergic neurotransmission, promoting glial reuptake of L-glutamate. A deficiency of guanosine could lead to dysregulated glutamatergic neurotransmission, including possible excitotoxic damage. This partly explains the mental retardation and some other neurological features.
3. Decreased GTP synthesis through salvage pathway reduces its availability for the enzyme GTP cyclohydrolase, an enzyme which initiates the synthesis of biopterins. The latter are essential for the synthesis of many neurotransmitters, e.g dopamine in the striatal dopaminergic pathways. This is thought to result in self-mutilation.

Diagnosis

i. Increase urinary urate/creatinine ratio.
ii. Absent/reduced enzyme activity in lymphocytes or fibroblasts.
iii. Mutation analysis of *HGPRTase* gene.

2. Salvage reactions are important in cells like **erythrocytes** which lack amidotransferase and cannot synthesize 5-phosphoribosylamine.

Interconversion of Purine Nucleotides

To meet their need, cells can interconvert adenine and guanine nucleotides and thus maintain a balance between the two purine nucleotides. For their interconversion, GMP or AMP is first degraded to IMP which then, depending upon the need of the cell, can resynthesize any of the two nucleotides:

- By reductive deamination, GMP is converted to IMP. The reaction is catalyzed by GMP reductase. GTP activates this step, whereas XMP competitively inhibits the reaction.
- Conversion of AMP to IMP is catalyzed by AMP deaminase (5′-AMP aminohydrolase). This reaction is activated by K^+ and ATP but inhibited by Pi, GDP and GTP (Fig. 7.20).

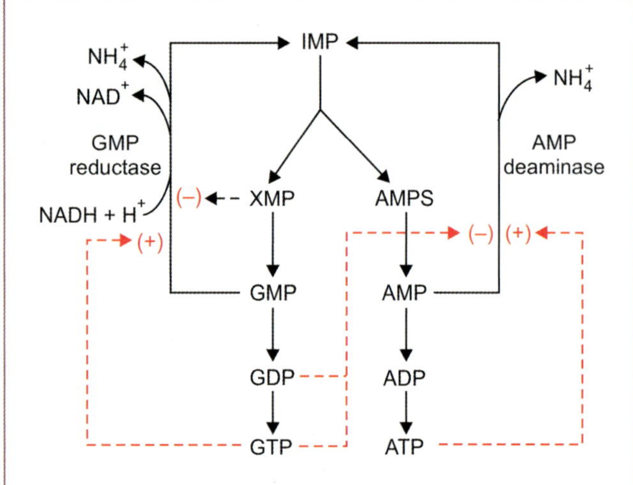

Fig. 7.20: Interconversion of purine nucleotides. (+) = Stimulation; (–) = Inhibition

Degradation of Purine Nucleotides

Degradation of purine nucleotides, i.e. AMP and GMP, leads to the formation of **uric acid**, in humans (Fig. 7.21).

Degradation of AMP

1. AMP is converted to adenosine, by 5'-AMP-nucleotidase which has high specificity for its substrate. Thereafter, adenosine deaminase (ADA) converts adenosine as well as deoxyadenosine to inosine. Alternatively, AMP deaminase, which is specific for AMP, removes ammonia and converts AMP to IMP. Subsequently, nucleotidase removes phosphoric acid and converts IMP to inosine.

   Activities of the above three enzymes, i.e. AMP-nucleotidase, ADA and AMP deaminase are several fold higher in muscle than in other tissues.
2. Purine nucleoside phosphorylase (PNP) then removes the ribose moiety from inosine and converts it to hypoxanthine.

Degradation of GMP

1. In the first step, phosphoric acid is removed by 5'-nucleotidase and GMP is converted to guanosine.
2. With the removal of the ribose moiety by PNP, guanosine is converted to guanine.
3. Guanase (an aminohydrolase) removes amino group from guanine and converts it to xanthine.

Immunodeficiency Diseases

Two distinct immunodeficiency diseases, i.e. **ADA deficiency** and **PNP deficiency** are associated with defects in the degradation of purine nucleosides (adenosine and guanosine; Chemistry to Clinics 7.4).

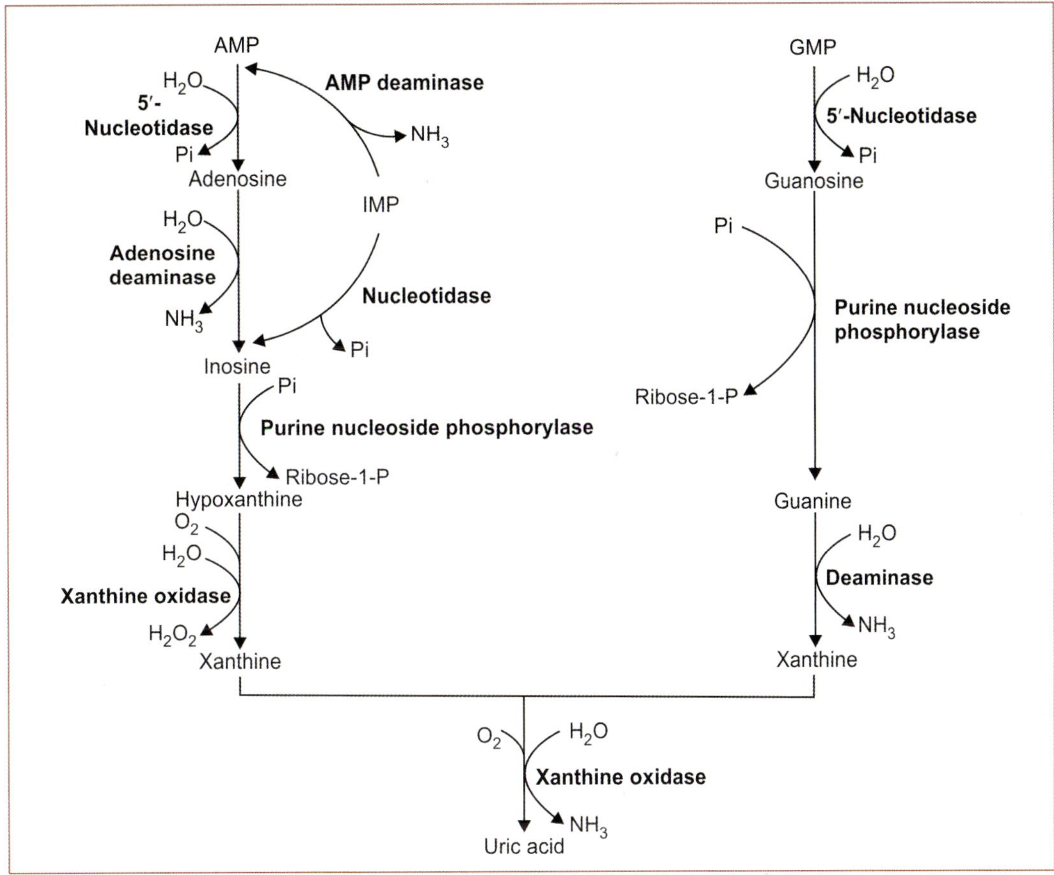

Fig. 7.21: Degradation of purine nucleotides

Chemistry to Clinics 7.4: Immunodeficiency Diseases Associated with Degradation of Purine Nucleosides

- **Severe Combined Immunodeficiency:** A deficiency in ADA is associated with severe combined immunodeficiency (SCID) involving both T-cell and B-cell functions. In ADA deficient patients, intracellular concentration of 2′-deoxyadenosine is increased leading to accumulation of dAMP and dATP. This not only decreases ATP synthesis but also blocks DNA replication by reducing the synthesis of other dNTPs. Thus, proliferation and differentiation of immune cells are compromised. Treatment of such children includes blood transfusion, bone marrow transplantation, enzyme replacement therapy with ADA-polyethylene glycol (the first successful application of enzyme replacement therapy for an inherited disease) and gene therapy. Recently, ADA gene has been successfully transfected into stem cells of ADA-deficient children.
- **Purine Nucleoside Phosphorylase Deficiency:** It is associated with immunodeficiency involving T-cell functions, i.e. a defective T-cell immunity but with normal B-cell functions. In both the conditions, i.e. SCID and PNP deficiency, there is a decrease in uric acid formation which is accompanied with increased levels of purine nucleosides and nucleotides. Overwhelming infection in such children results in death within 2 years of age.

Synthesis of Uric Acid

Hypoxanthine and xanthine, produced as above, are catabolized by the enzyme **xanthine oxidase** and are converted to uric acid (Fig. 7.21).

Xanthine oxidase occurs in the liver and small intestinal mucosa. It is a dimeric protein, which contains FAD, a Mo complex and two different Fe-S clusters. It also requires molecular oxygen as a substrate.

METABOLISM OF PYRIMIDINE NUCLEOTIDES

De novo Synthesis of Pyrimidine Nucleotides

A pyrimidine ring is synthesized by utilizing two amino acids, i.e. aspartate and glutamine as carbon and nitrogen donors, and respiratory CO_2 (HCO_3^-) as a carbon donor. The N1, C4, C5 and C6 of the pyrimidine ring are derived from aspartate, C2 from HCO_3^- and N3 from glutamine (Fig. 7.22).

In the *de novo* synthesis of pyrimidine nucleotides, a **pyrimidine ring is formed first**. Thereafter, ribose-5-phosphate is added via PRPP. This leads to the

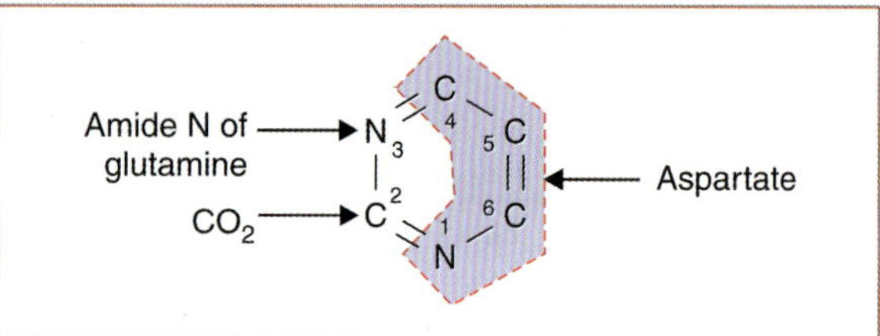

Fig. 7.22: Sources of carbons and nitrogens in pyrimidine ring

synthesis of UMP, which serves as a precursor for other pyrimidine nucleotides.

Synthesis of UMP

1. The first step in the synthesis of a pyrimidine ring is the synthesis of carbamoyl phosphate from glutamine and HCO_3^-. This reaction consumes two molecules of ATP.

   This is a regulated step in the pathway and is catalyzed by carbamoyl phosphate synthetase II (**CPS II**), in the cytosol.
2. In the next step, carbamoyl phosphate condenses with aspartate and forms carbamoyl aspartate. The reaction is catalyzed by aspartate transcarbamoylase (aspartate carbamoyltransferase). This is the **committed step** in the synthesis of pyrimidine nucleotides.
3. Dihydro-orotase results in ring closure and forms dihydro-orotate. In animals, activities of the 3 enzymes, i.e. CPS II, aspartate transcarbamoylase and dihydro-orotase are present on a single trifunctional protein, termed **CAD**.
4. Dihydro-orotate dehydrogenase, a mitochondrial enzyme, oxidizes dihydro-orotate to orotate.
5. Orotate phosphoribosyltransferase transfers ribose-5-phosphate from PRPP and converts the pyrimidine base orotate to its nucleotide, orotidine monophosphate (OMP).
6. OMP is converted to UMP by OMP decarboxylase (orotidylate decarboxylase; Fig. 7.23).

   Orotate phosporibosyltransferase and OMP decarboxylase activities are present on a single **bifunctional protein**, termed UMP synthase (Chemistry to Clinics 7.5).

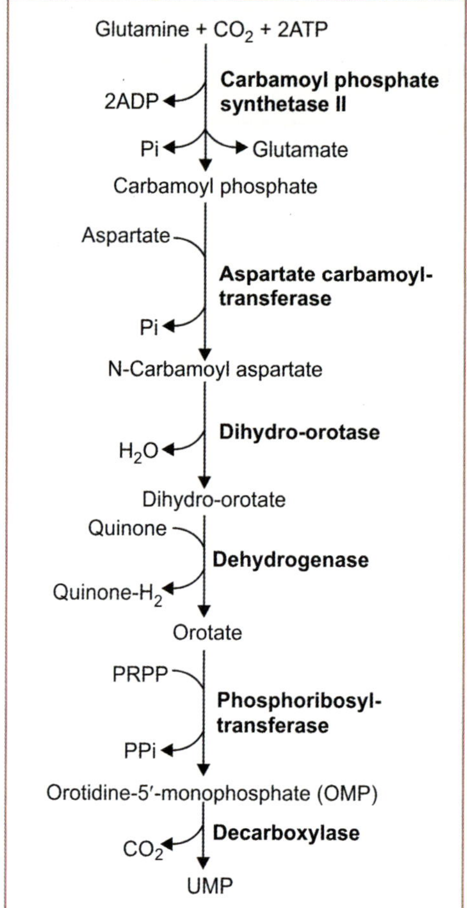

Fig. 7.23: Synthesis of UMP

Chemistry to Clinics 7.5: Orotic Aciduria

There are several types of the disease:

Type 1: It is due to a defect in *de novo* synthesis of pyrimidine nucleotides. There is a genetic deficiency of both the activities of the bifunctional protein UMP synthase, comprising of orotate phosphoribosyltransferase and OMP decarboxylase. High levels of orotic acid excretion in the urine and deficiency of enzymes in erythrocytes confirm the diagnosis.

Type 2: Reduced activity of OMP decarboxylase only.

Others

i. Ornithine transcarbamoylase (an enzyme of urea cycle) deficiency results in accumulation of carbamoyl phosphate which is channelized towards pyrimidine biosynthesis. Blood ammonia is increased, whereas urea is decreased, the two features not observed in type 1 and 2 orotic aciduria.
ii. Reye's syndrome.
iii. During allopurinol therapy.

Features

Megaloblastic anemia: Deficiency of UMP (precursor of UTP, CTP and TMP) leads to decreased nucleic acid synthesis in erythroid precursors in bone marrow, and megaloblastic anemia. It does not respond to vitamin B_{12} and/or folic acid.

Physical and mental retardation: This could be due to reduced supply of pyrimidine nucleosides in the neonatal period.

Treatment: It includes feeding uridine-rich diet which reduces formation of orotate and improves anemia. Uridine is taken up by the cells, salvaged to UMP and finally to UTP which inhibits CPS II, the regulatory step in pyrimidine biosynthesis. As a result, orotic acid synthesis is decreased. Exogenous uridine thus bypasses the defective step in pyrimidine biosynthesis and by its salvage utilization, uridine supplies UTP and CTP required by the cell.

Conversion of Nucleoside Monophosphates to Di- and Triphosphates

Various nucleoside monophosphates, i.e. AMP, GMP, CMP, UMP as well as dAMP, dGMP, dCMP and dTMP are sequentially converted to their nucleoside triphosphates.

- Firstly, a nucleoside monophosphate (NMP) is converted to the corresponding nucleoside diphosphate (NDP). The reaction is catalyzed by the base specific nucleoside monophosphate kinase.
- Thereafter, nucleoside diphosphate kinase converts a nucleoside diphosphate to the corresponding nucleoside triphosphate (Fig. 7.24).

Conversion of UTP to CTP

CTP synthetase catalyzes the formation of CTP from UTP by using glutamine as a donor of the amino group. ATP is used as a source of energy. CTP is a negative effector of the reaction (Fig. 7.25).

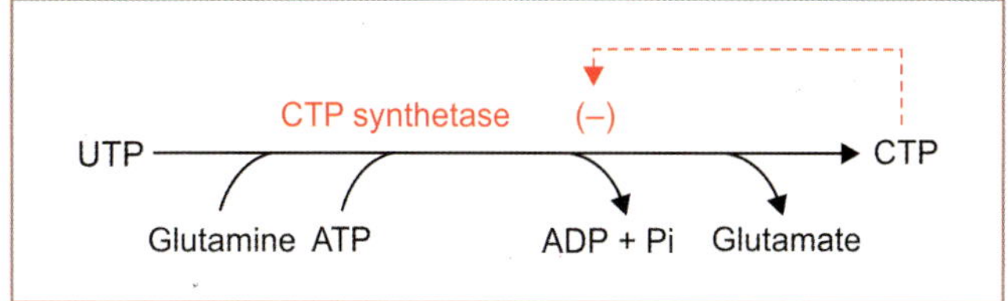

Fig. 7.25: Synthesis of CTP from UTP

Synthesis of TMP

Both UTP and CTP can serve as precursors of TMP. The two nucleoside triphosphates are first hydrolyzed to the corresponding nucleoside diphosphates, i.e. CDP and UDP which, in turn, act as precursors of dUMP.

Thereafter, thymidylate (deoxythymidylate, dTMP or TMP) is synthesized by methylation of the deoxyuridine monophosphate (dUMP). The reaction is catalyzed by thymidylate synthase. In this reaction, N^5, N^{10}-methylenetetrahydrofolate (N^5, N^{10}-methylene-FH_4) is used as a source of the methyl group (one carbon moiety) and also as a reducing agent. N^5, N^{10}-methylene-FH_4, in turn, is converted to FH_2 (*see* Figs 18.10 and 18.13).

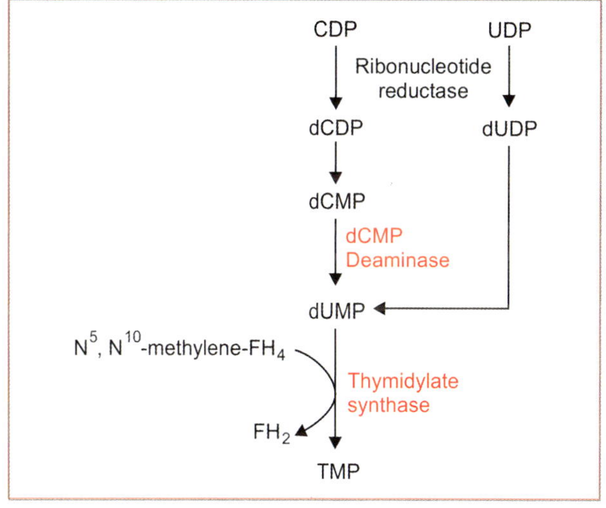

Fig. 7.26: Synthesis of TMP

Regulation of Biosynthesis of Pyrimidine Nucleotides

- Pyrimidine synthesis is regulated by CPS II. The enzyme is inhibited by CTP and is activated by ATP and PRPP (Fig. 7.27).

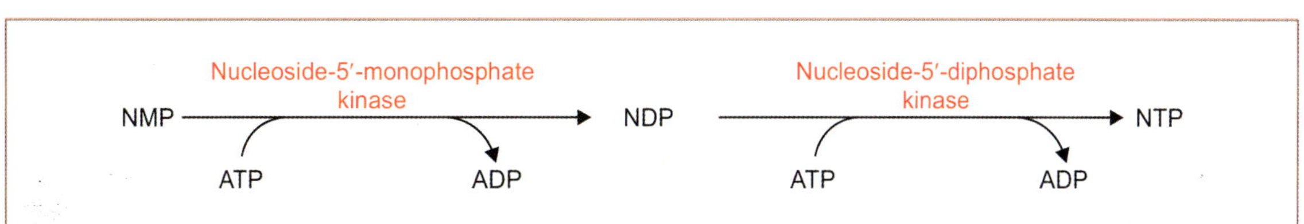

Fig. 7.24: Conversion of a nucleoside monophosphate to di- and triphosphate

7

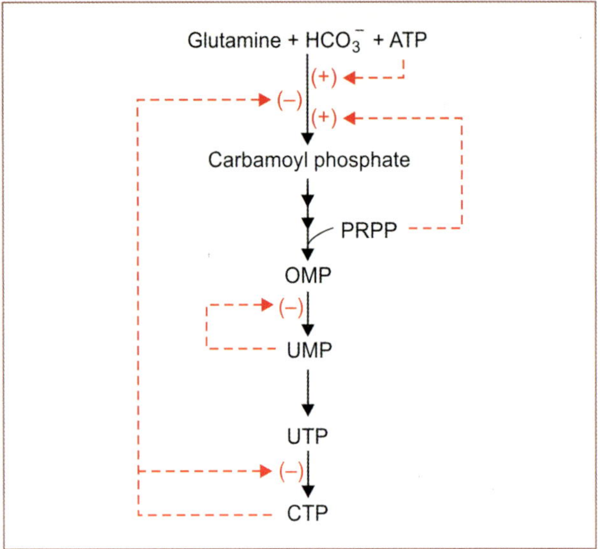

Fig. 7.27: Regulation of pyrimidine nucleotide biosynthesis
(+) = Stimulation; (–) = Inhibition

- OMP decarboxylase is competitively inhibited by UMP.
- CTP synthetase is inhibited by CTP. This is an example of feedback inhibition. This, in turn, regulates the conversion of UTP to CTP. Cells thus maintain a balance between uridine and cytidine nucleotides.

Importance of DHFR and Thymidylate Synthase

TMP (dTMP) synthesis is essentially required for rapidly proliferating cells, such as cancer cells, for DNA synthesis. Inhibition of thymidylate synthase, or of DHFR, blocks the synthesis of dTMP and thus kills cancer cells. Various inhibitors of these enzymes are known and are used as effective anticancer/antibacterial agents (Chemistry to Clinics 7.6 and 7.7).

Chemistry to Clinics 7.6: Suicide Inhibitors

Analogs of dUMP, such as 5-fluorodeoxyuridylate (FdUMP) are irreversible inhibitors of thymidylate synthase. FdUMP binds to the enzyme thymidylate synthase like dUMP and forms an enzyme-FdUMP-FH_4 ternary covalent complex. This, in turn, inactivates the enzyme after undergoing some of the normal catalytic reactions. Such enzyme inhibitors are called mechanism-based inhibitors or suicide inhibitors or suicide substrates, as they force the enzyme to commit suicide.

SALVAGE PATHWAY FOR PYRIMIDINE NUCLEOTIDES SYNTHESIS

Pyrimidine bases orotate, uracil and thymine, but not cytosine, can be salvaged and converted to the corresponding nucleotides by pyrimidine phosphoribosyltransferase. The enzyme utilizes PRPP as a source of ribose-5-phosphate (Fig. 7.28).

Chemistry to Clinics 7.7: Antifolates

Antimetabolites, such as methotrexate (amethopterin), aminopterin and trimethoprim are analogs of FH_2 and are called antifolates. These drugs inhibit dihydrofolate reductase and block the regeneration of FH_4. This, in turn, affects dTMP biosynthesis. These drugs are used as effective anticancer agents, particularly against childhood leukemias.

Trimethoprim binds more tightly to bacterial enzymes than to mammalian cells. It is, therefore, used as an important antibacterial agent. It is an active ingredient of the popular antibiotic 'Septran'.

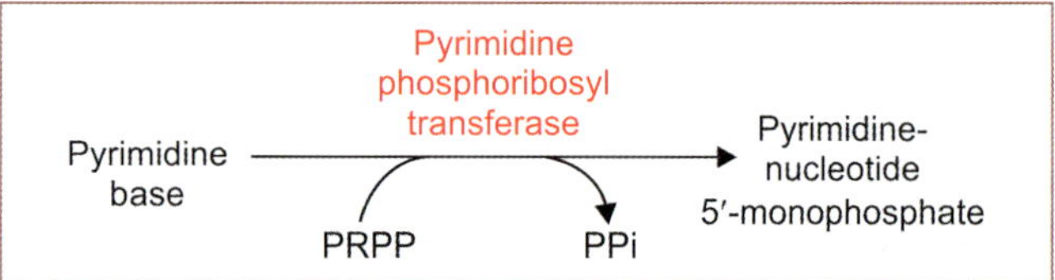

Fig. 7.28: Conversion of a pyrimidine base to a pyrimidine nucleotide

DEGRADATION OF PYRIMIDINE NUCLEOTIDES SYNTHESIS

Pyrimidine nucleotides are first converted to free bases which are then degraded to form the end products.

Degradation of Pyrimidine Nucleotides to the Free Bases

- Pyrimidine nucleotides (CMP, UMP, dCMP and dTMP), released as a result of the turnover of nucleic acids, are converted to the corresponding nucleosides by the nonspecific phosphatases.
- Cytidine and deoxycytidine are thereafter deaminated by pyrimidine nucleoside deaminase to uridine and deoxyuridine, respectively.
- Uridine, deoxyuridine and deoxythymidine are degraded by uridine phosphorylase and result in the formation of uracil (from uridine and deoxyuridine) and thymine (from deoxythymidine; Fig. 7.29).

Degradation of Pyrimidine Bases

Uracil and thymine produced as above are further degraded to β-alanine and β-aminoisobutyric acid, respectively (Fig. 7.30; Chemistry to Clinics 7.8).

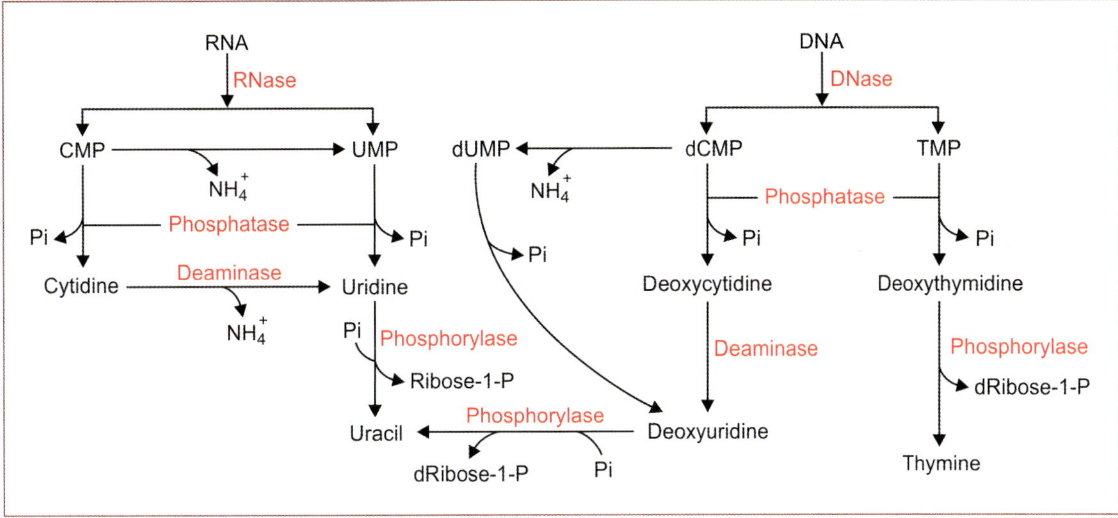

Fig. 7.29: Degradation of pyrimidine nucleotides

Chemistry to Clinics 7.8: β-Aminoisobutyric Acid

β-Aminoisobutyric acid is excreted in the urine and is a measure of turnover of DNA or thymine nucleotides. Its urinary excretion is increased in cancer patients undergoing chemotherapy or radiation therapy, due to the increased degradation of DNA.

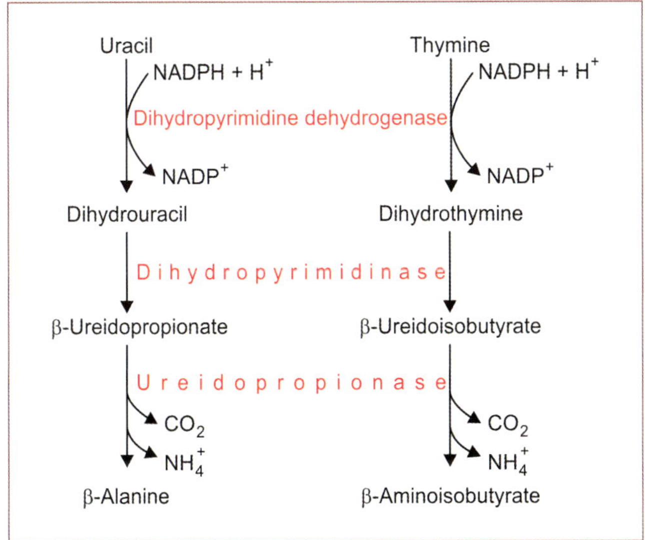

Fig. 7.30: Degradation of pyrimidine bases

CONVERSION OF RIBONUCLEOTIDES TO DEOXYRIBONUCLEOTIDES

Purine and pyrimidine ribonucleotides formed by the respective *de novo* pathways, are converted to their deoxyribonucleotides during **DNA replication**.

- Ribonucleoside diphosphates (NDPs), i.e. ADP, GDP, CDP and UDP are reduced at C2′ position to their deoxy forms, i.e. dADP, dGDP, dCDP and dUDP by ribonucleotide reductase (ribonucleoside diphosphate reductase). **Thioredoxin** (a peptide containing two cysteine residues) is used as a source of reducing equivalents. Reduced form of the coenzyme (reduced thioredoxin) gets oxidized and forms a disulfide bond.

  Mammalian ribonucleotide reductase is a heterodimer. The enzyme is under allosteric regulation where the products serve as potent negative effectors of the enzyme. dATP is a potent inhibitor of the reduction of all the four nucleoside diphosphates (CDP, UDP, GDP and ADP). dGTP inhibits the reduction of CDP, UDP and GDP while dTTP inhibits the reduction of CDP, UDP and ADP.
- The oxidized thioredoxin is then reduced by thioredoxin reductase which is a flavoprotein and contains FAD as a prosthetic group. NADPH + H^+ serves as the terminal reducing agent (Fig. 7.31).

  In place of thioredoxin, **glutaredoxin** can also be used which requires glutathione and glutathione reductase.
- Phosphorylation of dNDP produces dNTP which, in turn, is used in the biosynthesis of DNA. The reaction is catalyzed by nucleoside diphosphate kinase. Any of the NTP or dNTP, such as ATP, can function as the phosphoryl donor for this reaction (Fig. 7.32).

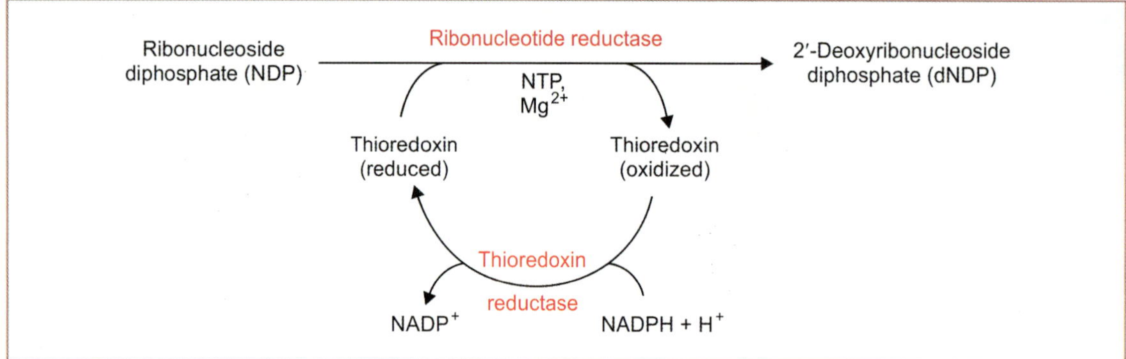

Fig. 7.31: Conversion of a ribonucleotide to deoxyribonucleotide

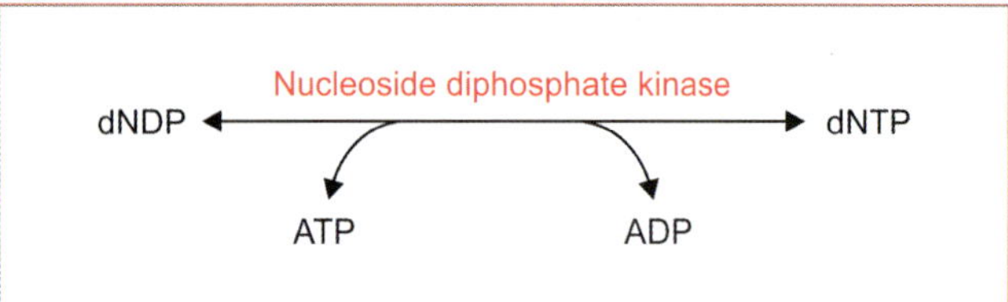

Fig. 7.32: Interconversion of dNDP and dNTP

ANALYTES ASSOCIATED WITH GOUT AND LESCH-NYHAN SYNDROME

As discussed above, Lesch-Nyhan syndrome is due to the deficiency of the enzyme HGPRTase, which, in turn, results in the accumulation of purines that are further degraded to **uric acid**. Thus, uric acid is, finally, the **analyte associated with gout** and **Lesch-Nyhan syndrome**.

Uric acid is sparingly soluble in an aqueous medium. **Normal serum uric acid concentration** is between **3 and 7 mg/dL**. Males have physiologically higher values because of higher rate of tubular urate reabsorption, and the uricosuric effect of estrogen in females.

Hyperuricemia

Elevated level of uric acid in the serum (>7 mg/dl, called hyperuricemia) is often asymptomatic. However, it may result in its deposition as sodium urate crystals primarily in the joints, in a clinical condition, called gout (Chemistry to Clinics 7.9).

There are two types of hyperuricemia:

- **Primary hyperuricemia:** This is due to some metabolic defect that results in increased synthesis of purine nucleotides via ***de novo*** pathway, such as:
  1. ***Increased PRPP synthetase activity:*** This results in increased intracellular concentration of PRPP which acts as a positive effector of the enzyme amidotransferase. This, in turn, increases *de novo* synthesis of purine nucleotides as well as their subsequent degradation to uric acid.
  2. ***HGPRTase deficiency:*** Deficiency of HGPRTase, such as in **Lesch-Nyhan syndrome**, causes a decrease in the salvage pathway of hypoxanthine and guanine to reform nucleotides. This, in turn, spares PRPP and results in overproduction of purine nucleotides and their degradation to uric acid.
  3. ***Glucose-6-phosphatase deficiency:*** Glucose-6-phosphatase deficiency, also known as **glycogen storage disease I** or **von Gierke's disease**, results in increased levels of glucose-6-phosphate which is diverted to HMP shunt. This, in turn, increases availability of ribose-5-phosphate and enhances the generation of PRPP. Raised levels of PRPP, increase ***de novo*** synthesis of purine nucleotides and the overproduction of uric acid. In addition, associated lactic acidosis elevates renal threshold for urate which further leads to hyperuricemia.

Chemistry to Clinics 7.9: Gout

Gout is characterized by elevated levels of uric acid in the blood (**hyperuricemia**) and its increased excretion in the urine (**uric aciduria**) due to a variety of metabolic abnormalities.

Most of the clinical conditions with hyperuricemia arise due to the poor aqueous solubility of uric acid. As a result of it sodium urate crystals are deposited in joints of the extremities (**gouty arthritis**) and/or in the renal interstitial tissue (**gouty nephropathy**). The crystals activate the complement pathway resulting in the recruitment of neutrophils, macrophages, release of inflammatory mediators and free radicals. In the affected joint, hyaluronic acid is reduced both due to decreased production and increased degradation. Hyperuricemia is, thus, associated with recurrent attacks of painful arthritic joints and inflammation, most often of big toe caused by the deposition of insoluble sodium urate crystals, called **tophi** (Fig. 7.33).

7

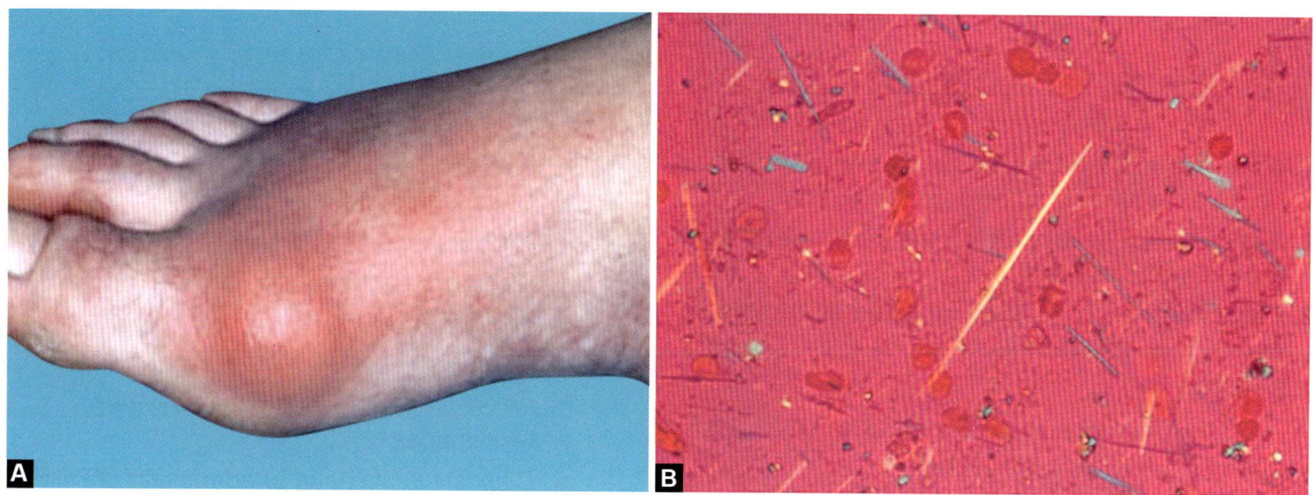

Fig. 7.33: Gout. (A) The condition most commonly affects the great toe (first metatarsophalangeal joint) when it is also called podagra; (B) Under polarized microscope, negatively birefringent needle-shaped monosodium urate crystals of various sizes and colors are seen in the joint aspirate

- **Secondary hyperuricemia:** It is secondary to some disease other than a metabolic disorder, such as a kidney disease or a disease associated with excessive cell turnover and increased breakdown of nucleic acids, e.g. radiation therapy/cancer chemotherapy, or psoriasis.

A better way of classifying hyperuricemia is based on its pathophysiology, i.e. overproduction of uric acid (e.g. in rapidly multiplying tumors, cancer chemotherapy), underexcretion (e.g. in lactic acidosis, diabetic ketoacidosis), or both (e.g. in alcoholism, von Gierke's disease).

Treatment: Most effective treatment of gout includes the use of **inhibitor of xanthine oxidase**, such as allopurinol or its metabolite alloxanthine. Allopurinol decreases both uric acid formation as well as ***de novo*** synthesis of purine nucleotides.

Some Important Questions

1. What are nucleotides? Explain the process of *de novo* synthesis of purine nucleotides.

2. Describe the process of the degradation of purine nucleotides.

3. Describe the process of *de novo* synthesis of pyrimidine nucleotides.

4. Explain:

i. Various nitrogenous bases found in nucleic acids
ii. Unusual nitrogenous bases

5. Describe briefly:

i. Synthesis of IMP
ii. Regulation of purine biosynthesis
iii. Interconversion of purine nucleotides
iv. Immunodeficiency diseases related to purines degradation
v. Formation of uric acid
vi. Primary hyperuricemia
vii. Secondary hyperuricemia

6. Write notes on:

i. Unusual nitrogenous bases
ii. Nucleosides
iii. Salvage pathway for purine nucleotides synthesis
iv. Lesch-Nyhan syndrome
v. Severe combined immunodeficiency
vi. Nucleotides
vii. Clinical significance of adenosine
viii. Purine/pyrimidine analogs of pharmacological significance
ix. Suicide inhibitors
x. Antifolates
xi. Gout
xii. Hereditary orotic aciduria
xiii. CAD
xiv. UMP synthase

Multiple Choice Questions

1. The first purine nucleotide synthesized *de novo* is:

A. AMP
B. GMP
C. IMP
D. None of the above

2. The following may be seen in Lesch-Nyhan syndrome:

A. Hyperuricemia
B. Mental retardation
C. Self-mutilation
D. All of the above

3. Adenosine deaminase (ADA) activity is highest in:

A. Muscles
B. Liver
C. Kidneys
D. Brain

4. Increased uric acid synthesis occurs in the following *except*:

A. ADA deficiency
B. HGPRTase deficiency
C. Increased activity of PRPP synthetase
D. Glucose-6-phosphatase deficiency

5. The following enzyme catalyzes the committed step in pyrimidine nucleotide biosynthesis:

A. PRPP synthetase
B. CPS II
C. Aspartate transcarbamoylase
D. CPS I

6. The methyl group donor in thymidylate synthesis is:

A. S-Adenosylmethionine
B. Betaine
C. N^5,N^{10}-Methylenetetrahydrofolate
D. N^5-Methyltetrahydrofolate

7. The following is a suicide substrate:

A. FdUMP
B. Allopurinol
C. Both
D. None of the above

8. The following is true for sodium urate:

A. Poor aqueous solubility
B. Precipitates in acidic pH
C. Dehydration promotes precipitation
D. All of the above

9. SCID is characterized by:

A. Decreased T-cell function, normal B-cell function
B. Decreased T-cell and B-cell function
C. Normal T-cell function, decreased B-cell function
D. Normal T-cell and B-cell function

10. The following is measured in urine to assess DNA turnover:

A. β-Alanine
B. Putrescine
C. β-Aminoisobutyric acid
D. Adenosine deaminase

CHAPTER 8

Vitamins

Competency Achievement: The student should be able to:

BI6.5	Describe the biochemical role of vitamins in the body and explain the manifestations of their deficiency
IM23.3	Discuss and describe the etiology, causes, clinical manifestations, complications, diagnosis and management of common vitamin deficiencies
PA15.1	Describe the metabolism of vitamin B_{12} and the etiology and pathogenesis of B_{12} deficiency
PE12.1	Discuss the (RDA), dietary sources of vitamin A and their role in health and disease
PE12.2	Describe the causes, clinical features, diagnosis and management of deficiency/excess of vitamin A
PE12.3	Identify the clinical features of dietary deficiency/excess of vitamin A
PE12.4	Diagnose patients with vitamin A deficiency, classify and plan management
PE12.5	Discuss the vitamin A prophylaxis program and their recommendations
PE12.6	Discuss the RDA, dietary sources of vitamin D and their role in health and disease
PE12.7	Describe the causes, clinical features, diagnosis and management of deficiency/excess of vitamin D
PE12.8	Identify the clinical features of dietary deficiency of vitamin D
PE12.9	Assess patients with vitamin D deficiency, diagnose, classify and plan management
PE12.11	Discuss the RDA, dietary sources of vitamin E and their role in health and disease
PE12.12	Describe the causes, clinical features, diagnosis and management of deficiency of vitamin E
PE12.13	Discuss the RDA, dietary sources of vitamin K and their role in health and disease
PE12.14	Describe the causes, clinical features, diagnosis, management and prevention of deficiency of vitamin K
PE12.15	Discuss the RDA, dietary sources of vitamin B and their role in health and disease
PE12.16	Describe the causes, clinical features, diagnosis and management of deficiency of B complex vitamins
PE12.17	Identify the clinical features of vitamin B complex deficiency
PE12.18	Diagnose patients with vitamin B complex deficiency and plan management
PE12.19	Discuss the RDA, dietary sources of vitamin C and their role in health and disease
PE12.20	Describe the causes, clinical features, diagnosis and management of deficiency of vitamin C (scurvy)
PE12.21	Identify the clinical features vitamin C deficiency
DR17.1	Enumerate and identify the cutaneous findings in vitamin A deficiency
DR17.2	Enumerate and describe the various skin changes in vitamin B complex deficiency
DR17.3	Enumerate and describe the various changes in vitamin C deficiency

Vitamins are organic constituents of food, called '**protective accessory food factors**'. These are essential for life and well-being. Vitamins, in general, cannot be synthesized by the body and have to be supplied in the diet though in very small quantities. Thus, they are **micronutrients**. Vitamins are divided into two groups:

1. Lipid-soluble vitamins, and
2. Water-soluble vitamins

LIPID-SOLUBLE VITAMINS

Lipid-soluble vitamins are vitamin A, vitamin D, vitamin E and vitamin K. Their general properties include:

- Dietary lipid-soluble vitamins are absorbed from the gastrointestinal lumen, in the presence of **lipids and bile salts**.
- Their precursors are called **provitamins** and are found mostly in plants.

- Due to their lipid solubility, they are **stored** in the liver, adipose tissue, etc.
- Because they can be stored, a dietary **deficiency takes time** to become manifest.
- Large doses, for a fairly long duration, may result in toxic symptoms (**hypervitaminosis**).

VITAMIN A

Vitamin A, also known as anti-nightblindness factor, has a characteristic 6-membered ring known as β-ionine ring attached with a long hydrocarbon side chain (Fig. 8.1).

Fig. 8.1: Vitamin A alcohol (retinol)

Vitamin A is an alcohol (**retinol**) but it may be converted into an aldehyde (**retinal**, also called retinene) or an acid (**retinoic acid**). All the three forms are found in different tissues. The main, naturally occurring form of vitamin A though contains β-ionine ring, a dehydro form, with two double bonds in the ring is also known to occur. This is called vitamin A_2. The β-ionone ring of vitamin A_2 thus contains two double bonds. The aldehyde form of vitamin A_2 is designated as 3-dehydroretinal.

PROVITAMIN A

Carotenoids are called provitamin A. These are found in plants and depending upon the presence of additional ionine ring(s), these provitamins are designated as α, β or γ-carotenes. Rich sources of carotenes are yellow-colored fruits and vegetables such as carrots, pumpkin, papaya, mango, etc. **Polar bear is the richest animal source.**

β-Carotene has highest vitamin A activity of all the natural carotenoids. Cleavage of the carotenes gives rise to vitamin A in the intestinal wall. Whereas β-carotene gives 2 molecules, α- and γ-carotenes, each give rise to only one molecule of vitamin A (retinol).

Conversion of β-carotene into retinal requires β-carotene dioxygenase, retinene reductase, molecular oxygen and bile salts (Fig. 8.2).

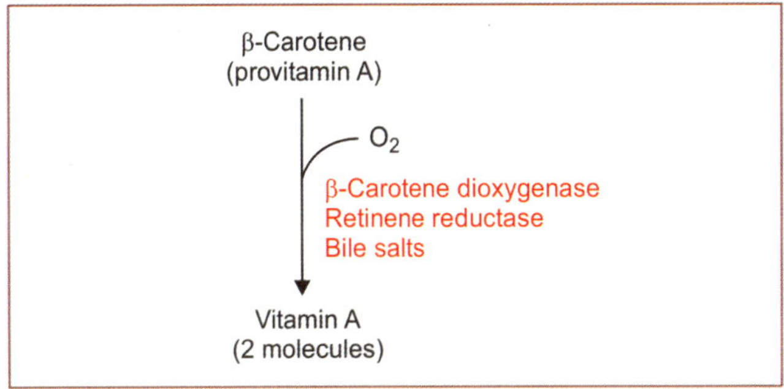

Fig. 8.2: Conversion of β-carotene to vitamin A

Conversion of Carotenes into Vitamin A

Provitamins (carotenoids) are, as such, absorbed in the gastrointestinal lumen and are converted into retinol in the intestinal epithelium. After its entry into the intestinal mucosa, retinol is re-esterified with long chain fatty acids and enters the lymphatics, in chylomicrons as retinyl esters. Most of the vitamin A esters are **stored in the liver**. When needed, retinol is released from the liver and is transported in the blood vessels bound to **retinol-binding protein (RBP)**. In the serum, RBP-retinol complex combines with transthyretin, another protein, which is also synthesized in the liver. Retinol-binding protein can transport retinol, retinoic acid and carotenes. Some of the retinoic acid is also transported, in circulation, by albumin.

The retinol is removed from the serum and is utilized by the target cells, such as retinol photoreactors and epithelial linings. In the retina, it is converted to retinal which is essential in visual functions, whereas in the epithelial tissues, retinol is converted to retinoic acid which is required for maintaining epithelial functions, i.e. growth and differentiation.

Absorption and Metabolism of Vitamin A

Nearly 50–90% of vitamin A is absorbed in the intestine and is released into the lacteals. The vitamin is absorbed in the esterified form (retinyl esters) in the presence of bile. Dietary absorption of vitamin A and its main metabolism is shown in Fig. 8.3.

ROLE OF VITAMIN A IN HEALTH AND DISEASE

Retinol, retinal and retinoic acid perform various physiological functions in the body:

1. **Biochemical role of vitamin A in vision:** On the basis of differences in the biochemical series of events, vision is of two types, i.e. scotopic and photopic.

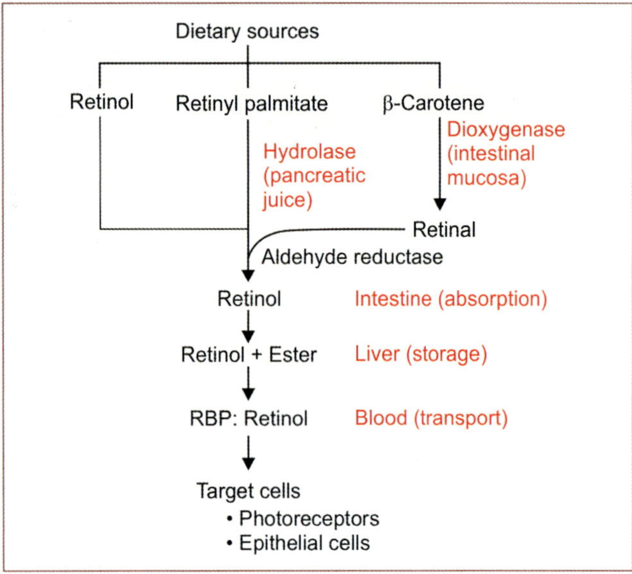

Fig. 8.3: Vitamin A metabolism

***Scotopic vision*:** It refers to vision in **dim light** that depends on the **rod cells** in the retina. Rods are of one type only and provide **monochromatic vision**. They contain a photopigment called **rhodopsin** made up of the glycoprotein opsin and the aldehyde derivative of vitamin A called retinal. In dim light or darkness, retinal has a bent shape and is called 11-*cis*-retinal, which fits with opsin. When it absorbs light, the molecule straightens to form all-*trans*-retinal. This *cis* to *trans* conversion (isomerization) is the first step in converting light to an electrical signal in the retina. In darkness, an enzyme reverses the process. The chain of events in the cells of the retina is known as **Wald's visual cycle** and is shown in Fig. 8.4.

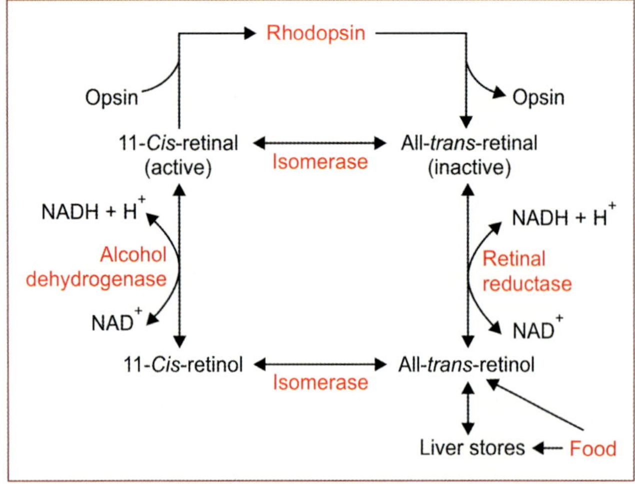

Fig. 8.4: Wald's visual cycle in rod cells

When light falls on the retina, rhodopsin is bleached and generates all-*trans* retinal which cannot form a complex with opsin. Visual excitation further changes the structural configuration of opsin that induces a decrease in permeability to sodium ions with consequent increased polarization of the retinal membrane, which in turn, generates nerve impulses. Transducin, a G-protein, also plays an important role in this sequence of events. All-*trans* retinal is immediately reduced to all-*trans* retinol by the enzyme, all-*trans* retinal dehydrogenase (retinal reductase). All-*trans* retinol is then transported to and stored in the liver where it is isomerized to 11-*cis* retinol by an isomerase. After its delivery to the retina, 11-*cis* retinol is again changed to 11-*cis* retinal which can conjugate with opsin to form rhodopsin, in dark.

***Photopic vision*:** It refers to vision in **bright light** that depends on the **cone cells** in the retina. Cones are of three types and provide **trichromatic vision**. Each cone type contains a specific photopigment made up of retinal and one of three opsins which filter the light before it reaches retinal. The 'red' photopigment (**porphyropsin**) responds best to yellow-orange light (558 nm), the 'green' photopigment (**iodopsin**) responds best to green light (531 nm) and the 'blue' photopigment (**cyanopsin**) responds best to blue light (420 nm). Although each cone type responds maximally to a particular wavelength, it does respond to other wavelengths as well. This means that for any given wavelength, all the three cone types get excited to different degrees. The final color sensation is determined by the pattern of the frequency of impulses generated by the three cone systems. When white light falls on the retina, they are stimulated in roughly equal proportions. As the intensity of light is reduced, the cones cease to respond and the rods take over. The various types of **color blindness** can be explained in terms of the absence or deficiency of one or more of the specific cone cell type (Chemistry to Clinics 8.1).

Chemistry to Clinics 8.1: Color Blindness

Color blindness is a genetic disease; however, severe vitamin A deficiency may result in acquired defects in the functioning of cones. It may be clinically difficult to diagnose because by this time, the corneal damage already interferes with vision. Chronic malabsorption is a frequent cause which is often over-looked, though it readily responds to vitamin A supplementation.

Light/dark adaptation: When a person passes from darkness to bright light he is dazzled, but shortly thereafter he sees well again. This adjustment or decrease in sensitivity on exposure to bright light is called light adaptation but is, strictly speaking, the disappearance of dark adaptation.

2. **Cell growth and differentiation:** Vitamin A, as **retinoic acid**, plays a key role in:
   i. Synthesis of membrane glycoproteins.
   ii. Synthesis of glycosaminoglycans that is important constituents of the extracellular matrix.
   iii. Formation of intercellular gap-junctions required for proper cell-to-cell communication.
   iv. Controlling the stepwise formation of particular cell types from precursor cells, i.e. differentiation.
   v. It has also been proposed that retinoylphosphate acts as a carrier of oligosaccharides across the lipid bilayer.

   Collectively, these actions ensure the maintenance of epithelial integrity.
3. **Immunity:** Since vitamin A is required to maintain the integrity of the tissues lining the eyes, the gastrointestinal tract, the genitourinary tract, the respiratory system, and skin, it ensures an optimal functioning of the immune system.
4. **Antioxidant:** Both, vitamin A and β-carotene detoxify free radicals, and are therefore, lipid-phase antioxidants. It can trap peroxy free radicals at low partial pressures of oxygen.
5. **Anticancer:** The ability of vitamin A to maintain epithelial integrity, to strengthen the immune response, to act as an antioxidant, and to regulate cell growth and differentiation, makes it an important anticancer vitamin.
6. **Intermediary metabolism:** Vitamin A favors synthesis of the steroid hormones particularly corticosterone and cortisol that, in turn, favor gluconeogenesis. Vitamin A also plays a role in cholesterol biosynthesis, i.e. in the final stage of cyclization of squalene to cholesterol.

DEFICIENCY MANIFESTATIONS OF VITAMIN A

Vitamin A deficiency is primarily due to its low dietary intake. It is aggravated by infections which reduce its absorption and utilization.

1. Vitamin A deficiency though affects many tissues; it is most detrimental for the **eyes** (Chemistry to Clinics 8.2).

> **Chemistry to Clinics 8.2: Ocular Effects of Vitamin A Deficiency**
>
> Deficiency of vitamin A results in **xerophthalmia**, i.e. drying of the conjunctiva and the cornea, followed by destruction of the cornea and blindness. The various stages are shown in Fig. 8.5.

It should be remembered that the initial symptoms (night blindness) are due to retinol/retinal deficiency in the visual pigments, whereas the later manifestations (Bitot's spots onwards) are due to a deficiency of retinoic acid and a consequent failure to maintain epithelial integrity.

Xerophthalmia occurs when body stores of vitamin A are exhausted and supply fails to meet requirement. The first symptom of xerophthalmia is **night blindness**, i.e. an individual cannot see to get around

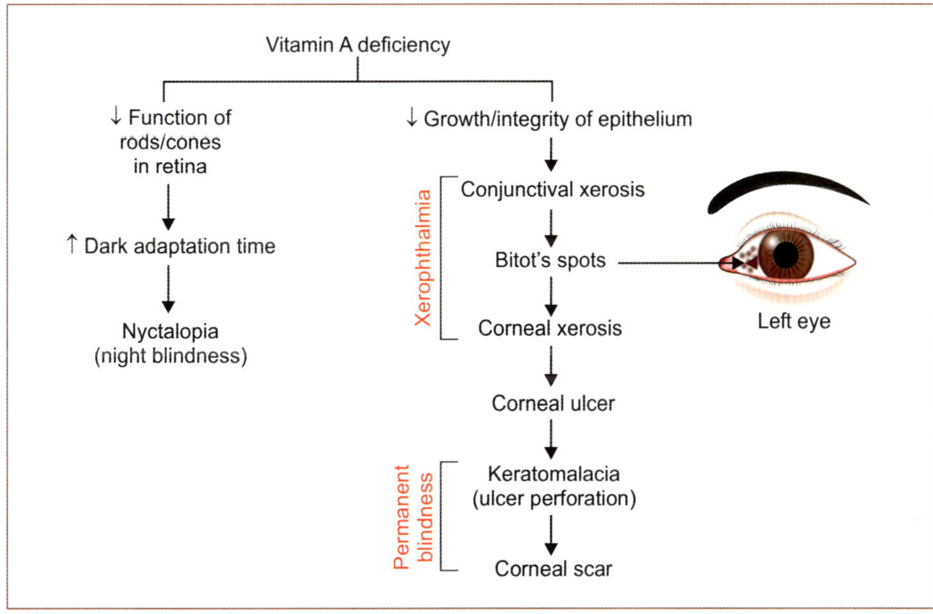

Fig. 8.5: Effect of vitamin A deficiency on the eyes

after dark or in a dark room. Since retinal is essential for the synthesis of rhodopsin by the rods, vitamin A deficiency interferes with the production of rhodopsin, impairs rod functions and results in night blindness. It responds rapidly to vitamin A therapy.

1. If untreated, **Bitot's spots** develop: Accumulation of foamy/cheesy material on the conjunctiva. Although these spots may differ in size, location and shape, they have a similar appearance. When the cornea becomes dry, the condition is called xerosis. If the disease is not treated, it can progress within hours to an ulcer of the cornea. A **corneal ulcer** can lead to melting or wasting of the cornea, called **keratomalacia**.

   It indicates destruction of a part or of the complete corneal stroma, resulting in permanent structural alteration. Keratomalacia can lead to perforation of the cornea. At this stage, a **corneal scar** remains in the eye. The sooner the disease is treated, the smaller the ulcer and smaller the scar which however, remains forever (Fig. 8.6).

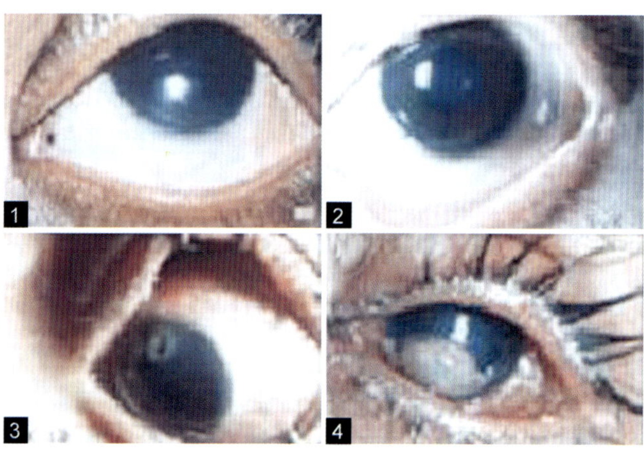

Fig. 8.6: Xerophthalmia. (1) Bitot's spot; (2) Corneal xerosis and ulceration; (3) Keratomalacia; (4) Corneal scar

2. Deficiency of vitamin A results in **xerosis and keratinization of various extraocular epithelial surfaces** including the mucous membrane, skin (**cutaneous findings** include dry and rough skin) and urogenital tract (chances of urolithiasis, infertility, degeneration of the testes, abortion and production of malformed off-springs), etc.
3. Increased susceptibility to infections, free radical mediated cytotoxicity and carcinogenesis.
4. Vitamin A deficiency also affects osteoblastic activity and results in defective resorption of the bone, thereby affecting growth of children.

DIETARY SOURCES OF VITAMIN A

Liver oil (especially fish-liver oil), eggs, milk and milk products are good sources of **vitamin A**.

Papaya, carrots, sweet potatoes and green-leafy vegetables are good sources of **carotenes**.

RECOMMENDED DAILY ALLOWANCES OF VITAMIN A

The recommended daily allowance (RDA) of vitamin A for an adult is 1000 μg/day.

One IU of vitamin A is the activity present in 0.3 μg of retinol.

One retinol equivalent is the activity present in 1 μg of retinol or 6 μg of β-carotene.

DIETARY EXCESS OF VITAMIN A

Since vitamin A is a lipid-soluble vitamin and is stored in the liver, so if taken in large quantities for a longer period (hypervitaminosis A), it may be toxic. **Vitamin A toxicity** symptoms include dry and rough skin, scaly dermatitis, besides headache, nausea, vomiting, loss of appetite, hepatomegaly, painful joints and bone abnormalities. In high doses, preformed vitamin A or retinol can be even teratogenic. It can cause birth defects (craniofacial abnormalities) and spontaneous abortions if taken during early stages of pregnancy. Because body converts carotenoids into vitamin A only when necessary, thus taking large quantities of carotenes do not cause vitamin A toxicity and there is no risk of its overdose.

VITAMIN A PROPHYLAXIS PROGRAM

As discussed above, vitamin A is essential for normal vision. It also maintains integrity of the epithelial cells and is required for many metabolic functions. **Vitamin A deficiency** (VAD) delayed dark adaptation and lowers the resistance to infections. Prolonged deficiency of the vitamin may produce blindness, a permanent disability.

In India, VAD is most common, in underprivileged population. Young children below the age of 3 years, and pregnant and lactating women are most vulnerable to VAD. Prevalence of VAD is more pronounced in several states, like Rajasthan, Bihar, Madhya Pradesh, Orissa, UP, Tamil Nadu, Karnataka and Andhra Pradesh. VAD was recognized as a major public health problem in 1970, when it was estimated that nearly 30,000–40,000 children could lose their eye sight, due to VAD.

To overcome the problem of VAD, Ministry of Health and Family Welfare launched **vitamin A prophylaxis for prevention of nutritional blindness**, or **vitamin A deficiency program**, in 1970, as a component of **National Program for Control of Blindness** (NPCB).

Aim of the Program

To prevent nutritional blindness due to VAD, leading to keratomalacia in children, under 5 years of age.

There were two strategies:

- **Short-term strategy** included the administration of vitamin A to young children, below 5 years of age (**vitamin A supplementation**), and
- **Long-term strategy** was suggested as ultimate solution for prevention of vitamin A deficiency, by regular consumption of vitamin A-rich foods, which are cheap and locally available (**food-based approach**).

Beneficiaries

All children in 6 months to 5 years of age.

Services and Recommendations

- **Administration of supplemental dose of vitamin A:**
  - 6–11months-1 dose of 1 lac IU
  - 1–5 years-2 lac IU, bianually
- **Long-term strategy:**
  - Promotion of regular intake of vitamin A-rich food
  - Feeding locally available food
  - Kitchen gardening of vitamin A-rich food
- **Treatment of vitamin A deficiency**:
  - Immediately after diagnosis-2 lac IU, followed by another dose of 2 lac IU 1–4 weeks later.

VITAMIN D

Vitamin D, also known as calciferol, anti-rickets factor, sunshine vitamin, is a **sterol** and a **prohormone,** present in nature in several forms. Two common forms are:

- **Vitamin D_2 (ergocalciferol):** It is of **plant origin**, obtained from the ergot plant. It can also be synthesized in the laboratory, by irradiating ergosterol. Note that vitamin D_1 is a complex of ergocalciferol and lumisterol.
- **Vitamin D_3 (cholecalciferol):** It is of **animal origin**, the natural substance obtained from fish oil or derived from 7-dehydrocholesterol by ultraviolet irradiation in the skin (Fig. 8.7).

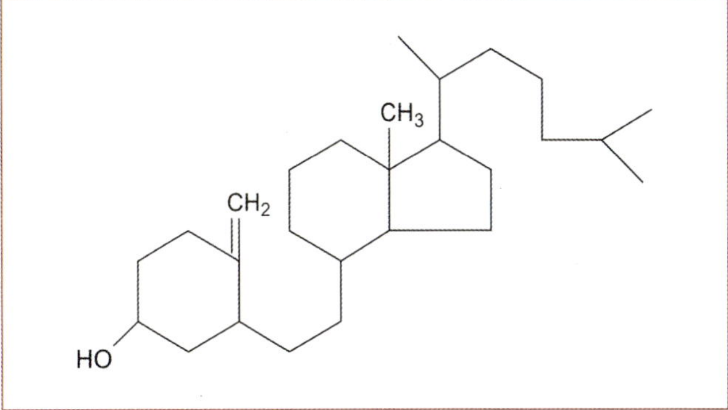

Fig. 8.7: Vitamin D_3 (cholecalciferol)

Interestingly, vitamin D_3 and its active metabolites have also been obtained from some plant sources, particularly from tomato leaves.

Both vitamin D_2 and D_3 are **secosteroids** (steroid with an open 'B' ring) and are metabolically activated to carry out their functions.

Provitamin D and Previtamin D

7-Dehydrocholesterol is a precursor of vitamin D_3 in animals and is called **provitamin D_3.** It is synthesized in human beings in the intestinal mucosa. By the action of UV light in the skin, 7-dehydrocholesterol is converted into an intermediate called **previtamin D_3** which is spontaneously isomerized to vitamin D_3 (cholecalciferol). In this process (photobiogenesis), the UV rays of sunlight with a wavelength of **290–315 nm** (the UV-B range), initiates photoconversion (Fig. 8.8).

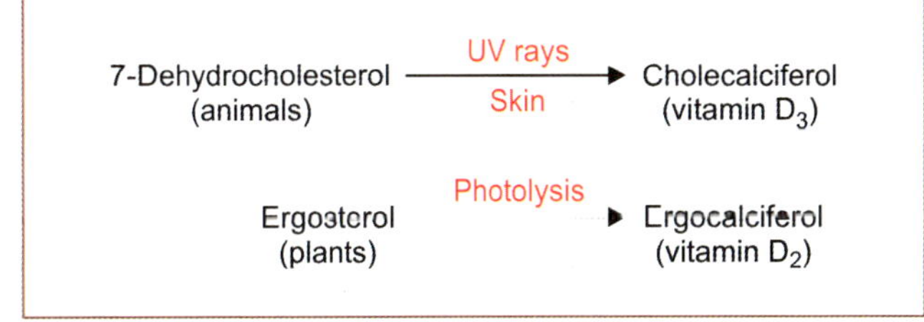

Fig. 8.8: Conversion of provitamin D to vitamin D

On the other hand, ergosterol is the provitamin D_2 in plants. In the presence of light, by the process of photolysis, ergosterol is converted to previtamin D_2 which is isomerized to ergocalciferol (vitamin D_2).

Absorption and Metabolism

In addition to its endogenous synthesis, vitamin D is also absorbed from diet. Maximum absorption of vitamin D_3 occurs in the jejunum. After its absorption from the intestine or following formation in the skin, vitamin D_3 binds to a specific globulin termed

vitamin D binding-protein (DBP, also called transcalciferrin) in the plasma and transported to the liver.

Metabolic Activation of Vitamin D

Activation of vitamin D takes place partly in the liver and partly in the kidney.

The first metabolic step occurs in the liver where vitamin D is hydroxylated by the cytochrome P450-dependent enzyme 25-hydroxylase, to 25-hydroxycholecalciferol [$25(OH)D_3$]. This is also the storage form of the vitamin in the liver. The circulating level of **$25(OHD_3)$** also reflects **vitamin D nutritional status**. It is an immediate precursor of the **active vitamin D (calcitriol)**.

From liver, 25-hydroxycholecalciferol is transported to the kidneys, where it is further hydroxylated at position 1, by the mitochondrial enzyme 1-α-hydroxylase, and is converted to 1,25-dihydroxycholecalciferol **[$1, 25(OH)_2D_3$]**. This is the **physiologically active form of the vitamin**. This metabolite functions as a hormone and is essential in calcium homeostasis. Further, due to the presence of 3-OH groups, active form of vitamin D, i.e. $1,25(OH)_2D_3$ is also called **calcitriol**. Alternatively, $25(OH)D_3$ may also be converted to the inactive 24, $25(OH)_2D_3$ (Fig. 8.9).

Regulation of 1-α-hydroxylase: The enzyme 1-α-hydroxylase is present in renal tubules, bone and placenta. The enzyme is regulated by parathormone (parathyroid hormone or **PTH**), which is required for the conversion of 25-hydroxycholecalciferol to calcitriol. Besides PTH, 1-α-hydroxylase is also regulated by serum **phosphorus** as well as by calcitriol itself (**autoregulation**). The production of $1,25(OH)_2D_3$ is also enhanced or suppressed under the conditions of low or high serum calcium, respectively.

ROLE OF VITAMIN D IN HEALTH AND DISEASE

1. **Skeletal effects:** The most important biological role of calcitriol is the regulation of serum calcium and phosphorus levels. The net result is achieved through its action in the intestine, bone and kidneys:
   - ***In the intestine***: Calcium absorption from the intestine occurs in **three steps**: Release of calcium from its bound forms in the food such as calcium phosphate; sequestering calcium in the cytosol by binding it to specific proteins; and energy-dependent exit of calcium from the cells into the circulation. Calcitriol induces the synthesis of alkaline phosphatase, calcium binding proteins

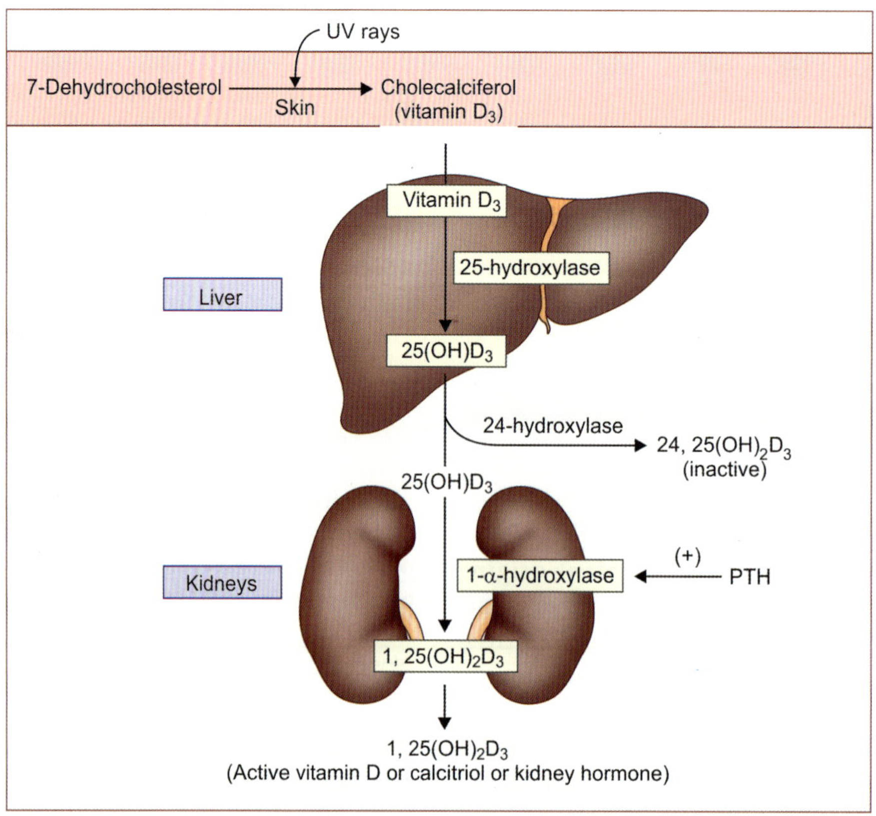

Fig. 8.9: Activation of vitamin D

8

such as calmodulin, and Ca^{2+}-dependent ATPase to increase the efficiency of absorption of calcium as well as phosphorus at each step.

- *In bones*: Bone remodeling is a **dynamic and continuous** process. Bone formation is carried out by cells called osteoblasts, whereas the opposite process, bone resorption, is performed by osteoclasts. Calcitriol stimulates the synthesis of the proteins osteocalcin and osteopontin in the osteoblasts; these proteins become a part of the bone matrix (osteoid) and bind calcium. Thus, calcitriol favors mineralization when serum calcium is normal or rising (as after a meal). However, when serum calcium tends to fall, calcitriol promotes the differentiation of pre-osteoclasts to osteoclasts which in turn mobilize calcium from the bone, i.e. causes demineralization of the bone and restores normocalcemia.
- *In kidneys*: Calcitriol increases the tubular reabsorption of calcium and excretion of phosphorus.

  The overall effect of calcitriol therefore is to maintain **calcium/phosphorus homeostasis** and its actions on individual target tissues are dictated by the serum calcium/phosphorus levels. It should be remembered that calcitriol always works in **collaboration with PTH and calcitonin**.

2. **Nonskeletal effects:** Contrary to popular belief, the nonskeletal actions of vitamin D are **as important** as the skeletal ones. The major aspects regulated by vitamin D include:
   - Cell proliferation and differentiation
   - Insulin release
   - Action of growth hormone
   - Immune response
   - Fertility

Significance of 25-hydroxyvitamin D: Serum 25(OH)D_3 is an indicator of an individual's **vitamin D status** in the body; normal range 25–30 ng/ml although some consider that it should be >30 ng/ml.

DEFICIENCY MANIFESTATIONS OF VITAMIN D

Deficiency of vitamin D generally does not occur as it can be synthesized in the body. Deficiency may however, occurs due to lack of sunshine.

- ***Skeletal effects of vitamin D deficiency:*** A deficiency of vitamin D leads to **rickets in children.** Rickets is of several types (Fig. 8.10).

  In adults, deficiency of vitamin D leads to **osteomalacia**, also called adult rickets. Osteomalacia is different from osteoporosis (Fig. 8.11).

  Table 8.1 shows differences between three different types of rickets, osteomalacia and osteoporosis.

  It should be remembered that serum alkaline phosphatase is normally elevated in growing children and may also be raised in unrelated diseases in adults because of the existence of isoenzymes, hence it is useful to measure calcium × phosphate product (Chemistry to Clinics 8.3).

Chemistry to Clinics 8.3: Calcium × Phosphate Product

Product of serum calcium and inorganic phosphorus which is normally 40 (10 mg calcium × 4 mg phosphorus), may decrease to <30 in rickets and osteomalacia. Administration of vitamin D in therapeutic doses and/or exposure to sunlight corrects the deficiency.

- ***Nonskeletal effects of vitamin D deficiency***: Vitamin D deficiency may also lead to defects in insulin secretion and impaired glucose tolerance; impaired immunity; carcinogenesis, etc.

DIETARY SOURCES OF VITAMIN D

Vitamin D can be synthesized in the body by the action of ultraviolet light on the skin: 10–20 minutes of daily exposure to the midnoon/afternoon sunshine is adequate to meet the daily needs of vitamin D. However, some researchers recommend a much longer exposure.

Rich dietary sources are milk, butter, egg yolk, fish oil and liver oil.

RDA OF VITAMIN D

The RDA for vitamin D is 600 IU/d.

DIETARY EXCESS OF VITAMIN D

Dietary excess of vitamin D (in extremely large doses or hypervitaminosis D) can cause hypercalcemia, hyperphosphatemia, anorexia, nausea, vomiting and diarrhea, besides bone pain and metastatic calcification of the soft tissues including the kidney, the myocardium, the pancreas and the uterus.

VITAMIN E

Several compounds belonging to the group of **tocopherols**, such as α, β, γ and d tocopherols have been

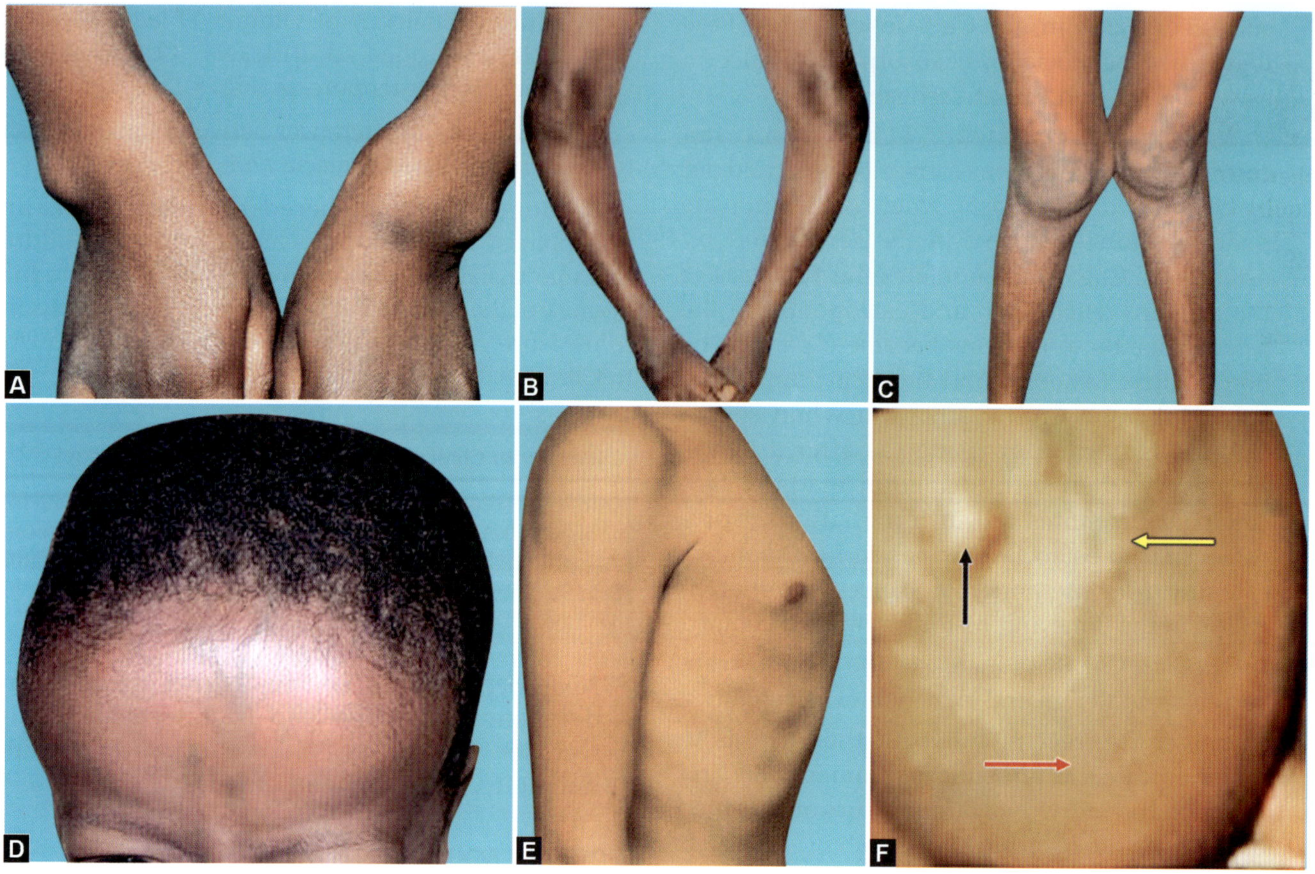

Fig. 8.10: Salient clinical features of rickets. (A) Enlarged wrists; (B) Bow legs (genu varum); (C) Knock-knees (genu valgum); (D) Frontal bossing; (E) Pigeon chest (pectus carinatum, protrusion of the sternum and ribs); (F) Rachitic rosary (prominence of costochondral junctions, black arrow), Harrison's sulcus (horizontal groove corresponding to the indentation of lower ribs at the diaphragmatic attachment, yellow arrow) and pot belly (red arrow)

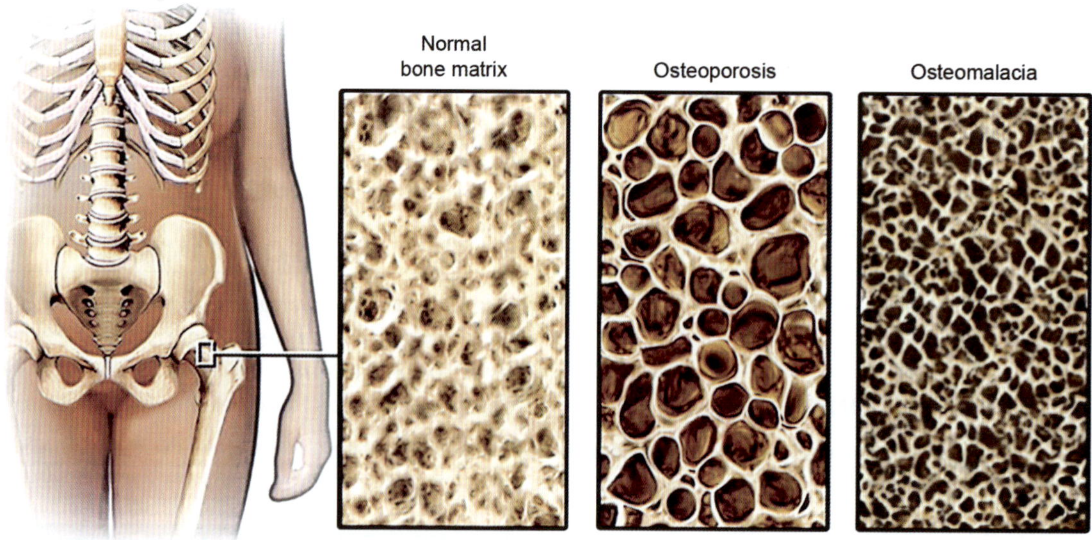

Fig. 8.11: **Osteoporosis** is characterized by a decrease in bone density (mass per unit volume) and occurs in a fully developed bone. It appears like 'pores' in the bone, hence the name. **Osteomalacia** is a defect in bone mineralization in a developing or developed bone. The osteoid is generally preserved. It is the adult counterpart of rickets

Table 8.1: Comparison between the various types of rickets, osteomalacia and osteoporosis

Parameter	Vitamin D-responsive rickets	Vitamin D-resistant rickets	Renal rickets	Osteomalacia (adult rickets)	Osteoporosis
Inherited/ acquired	Acquired	Inherited	Acquired	Acquired	Acquired
Age	Infancy/childhood	Infancy/ childhood	Any	Adult and elderly	Adult and elderly
Cause	↓Dietary vitamin D and/or ↓exposure to sunlight	↓Renal 1-α-hydroxylase	↓Functional renal mass, e.g. chronic renal failure due to diabetes mellitus, hypertension, etc.	↓Dietary vitamin D and/or ↓exposure to sunlight (females during pregnancy and lactation; women who are protected from sunlight, such as those observing purdah; prolonged bed-ridden patients)	Multifactorial-↓dietary calcium, ↓estrogen, prolonged bed-ridden patients, drug induced, e.g. corticosteroids
Bone structure	Osteoid matrix of developing bone fails to get properly mineralized	As in vitamin D-responsive rickets	Bone healthy initially; demineralization of osteoid later in life, coinciding with the phase of renal disease	Bone healthy since childhood; extensive demineralization of normal osteoid later in life, coinciding with the phase of vitamin D deficiency	Bone healthy since childhood; ↓osteoid formation plus ↓mineralization leads to ↓bone density (mass per unit volume) later in life
Common clinical presentation	Enlarged wrists and ankles, bowed-legs, knock-knees, delayed dentition	As in vitamin D-responsive rickets	Features of the specific disease that resulted in chronic renal failure	Weakness, bone pain, delayed parturition (in females due to pelvic bone deformities)	Weakness, bone pain, fracture(s)
Biochemical findings in serum	↓Calcium, ↓vitamin D, ↓Ca × P product, ↓alkaline phosphatase, ↑PTH	As in vitamin D-responsive rickets	As in vitamin D-responsive rickets; plus features of the specific disease that resulted in chronic renal failure	As in vitamin D-responsive rickets	Normal calcium and vitamin D, normal or ↓alkaline phosphatase, normal PTH, ↓estrogen (postmenopausal)
Treatment	Vitamin D, sunlight	Calcitriol	Calcitriol	Vitamin D, sunlight	Calcium, vitamin D, estrogen replacement (postmenopausal)

shown to exhibit vitamin E activity but **α-tocopherol has the highest biological activity** and widest distribution. α-Tocopherol is an alcohol which has phytol and trimethylhydroquinone in its structure (Fig. 8.12).

Fig. 8.12: α-Tocopherol (vitamin E)

Commercially, vitamin E is available both as a natural substance as well as a synthetic compound. Natural vitamin E is d-α-tocopherol and is a single stereoisomer. On the other hand, synthetic vitamin E is d-α-tocopherol which is produced commercially.

Absorption and Metabolism

Vitamin E is readily absorbed from the gastrointestinal tract with the dietary lipids and is transported in lipoproteins to the liver and peripheral tissues. Compared to synthetic vitamin E, natural form is retained better by the body. It is also concentrated in phospholipids. The levels of vitamin E in plasma lipoproteins and phospholipids depend upon the dietary levels of vitamin E, various pro- and antioxidants, selenium and sulfur-containing amino acids. High doses of vitamin C may decrease vitamin E absorption.

ROLE OF VITAMIN E IN HEALTH AND DISEASE

- All **unsaturated fatty acids**, especially, those containing more than two double bonds, are sensitive to the attack by oxygen and form lipid peroxides. The process, designated as peroxidation, is initiated by free radicals. Once initiated, **lipid peroxidation process is a chain reaction** and is a potential source of damage to the cell membrane and other components. The products of lipid peroxidation, such as malondialdehyde can cross-link several biological molecules. Vitamin E is the major lipid soluble antioxidant in cell membrane that breaks the chain of lipid peroxidation and, thus, it acts as **chain-breaking antioxidant** (Fig. 8.13).
- It protects readily oxidizable molecules in the cells, such as polyunsaturated fatty acyl components of phospholipids of the cell membrane, and vitamin A esters.
- Through its ability to quench free radicals generated by metabolic processes and environmental pollutants, vitamin E can help protect cells and other components of the body from several diseases, such as cancer, heart diseases and premature aging.

DEFICIENCY MANIFESTATIONS OF VITAMIN E

Unlike other vitamins, deficiency of vitamin E does not produce a specific disease with rapidly progressing symptoms. Instead, the results of vitamin E deficiency usually take years to develop:

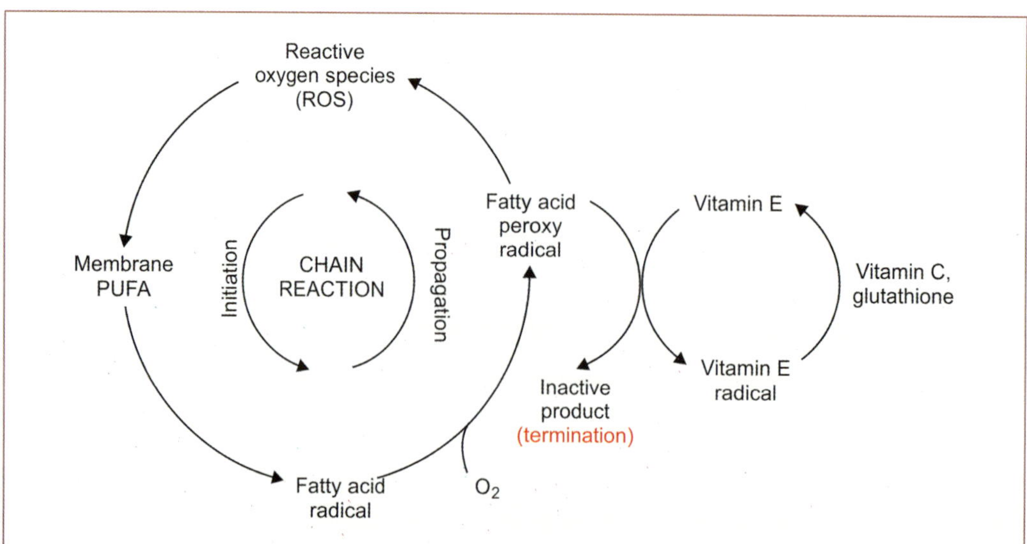

Fig. 8.13: Vitamin E: A chain-breaking antioxidant

1. Low blood levels of vitamin E have been reported in acne, anemia, infections, cancers, periodontal disease, neuromuscular diseases and Alzheimer's disease.
2. Vitamin E deficiency is seen in patients with abetalipoproteinemia. Such individuals are unable to form chylomicrons and VLDL, as a consequence of which vitamin E is neither absorbed nor distributed.
3. Deficiency of vitamin E is seen in children with fat malabsorption. In newborn infants, sprue, creatinuria, peptic ulceration, red cell hemolysis, etc, is common. Such children show signs of severe progressive neuropathy and retinopathy.
4. Other deficiency symptoms, observed in various animal species include certain reproductive defects such as sterility, degeneration of the testes, regression in the fetal resorption besides hepatic necrosis, muscular dystrophy and vascular system defects. Axonal degeneration of the large myelinated axons results in posterior column and spinocerebellar symptoms such as ataxia, decreased vibration and position sensation.

Clinical use of vitamin E: Contrary to common practice, clinical use of vitamin E should be limited (Chemistry to Clinics 8.4).

Chemistry to Clinics 8.4: Prescribing Vitamin E as a general health supplement

The common practice of prescribing vitamin E as a general health supplement should be discouraged. Since a clear-cut clinical deficiency of vitamin E is not seen, its use is limited and may show response in:

1. Fibrocystic breast disease (episodes of tightness or pain in the breasts at specific periods of the menstrual cycle).
2. Intermittent claudication (episodes of tingling, numbness and pain in the legs due to ischemia).
3. Patients at high risk of free radical-mediated injury (prescribed along with other antioxidants).

DIETARY SOURCES OF VITAMIN E

Oils such as corn oil, cotton seed oil and sunflower oil are the richest sources of vitamin E.

Tocopherols are present in small quantities in green-leafy vegetables (spinach and lettuce), milk products and egg yolk.

RDA OF VITAMIN E

Requirement of vitamin E however, varies from individual to individual, depending on the level and nature of activity, diet, exposure to psychological stress and polluted environment, and on the intake of polyunsaturated fatty acids (PUFA). As per ICMR-NIN (2020), 0.8 mg of vitamin E is required per g of PUFA.

The RDA of vitamin E in adults is 8–10 mg per day.

VITAMIN K

The name vitamin K (**Koagulation** factor) has been derived from the Danish word Koagulation since it has an important role in blood clotting. Various compounds related to 2-methyl-1,4-naphthoquinone have been described to have vitamin K activity.

The most important form which occurs naturally is **vitamin K_1** (phylloquinone). It is found in **plants** and has a phytyl side chain (Fig. 8.14).

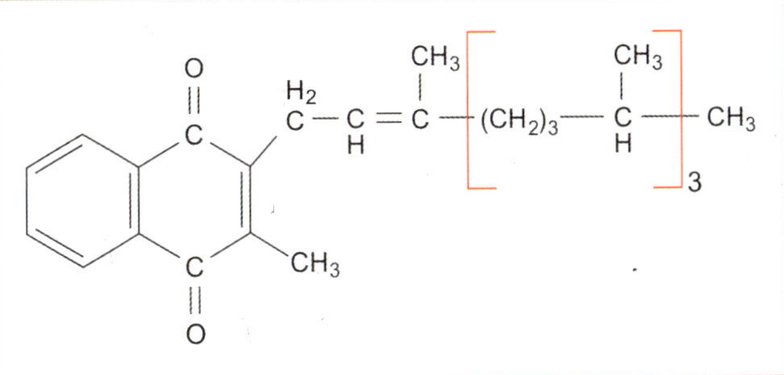

Fig. 8.14: Vitamin K_1 (phylloquinone)

Vitamin K_2 (menaquinone or farnequinone) is synthesized by the **intestinal bacteria** and has a farnesyl side chain (the chain with 7 isoprenoid units).

Vitamin K_3 (menadione) is a **synthetic** compound available commercially for therapeutic uses. It is water soluble and gets easily absorbed on parenteral administration.

Absorption of Vitamin K

Vitamin K is absorbed with dietary lipids in the presence of bile salts and is utilized in the liver.

ROLE OF VITAMIN K IN HEALTH AND DISEASE

Vitamin K is essential for the maintenance of normal levels of some of the blood clotting factors such as **factor II (prothrombin), factor VII, factor IX and factor X.** These proteins are synthesized in the liver in their **inactive forms** and are converted into their **biologically active forms** in the presence of vitamin K.

Prothrombin is rich in glutamate residues (**Glu**). During post-translational changes, several of the Glu are carboxylated into γ-carboxyglutamate (**Gla**) and form the sites of Ca^{2+} binding on a prothrombin molecule. The reduced form of vitamin K is essential for the introduction of carboxylate groups into Glu and thus converts them into Gla. For this process, O_2 is also necessary. Vitamin K, in turn, gets oxidized to vitamin K epoxide, which is reduced back by epoxide reductase (Fig. 8.15).

Besides prothrombin, clotting factors VII, IX and X also undergo carboxylation of their Glu.

DEFICIENCY MANIFESTATIONS OF VITAMIN K

Deficiency of vitamin K is seen in newborns due to sterile intestine, particularly the premature infants. It is also common in patients with malabsorption (sprue), obstructive jaundice, advanced hepatic damage (liver carcinoma, cirrhosis, etc.), in subjects on prolonged antibiotics or anticoagulant therapy (Chemistry to Clinics 8.5).

DIETARY SOURCES OF VITAMIN K

Vitamin K is found in abundance in green-leafy vegetables such as spinach, lettuce and cabbage. Besides, fish, liver and skeletal muscle are also good sources of vitamin K.

RDA OF VITAMIN K

The RDA of vitamin K is 55 μg/d. However, it is advised to administer a **single prophylactic dose of 1 mg of vitamin K_3 to the newb orn on the first day of life.**

Table 8.2 lists various lipid-soluble vitamins, their role in health and disease, deficiency manifestations, dietary sources and RDA.

Chemistry to Clinics 8.5: Vitamin K Antagonists

Due to structural similarity to vitamin K, dicumarol and warfarin act as antagonists to vitamin K. They act as competitive inhibitors of the enzymes concerned with the activation of prothrombin and other coagulation factors which require vitamin K as the coenzyme. Warfarin inhibits the conversion of vitamin K epoxide to vitamin K as well as the conversion of preprothrombin precursor to active prothrombin.

Common deficiency symptoms include cutaneous and intramuscular **hemorrhages** with bluish-red coloration in different parts of the body. There is a decrease in the levels of plasma vitamin K. **Prothrombin time is increased.**

WATER-SOLUBLE VITAMINS

Water-soluble vitamins include vitamin B complex and vitamin C. Their general properties include:

- Dietary water-soluble vitamins are absorbed rapidly from the gastrointestinal lumen, **irrespective of the presence of lipids.**
- Most of them are converted into **coenzymes** for various metabolic reactions.
- Vitamin status of the body can be **assessed** by measuring one or more **enzyme activities** in the **isolated red blood cells.**
- Due to their water solubility, they **cannot be stored** to any significant extent.
- Because they cannot be stored, a dietary **deficiency quickly becomes manifest.** Typical deficiency symptoms for most of the water-soluble vitamins, particularly those of vitamin B complex, include dermatitis, glossitis, cheilosis and diarrhea besides

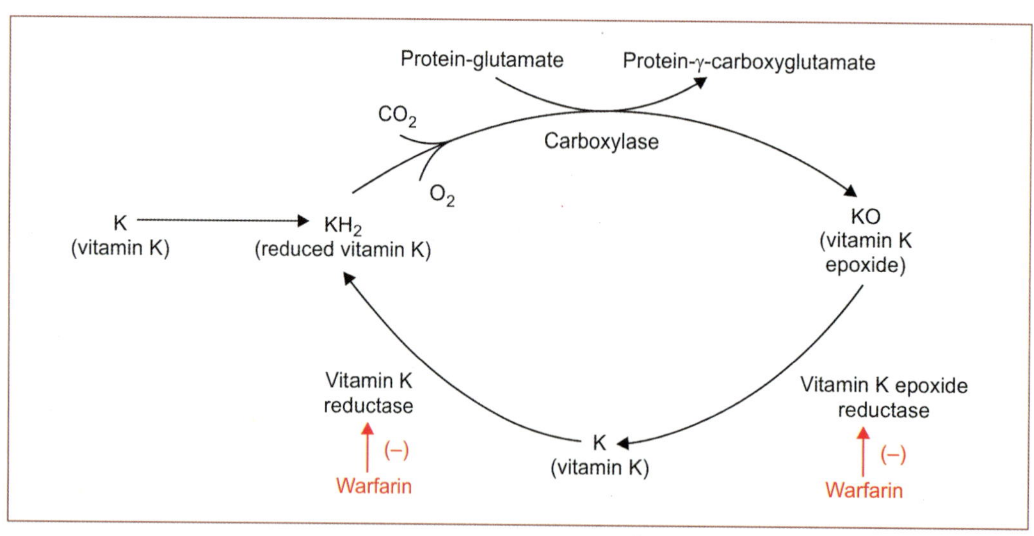

Fig. 8.15: Vitamin K cycle

Table 8.2: Lipid-soluble vitamins, their biological functions and RDA

Vitamin	Provitamin	Biological functions	Deficiency disorders	Sources	RDA*
A (Retinol)	Carotenoids (Carotenes)	In vision, epithelial integrity	Night blindness, disorders of epithelium and mucus membrane	Animal, fish and vegetable oils	1000 µg
D (Calciferol)	7-Dehydrocholesterol	Calcium/phosphate homoeostasis	Rickets, osteomalacia	Fish oil, UV rays	600 IU
E (Tocopherol)	–	As antioxidant	Hemolytic anemia in infants	Plant oils	8–10 mg
K	–	In blood coagulation	Bleeding disorder	Plant oils, intestinal bacteria	55 µg

*ICMR-NIN (2020)

some of the neurological symptoms, such as peripheral neuropathy and malaise.

- Large doses are excreted in the urine and **rarely result in toxicity**.

VITAMIN B COMPLEX

Vitamins of the B complex group include a group of compounds, most of which can also be synthesized in the gastrointestinal tract by the microbial flora. Most of the components of vitamin B complex group are **heat stable, except vitamin B_1 which is heat labile**.

VITAMIN B_1

Vitamin B_1 is the name given to **thiamin.** Since thiamin was the first member of the vitamin B complex, it is referred to as **vitamin B_1**. Further, due to its role in the prevention of beriberi, it is called **anti-beriberi factor**. Also, as this vitamin has an important role in the nervous system, it is also called **aneurine**.

Structurally, a thiamin molecule consists of a pyrimidine ring, which in turn, is linked to a thiazole ring (Fig. 8.16).

Thiamin occurs as thiamin hydrochloride. Though thiamin is heat labile, it is quite stable in the acidic medium. Tea, coffee, raw-fish and shellfish contain **thiaminase** which can destroy the vitamin.

Biochemical Role of Vitamin B_1

In its diphosphorylated form, i.e. as thiamin pyrophosphate (**TPP**), it acts as a coenzyme. It is important in carbohydrate metabolism. The reactions where TPP is used as a coenzyme include:

1. **Oxidative decarboxylation** of α-ketoacids, e.g. of pyruvate to acetyl-CoA by pyruvate dehydrogenase complex, and α-ketoglutarate to succinyl-CoA by α-ketoglutarate dehydrogenase complex, in the citric acid cycle (Fig. 8.17).
2. TPP is also a coenzyme for **transketolase** in the hexose monophosphate shunt. RBC transketolase activity is measured to assess thiamin status of the body.

Fig. 8.16: Thiamin (vitamin B_1)

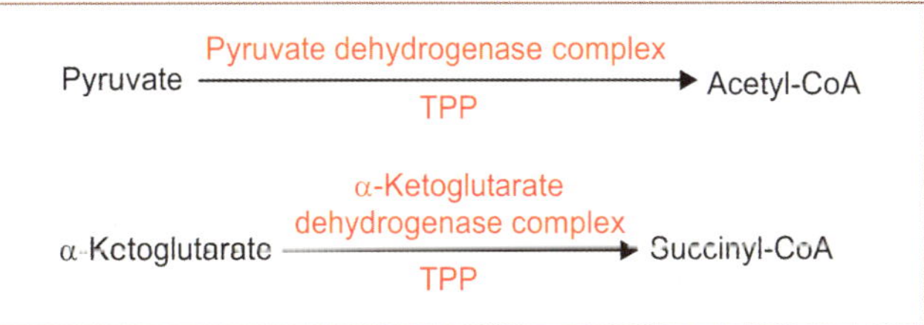

Fig. 8.17: Biochemical functions of TPP

Deficiency Manifestations of Vitamin B_1

Thiamin deficiency results in beriberi (Chemistry to Clinics 8.6).

Chemistry to Clinics 8.6: Beriberi

Deficiency of thiamin commonly occurs in:

1. Areas where people consume polished-rice; it results in loss of available thiamin. The loss can be decreased by using unpolished or parboiled rice or whole wheat flour.
2. Consumption of raw fish in large quantities
3. Chronic alcoholics.

Deficiency of thiamin causes beriberi. Signs and symptoms, however, vary according to duration and severity of the disease as well as the predominant organs involved. It is classified into:

1. **Wet beriberi:** It affects the cardiovascular system, and results in edema and dilated heart.
2. **Dry beriberi:** It affects the nervous system and causes peripheral neuropathy with myelin degeneration, leading to foot-drop, wrist-drop and sensory changes (Fig. 8.18).

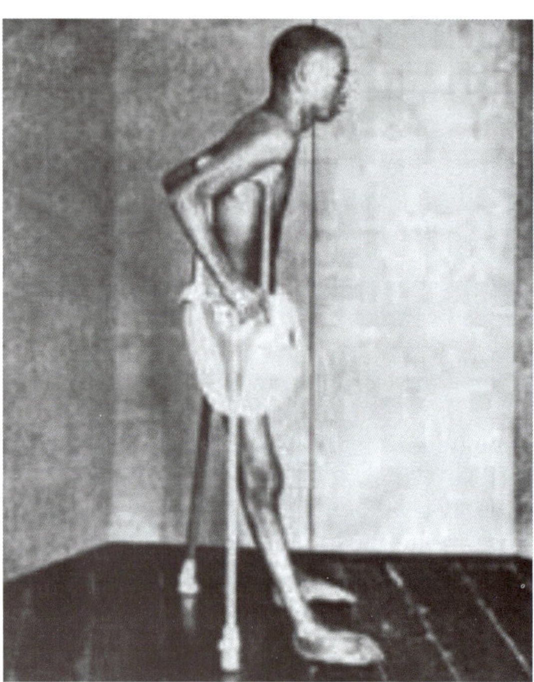

Fig. 8.18: Beriberi

3. **Wernicke's encephalopathy:** Alcoholic patients with chronic thiamin deficiency may also have CNS manifestations, ophthalmoplegia, cerebellar ataxia and mental impairment.

RBC transketolase activity is reduced in beriberi. Blood pyruvic acid concentration is raised.

Dietary Sources of Vitamin B_1

Though widely distributed; rich sources of vitamin B_1 are cereal grains, yeast, liver, kidney and heart.

RDA of Vitamin B_1

Average daily requirement of vitamin B_1 is **1.4–2.3 mg/day.** Its RDA depends upon carbohydrate intake of the individual. Requirement is increased in fever, hyperthyroidism, alcoholics and pregnant woman.

VITAMIN B_2

Vitamin B_2 is also called riboflavin or lactoflavin, due to its high content in milk. The vitamin is sensitive to light and ultraviolet irradiation but is stable in acidic and neutral medium. The structure contains an isoalloxazine ring with a ribitol side chain (Fig. 8.19).

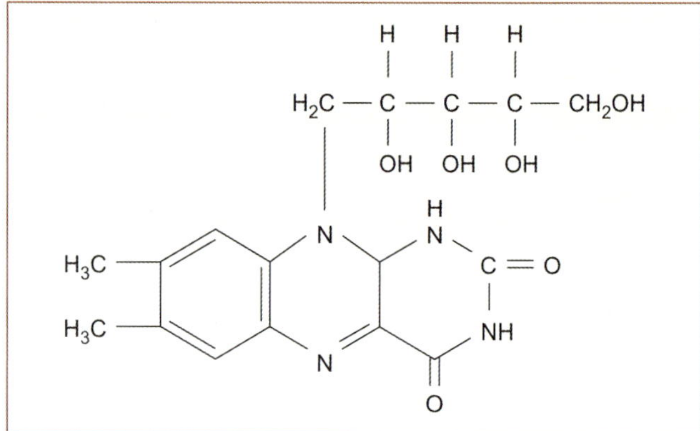

Fig. 8.19: Riboflavin (vitamin B_2)

Biochemical Role of Vitamin B_2

Riboflavin with phosphoric acid forms flavin mononucleotide (FMN) which is a coenzyme form of the vitamin. The other coenzyme form of riboflavin is flavin adenine dinucleotide (FAD). It is a dinucleotide of FMN and AMP (Fig. 8.20).

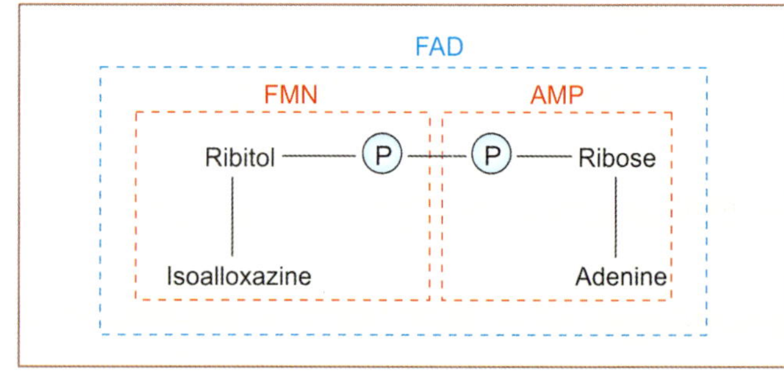

Fig. 8.20: FMN and FAD

The two coenzymes form an integral part of the flavoprotein containing enzymes and are important in oxidation-reduction reactions, requiring **oxidoreductases**. The isoalloxazine ring serves as an acceptor of the two hydrogens, and in turn, gets reduced (Fig. 8.21).

FMN is an important coenzyme of cytochrome c reductase and L-amino acid oxidases. FAD is a coenzyme of succinate dehydrogenase, glycerol-3-phosphate dehydrogenase, xanthine oxidase, glycine

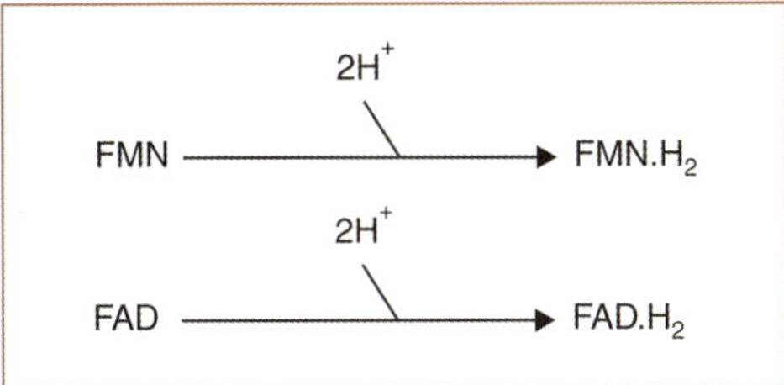

Fig. 8.21: Biochemical functions of FMN and FAD

oxidase, sphingosine reductase and D-amino acid oxidases. It is an integral part of acyl-CoA dehydrogenase. It is thus important in the metabolism of carbohydrates, lipids as well as proteins.

Deficiency Manifestation of Vitamin B_2

It is uncommon but may be associated with niacin or iron deficiency. Symptoms include cheilosis (lesions of the angles of the mouth), glossitis, dermatitis, photophobia and lacrimation (Fig. 8.22).

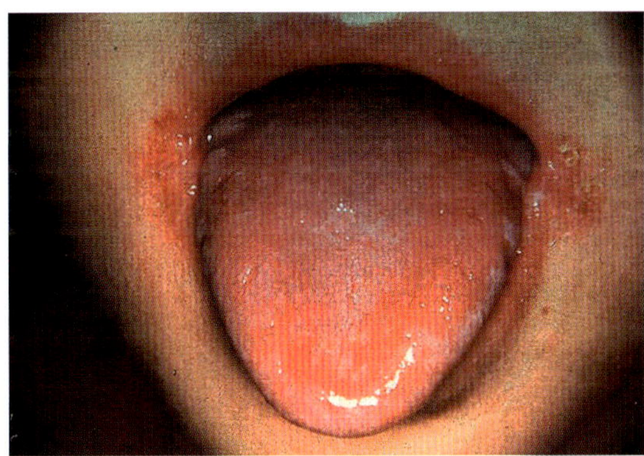

Fig. 8.22: Angular cheilosis

Erythrocyte glutathione reductase activity is used as an assay of riboflavin status of the body.

Dietary Sources of Vitamin B_2

It is though widely distributed in nature, milk, liver and kidneys are rich sources of riboflavin.

RDA of Vitamin B_2

The RDA of vitamin B_2 is **1.9–3.1 mg/day.**

NIACIN

Niacin is also known as **pellagra preventive factor** or anti-pellagra factor because of its role in the prevention of pellagra. Sometimes it is also referred to as vitamin B_3. Niacin is a generic name given to two compounds having pyridine ring with a carboxyl group, i.e. **nicotinic acid** and its amide, called **nicotinamide** (Fig. 8.23).

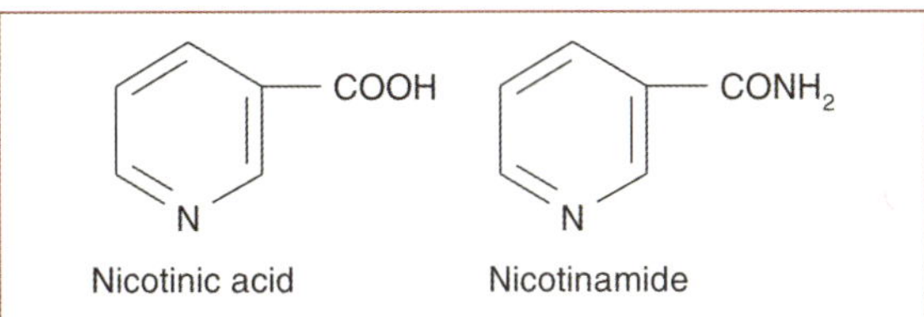

Fig. 8.23: Niacin vitamins

Nicotinic acid has a clinical significance (Chemistry to Clinics 8.7).

Chemistry to Clinics 8.7: Niacin Flush

Nicotinic acid, derived from the vitamin niacin, is clinically used as a hypolipidemic agent to reduce high blood cholesterol levels. Large amounts of nicotinic acid dilate the capillaries so that the patient may complain of tingling sensations that could be painful. This is known as 'niacin flush'. Interestingly, another niacin derivative called nicotinamide, neither exhibits niacin flush nor it reduces blood cholesterol.

Besides its absorption by the intestine, niacin is also synthesized in the body from an essential amino acid **tryptophan**.

Biochemical Role of Niacin

Niacin is an important constituent of two coenzymes, i.e. nicotinamide adenine dinucleotide (NAD^+) and its phosphorylated form called nicotinamide adenine dinucleotide phosphate ($NADP^+$). Both the coenzymes contain two nucleotides (each of pyridine and adenine), which are linked together. In both the forms, i.e. NAD^+ as well as $NADP^+$, since the nitrogen atom of the pyridine ring is in the oxidized state, they have a positive charge. These coenzymes are important in **oxidation-reduction reactions** and are used with dehydrogenases where they act as electron acceptors.

NAD^+ is used as a coenzyme with malate dehydrogenase (in the conversion of malate to oxaloacetate) and lactate dehydrogenase (LDH) which converts lactate to pyruvate (Fig. 8.24).

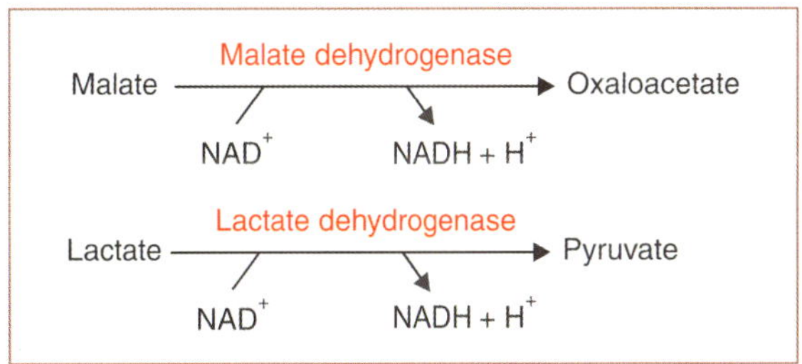

Fig. 8.24: Biochemical functions of NAD

$NADP^+$ is used as a coenzyme with isocitrate dehydrogenase and glucose-6-phosphate dehydrogenase (Fig. 8.25).

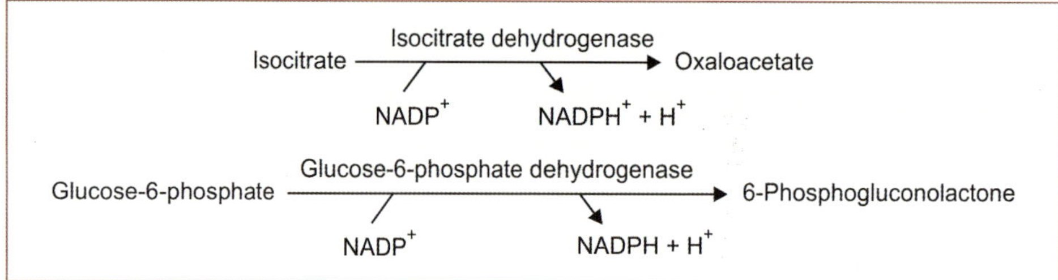

Fig. 8.25: Biochemical functions of NADP

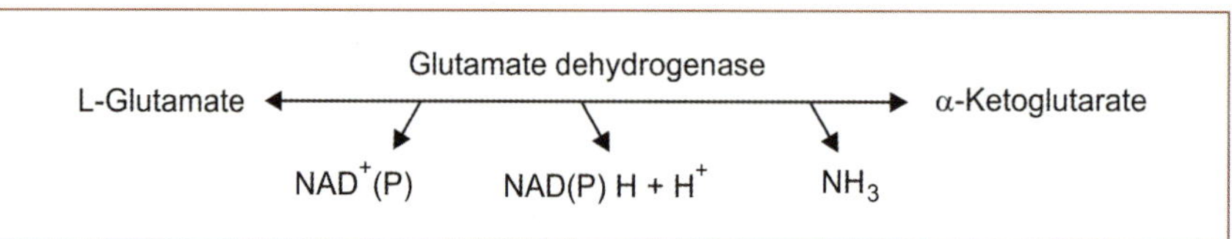

Fig. 8.26: Glutamate dehydrogenase reaction

Glutamate dehydrogenase, however, can use both, i.e. either NAD^+ or $NADP^+$ (Fig. 8.26).

Deficiency Manifestations of Niacin

Niacin deficiency results in pellagra (Chemistry to Clinics 8.8).

Chemistry to Clinics 8.8: Pellagra

Deficiency of niacin is not usually observed since it can be synthesized in the body from tryptophan (an essential amino acid). Its deficiency, however, may occur in:

1. People whose staple food is maize or sorghum (jowar). These cereals are rich in leucine but are deficient in tryptophan; the amino acid imbalance affects tryptophan-niacin pathway, and in turn, reduces the biosynthesis of niacin (normally 60 mg tryptophan forms 1 mg niacin). Leucine itself also inhibits endogenous biosynthesis of niacin.
2. Patients taking isonicotinic acid hydrazide (INH), an antitubercular drug (along with the deficiency of vitamin B_6).
3. Patients with Hartnup's disease which is due to a defect in tryptophan absorption.

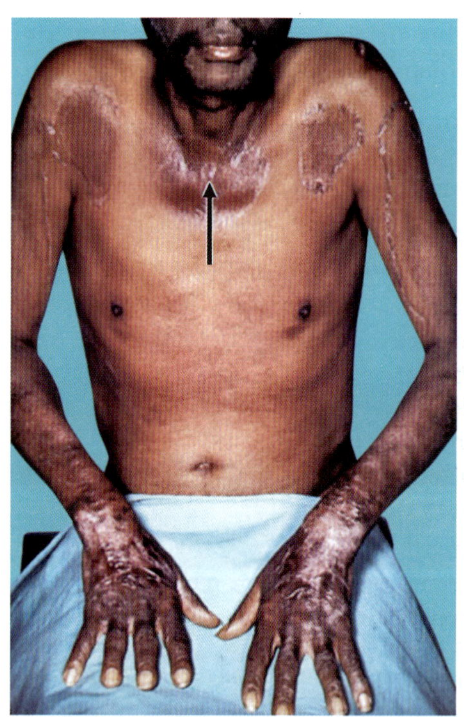

Fig. 8.27: Pellagra with characteristic dermatologic features: Desquamation, erythema, scaling and keratosis of sun-exposed parts. The skin lesion may surround the neck, the so-called Casal's necklace (arrow)

Deficiency of niacin leads to pellagra, a disease characterized by 3Ds, i.e. **d**ermatitis, **d**iarrhea and **d**ementia:

1. **Dermatitis:** It results in pain in those parts of the body which are exposed to sunlight, such as face, neck, hands and feet. These parts become bronze-colored resembling sunburn and later become thickened (Fig. 8.27).
2. **Diarrhea:** It is accompanied with anorexia and other abdominal discomforts.
3. **Dementia:** It is due to impaired ability of the brain to utilize carbohydrates. Symptoms like depression, confusion and psychosis are commonly observed which are due to decreased synthesis of tryptophan-derived neurotransmitters.

Prolonged deficiency of niacin may ultimately result in **d**eath, the fourth 'D' of pellagra.

Dietary Sources of Niacin

Rice polish, yeast, liver, poultry and green vegetables are good sources of niacin. Milk and milk products though are not common sources of niacin but are important pellagra preventive factors due to their high content of tryptophan.

RDA of Niacin

Daily requirement of niacin is related to the intake of tryptophan. The RDA for niacin is **11-23 mg per day.**

Niacin can be synthesized by human beings from tryptophan provided other B complex vitamins are adequate in the diet. Biosynthesis of niacin requires pyridoxal phosphate. **60 mg of tryptophan can form 1 mg of niacin**.

PYRIDOXINE

Pyridoxine is also called **vitamin B_6**. It is a group of 3 compounds, i.e. **pyridoxine, pyridoxal and pyridoxamine,** which contain a pyridine ring (Fig. 8.28).

Biochemical Role of Vitamin B_6

The vitamin is transported in the blood in its coenzyme form, i.e. pyridoxal-5-phosphate or **PLP** (Fig. 8.29).

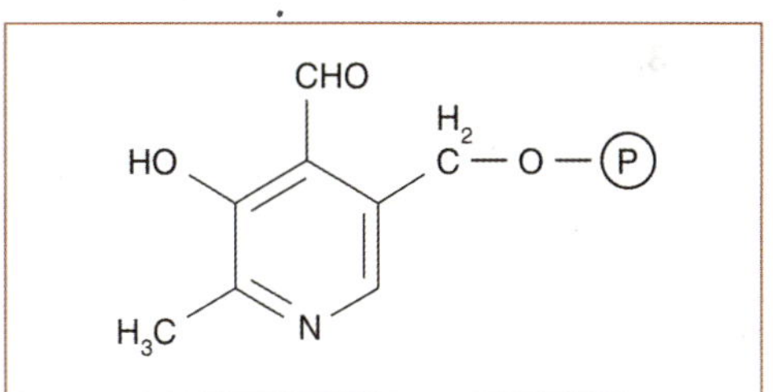

Fig. 8.29: Pyridoxal-5-phosphate

1. **Transamination:** With transaminases, PLP acts as an acceptor of the amino group from an amino acid, thereby forming the corresponding α-keto acid and pyridoxamine phosphate. Followed by reversal of the process, pyridoxamine releases amino group to the other α-keto acid, for the formation of the corresponding amino acid (Fig. 8.30).

   During this process, PLP forms a Schiff's base with α-amino acid through a bond between aldehyde group of PLP and α-amino group of the amino acid.

   Pyridoxal phosphate is used as a coenzyme for glutamate pyruvate transaminase (GPT) also called alanine aminotransferase (ALT), glutamate oxaloacetate transaminase (GOT) also called aspartate aminotransferase (AST), tyrosine transaminase, etc.

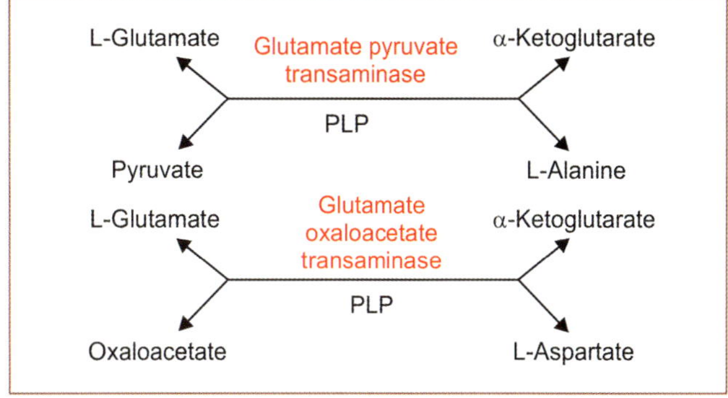

Fig. 8.30: Biochemical functions of PLP

2. **Dehydratases and desulfhydrases:** These enzymes require PLP for the metabolism of hydroxyamino acids and sulfur-containing amino acids.
3. **Decarboxylation:** Pyridoxal phosphate is a coenzyme for decarboxylases. The PLP thus regulates neuronal activity since it is important in the synthesis of many biogenic amines that are neurotransmitters (Table 8.3).
4. **Niacin synthesis:** Pyridoxal phosphate, as a coenzyme is required for kynureninase in the conversion of tryptophan to niacin. In pyridoxine deficiency, instead of niacin, tryptophan is converted to xanthurenic acid, which is excreted in the urine. Deficiency of pyridoxine thus can be **diagnosed by**

Fig. 8.28: Compounds having vitamin B_6 activity

Table 8.3: Neurotransmitters (biogenic amines) synthesized by vitamin B_6-dependent decarboxylation reactions

Substrate	Enzyme	Product (neurotransmitter)
Glutamic acid	Glutamate decarboxylase	γ-Aminobutyric acid (GABA)
DOPA	DOPA decarboxylase	Dopamine
5-Hydroxytryptophan	5-Hydroxytryptophan decarboxylase	5-Hydroxytryptamine (serotonin)
Histidine	Histidine decarboxylase	Histamine
Tyrosine	Tyrosine decarboxylase	Tyramine
Kynurenic acid	Kynurenic acid decarboxylase	kynurenine

measuring urinary excretion of xanthurenic acid, following a test dose of tryptophan.

5. **Heme synthesis:** Pyridoxal phosphate is required as a coenzyme in the synthesis of heme, i.e. for the formation of δ-aminolevulinic acid from glycine and succinyl-CoA, by δ-aminolevulinic acid synthase. It is also important for the incorporation of iron into hemoglobin. Hence, PLP is an accessory hemopoietic vitamin.
6. **Glycogen metabolism:** Pyridoxal phosphate is essential in glycogen metabolism in muscle and liver since it acts as a coenzyme for phosphorylase.
7. **Fatty acid chain elongation:** Vitamin B_6 is essential in chain elongation of unsaturated fatty acids, e.g. in the conversion of linoleic acid to arachidonic acid.
8. **Amino acid absorption:** Vitamin B_6 is required for the absorption of dietary amino acids.

Deficiency Manifestations of Vitamin B_6

Deficiency symptoms include cheilosis, glossitis and hypochromic anemia. In infants, deficiency of B_6 affects central nervous system and results in convulsions, demyelination of the peripheral nerves and degeneration of axons. Practically, however, the important causes include:

1. **Tuberculosis:** Deficiency of vitamin B_6 may occur in patients with tuberculosis who are taking the antitubercular drug isonicotinic acid hydrazide (isoniazid or **INH**) which acts as an antagonist to vitamin B_6 (Fig. 8.31).
2. **Oral contraceptive pills (OCP):** In the past, the use of OCP with high estrogen content led to a vitamin B_6 deficiency state. This is because estrogen stimulates tryptophan catabolism, that in turn, requires vitamin B_6. Currently, OCP are formulated with low to moderate estrogen content.

Clinical uses of pyridoxine: Several clinical situations mandate the use of pyridoxine (Chemistry to Clinics 8.9).

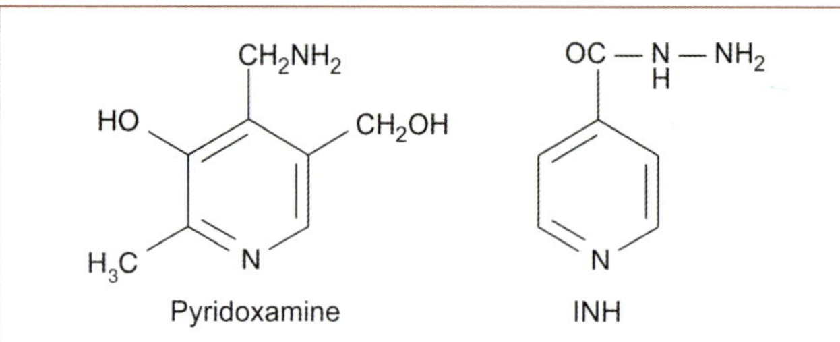

Fig. 8.31: Vitamin B_6 and INH

Chemistry to Clinics 8.9: Prescribing Pyridoxine

1. Along with isoniazid-containing antitubercular regimen.
2. Supportive treatment of hyperemesis gravidarum, an extreme form of nausea and vomiting during the first trimester of pregnancy.
3. During radiation therapy for cancer.
4. Muscular dystrophy.
5. A general supplement for various neurological disorders.

Dietary Sources of Pyridoxine

Rich sources are egg, fish, green-leafy vegetables and cereals. Besides, it is also produced by microflora of the intestinal tract.

RDA for Pyridoxine

Since vitamin B_6 is important in the metabolism of several amino acids, its requirement depends upon dietary intake of protein. The RDA is 1.9-3.1 mg per day.

PANTOTHENIC ACID

Pantothenic acid contains a molecule of pantoic acid and β-alanine (Fig. 8.32).

It is heat stable in acidic medium.

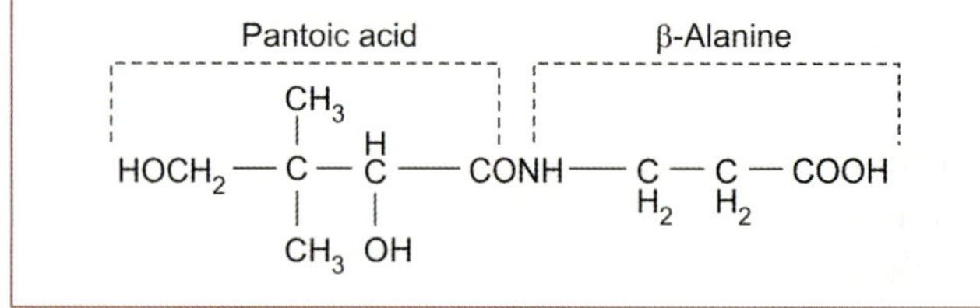

Fig. 8.32: Pantothenic acid

Biochemical Role of Pantothenic Acid

Pantothenic acid is an important constituent of **coenzyme A.** Besides pantothenic acid, coenzyme A contains a nitrogenous base adenine in the form of its nucleotide (AMP). Formation of coenzyme A therefore requires ATP. Coenzyme A also has a sulfhydryl group (–SH) which is contributed by β-mercaptoethanolamine (thioethanolamine). Due to the presence of –SH group, coenzyme A is also written as **HS-CoA** or simply as **CoA** (Fig. 8.33).

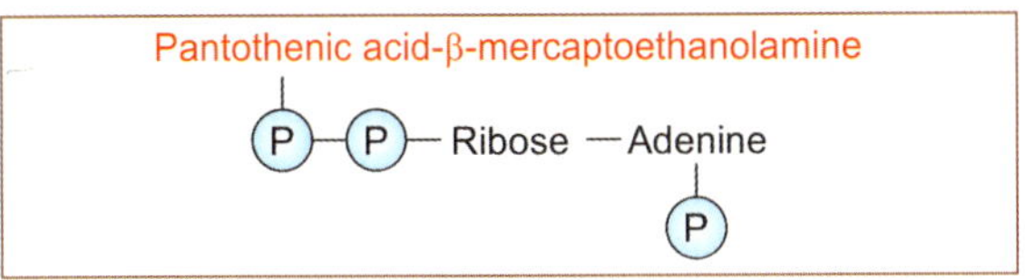

Fig. 8.33: Coenzyme A

1. The most important function of CoA is that it acts as a carrier for acetate by forming **acetyl-CoA (active acetate)**.
   - Active acetate is used in the synthesis of citrate and enters Krebs cycle.
   - Active acetate is also used in the synthesis of acetylcholine, a neurotransmitter.
   - Acetyl-CoA is also a precursor of cholesterol and steroid hormones in the adrenal cortex.
2. Pantothenic acid, as 4-phosphopantothenic acid, forms a prosthetic group of the acyl carrier protein and thus participates in fatty acid synthesis.
3. Activation of fatty acids to form fatty acyl-CoA and for their subsequent oxidation to give 2-carbon fragments (acetyl-CoA).
4. Oxidative decarboxylation of pyruvate which is converted to acetyl-CoA and enters Krebs cycle (Fig. 8.34).

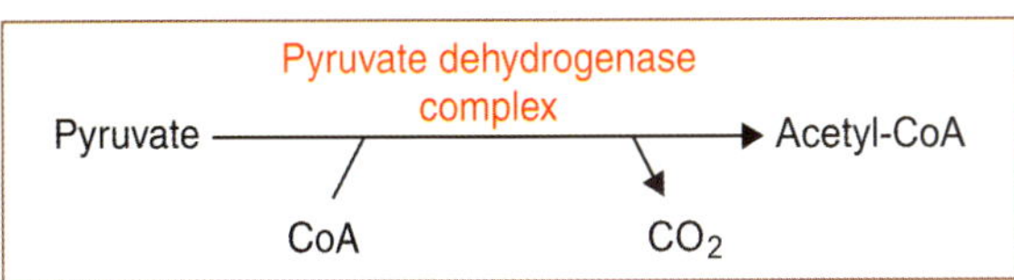

Fig. 8.34: Biochemical role of CoA

5. Metabolism of branched chain amino acids (valine, leucine and isoleucine) and forms CoA derivatives of their α-keto acids.
6. Activation of succinic acid, and therefore, is also used in the biosynthesis of heme. Hence, pantothenic acid is an accessory hemopoietic vitamin.

Deficiency Manifestations of Pantothenic Acid

Pantothenic acid deficiency in human beings affects both, the nervous system as well as the digestive system. Its deficiency has also been shown to result in adrenal insufficiency. Deficiency symptoms include headache, fatigue, impaired motor activity, muscle cramps and gastrointestinal disturbances.

It has been used with limited success in the treatment of **burning feet syndrome** and in the healing of ulcers and bedsores.

Dietary Sources of Pantothenic Acid

Pantothenic acid occurs in all animals and plant tissues. Rich sources are yeast, liver, egg, potato, whole cereals and legumes.

RDA of Pantothenic Acid

The RDA is 5 mg per day.

BIOTIN

Biotin is also called anti-egg white injury factor, since it protects animals against the toxicity of raw-egg white. Raw-egg white contains a protein **avidin** which acts as an antagonist to biotin and forms avidin–biotin complex. On cooking the egg white, avidin gets inactivated and cannot bind biotin.

Structurally, biotin is a cyclic derivative of urea with a thiophene ring (Fig. 8.35).

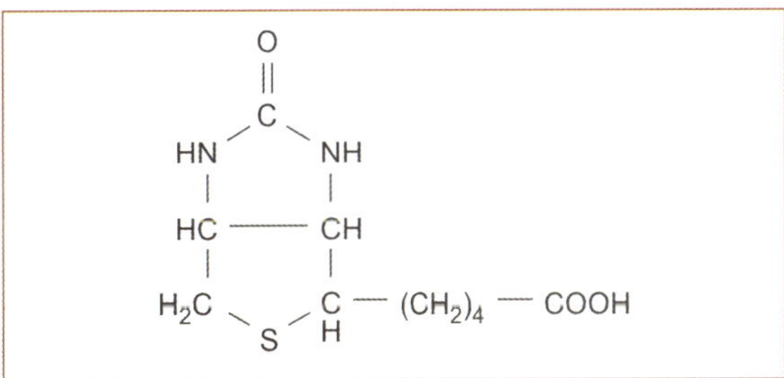

Fig. 8.35: Biotin

Biochemical Role of Biotin

Biotin coenzyme, as a prosthetic group, binds by an amide linkage to the ε-amino group of the lysyl residue of the apoenzyme and forms biotin–enzyme complex (holoenzyme), called **biocytin**. Biocytin accepts carboxylate group from bicarbonate and forms **carboxy biocytin–enzyme complex**, called **active biotin** (Fig. 8.36).

Biotin (as active biotin) is required as a coenzyme by **carboxylases** and is important in several reactions involving CO_2 fixation, such as:

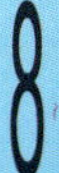

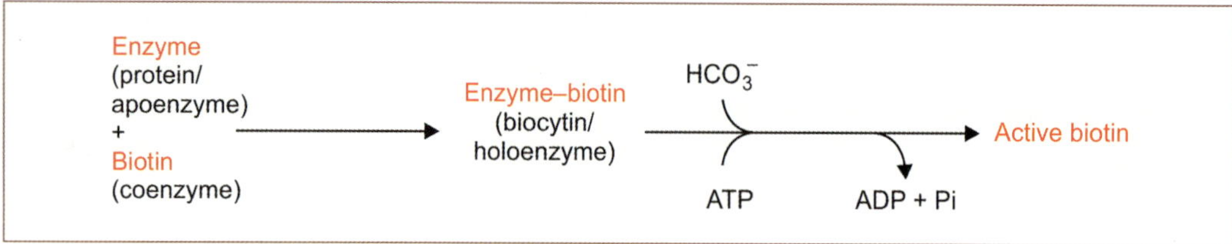

Fig. 8.36: Activation of biotin

- In the carboxylation of pyruvate to form oxaloacetate with the enzyme pyruvate carboxylase.
- For the conversion of propionic acid (propionyl-CoA) to succinic acid via methylmalonyl-CoA with the enzyme propionyl-CoA carboxylase.
- In the conversion of acetyl-CoA to malonyl-CoA (required in the formation of long-chain fatty acids) with the enzyme acetyl-CoA carboxylase.
- In transcarboxylation reaction, i.e. in the catabolism of branched-chain amino acids.

Deficiency Manifestations of Biotin

Biotin deficiency is not generally seen as it can be synthesized by the intestinal flora. Consumption of raw-egg white, however, can produce neurological abnormalities by inhibiting the absorption of biotin. Deficiency may cause mild dermatitis, nausea, loss of appetite, muscular pain and anemia.

Dietary Sources of Biotin

Rice polish, whole cereals, milk, yeast and meat (liver, kidney) are good sources of biotin.

RDA of Biotin

The RDA is 25 μg/day.

CHOLINE

Choline is trimethylethanolamine (Fig. 8.37).

$$HO-\underset{H_2}{C}-\underset{H_2}{C}-\overset{+}{N}-(CH_3)_3$$

Fig. 8.37: Choline

Biochemical Role of Choline

Choline has several important biochemical functions in the body:

- It is converted to betaine which is used as a methyl group donor for several transmethylation reactions.
- Choline is acetylated and is converted to acetylcholine, a neurotransmitter.
- It has lipotropic activity and thus prevents fatty liver (accumulation of abnormal quantities of fat in the liver).

Deficiency Manifestations of Choline

Choline deficiency is not generally observed since it is widely distributed in nature, as a constituent of phospholipids. Moreover, it can also be synthesized in the liver if adequate amounts of methyl donors, such as betaine and methionine are present. Deficiency may be associated with fatty liver and hemorrhagic necrosis of kidneys.

Choline as a drug: As choline salicylate, it is a part of topical preparations for the treatment of **aphthous ulcers** (small, painful mouth sores).

Dietary Sources of Choline

Egg yolk, several animal tissues, cereals and vegetables are good sources.

RDA for Choline

The RDA is 0.3–1.0 g.

LIPOIC ACID

Chemically, lipoic acid is a **sulfur**-containing fatty acid and is also called **thioctic acid** (Fig. 8.38).

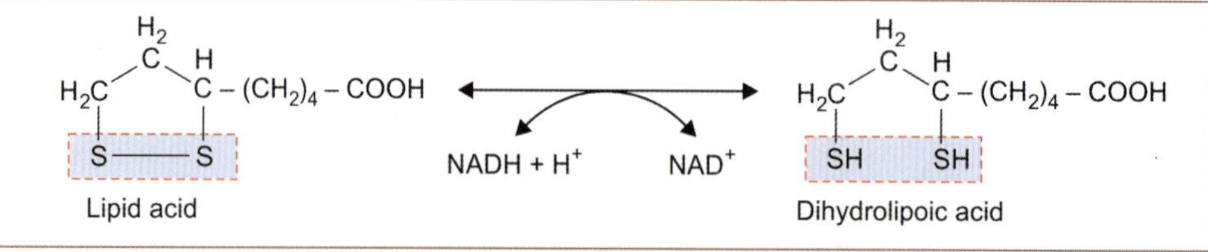

Fig. 8.38: Lipoic acid

Biochemical Role of Lipoic Acid

Lipoic acid mediates the transfer of electrons and activated acyl group which is released after decarboxylation and oxidation of α-keto acids, within the multienzyme complex. Lipoic acid, in turn, undergoes reversible oxidation and reduction. It is reduced to **dihydrolipoic acid** which acts as an acceptor of the activated acyl group.

Lipoic acid is used as a coenzyme with several other coenzymes, such as TPP, NAD^+, FAD, and CoA, in the oxidative decarboxylation of α-keto acids, e.g. in the conversion of pyruvate to acetyl-CoA by pyruvate dehydrogenase complex or in the conversion of α-ketoglutarate to succinyl-CoA by α-ketoglutarate dehydrogenase complex, in the citric acid cycle.

Dietary Sources of Lipoic Acid

Since lipoic acid is widely distributed in all natural foods, deficiency symptoms as well as requirements have not been well established.

FOLIC ACID

Folic acid and related compounds with folic acid activity are given the generic name **folacin**, a word derived from 'folium' meaning leaf. Folic acid is also called **pteroylglutamic acid**. It contains a pteridine nucleus, a molecule of *p*-aminobenzoic acid (PABA) and 1, 3 or 7 glutamate molecules (Fig. 8.39).

Biochemical Role of Folic Acid

Folic acid (folate) is reduced to its coenzyme form called **tetrahydrofolic acid (FH_4)**, by NADPH-dependent reactions. Firstly, folate is reduced by folate reductase to dihydrofolate (FH_2) and subsequently, by dihydrofolate reductase to the active coenzyme, i.e. FH_4 (Fig. 8.40).

One Carbon Metabolism

Tetrahydrofolate (FH_4) serves both as acceptor as well as donor of one carbon (1C) unit, in a variety of reactions involved in amino acid and nucleotide metabolism:

1. Folic acid is converted to N^5-formyltetrahydrofolic acid (N^5-CHO-FH_4) or folinic acid in the liver and is thus used in the transfer of one carbon group (one carbon moiety) from a donor to the acceptor molecule (Fig. 8.41).
   Besides formyl (–CHO), 1C moiety may participate in the form of formate ($-HCOO^-$), methenyl (=CH–), methylene ($-CH_2-$), methyl ($-CH_3$), hydroxymethyl ($-CH_2OH$) or formimino (–CH=NH) groups. The various forms are interconvertible to one another by $NADP^+$ or NAD^+ dependent dehydrogenases.
   The sources of one carbon moiety may be histidine (formimino group), β-carbon of serine (hydroxymethyl group) or choline, thymine and methionine (methyl group).

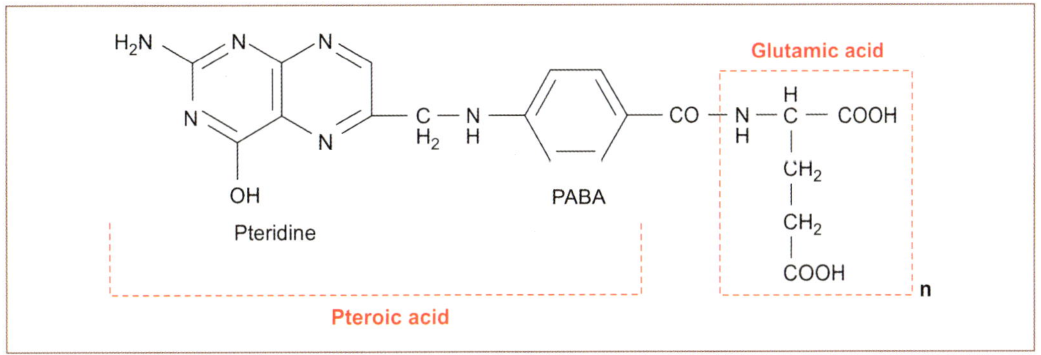

Fig. 8.39: Folic acid (pteroyl glutamic acid)

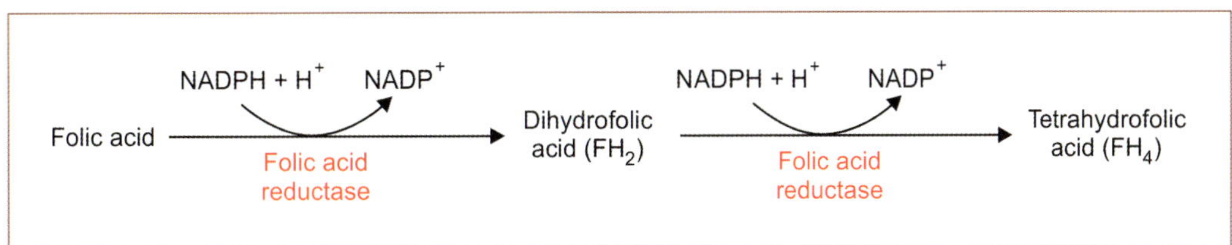

Fig. 8.40: Formation of active folate (FH_4)

8

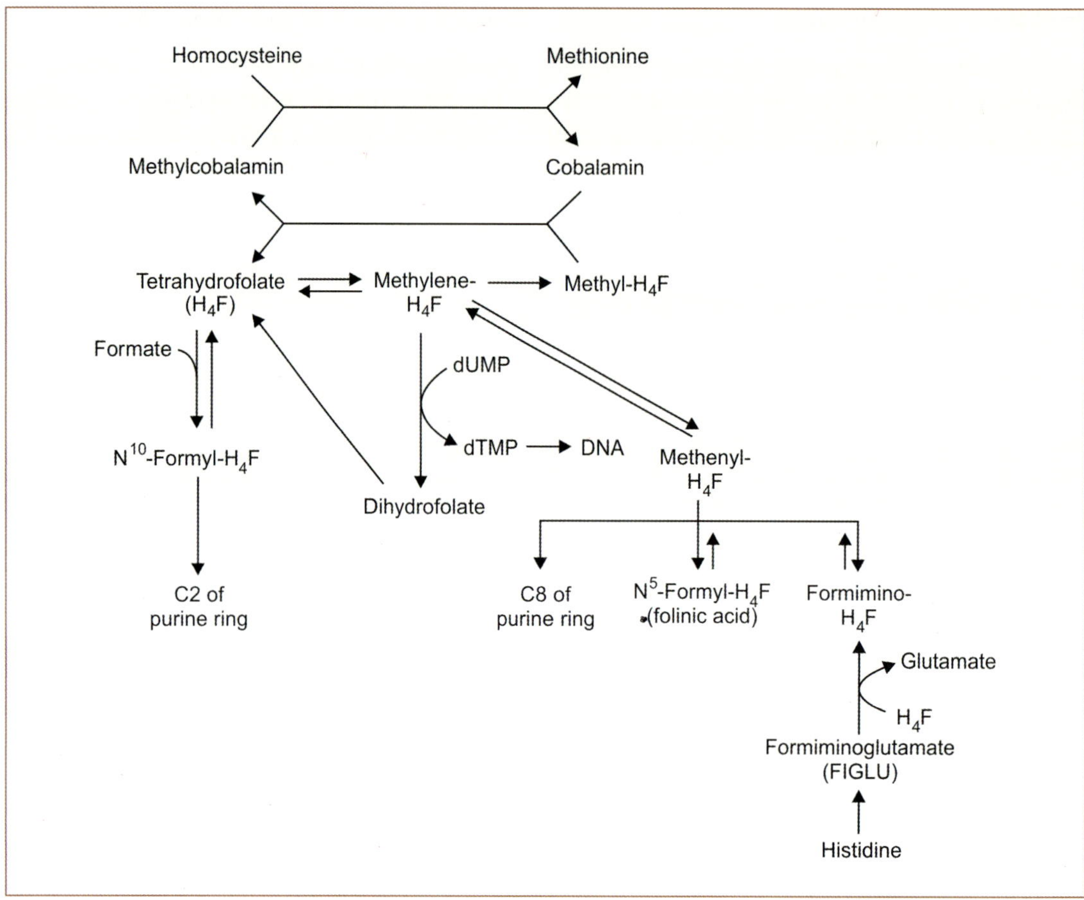

Fig. 8.41: Interrelationships between cobalamin, folate and 1 'C' metabolism

2. One carbon moiety carried by FH_4 may be utilized in many reactions, such as it acts as a donor of carbon atom 2 and 8 in the biosynthesis of a purine ring, in the conversion of glycine to serine, uracil to thymine, homocysteine to methionine, and in the biosynthesis of choline.

   In some of these reactions, vitamin B_{12} (cobalamin) is also required.

Deficiency Manifestations of Folic Acid

Folic acid deficiency is not generally observed as it can be synthesized by the intestinal flora. Deficiency may occur in stressful conditions, during pregnancy, intestinal malabsorption (such as steatorrhea or due to antibiotic therapy) and may result in:

Macrocytic (megaloblastic) anemia: It may be accompanied by leucopenia. It is based on the 'methyl folate trap hypothesis' (discussed below under 'hemopoietic 'vitamins').

Neural tube defects: Folic acid deficiency in early pregnancy has been implicated in neural tube defects. Folate deficiency impairs nucleotide biosynthesis; hence, it reduces the efficiency of both DNA as well as RNA synthesis and thus affects growth. Folic acid supplementation is therefore routinely done in pregnant women.

Deficiency of folic acid can be **diagnosed by measuring urinary excretion of formiminoglutamic acid (FIGLU**; Chemistry to Clinics 8.10).

Chemistry to Clinics 8.10: FIGLU Test

Histidine is catabolized in the liver and releases formiminoglutamic acid (FIGLU), which in the presence of FH_4, forms N^5-formiminotetrahydrofolic acid and glutamic acid.

In folic acid deficiency, FIGLU is excreted in large quantity in the urine following a test dose of histidine.

Folic Acid Antagonists

Interestingly, folate antagonists are useful anticancer drugs (Chemistry to Clinics 8.11).

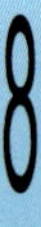

> **Chemistry to Clinics 8.11: Folic Acid Antagonists**
>
> Certain compounds interfere with the metabolic functions of folic acid and are called folic acid antagonists. Most potent of these are aminopterin and amethopterin. These are the competitive inhibitors of dihydrofolate reductase and are used as anticancer agents, e.g. in childhood leukemias.

Aminopterin (4-aminofolic acid) inhibits the conversion of folic acid to folinic acid and thus blocks the biosynthesis of nucleic acids.

Amethopterin (N^{10}-methylfolic acid or methotrexate) inhibits folic acid reductase, thus affects the conversion of folic acid to FH_4.

Dietary Sources of Folic Acid

Folic acid is present in green leafy vegetables such as spinach and cabbage, besides yeast, liver and kidney.

RDA for Folic Acid

The RDA is 220–300 µg/day.

VITAMIN B_{12}

Vitamin B_{12} is also known as **Castle's extrinsic factor**. It is also referred to as **cyanocobalamin** due to the presence of a cyano group and a cobalt atom. The central ring structure of vitamin B_{12} has a corrin nucleus which is similar to a porphyrin but with a central cobalt atom. Cobalt is linked to a cyano group and to a nitrogen of the imidazole ring which is esterified through aminopropanol and propionic acid to ring IV of the corrin nucleus (Fig. 8.42).

The cyano group may be replaced by nitrate ($-NO_2$) or hydroxyl group (–OH) to give **nitrosocobalamin** or **hydroxycobalamin**, both of which are hemopoietically active forms of the vitamin.

Absorption, Storage and Transport

Dietary cobalamin (Cbl) initially binds to specific '**R-proteins**' in the stomach in the presence of HCl. There are two sources of R-proteins: The saliva and the gastric secretions. Another protein, **Castle's intrinsic factor** (IF), is secreted from the gastric parietal cells which replaces R-proteins and binds to Cbl (the '**extrinsic factor**') in the duodenum. The IF-Cbl complex is carried over to the ileum where it is recognized by specific receptors. Here, Cbl is absorbed leaving IF in the lumen. In pernicious anemia, autoantibodies interfere with the handling of Cbl resulting in Cbl deficiency despite adequate dietary intake of Cbl (Fig. 8.43).

Fig. 8.42: Vitamin B_{12}

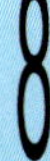

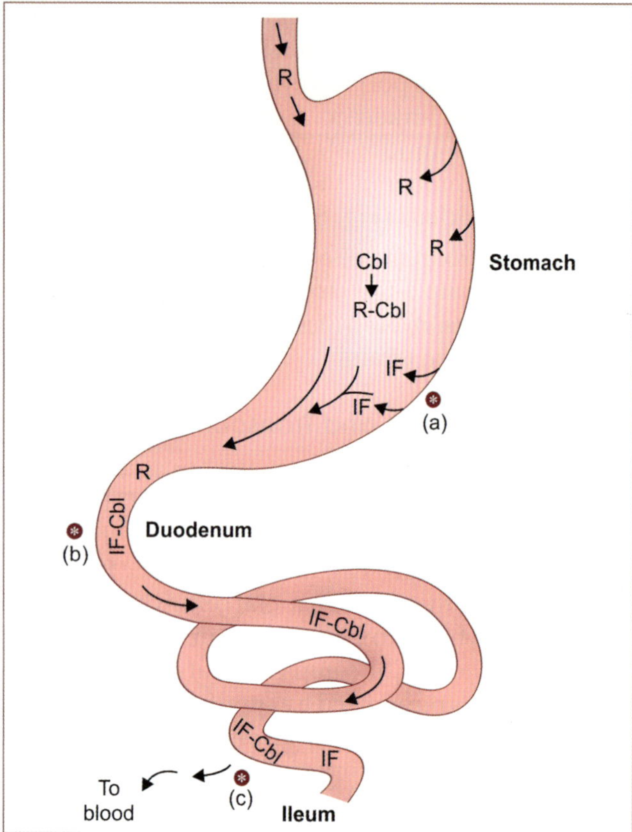

Fig. 8.43: Mechanism of handling of cobalamin (Cbl) in the gastrointestinal tract. ⊛ Indicates the three types of auto-antibodies found in pernicious anemia: (a) Antibodies against parietal cells, (b) blocking antibodies prevent formation of IF-Cbl complex, and (c) antibodies against IF-Cbl ileal receptors

Vitamin B_{12} is transported in the blood by two proteins which are designated as transcobalamin I and transcobalamin II. They deliver Cbl from the liver to various tissues as hydroxycobalamin which is either converted to methylcobalamin or to deoxyadenosylcobalamin. **Vitamin B_{12} activity is thus present in methylcobalamin, nitrosocobalamin as well as hydroxycobalamin.**

Vitamin B_{12} is excreted in the urine as well as in the feces.

Biochemical Role of Vitamin B_{12}

Both **methylcobalamin** as well as **deoxyadenosylcobalamin** act as B_{12} coenzymes and are called **cobamides**.

1. **Collaborative action with folic acid (as methylcobalamin):** Required for the formation of methionine from homocysteine.

   The vitamin, thus, maintains methionine stores in the body and spares FH_4 for the biosynthesis of purine and pyrimidine bases for nucleic acids.
2. **Metabolism of branched-chain amino acids (as deoxyadenosylcobalamin).**
3. **Metabolism of fatty acids containing odd number of carbon atoms (as deoxyadenosylcobalamin):** Required for the conversion of methylmalonyl-CoA to succinyl-CoA catalyzed by methylmalonyl-CoA isomerase.

Deficiency Manifestations of Vitamin B_{12}

Vitamin B_{12} deficiency is not generally observed, due to its widespread distribution in animal tissue and synthesis by the microbial flora, except in geriatric cases or in strict vegetarians because plants do not synthesize vitamin B_{12}.

- Deficiency can occur because of prolonged reduced intake, intestinal malabsorption, atrophy of the gastric mucosa or deficiency of the intrinsic factor (e.g. in **pernicious anemia**). In pernicious anemia, any of three different types of antibodies may be found in the serum.
- The clinical outcomes are **megaloblastic anemia** and **subacute combined degeneration of the spinal cord** (discussed later under 'hemopoietic vitamins').
- Vitamin B_{12} deficiency also results in **methylmalonic aciduria**. Measurement of the urinary excretion of methylmalonic acid thus is also used to confirm the deficiency of vitamin B_{12}.

Methyl Folate Trap Hypothesis: Megaloblastic Anemia

The metabolism of methylcobalamin and folate is closely linked as far as hemopoiesis is concerned. Therefore, in vitamin B_{12} or folate deficiency, folate is '**trapped**' in the form of **methyltetrahydrofolate** since it fails to get converted into tetrahydrofolate which is the functionally active form of folate. As a result, deoxythymidylate cannot be synthesized which means that **DNA cannot be synthesized** in the bone marrow erythroid precursor cells. However, **protein synthesis continues** in the cytosol from the pre-existing mRNA so that the cells become enlarged though they fail to divide. These cells are appropriately called '**megaloblasts**' instead of normoblasts, since they mature into large, fragile, short-lived RBC called '**macrocytes**' (Fig. 8.44).

The condition is called **megaloblastic or macrocytic anemia** characteristic of vitamin B_{12} or folate deficiency. In addition, an interesting observation is the neurological manifestations of vitamin B_{12} (but not folate) deficiency (Chemistry to Clinics 8.12).

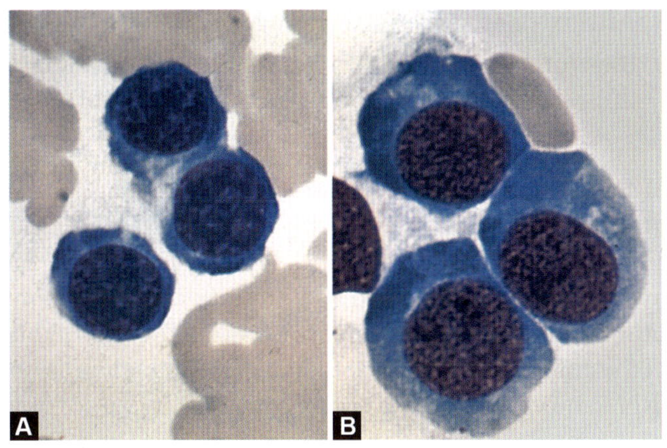

Fig. 8.44: Comparison of normoblasts (A) and megaloblasts (B) in a bone marrow aspirate. The **megaloblast** is an abnormal immature red cell precursor and is the equivalent of the normoblast in normal red cell production (the general term 'erythroblast' covers both normoblasts and megaloblasts). The megaloblast is characterized by its larger size, abundant cytoplasm and the fine reticular nuclear structure in comparison with the very coarse reticular nuclear structure of a normoblast at the same stage of cytoplasmic hemoglobinization. Thus, a megaloblast is characterized by nucleocytoplasmic dissociation

Chemistry to Clinics 8.12: Neurological Manifestations of Vitamin B_{12} Deficiency

This is explained by the combined deficiency of both cobamide forms of B_{12}, i.e. deoxyadenosylcobalamin and methylcobalamin:

1. Deficiency of deoxyadenosylcobalamin results in accumulation of methylmalonyl-CoA thereby competitively inhibiting the utilization of malonyl-CoA in the synthesis of fatty acids with even number of carbon atoms.
2. Propionyl-CoA also accumulates and is directed towards the synthesis of fatty acids with odd number of carbon atoms.
3. Lack of methylcobalamin results in decreased formation of methionine from homocysteine. The active form of methionine, S-adenosyl methionine or SAM, is required for the synthesis of choline and hence choline-containing phospholipids.

The net result of all these factors is an inappropriate synthesis of myelin sheath and subacute combined degeneration of spinal cord that results in neurological manifestations.

The biochemical diagnosis of vitamin B_{12} or folate deficiency is given in Table 8.4.

Dietary Sources of Vitamin B_{12}

Primary source of vitamin B_{12} is its synthesis by the intestinal microbial flora. Besides liver, kidney, egg, fish and milk are good sources.

Table 8.4: Biochemical diagnosis of vitamin B_{12} and folate deficiencies

Vitamin B_{12} deficiency	Folate deficiency
• Low serum B_{12}	• Low RBC folate
• Increased urinary methylmalonic acid	• Increased urinary FIGLU with histidine challenge (FIGLU test)
• Demonstration of serum autoantibodies in case of pernicious anemia	

RDA for Vitamin B_{12}

Amongst various vitamins of the B complex group, it has the lowest RDA of 2.2 µg/day.

VITAMIN C

The most important compound with vitamin C activity is **L-ascorbic acid**. Due to its role in the treatment of scurvy, it is also called antiscorbutic factor.

The enediol groups at the second and the third carbon atoms of the molecule are sensitive to oxidation. The oxidation of ascorbic acid converts it to **dehydroascorbic acid** (Fig. 8.45).

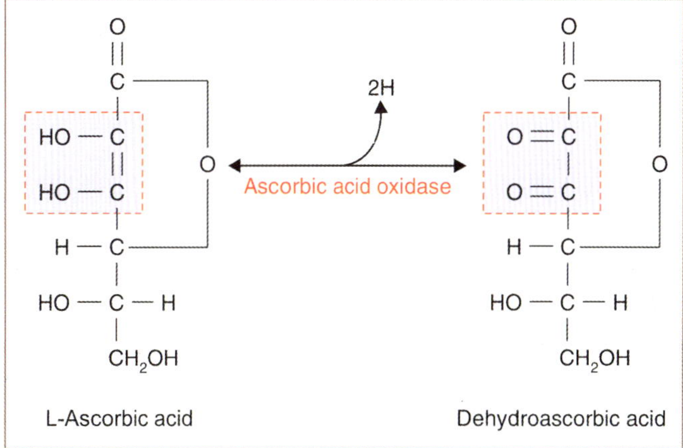

Fig. 8.45: Vitamin C

Vitamin C is easily destroyed by heat especially in an alkaline medium.

Majority of the animals can synthesize ascorbic acid from glucuronate but **humans, primates and guinea pigs cannot synthesize** it and depend upon its exogenous supply.

Dietary vitamin C is readily absorbed from the intestinal tract. Its absorption is reduced in gast-

8

rointestinal infections and in achlorhydria. It is stored in the liver and the adrenals. **Highest concentration is found in the adrenal cortex.**

Role of Vitamin C in Health and Disease

Due to its **oxidation-reduction properties,** ascorbic acid is important for a number of biological functions:

1. **Hydroxylation reactions**
   - Hydroxylation of amino acids (particularly aromatic amino acids).
   - Hydroxylation of steroid hormones in the adrenal cortex which are synthesized from cholesterol.
   - Repair of the ground substance present in the tissues, due to its role in the hydroxylation of proline and lysine in the collagens.
2. **Hemopoiesis:** It ensures the availability of iron. As a powerful reducing agent, vitamin C reduces most of the inorganic iron present in the ferric form to the ferrous state which is absorbed more efficiently. Ascorbic acid also helps in the release of iron from ferritin.
3. **Conversion** of FH_4 to folinic acid.
4. **Immunity:** Stimulating effects on the phagocytic activity of the leukocytes and in the formation of antibodies. It thus provides resistance to the body.
5. **Antioxidant** and anticancer agent.
6. **Biosynthesis of bile acids from cholesterol:** Vitamin C thus also helps in lowering blood cholesterol level.

Vitamin C and collagen(s) biosynthesis: The chains of the intracellular precursors of collagens are called **protocollagens** which are synthesized on the ribosomes and are rich in proline and lysine. However, the hydroxylated forms of these amino acids (hydroxyproline and hydroxylysine) are essential components of the collagen fiber. Since there are neither codons nor tRNA molecules for hydroxyproline and hydroxylysine, **proline and lysine are hydroxylated** within the protocollagens to form collagens (**post-translational modifications**).

Ascorbic acid is essentially required for the hydroxylation of these two amino acids and thus plays an important role in collagen biosynthesis.

Deficiency Manifestations of Vitamin C

1. **Scurvy:** Prolonged deficiency of vitamin C causes scurvy (Fig. 8.46).

   Scurvy is due to impaired collagen formation and poor blood vessel support. Bleeding gums are a characteristic feature (Fig. 8.47).

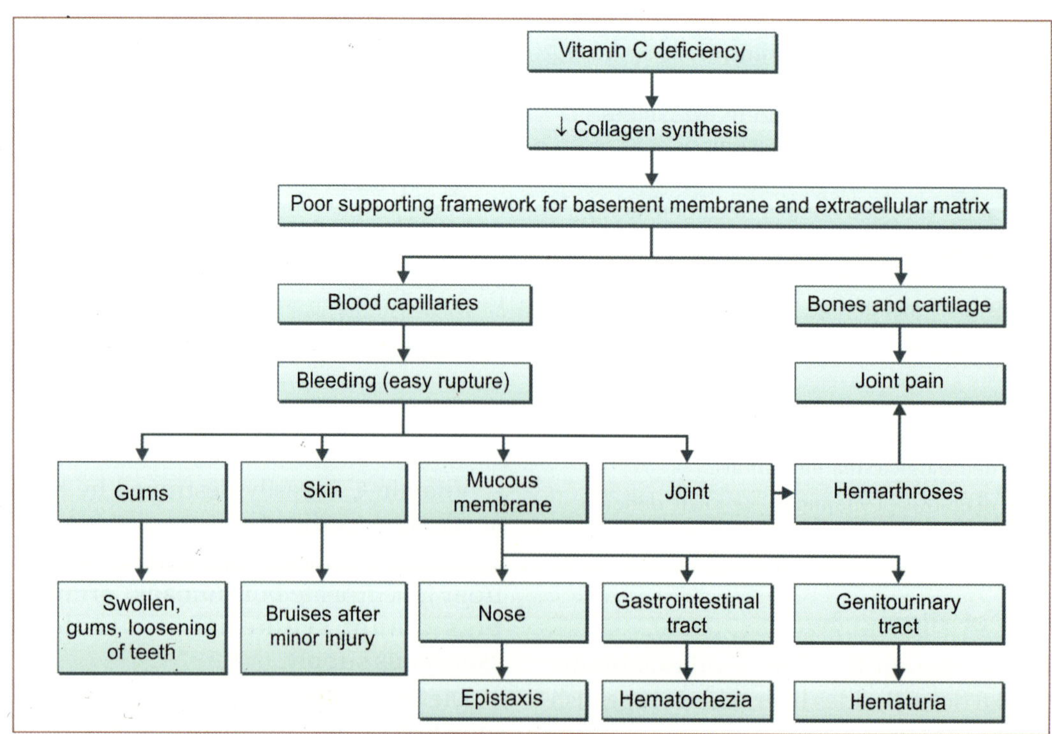

Fig. 8.46: Biochemical-clinical correlations in scurvy

8

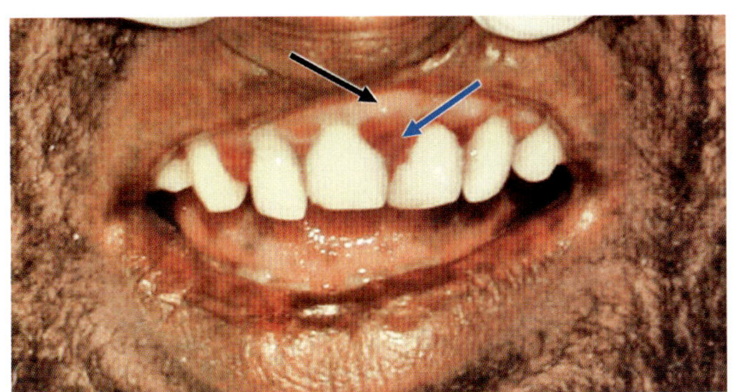

Fig. 8.47: Scurvy: Gingival swelling (black arrow) and hemorrhage (blue arrow)

Scurvy may also be observed in infants and is called **infantile scurvy**. Infants loose appetite and weight with painful tenderness of the extremities, and bleeding from gums and mucous membrane. In addition, long bones show cessation of osteogenesis.

2. **Microcytic anemia:** Because of the role of vitamin C in absorption, transport and storage of iron, deficiency of vitamin C may also lead to anemia (microcytic anemia). The accompanying loss of blood may aggravate the anemia.

An early diagnosis of vitamin C deficiency can be made by **ascorbic acid saturation test, in platelets**.

Dietary Sources of Vitamin C

Vitamin C is widely distributed in **citrus fruits**, green chillies, guava and tomato. **Amla (Indian gooseberry) is the richest source** of vitamin C.

RDA for Vitamin C

Amongst the various water-soluble vitamins ascorbic acid has the highest RDA of 65–80 mg/day.

HEMOPOIETIC VITAMINS

These include methylcobalamin, folate, vitamin C, pyridoxine, biotin, deoxyadenosylcobalamin and pantothenic acid (Fig. 8.48).

Various water-soluble vitamins, their coenzyme form, biochemical role, deficiency manifestations and daily requirement are given in Table 8.5.

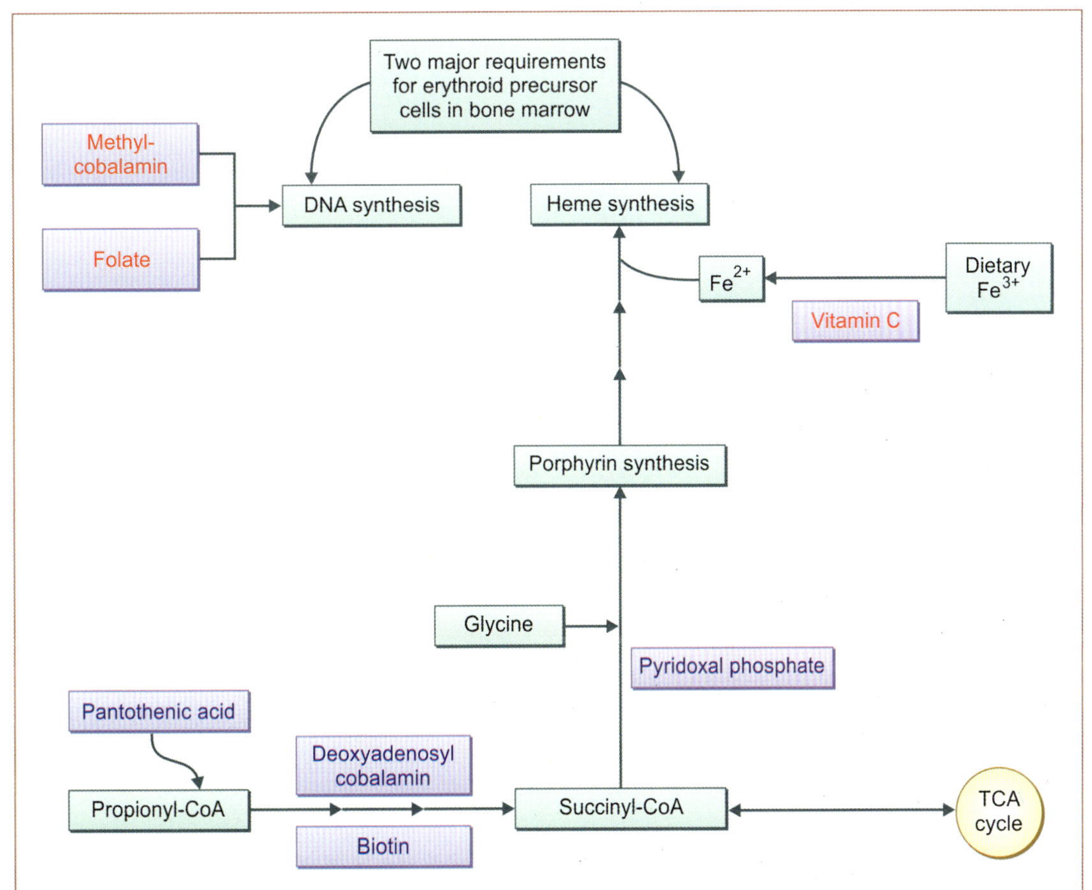

Fig. 8.48: Major (red) and accessory (blue) **hemopoietic** vitamins

8

Table 8.5: Water-soluble vitamins, their coenzyme forms, biochemical functions, deficiency disorders and RDA

Vitamin	Coenzyme	Biochemical function	Deficiency disorders	RDA*
B Complex				
Thiamin (B_1)	TPP	Oxidative decarboxylation	Beriberi	1.4–2.3 mg/d
Riboflavin (B_2)	FMN, FAD	Oxidation-reduction with flavoproteins	Cheilosis, lesions on the lips	1.9–3.2 mg/d
Niacin	NAD^+, $NADP^+$	Hydrogen acceptor for dehydrogenases	Pellagra	11–23 mg/d
Pyridoxine (B_6)	PLP	Transamination, decarboxylation	Peripheral neuritis	1.9–3.1 mg/d
Pantothenic acid	Coenzyme A	Formation of CoA derivative, component of acyl carrier protein	Muscle cramps, burning feet	5 mg/d
Biotin	Carboxybiocytin	Carrier of CO_2 for carboxylases	Anemia, dermatitis	25 µg/d
Folic acid	FH_4	Carrier of 1-C moiety	Megaloblastic macrocytic anemia	220–300 µg/d
Cobalamin (B_{12})	Cobamides	Transmethylation with FH_4	Pernicious anemia, megaloblastic anemia, subacute combined degeneration of spinal cord	2.2 µg/d
Vitamin C (Ascorbic acid)	L-Ascorbate	Hydroxylation	Scurvy	65–80 mg/d

*ICMR-NIN (2020)

Some Important Questions

1. Name Lipid-soluble vitamins. Mention their dietary sources, functions and associated deficiency disorders.

2. Describe chemistry, functions and deficiency manifestations of vitamin A.

3. How is vitamin D activated in the body? Describe its biochemical role.

4. Describe sources, functions and deficiency manifestations of folic acid and vitamin B_{12}.

5. Give an account of chemistry, sources, functions and deficiency manifestations of vitamin C.

6. Describe the coenzyme form and biochemical role of:

i. Riboflavin
ii. Pantothenic acid
iii. Biotin
iv. Vitamin B_6
v. Thiamin
vi. Niacin

7. Write notes on:

i. Keratomalacia
ii. Pellagra
iii. Beriberi
iv. Scurvy
v. Cobamide coenzymes
vi. Calcitriol
vii. β-Carotene

8. Discuss briefly:

i. Role of pyridoxal phosphate in amino acid metabolism
ii. Structure and functions of vitamin D
iii. Role of vitamin A in vision
iv. Methyl folate trap hypothesis
v. Megaloblastic anemia
vi. Pernicious anemia

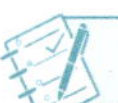

Multiple Choice Questions

1. Vitamin A is stored in the liver as:

A. All *trans*-retinol and 11-*cis*-retinal
B. All *trans*-retinal and 11-*cis*-retinol
C. β-Carotene
D. None of the above

2. During hypocalcemia, calcitriol:

A. Promotes bone mineralization
B. Promotes bone resorption
C. Inhibits renal calcium reabsorption
D. Inhibits intestinal calcium absorption

3. The activation of vitamin D sequentially involves:

A. Skin, liver, kidneys
B. Liver, skin, kidneys
C. Skin, kidneys, liver
D. Kidneys, skin, liver

4. Decreased serum vitamin E may be associated with:

A. Acne
B. Abetalipoproteinemia
C. Anemia
D. All of the above

5. Warfarin inhibits:

A. Vitamin K epoxide reductase
B. Vitamin K carboxylase
C. Factor VIII
D. Fibrinogen

6. Thiamin deficiency is confirmed by:

A. Increased RBC transketolase, increased plasma pyruvate
B. Decreased RBC transketolase, decreased plasma pyruvate
C. Increased RBC transketolase, decreased plasma pyruvate
D. Decreased RBC transketolase, increased plasma pyruvate

7. Prolonged consumption of sorghum as staple food may cause:

A. Beriberi

B. Pellagra

C. Megaloblastic anemia

D. Burning feet syndrome

8. Vitamin B_6 deficiency may occur in women using oral contraceptive pills containing:

A. No estrogen B. Low estrogen

C. High estrogen D. All of the above

9. The following condition may partly respond to pantothenic acid supplementation:

A. Burning feet syndrome

B. Adrenal insufficiency

C. Muscle cramps

D. All of the above

10. Vitamin B_{12} deficiency may result in:

A. Subacute combined degeneration of spinal cord

B. Megaloblastic anemia

C. Methylmalonic aciduria

D. All of the above

CHAPTER 9

Biochemical Processes Involved in Generation of Energy in Cells

Competency Achievement: The student should be able to:

BI6.6 Describe the biochemical processes involved in generation of energy in cells

Most chemical changes in a cell result from chains and cycles of biochemical reactions, with each step controlled by a separate specific enzyme. The totality of the chemical reactions which occur within a cell is referred to as **metabolism**.

TYPES OF METABOLIC REACTIONS

Metabolic reactions can be divided into two types:

- **Anabolic reactions** involve the **synthesis of complex molecules** from simpler ones and, usually, **require energy** to form new bonds, also referred to as **endergonic reactions**.
- **Catabolic reactions** involve the **breakdown of complex molecules** into simpler ones and, usually, **release energy** from breaking bonds, also referred to as **exergonic reactions**.

ADENOSINE TRIPHOSPHATE (ATP)

Energy, in living cells, is stored and released in the chemical form of **ATP** (adenosine triphosphate), which is made up of a ribonucleotide (with base adenine) bonded to two additional phosphate groups (Fig. 9.1).

These two additional phosphates are connected by high energy bonds that release a large amount of free energy when hydrolysed (Fig. 9.2).

Fig. 9.1: ATP (~ = High energy bonds)

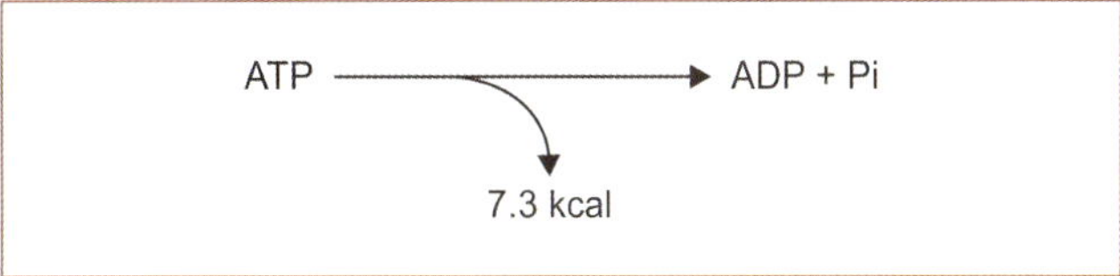

Fig. 9.2: Hydrolysis of ATP with release of energy

Utilization of Energy in the Cell

The energy released from ATP is utilized in several biochemical processes in the cell, which include:

- **Growth and repair:** Increase of cell size and replacement of the damaged tissue requires ATP.
- **Movement:** The contraction of muscle fibers, in order to generate movement in organisms, also requires ATP.
- **Nerve transmissions:** The generation and transmission of a nerve impulse (action potential) too needs ATP.
- **Active transport:** Moving molecules against their concentration gradient, or by cytosis, also require ATP.
- **Biosynthesis of macromolecules:** Building complex organic molecules from the simpler subunits (anabolism) also require ATP.
- **Emission of light:** Some of the cells may be capable of luminescence, and this process also requires ATP.

Universal Cellular Energy Currency

ATP occupies a middle rank with respect to the standard free energy of phosphate hydrolysis of various high energy phosphorylated compounds, since it is continually hydrolyzed as well as regenerated. After the phosphoanhydride hydrolysis of ATP, it can be regenerated by coupling its formation to a more exergonic metabolic process, such as by the direct transfer of a phosphoryl group from another high-energy compound like phosphoenolpyruvate (Table 9.1).

Thus, there is a flow of energy from high energy phosphate compounds (such as 1,3-bisphosphoglycerate) to form ATP, and from ATP to form low energy phosphate compounds (such as glucose-6-phosphate and glycerol-3-phosphate) whose free energy of hydrolysis is much below than the preceding high energy compound.

Table 9.1: Phosphorylated compounds of biological significance

Phosphorylated compound	Free energy of hydrolysis ($\Delta G^{o\prime}$/kcal/mol)
Phosphoenolpyruvate	14.8
1,3-Bisphosphoglycerate	11.8
Creatine phosphate	10.5
ATP	**7.3**
Glucose-1-phosphate	5.0
Glucose-6-phosphate	3.3
AMP	2.2

*ATP occupies a central position, hence it is called the universal cellular energy currency.

SYNTHESIS OF ATP

ATP can be **synthesized** by the transmembrane enzyme ATP synthase, via cell respiration.

BIOCHEMICAL PROCESSES INVOLVED IN GENERATION OF ENERGY IN CELLS

The complex organic food macromolecules, i.e. carbohydrates, lipids and proteins, are the rich sources of energy for cells, because much of the energy used to form these molecules is, literally, stored within the chemical bonds that hold them together. Cells release this energy (stored in the food molecules) through a series of metabolic processes.

Eukaryotic cells use three major processes to transform the energy held in the chemical bonds of food molecules into more readily usable forms, often energy-rich carrier molecules.

1. **The first process in the eukaryotic energy pathway is glycolysis**, which, literally, means sugar splitting. During glycolysis, single molecules of **glucose** are split and, ultimately, **converted into** two molecules of a substance called **pyruvate** (*see* Chapter 3).

   Glycolysis is actually a series of ten chemical reactions that requires the input of two ATP molecules. This input is used to generate four new ATP molecules, which means that glycolysis results in a net gain of **two ATP**. Besides, **two NADH molecules** are also produced, which serve as electron carriers for other biochemical reactions in the cell (*see* Fig. 3.13).
2. When oxygen is available, the pyruvate produced by glycolysis becomes the input for the next portion of the eukaryotic energy pathway. During this stage:
   i. **Each pyruvate molecule from the cytoplasm enters the mitochondrion**, where it is **converted into acetyl-CoA** (two-carbon energy carrier). The third carbon of pyruvate combines with oxygen and is released as carbon dioxide. At the same time, an **NADH** carrier is also generated (Fig. 3.14).
   ii. Acetyl CoA then enters a pathway called the **citric acid cycle**, which is the **second major energy process used by cells**. In eight steps, citric acid cycle generates three NADH, one $FADH_2$ and one GTP (*see* Fig. 3.41 and Table 3.7).
3. The third major process in the eukaryotic energy pathway involves an **electron transport chain** (described below), catalyzed by several protein complexes located in the mitochondrional inner membrane. This process, called **oxidative phosphorylation, transfers electrons from NADH and $FADH_2$** through the membrane protein complexes, and ultimately to oxygen, where they combine to form water. As electrons travel through the protein complexes in the chain, a gradient of hydrogen ions, or protons, is formed across the mitochondrial membrane. Cells harness the energy of this proton gradient to create three additional ATP molecules for every electron that travels along the chain.

   Together, these processes that occur inside the mitochondrion, the citric acid cycle and oxidative phosphorylation, are referred to as **respiration**, a term used for processes that couple the uptake of oxygen and the production of carbon dioxide.

TRANSFER OF ELECTRONS FROM NADH AND $FADH_2$ THROUGH THE MEMBRANE PROTEIN COMPLEXES

Electrons from NADH and $FADH_2$ (generated during the processes of glycolysis and citric acid cycle) are transferred into the inner mitochondrial membrane through membrane protein complexes, which comprise malate-aspartate shuttle and glycerol phosphate shuttle.

Malate-aspartate Shuttle

- Firstly, pyruvate, formed in the cytosol during glycolysis is converted to oxaloacetate.
- Thereafter, with the help of NADH, oxaloacetate is reduced and converted to malate.
- Malate is transported into the inner mitochondrial membrane.
- In the matrix, malate is reconverted back to oxaloacetate with the help of NAD^+ within the mitochondria. During this reaction, NAD^+ is converted to NADH, which enters the electron transport chain.
- Since oxaloacetate cannot be transferred from the matrix back to the cytosol, it is converted to aspartate.
- Aspartate is transferred to the cytosol and is reconverted back to oxaloacetate, to re-enter the shuttle.
- Thus, the malate-aspartate shuttle transfers electrons from NADH into the inner mitochondrial membrane, for their use in the electron transport chain (Fig. 9.3).

Glycerol Phosphate Shuttle

It helps in the transfer of electrons from $FADH_2$ into the inner mitochondrial membrane, for their use in the electron transport chain (Fig. 9.4).

ELECTRON TRANSPORT CHAIN

Electron transport chain has various components, which include NAD-linked dehydrogenase, flavin-linked dehydrogenase, iron-sulfur proteins, coenzyme Q and various cytochromes.

Components of Electron Transport Chain

1. **NAD-linked dehydrogenase:** NAD-linked dehydrogenase reaction reduces NAD to NADH, and, in turn, converts a reduced member of the oxidation-reduction reaction to the oxidized form such as malate to oxaloacetate (Fig. 9.5).

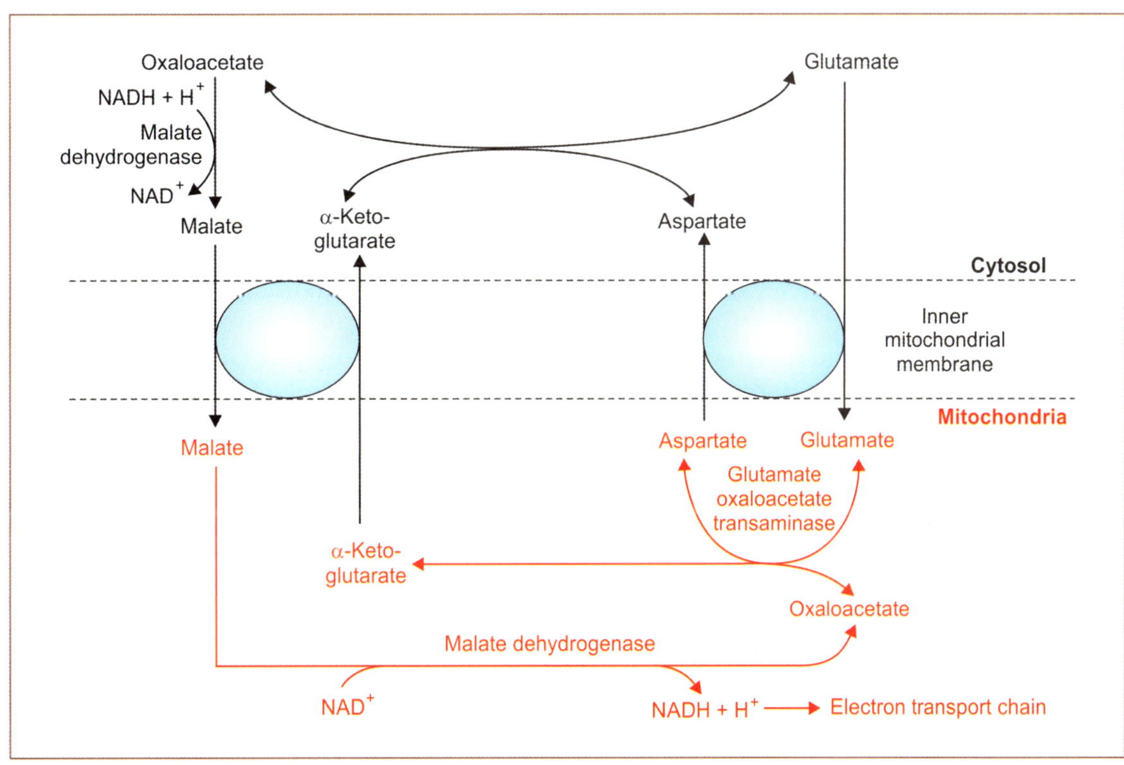

Fig. 9.3: Malate-aspartate shuttle

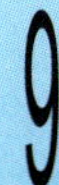

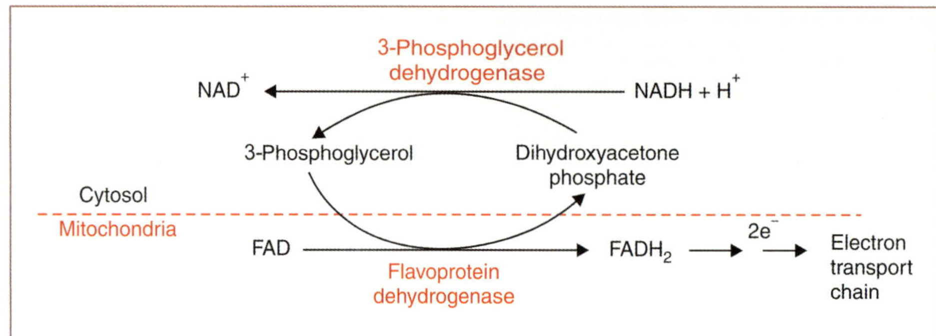

Fig. 9.4: Glycerol phosphate shuttle

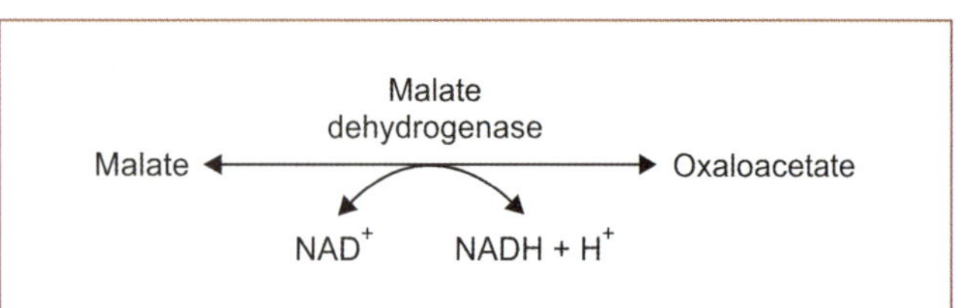

Fig. 9.5: Malate dehydrogenase, an NAD-linked dehydrogenase

In this process, **two electrons** and two protons are removed, out of which both the electrons **and one of the protons are transferred to NAD$^+$**. Since only one of the protons, as an anhydride ion (H^- which has a hydrogen atom and an electron), is accepted by NAD$^+$, the second proton (H^+) is released free into the aqueous environment.

2. **Flavin-linked dehydrogenase:** NADH (which is produced as a result of the NAD-linked dehydrogenase reaction) is oxidized by the FMN-linked NADH dehydrogenase.

   In this process, isoalloxazine ring of **FMN accepts two electrons and one proton from NADH** plus **one proton from the aqueous environment**, and pass them on to coenzyme Q.

   This type of reaction employs a flavin nucleotide as an electron acceptor which forms a part of the flavin-linked dehydrogenase. Either FMN or FAD can be used in the oxidation-reduction reaction.

   FMN-linked NADH dehydrogenase is a complex enzyme, which has a **flavoprotein** and at least four **iron-sulfur centers**. Some of the flavin-linked dehydrogenases include NADH dehydrogenase, succinate dehydrogenase, etc.

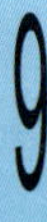

3. **Iron-sulfur centers:** Iron-sulfur centers, also called **iron-sulfur clusters**, form prosthetic group of the iron-sulfur protein (a nonheme iron protein). Iron component of the iron-sulfur center is bound to the cysteine residue of the protein as well as to the acid labile sulfur. Iron-sulfur centers undergo one electron oxidation-reduction.

   In this process of the transfer of reducing equivalents, **iron is converted from Fe^{3+} to Fe^{2+}**, on and off the flavin moiety. Iron-sulfur centers function in the **transfer of electrons from FMN-H_2 to coenzyme Q** and **from cytochrome *b* to cytochrome c_1**.

4. **Coenzyme Q:** Acceptor of the electrons, and protons, from NADH dehydrogenase is coenzyme Q (**CoQ**), also called **ubiquinone**. It is neither a protein nor a nucleotide, but is **a lipophilic electron carrier**. It serves as a mobile electron transporter within the mitochondrial membrane and operates between flavin-linked dehydrogenase and cytochrome *b*.

   With the addition of two reducing equivalents ($2H^+ + 2e^-$), **CoQ is reduced to CoQ-H_2. Hydrogen atoms** collected by CoQ **are released into the mitochondrial matrix and ultimately form water, with the molecular oxygen**.

5. **Cytochromes:** Cytochromes are a class of proteins containing heme as a prosthetic group and are called **hemoproteins**. Various cytochromes of the mammalian mitochondria are designated as **cytochrome *a* (cyt *a*), cyt *b*, cyt *c***, etc. Cytochromes **carry electrons from CoQ to molecular oxygen**, sequentially, and thus, act as **transelectronases**.

   Each cytochrome **accepts a pair of electrons** from its predecessor, **converting Fe^{3+} to Fe^{2+}**. Transfer of electrons **from one cytochrome to another**, and eventually, **to cytochrome oxidase**, accomplishes regeneration of Fe^{3+}. **No hydrogen transfer takes place** in this segment of the electron transport chain.

Cytochrome *a*-a_3, also called **cytochrome oxidase**, is a **terminal unit of the electron transport chain**.

- It has both iron and copper.
- This component functions in the **transport of electrons by the reversible oxidation and reduction of its iron**.

- **Copper ions are involved in the transfer of electrons from the cyt *a* to the cyt a_3.**
- The cyt a_3 **component**, finally, **reacts with oxygen.**
  Note: NAD-linked dehydrogenase, flavin-linked dehydrogenase and CoQ are involved in the transfer of both, hydrogen and electrons. Electron transfer reactions from NADH through CoQ involves transport of two e^-, whereas reactions between CoQ and O_2, involving various cytochromes, are one e^- transfer reactions.

Organization of the Electron Transport Chain

Above components of the electron transport chain are arranged in the inner mitochondrial membrane. They participate in a sequential manner, in **four complexes,** which contain redox centers with progressively increasing affinity for electrons, i.e. with the increasing standard redox potentials. Electrons travel through this chain from lower to higher standard redox potential, and are carried from complex II to complex III by CoQ and from complex III to IV by cyt *c* (Fig. 9.6).

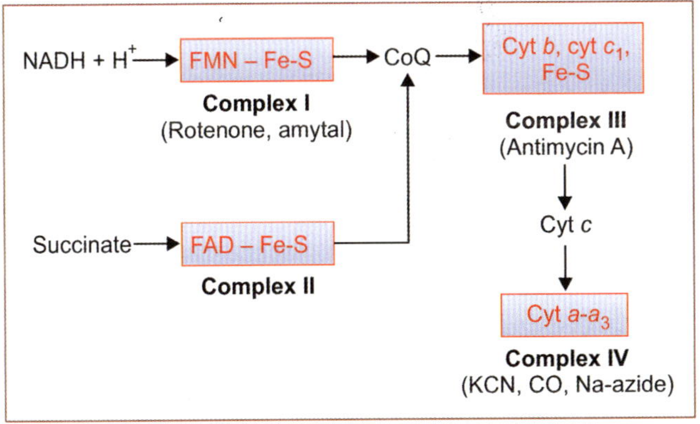

Fig. 9.6: Four complexes in the electron transport chain (inhibitors are shown in parentheses)

Complex I: It is also called **NADH dehydrogenase complex (NADH-CoQ reductase)**. It catalyzes the first reaction in which **protons and electrons are accepted from NADH + H⁺**, and **transferred to CoQ**.

Thus, complex I catalyzes the **oxidation of NADH,** by the **reduction of CoQ**. This is a protein complex that is tightly bound to the inner mitochondrial membrane.

- Complex I contains a flavoprotein (Fp), consisting of one molecule of FMN as the prosthetic group, and an iron-sulfur protein (Fe-S). NADH transfers electrons to FMN and converts it to $FMN\text{-}H_2$.

$$NADH + H^+ + FMN \rightarrow NAD^+ + FMN\text{-}H_2$$

- Electrons from $FMN\text{-}H_2$ are then transferred, via Fe-S, to CoQ.
- Thus, complex I accepts the pair of electrons from NADH and transfer them to CoQ. As a result of it, NADH is oxidized to NAD^+, whereas CoQ is reduced to $CoQ\text{-}H_2$.

$$NADH + H^+ + CoQ \rightarrow NAD^+ + CoQ\text{-}H_2$$

- This, in turn, results in large negative free energy change, which is utilized to translocate **(pump out) four protons out of the mitochondria** (Fig. 9.7).

Complex II: It is also called **succinate-CoQ reductase.** It accepts reducing equivalents from succinate, via FAD.

- FAD is reduced to $FAD\text{-}H_2$ and these electrons (from $FAD\text{-}H_2$) enter electron transport chain, via glycerol-phosphate shuttle, at the level of CoQ.

$$FAD\text{-}H_2 + CoQ \rightarrow FAD + CoQ\text{-}H_2$$

- Thus, CoQ facilitates the transfer of electrons from NADH through complex I or $FAD\text{-}H_2$ through complex II, to complex III.

Complex III: It is also called **cytochrome reductase.** It consists of Fe-S protein, cyt *b* and cyt c_1. It catalyzes oxidation of $CoQ\text{-}H_2$ and converts it to CoQ.

- In this process, cyt *c* receives electrons from complex III and delivers them to complex IV.
- During the process of the transfer of electrons, iron (in the heme group) shuttles between Fe^{3+} and Fe^{2+}.

$$CoQ\text{-}H_2 + Cyt\ c\ (Fe^{3+}) \rightarrow CoQ + Cyt\ c\ (Fe^{2+})$$

- This, in turn, also results in large negative free energy change, which is utilized to translocate **(pump out) four protons, which are moved out of the mitochondria.**

Complex IV: It is also called **cytochrome oxidase.** It is the terminal acceptor of electrons and is tightly bound to the mitochondrial membrane. It catalyzes oxidation of the reduced cyt *c* by molecular oxygen ($\frac{1}{2}O_2$). Its functional unit is referred to as cytochrome *a*-a_3 that contains two heme groups and two copper ions.

In this complex, two electrons are accepted from cyt *c* and pass on to the molecular oxygen.

$$Cyt\ c\ (Fe^{2+}) + \tfrac{1}{2}O_2 \rightarrow Cyt\ c\ (Fe^{3+}) + H_2O$$

In addition, **two proto ns are pumped out of the mitochondria.**

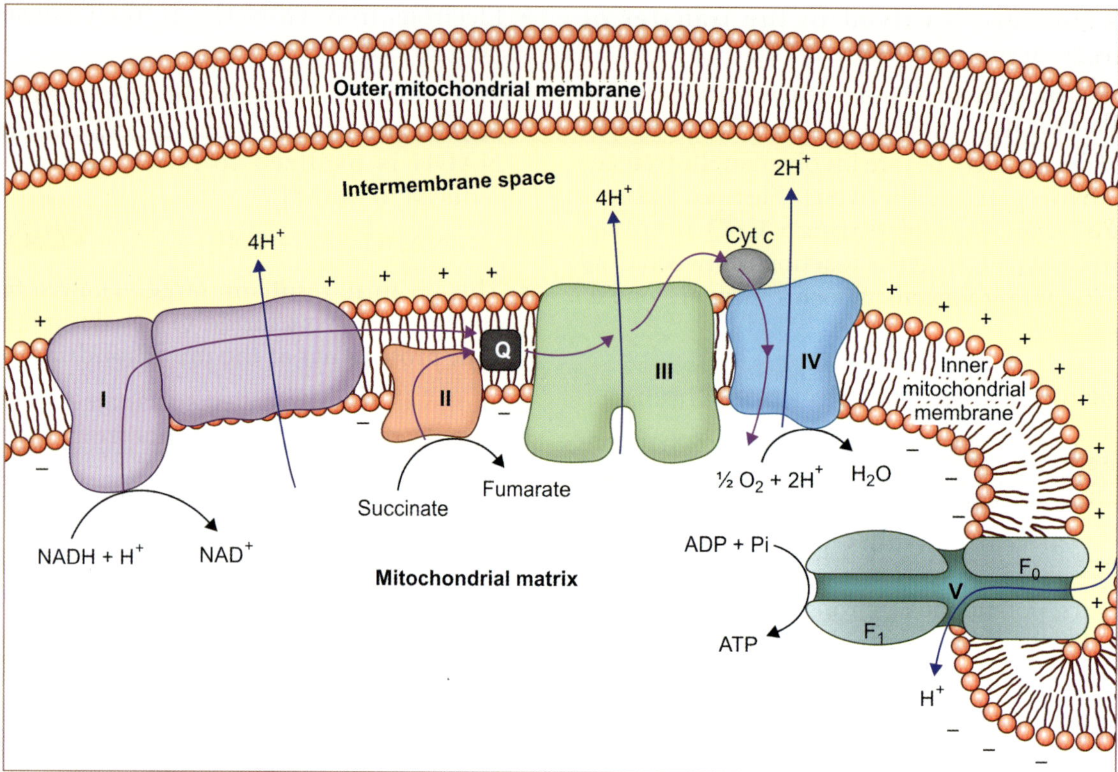

Fig. 9.7: Chemiosmotic theory of oxidative phosphorylation

Inhibitors of the Electron Transport Chain

Several compounds are known to inhibit electron transport chain at the specific sites. They block the transport of electrons; inhibit oxygen consumption and synthesis of ATP. These include:

- **Rotenone** (a fish poison), barbiturates (such as **amytal**) and certain antibiotics, like **piericidin A**, which inhibit the flow of electrons through complex I.
- Antibiotics, such as British antilewisite (**BAL**) and **antimycin A**, inhibit complex III.
- **Cyanide**, **azide**, carbon monoxide (**CO**) and hydrogen sulfide (**H_2S**) act at complex IV. Cyanide and azide bind to Fe^{3+}, whereas CO binds to Fe^{2+}.

Inhibition of the mitochondrial electron transport chain results in an impairment of its normal energy-generating function and may cause death of the organism (Chemistry to Clinics 9.1).

Chemistry to Clinics 9.1: Cyanide Poisoning

Mechanism: Ingestion of potassium cyanide or inhalation of hydrogen cyanide gas causes a rapid and extensive inhibition of the mitochondrial electron transport chain at the cytochrome oxidase step. Cyanide binds to Fe^{3+} in the heme of cytochrome a-a_3 component at the terminal step in the electron transport chain and prevents oxygen from reacting with the cyt a-a_3 as the final electron acceptor. As a result, mitochondrial respiration and energy production is stopped and cell death occurs rapidly from tissue hypoxia, particularly, of the central nervous system.

Emergency Management

1. **Nitrites:** They convert oxyhemoglobin to methemoglobin, by converting Fe^{2+} of oxyhemoglobin to Fe^{3+} in methemoglobin. Methemoglobin (Fe^{3+}) competes with cyt a-a_3 (Fe^{3+}) for cyanide, forming a methemoglobin-cyanide complex. Administration of thiosulphate at this stage causes cyanide to react with the enzyme rhodanese, forming a nontoxic excretory compound thiocyanate.
2. **Hydroxocobalamin:** A form of cobalamin (vitamin B_{12}) which binds with plasma as well as intracellular cyanide to form cyanocobalamin. The latter is excreted in the urine.

OXIDATIVE PHOSPHORYLATION

Generation of ATP from ADP and Pi is termed **phosphorylation**. When phosphorylation is coupled with biological oxidation, the process is called **oxidative phosphorylation**, whose salient features are:

- As discussed above, during electron transfer, protons are also expelled from the mitochondria, thereby,

9

producing a proton gradient across the mitochondrial membrane. Free energy, stored in this electrochemical gradient, is used for the synthesis of ATP. The term oxidative phosphorylation, thus, is a descriptive blend of the two processes operating simultaneously, i.e. the **oxidation of a metabolite by oxygen via electron transport chain** and the **phosphorylation of ADP**.

- Oxidative phosphorylation is the **major route for ATP production** in a cell.
- During the transfer of electrons from NADH-NAD^+ redox couple (E_0' = –0.32 volt) to molecular oxygen (E_0' = +0.82 volt), there occurs a redox potential decrease of 1.14 volts. Within this sequential process there are **three different sites** with a decrease of at least 0.3 volt in the potential at each site. This release of energy is sufficient enough for the phosphorylation of ADP (Table 9.2).
- **P/O ratio:** It is the ratio of the number of moles of ATP generated to the number of atoms of oxygen reduced by the electron transport chain. It is used to express the efficiency of oxidative phosphorylation of the system. Since, there are 3 sites of generation of ATP in the electron transport system, thus, the P/O ratio is 3, if reducing equivalents enter the electron transport chain through NADH. On the other hand, for the FAD-H_2 requiring reactions P/O ratio is only 2.

  However, based on the **recent experimental evidences**, it has now been suggested that instead of 3 for NADH and 2 for FAD-H_2, the values are actually **2.5** and **1.5,** respectively. The new values should be followed in all energy-based calculations involving the electron transport chain, e.g. the energy yield during glycolysis, Krebs cycle, β-oxidation of fatty acids, etc.

Table 9.2: Redox potentials of some redox systems

Redox system	E_0' (Volt)
NADH/NAD^+	–0.32
Succinate/fumarate	–0.03
$FADH_2$/FAD	0.0
Coenzyme QH_2/CoQ	0.10
Cytochrome *b* (Fe^{2+}/Fe^{3+})	0.12
Cytochrome c_1 (Fe^{2+}/Fe^{3+})	0.22
Cytochrome *a* (Fe^{2+}/Fe^{3+})	0.29
Cytochrome a_3 (Fe^{2+}/Fe^{3+})	0.39
$H_2O/½O_2$	0.82

Mechanism of Oxidative Phosphorylation

Most accepted theory of oxidative phosphorylation is referred to as chemiosmotic theory. According to this theory:

1. In the first step, two electrons and a proton from NADH, in addition to one proton from the aqueous matrix, are added to FMN of the NADH dehydrogenase (**complex I**), thereby, reducing the prosthetic group FMN to FMN-H_2. Two electrons from FMN-H_2 are then accepted by the iron-sulfur centers, which cycle electrons back across the membrane, to the interior. Two electrons from Fe-S centers are now transferred to CoQ, accompanied by $2H^+$ derived from the aqueous matrix.
2. The reduced CoQ-H_2 donates two electrons to cyt *b* and the protons are released into the medium. Then, the electrons from cyt *b* are returned to the inner surface, where together with $2H^+$ from the matrix, they again join CoQ. This is called the **Q cycle**.
3. In the next step, electrons are donated to cyt c1 and then to cyt *c* on the outer membrane surface. These electrons are then accepted by cyt *a*, and cross the membrane. On the matrix side, electrons are transferred by cyt a_3 to an atom of oxygen. With the acquisition of two protons, a molecule of water is formed.
4. Complexes I and III each transfer four protons across the membrane per pair of electrons. In complex IV, two protons per pair of electrons are pumped across the membrane and another two protons per pair of electrons are combined with oxygen to form water within the matrix. Thus, the equivalent of four protons per pair of electrons is transported out of the mitochondrial matrix at each of these three complexes.
5. Complex II receives electrons from succinate (an intermediate of the Krebs cycle). These electrons are transferred to FAD-H_2, rather than to NADH, and then to coenzyme Q. From coenzyme Q, electrons are transferred to complex III and then to complex IV, as described above.
6. During the flow of electrons from NADH or FAD-H_2 to $½O_2$, protons (H^+) are transported across the membrane into the intermembrane space, creating H^+-gradient across the membrane. Because protons are electrically charged particles, the potential energy stored in the proton gradient is electrical as well as chemical in nature **(proton-motive force or electrochemical gradient)**.
   - The **chemical component** is the proton concentration (or pH) gradient, which corresponds to

about a tenfold higher concentration of protons on the outer side of the inner mitochondrial membrane (i.e. a difference of one pH unit).
- In addition, there is an **electric potential** across the membrane, resulting from the net increase in positive charge on the outer side (intermembrane space). This electrical component corresponds to the voltage difference across the inner mitochondrial membrane.

7. Once the gradient is established, H^+ flow back, **spontaneously, downhill** across the membrane. The potential energy stored in this gradient is harvested by a fifth protein complex, referred to as complex V (Fig. 9.7).

Complex V

Complex V couples the energetically favorable flow of protons back across the membrane to the generation of ATP. In the complex V, protons traverse the membrane at certain sites, designated as F_0 protein of the **F_1–F_0 complex** ('0' indicates 'oligomycin-sensitive'). Two protons enter the **F_0 protein**, which provides an ion channel through the lipid bilayer, into the headpiece F_1. The **F_1** has binding sites for inorganic phosphate, near the proton channel. The energy of proton gradient and also the membrane potential, promotes a reaction of two protons with oxygen of the phosphate. Water is eliminated and the resulting highly reactive phosphate group (Pi) joins ADP, to generate ATP (Fig. 9.7).

Inhibitors and Uncouplers of Oxidative Phosphorylation

Inhibitors and uncouplers of oxidative phosphorylation stop ATP synthesis:

- **Inhibitors:** Oligomycin binds to the F_0 subunit of the mitochondrial F_1-F_0-ATPase, suppresses oxygen consumption and thus the phosphorylation of ADP to ATP.
- **Synthetic uncouplers:** 2,4-Dinitrophenol is a proton ionophore which uncouples phosphorylation from electron transport, resulting in the accumulation of ADP. The energy, normally conserved as ATP, is lost as heat. In this situation, electron transport may continue but without the generation of ATP.
- **Physiological uncouplers:** They dissipate the chemical energy of ATP in the form of heat and are one of the mechanisms for thermoregulation (Table 9.3).

Table 9.3: Physiological uncouplers

• Uncoupling protein 1 (thermogenin)
• Unconjugated bilirubin
• Free fatty acids
• Thyroxine
• Estrogen

Many uncoupling proteins have been identified and found to perform various functions in several tissues (Table 9.4).

One such protein called thermogenin or uncoupling protein 1 (UCP1) is found in mitochondria of the brown adipose issue that is more important in neonates (Chemistry to Clinics 9.2).

Table 9.4: Major uncoupling proteins

Type of uncoupling protein (UCP)	Major location	Major function
UCP1 (thermogenin)	Brown adipose tissue of human infants and hibernating mammals	Nonshivering thermogenesis to maintain body temperature
UCP2	Many tissues	Control of mitochondria-derived species, immunity, regulation of glucose sensing in brain and pancreas
UCP3	Skeletal muscle, brown adipose tissue	Control of mitochondria-derived reactive oxygen species during exercise
UCP4	CNS	Energy homeostasis, protect against neurotoxins, regulate intracellular Ca^{2+} concentration, regulate gene expression
UCP5	CNS	–Do–

Chemistry to Clinics 9.2: Beige Fat

Adipose tissue containing cells resembling brown adipocytes (but genetically distinct, expressing low levels of UCP1 compared with brown adipocytes) have been discovered in the subcutaneous tissue near the clavicle and along the spine of adult humans. This is called **beige fat**, also referred to as **brite fat** or **inducible thermogenic adipose tissue**. A hormone called **irisin** produced by exercising muscles, promotes the conversion of white fat into beige fat. Thus, with the help of novel drugs, it may be possible to further convert beige fat into brown fat with high expression of UCP1, with the potential to treat overweight/obesity and diabetes mellitus.

SUBSTRATE LEVEL PHOSPHORYLATION

In addition to oxidative phosphorylation, some ATP is also generated in the cytosol, within certain individual steps of a metabolic pathway. This process of the transfer of a phosphate group from a very high energy phosphate donor to ADP is called substrate level phosphorylation, e.g. two reactions of the glycolytic process, which are catalyzed by phosphoglycerokinase and pyruvate kinase.

Phosphorylation of ADP by creatine phosphate, catalyzed by creatine kinase, also represents an important mode of ATP generation in the muscle. Besides, succinate thiokinase catalyzed reaction in Krebs cycle is also an example of substrate level phosphorylation (Fig. 9.8).

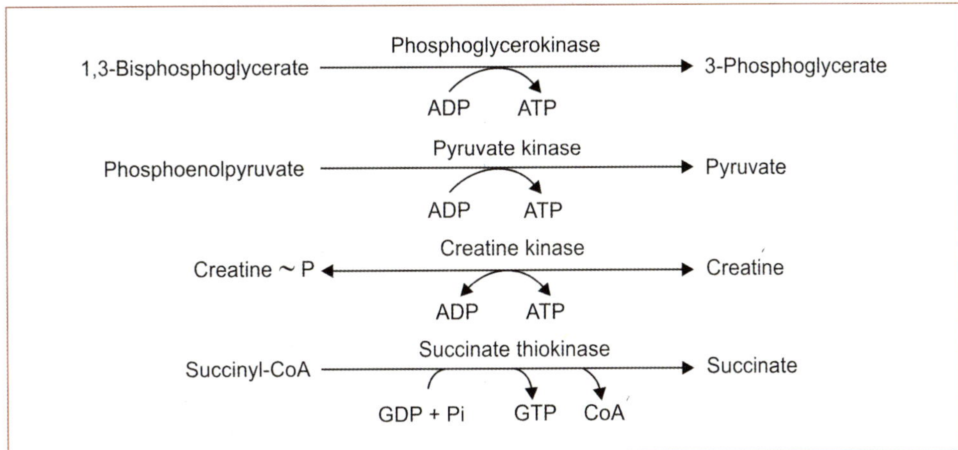

Fig. 9.8: Substrate level phosphorylation

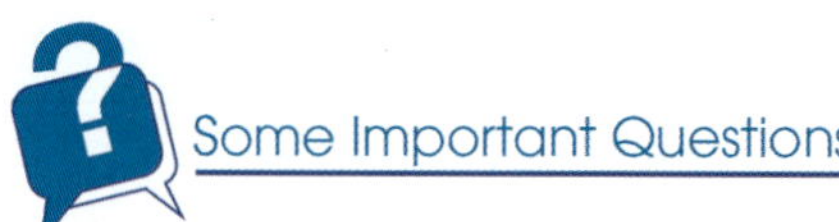

Some Important Questions

1. Explain oxidative phosphorylation and its inhibitors.

2. Descibe the components of the electron transport chain and its inhibitors.

3. Write notes on:

i. ATP
ii. ATP as cellular currency of energy
iii. Oxidative phosphorylation
iv. Substrate level phosphorylation
v. Iron-sulfur centers
vi. Cytochromes
vii. Cyanide poisoning
viii. P/O ratio

4. Discuss briefly:

i. Oxidative phosphorylation and uncouplers
ii. Diagrammatic representation of the electron transport chain
iii. Theory of oxidative phosphorylation
iv. Malate-aspartate shuttle
v. Glycerol phosphate shuttle
vi. Inhibitors of oxidative phosphorylation
vii. Beige fat

Multiple Choice Questions

1. The free energy of hydrolysis is maximum for:

A. Phosphoenolpyruvate
B. ATP
C. Creatine phosphate
D. 1,3-BPG

2. During catabolism, more reducing equivalents are extracted from:

A. Carbohydrates B. Lipids
C. Proteins D. Same for all

3. The inner mitochondrial membrane is impermeable to:

A. Glutamate B. Oxaloacetate
C. Malate D. Aspartate

4. Flavoprotein dehydrogenase is located in:

A. Outer surface of outer mitochondrial membrane
B. Outer surface of inner mitochondrial membrane
C. Inner surface of inner mitochondrial membrane
D. Mitochondrial matrix

5. In the electron transport chain (ETC), the following reacts directly with oxygen:

A. Coenzyme Q
B. Cytochrome *b*
C. Cytochrome *c*
D. Cytochrome a_3

6. Cytochrome a-a_3 requires:

A. Cu^{2+} B. Mg^{2+}
C. Mn^{2+} D. Ca^{2+}

7. Iron-sulfur proteins are absent in:

A. Complex I B. Complex II
C. Complex III D. Complex IV

8. The following inhibit complex IV by binding to Fe^{3+}-heme *except*:

A. Carbon monoxide
B. Sodium azide
C. Potassium cyanide
D. None of the above

9. The following is not a physiological uncoupler:

A. Free fatty acid
B. Thyroxine
C. Insulin
D. Unconjugated bilirubin

10. The following is not an example of substrate level phosphorylation:

A. Phosphoglycerokinase and pyruvate kinase reactions of glycolysis
B. Creatine kinase reaction
C. Succinate thiokinase reaction of TCA cycle
D. Oxidative phosphorylation

CHAPTER

10

pH, Water, Electrolytes and Acid–Base Balance

Competency Achievement: The student should be able to:

BI6.7 Describe the processes involved in maintenance of normal pH, water and electrolyte balance of body fluids and the derangements associated with these.

BI6.8 Discuss and interpret results of arterial blood gas (ABG) analysis in various disorders

PY1.6 Describe the fluid compartments of the body, its ionic composition and measurements

PY1.7 Describe the concept of pH and buffer systems in the body

The pH is defined as the negative logarithm to the base 10, of the molar concentration of hydrogen ions (H^+) in a solution:

$$pH = -\log[H^+] = \log(1/[H^+])$$

The pH of a solution thus is **inversely related to free H^+ concentration [H^+]**. A low pH indicates high H^+ concentration while a high pH indicates low H^+ concentration.

If we add a strong base such as NaOH to water, the OH– will combine with H^+ supplied by the water. This, in turn, shifts the equilibrium towards the undissociated water and lowers free H^+ ion concentration, thereby resulting in an increase in pH.

The scale of pH measurement varies from 0 to 14. If pH of a solution is <7, the solution is said to be **acidic**; if pH of the solution is equal to **7**, it is referred to as **neutral**; and if pH is **>7**, the solution is said to be **alkaline or basic** in nature.

Acid

An acid is a substance whose dissociation in water releases hydrogen ions (H^+). An H^+ since does not contain any neutron and is essentially equivalent to a proton, an acid, therefore, is often referred to as a **proton donor**. Addition of an acid to a solution thus increases the concentration of free H^+ in the solution and results in a decrease in pH. An acid, e.g. HA in aqueous solution, reversibly dissociates into **H^+** and a **conjugate base** (A^-):

$$HA \rightarrow H^+ + A^-$$

This tendency of an acid to give up H^+ depends upon its **strength**. A **strong acid** such as HCl, completely dissociates in an aqueous solution:

$$HCl \rightarrow H^+ + Cl^-$$

On the other hand, a **weak acid** gives up H^+ less rapidly and does not dissociate completely. A solution of a weak acid thus contains both dissociated (ions) as well as the undissociated molecules. Most of the acids produced in living systems are weak acids.

Base

A base releases hydroxyl ions (OH^-) in an aqueous solution and decreases its H^+ concentration by accepting or binding with the free H^+, resulting in an increase in pH of the solution. A **strong base** such as sodium hydroxide (NaOH), dissociates completely:

$$NaOH \rightarrow Na^+ + OH^-$$

The OH^- so produced accepts H^+ and results in the formation of water. This, in turn, lowers the concentration of H^+ in the solution. A **weak base** such as bicarbonate (HCO_3^-) can also utilize H^+ and thus raises the pH of the solution.

AMPHOTERIC SUBSTANCES

Some chemical substances such as amino acids and proteins can function both as an acid as well as a base. These substances are referred to as amphoteric substances or **ampholytes**. For example, an amino acid such as glycine, at physiological pH, acts as an acid when the ammonium group (NH_3^+) of glycine donates its H^+ to the OH^- of a base (Fig. 10.1).

$$H_2N-CH_2-COOH \rightleftharpoons H_3N^+-CH_2-COO^-$$

$$H_3N^+-CH_2-COO^- \xrightarrow[OH^- \quad H_2O]{} H_2N-CH_2-COO^-$$

$$H_3N^+-CH_2-COO^- \xrightarrow[H^+]{} H_3N^+-CH_2-COOH$$

Fig. 10.1: Glycine as an ampholyte

On the other hand, glycine also acts as a base when its carboxylate group (COO^-) accepts H^+ from an acid.

Henderson-Hasselbalch Equation

Weak acids, when dissolved in water, do not dissociate totally, but establish equilibrium between the undissociated compound and the dissociated ions. The concentration of the ionic species can be determined from the equilibrium equation, where K_{eq} is the equilibrium constant, $[H^+]$, $[A^-]$ and [HA] indicate the concentrations of the dissociated cations (H^+), anions (A^-, the conjugate base) and the undissociated weak acid, respectively (Fig. 10.2).

$$HA \rightleftharpoons H^+ + A^-$$

$$K'_{eq} = \frac{[H^+][A^-]}{[HA]}$$

Fig. 10.2: Equilibrium constant for the dissociation of a weak acid

K_{eq} is a function of temperature of the system and increases with the increasing temperature. On rearranging the equation, we get:

$[H^+] = K_{eq} \times ([HA]/[A^-]) = K_{eq} \times$ ([acid]/[conjugate base])

Multiplying the equation by –1, this equation can be written as:

$$-[H^+] = -K_{eq} \times ([acid]/[conjugate\ base])$$

The **logarithmic form** of the above equation is known as Henderson-Hasselbalch equation.

It is derived as follows

$-\log[H^+] = -\log K_{eq} + \log$ ([conjugate base]/[acid])

Since $-\log[H^+]$ = pH, and –logKa = pKa, the above equation can be rewritten as:

pH = pKa + log ([conjugate base]/[acid])

When half of the acid is present in its dissociated form, i.e. when $[A^-]$ = [HA], the pH of the solution is equal to its pKa. Thus, Henderson-Hasselbalch equation is a mathematical rearrangement of the fundamental equilibrium equation which states that there is a direct relationship between pH and ratio of the concentration of conjugate base to the concentration of undissociated weak acid.

BUFFER

Something that **tends to resist** a shock and thereby promotes relative stability is defined as a buffer. A buffer **minimizes the change in pH** when either an acid or a base is added to a solution. A chemical buffer consists of a weak acid (HA) and its conjugate base (A^-), or a weak base and its conjugate acid (Fig. 10.3).

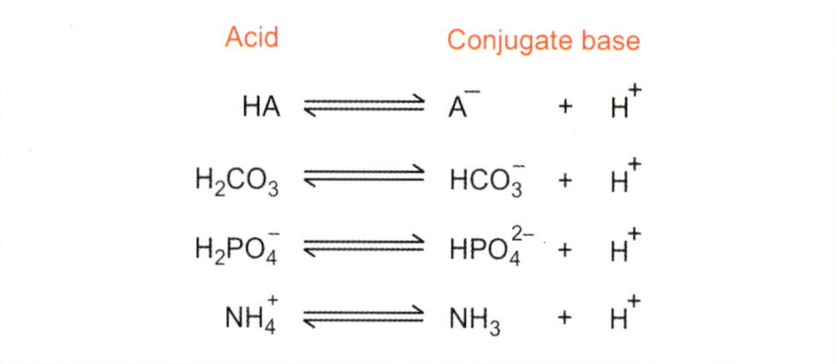

Fig. 10.3: Weak acids and their conjugate bases

The **effectiveness of a buffer**, in minimizing changes in pH, depends upon two factors:

1. The **pKa** of the buffer in relation to the desired pH, e.g. the pKa of the imidazole group of histidine in hemoglobin is close to 7.4 and thus it is an ideal buffer in the blood.
2. The **amount or concentration** of the buffer. The greater the concentration of a buffer, the greater is its ability to bind or release H^+.

Ionization Constant

Strong acids dissociate completely, i.e. do not bind H^+, hence they are not effective buffers. Weak acids strongly bind H^+, hence they are also inefficient buffers. Thus, the inherent strength or tendency of an acid to ionize, determines its **buffering capacity**. The **ionization constant** (K_{eq}) is a measure of this strength, expressed as its negative logarithm (pKa). The most effective buffers have **pKa close to the physiological pH**.

EFFECT OF DIET ON BLOOD AND URINE pH

A diet containing both meat and vegetables results in a net production of acids, largely from protein oxidation. To some extent, acid-consuming metabolic reactions balance H^+ production. Food also contains basic anions such as citrate, lactate and acetate. When these are oxidized to CO_2 and water, H^+ are consumed (i.e. HCO_3^- is produced).

A balance of acid-forming and acid-consuming metabolic reactions results in a net production of about 1 mEq H^+/kg body weight per day in an adult person, on a mixed diet. Vegetarians, generally, have less of a dietary acid burden and a more alkaline urine pH than nonvegetarians, because most fruits and vegetables contain large amounts of organic anions that are metabolized to HCO_3^-.

Whether a particular food has an acidifying or an alkalinizing effect, depends on whether and how its constituents are metabolized. For example, cranberry juice has an acidifying effect because of its content of benzoic acid that cannot be broken down in the body. On the other hand, orange juice has an alkalinizing effect despite its acidic pH of about 3.7, because it contains citrate, which is metabolized to HCO_3^-. The citric acid in lemons and pickles is converted to CO_2 and water, therefore, hardly affect blood and urine pH.

PROCESSES INVOLVED IN MAINTENANCE OF NORMAL pH OF BODY FLUIDS

As we know, acids are continuously produced in the body, and threaten normal pH of the extracellular and intracellular fluids. However, despite constant threats to acid–base homeostasis, a healthy person maintains normal blood pH, because of the **chemical buffers** along with the role played by the **lungs and the kidneys** (Fig. 10.4).

1. BODY BUFFERS: THE FIRST LINE OF DEFENSE

Chemical buffers, present in the extracellular and intracellular fluids as well as in the bones, minimize a change in pH, but they do not remove an acid or a base from the body (Table 10.1).

The main chemical buffer pair in the ECF is HCO_3^-/CO_2, while cells are rich in proteins and organic phosphate buffers. Bone contains large buffer stores, specifically, salts of phosphate and carbonate. Buffering in ECF occurs rapidly in minutes. Acids or bases also enter cells and bone but this, generally, occurs more slowly, may be over hours.

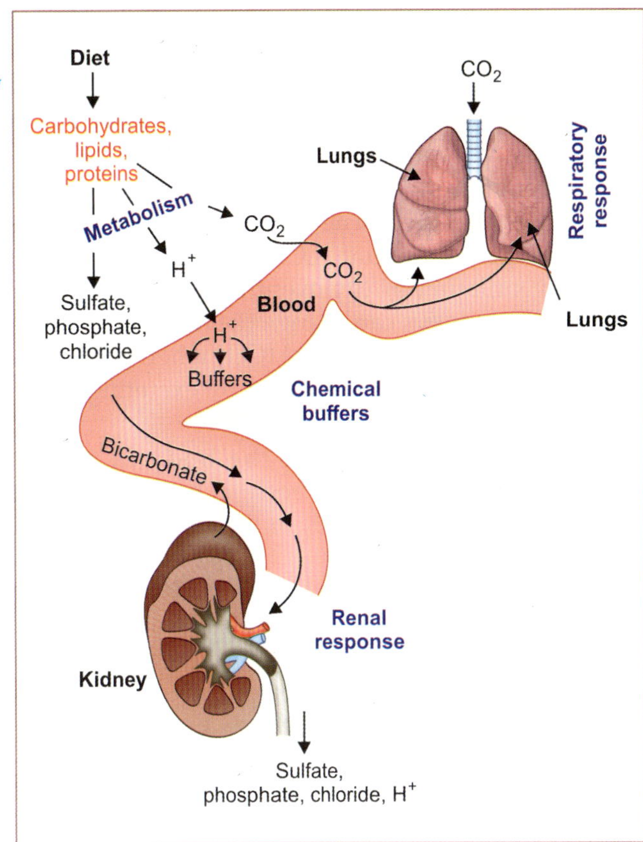

Fig. 10.4: The three major buffering mechanisms

Table 10.1: Major body buffers

Buffer	Reaction
Extracellular fluid	
Bicarbonate/CO_2	$CO_2 + H_2O \rightleftharpoons H_2CO_3 \rightleftharpoons H^+ + HCO_3^-$
Inorganic phosphate	$H_2PO_4^- \rightleftharpoons H^+ + HPO_4^{2-}$
Plasma proteins (Pr)	$HPr \rightleftharpoons H^+ + Pr^-$
Intracellular fluid	
Cell proteins, e.g. hemoglobin (Hb)	$HHb \rightleftharpoons H^+ + Hb^-$
Organic phosphates	Organic-$HPO_4 \rightleftharpoons H^+ +$ organic-PO_4^{2-}
Bicarbonate/CO_2	$CO_2 + H_2O \rightleftharpoons H_2CO_3 \rightleftharpoons H^+ + HCO_3^-$
Bone	
Mineral phosphates	$H_2PO_4^- \rightleftharpoons H^+ + HPO_4^{2-}$
Mineral carbonates	$HCO_3^- \rightleftharpoons H^+ + CO_3^{2-}$

Bicarbonate/CO_2 Buffer

For several reasons, the HCO_3^-/CO_2 buffer pair is of **prime importance** in acid–base regulation:

1. **High concentration:** Its components are abundant, i.e. the concentration of **HCO_3^- in plasma** or ECF, normally, averages **24 mmol/L** and metabolism generates an unlimited supply of CO_2.

10

2. **Open system:** Despite a pKa of 6.10, a little far from the desired plasma pH of 7.40, it is effective because the HCO_3^-/CO_2 buffer system is open, i.e. its **both the components can be added to or removed from the body**, at controlled rates, as discussed below.
3. **Dual regulation:** Further, it is **controlled**, both, **by the lungs** and **the kidneys**. The respiratory system can change the amount of CO_2 in the body fluids by hyperventilation or hypoventilation. On the other hand, the kidneys can change the amount of HCO_3^- in the ECF by forming new HCO_3^- when excess acid has been added to the body or by excreting HCO_3^- when excess base has been added.

   Carbon dioxide exists in the body in several forms—CO_2 exists in the body in several different forms, i.e. as **gaseous CO_2 in the lung alveoli**, and as **dissolved CO_2, H_2CO_3, HCO_3^-, carbonate** and **carbamino compounds in the body fluids.** The solubility coefficient for CO_2 in plasma at 37°C is 0.03 mmol CO_2/L per mm Hg. The normal pCO_2 is known to be 40 mm Hg. Therefore, the concentration of dissolved CO_2, represented as CO_2(d), is $0.03 \times 40 = 1.2$ mmol/L.

Role of carbonic anhydrase: In aqueous solution, the CO_2(d) forms carbonic acid:

$$CO_2(d) + H_2O \rightarrow H_2CO_3$$

The reaction to the right is called **hydration reaction** while reaction to the left is called **dehydration reaction**. These reactions are slow, if uncatalyzed. In many tissues such as the kidneys, pancreas, stomach and RBC, these reactions are catalyzed by carbonic anhydrase, a **zinc-containing** enzyme.

At equilibrium and at 37°C, the CO_2(d) is greatly favored so that the **ratio** of CO_2(d) to H_2CO_3 **is 400:1**. Therefore, although H_2CO_3 is a fairly strong acid (pKa = 3.5; $H_2CO_3 \rightarrow H^+ + HCO_3^-$), its low concentration in body fluids lessens its impact on acidity. Because plasma H_2CO_3 is so low and difficult to measure and that the ratio of $CO_2(d)/H_2CO_3$ is 400:1, we can use CO_2(d) to represent the acid in the Henderson-Hasselbalch equation.

Phosphate Buffer

The pKa for the phosphate buffer, i.e. $H_2PO_4^- \rightarrow H^+ + HPO_4^{2-}$, is 6.8, which is close to the desired blood pH of 7.4. So, phosphate is a good buffer. In the **ECF**, phosphate is present as inorganic phosphate. Its concentration, however, is low so it plays a minor role in extracellular buffering. However, phosphate is an important **intracellular buffer** for two reasons.

- First, cells contain large amounts of phosphate in such organic compounds as adenosine triphosphate (ATP), adenosine diphosphate (ADP) and creatine phosphate. Although these compounds primarily function in energy metabolism, they also act as pH buffers.
- Second, intracellular pH is generally lower than the pH of ECF and is closer to the pKa of phosphate.

Protein Buffer

Proteins are the **largest buffer pool** in the body and are excellent buffers. Proteins can function as both acids and bases, i.e. they are **amphoteric**. They contain many ionizable groups which can release or bind H^+. Plasma albumin and globulins are the major extracellular protein buffers. Cells also have large protein stores including the **hemoglobin** present in RBC.

Hemoglobin Buffer

Oxyhemoglobin is a stronger acid than deoxyhemoglobin. Therefore, in the tissues where CO_2 and hence H_2CO_3 are generated, the following reaction occurs in RBC:

$$KHbO_2 + H_2CO_3 \rightarrow H.Hb + KHCO_3 + O_2$$

HCO_3^- exchanges with Cl^- (chloride shift), while O_2 is delivered to the cells. This reaction is reversed in the lungs.

2. RESPIRATORY RESPONSE: THE SECOND LINE OF DEFENSE

Normally, CO_2 is expired at the same rate at which it is produced and thus pCO_2 is maintained.

- **If blood becomes acidic** by the addition of fixed acids, pulmonary ventilation is increased and CO_2 is flushed out at a rate greater than the rate at which it is produced. Consequently, pCO_2 falls and results in a decrease in H^+ concentration of the blood, and the reactions are pulled to the left (Fig. 10.5).

$$CO_2 + H_2O \rightleftharpoons H_2CO_3 \rightleftharpoons H^+ + HCO_3^-$$

Fig. 10.5: The equilibrium is pulled to the left during hyperventilation

  This, in turn, lowers the HCO_3^- concentration and reduces acidic shift in the blood.
- On the other hand, **if blood becomes more alkaline**, changes occur in the opposite direction. Accordingly, hypoventilation takes place, CO_2 is not removed at

an adequate rate, blood pCO_2 rises and the reactions are pushed to the right (Fig. 10.6).

$$CO_2 + H_2O \rightleftharpoons H_2CO_3 \rightleftharpoons H^+ + HCO_3^-$$

Fig. 10.6: The equilibrium is pushed to the right during hypoventilation

This results in a higher carbonic acid concentration in the blood and a less alkaline shift in blood pH. Hypoventilation, however, is limited because it causes retention of CO_2 which further stimulates ventilation.

Buffering of acid–base disturbances by the respiratory response although is **rapid** but is relatively coarse. It brings blood pH back, close to normal but **cannot eliminate a fixed acid or base** from the body and so it cannot restore pH to normal.

3. RENAL RESPONSE: THE THIRD LINE OF DEFENSE

Renal responses, in contrast to other buffering mechanisms, are **slow but more complete**; full renal compensation may take 1 to 3 days. The kidney regulates acid–base balance by controlling bicarbonate reabsorption and secreting acid. The kidneys also excrete the anions (phosphate, chloride, sulfate) that are liberated from strong acids.

In the basic ion exchange mechanism, H^+ formed in the reaction is actively secreted into the tubular fluid in exchange for Na^+. Within the tubule cell, Na^+ combines with HCO_3^- and generates sodium bicarbonate which is pumped out of the cell into the interstitial fluid and equilibrates with the plasma (Fig. 10.7).

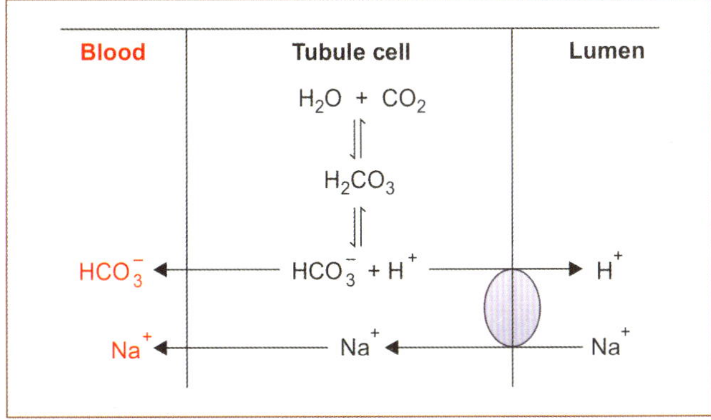

Fig. 10.7: Basic ion exchange mechanism

Sodium uptake by the tubular cell is partly passive with Na^+ flowing down the electrochemical gradient and partly active via Na^+/H^+-antiport system, in exchange for H^+.

MECHANISMS OF H^+ SECRETION

H^+ secreted into the tubular fluid can have one of the three fates, suggesting that three processes are involved in the acidification of urine:

1. Reabsorption of the filtered bicarbonate.
2. Excretion of the titratable acid.
3. Excretion of ammonia

All the three mechanisms involve H^+ secretion and are associated with the addition of bicarbonate to the peritubular capillary blood by the kidney tubules.

Reabsorption of Filtered Bicarbonate

H^+ that are secreted into the tubules in exchange for Na^+, combine with bicarbonate that has been filtered by the glomeruli. This, in turn, leads to the formation of carbonic acid in the tubular urine. The dissociation of this acid to CO_2 and water is catalyzed in the proximal convoluted tubule lumen by carbonic anhydrase within the brush border membrane. CO_2 rapidly diffuses through the cell membrane where it combines with water and forms carbonic acid, which in turn, gets dissociated into hydrogen and bicarbonate ions. The H^+ are secreted into the lumen while the bicarbonate ions exit from the basolateral membrane along with the sodium ions.

The filtered HCO_3^- thus is not reabsorbed by direct transport out of the tubular urine rather it is reabsorbed indirectly by the secretion of the hydrogen ions (Fig. 10.8).

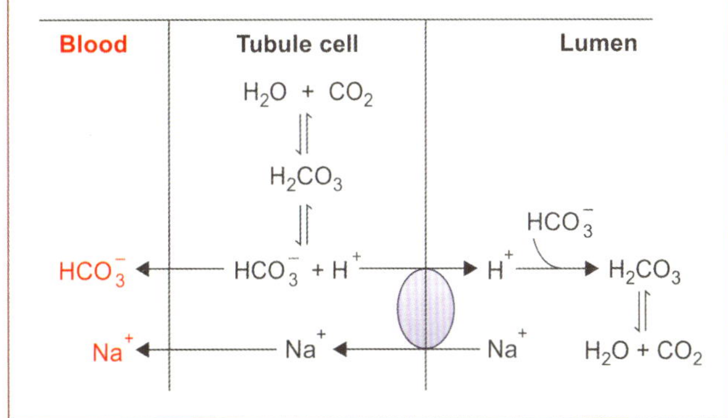

Fig. 10.8: Reabsorption of bicarbonate

The overall effect is to move sodium bicarbonate from the tubular fluid, back into the interstitial fluid.

Excretion of Titratable Acid

As reabsorption of sodium bicarbonate proceeds, the tubular fluid becomes depleted of HCO_3^- and the pH drops. At this stage, the H^+ are taken up by the phosphate buffer. Hydrogen ions that are secreted into the tubular urine in exchange for Na^+, titrate phosphate buffer in the urine in the acidic direction:

$$HPO_4^{2-} + H^+ \rightarrow H_2PO_4^-$$

As a result, the basic form of the phosphate (HPO_4^{2-}) is converted to its acidic form $H_2PO_4^-$.

Besides phosphate, which is the most important buffer in the urine, other ions are also significant in the excretion of H^+. For example, in diabetic ketoacidosis, when pH of the urine reaches its minimum ≈4.4), acetoacetate and β-hydroxybutyrate pass through the glomerular filtrate and appear in the tubular fluid. Under these conditions, these ions also serve as buffers.

Thus, excretion of titratable acids not only eliminates H^+ from the body but also restores the depleted plasma bicarbonate reserves since for each mEq of H^+ excreted as titratable acid, a new HCO_3^- is added to the blood (Fig. 10.9).

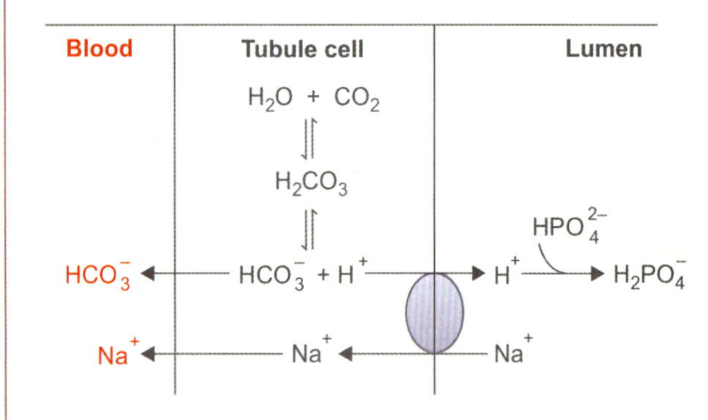

Fig. 10.9: Excretion of titratable acid

Titratable acidity of the urine: The amount of acid excreted (as the acid component of a urinary buffer) can be measured by the titration of urine, back to the normal pH of the plasma (to pH 7.4). The quantity of the base so required is equivalent to the quantity of the acid excreted and is referred to as titratable acidity of the urine. Most of the titratable acid normally, is inorganic phosphate. The formation of titratable acidity accounts for nearly one-third to one-half of our normal daily acid excretion.

Excretion of Ammonia

10 The third fate of H^+ in the tubular fluid is its neutralization by NH_3 which is mainly synthesized in the proximal tubule from amino acids, predominantly from glutamine. The ability of the kidney to synthesize NH_3 from glutamine is increased under conditions of excess acid in the body. Ammonia readily diffuses through the cell membrane and combines with the secreted H^+ and forms NH_4^+, which is usually accompanied by an anion, e.g. chloride, in the urine. For each H^+ excreted in the urine as NH_4^+, an equivalent quantity of HCO_3^- is added to the blood (Fig. 10.10).

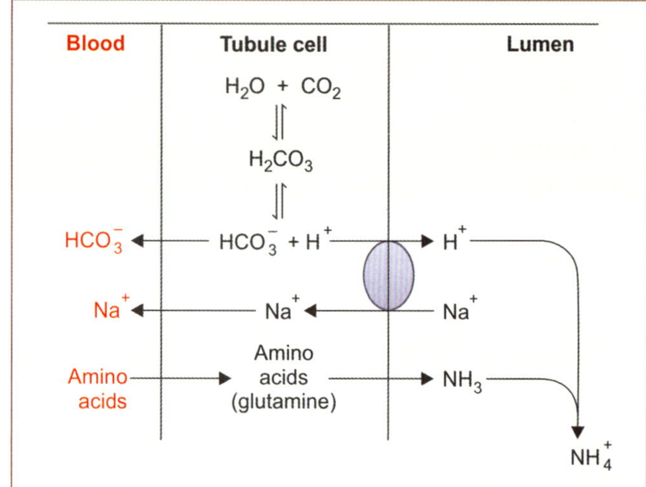

Fig. 10.10: Excretion of ammonia

Nearly, one-half to two-thirds of our daily acid load is excreted as NH_4^+.

Role of Collecting Duct in Acid–Base Regulation

The intercalated cells of the collecting duct are involved in acid–base transport and are of two types, i.e. **acid-secreting α-intercalated cells** and **bicarbonate-secreting β-intercalated cells**. The α-intercalated cells have vacuolar type of H^+-ATPase (the same kind as is found in lysosomes, endosomes and secretory vesicles) and a H^+/K^+-ATPase (similar to that found in stomach and colon epithelial cells) in the luminal cell membrane. The basolateral cell membrane contains the Cl^-/HCO_3^- exchanger. The β-intercalated cells have the opposite polarity.

Total acidity of urine: The sum of the titratable acidity and NH_4^+ comprises the total acidity of urine (total acid excretion).

REGULATION OF INTRACELLULAR pH

With the help of a combination of ion transport, buffering mechanisms and metabolic reactions, cells ensure a relatively stable intracellular pH as discussed below:

1. The intracellular and extracellular fluids are linked by **exchanges across cell membranes** of H^+, HCO_3^-, CO_2 and various other acids and bases. By stabilizing the ECF pH, the body helps to protect the ICF pH.
2. The protons (H^+) continuously tend to diffuse into cells down their concentration gradient. However, the H^+ is extruded by Na^+/H^+ exchangers (**NHE**) which are present in nearly all body cells. Eight different isoforms of these exchangers (designated NHE1, NHE2, etc.) with different tissue distributions have been identified. These transporters exchange one H^+ for one Na^+ and thus function in an electrically neutral fashion. The activity of the NHE is regulated by the intracellular pH itself as well as a variety of hormones and growth factors.
3. In some cells, various **HCO_3^- transporters** are present in the plasma membrane. These include Na^+-dependent and Na^+-independent Cl^-/HCO_3^- exchangers, and the electrogenic Na^+/HCO_3^- cotransporters.
4. Cells have **large stores of protein and organic phosphate buffers** which can bind or release H^+.
5. Various **chemical reactions** in cells can also use up or release H^+. For example, the conversion of lactic acid to CO_2 and water or to glucose effectively disposes of the acid.
6. Various cell **organelles may sequester H^+**. For example, H^+-ATPases in endosomes and lysosomes pump H^+ out of the cytosol into these organelles.

PROCESSES INVOLVED IN MAINTENANCE OF WATER AND ELECTROLYTE BALANCE OF BODY FLUIDS

Water is a very special kind of nutrient since:

- Water is consumed at more frequent intervals and in greater amounts as compared to other nutrients.
- It is the most abundant substance presents in the body.
- It is more important than food, as if one is given water but no food, the individual may survive for several weeks inspite of the loss of most of the body fat and 50% of the tissue proteins. On the other hand, a loss of about 10% of the body water may cause illness, whereas a further loss of 10% of body water may even cause death.
- Increased fluid intake is very beneficial for individuals with renal calculi, urinary tract infections and chronic obstructive respiratory disease.

Human body consists of about 50–70% of its weight as water. At birth, about 75% of total body mass is water which is reduced to nearly 60% for an average adult male. The value falls to about 50% thereafter. Due to relatively high fat content, females have nearly 5% less water.

Most tissues contain more than 70% water though bone and adipose tissue contain relatively lesser amounts. This is due to the reason that the proportion of water in a tissue or in the whole body depends upon the proportion of fat in the tissue (Table 10.2).

Table 10.2: Average water content of different tissues

Tissue	Water content (% of total weight)
Whole body	60–70
Muscles	75–80
Nervous tissue	70–85
RBC	60
Bones	25
Adipose tissue	20

BIOLOGICAL FUNCTIONS OF WATER

Water is needed for various physicochemical processes in the body:

1. It is a common solvent in which most of the chemical reactions of the body occur.
2. It participates in various metabolic processes within the cell.
3. It transports vital substances via blood, lymph and other body fluids.
4. It is also essential for the elimination of waste products from the body.
5. Water intake helps to maintain water content of the feces and thus promotes regular bowel movement.
6. Increased water intake prevents urinary tract infections and kidney stones by increasing the flow of urine.
7. It helps to provide lubrication in various strategic locations of the body, e.g. synovial fluid between the joints, mucus in the respiratory passage, etc.
8. As the latent heat of evaporation of water is high, it assists in the regulation of body temperature.

DISTRIBUTION OF WATER IN DIFFERENT COMPARTMENTS

Total body water can be divided into two major compartments, i.e. the intracellular fluid (ICF) and the extracellular fluid (ECF).

- **Intracellular fluid: ICF** is composed of the fluid within the trillions of cells in our body.
- **Extracellular fluid: ECF** is composed of fluid outside the cells. In a young adult man, two-thirds of the body water is in the ICF and one-third is in the ECF (Fig. 10.11).

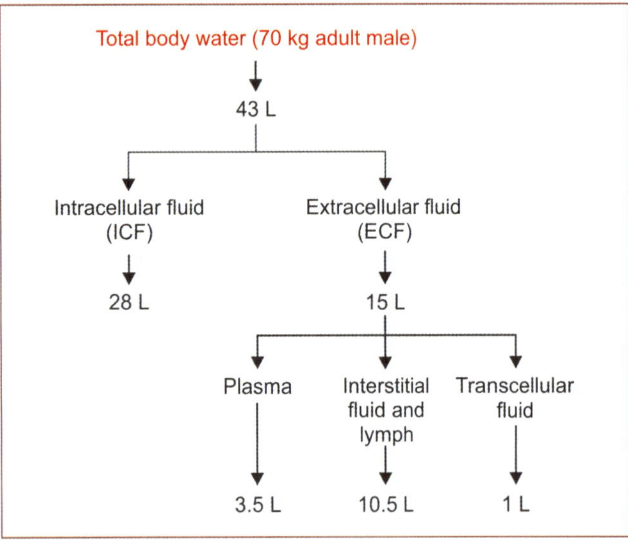

Fig. 10.11: Distribution of body water in different compartments

The fluids in the two compartments differ strikingly in terms of their electrolyte composition. Their total solute concentrations (osmolalities), however, are equal because of the high water permeability of most cell membranes so that an osmotic difference between cells and ECF rapidly disappears.

The ECF can be **further subdivided into** two sub-compartments, which are separated from each other by the endothelium of blood vessels as **plasma,** and the **interstitial fluid** and **lymph.**

- **Plasma** is the ECF found within the vascular system. It is the fluid portion of the blood in which blood cells are suspended. The plasma water comprises about 3.5 L for an average 70 kg man (Fig. 10.11).
- The **interstitial fluid** and **lymph** are considered together because they cannot be separated easily. Both are ultrafiltrates of plasma. The interstitial fluid directly bathes most body cells and the lymph is the fluid within lymphatic vessels. The water of the interstitial fluid and lymph comprises 10.5 L of the ECF.

  The plasma, interstitial fluid and lymph are nearly identical in composition except for the higher protein concentration in the plasma. Plasma is separated from the interstitial fluid by the endothelial lining of the capillaries which acts as a semipermeable membrane and allows the passage of water and diffusible solutes but not the large molecular weight substances, such as proteins (Chemistry to Clinics 10.1).

> **Chemistry to Clinics 10.1: Shock**
>
> In pathological conditions causing shock such as bacterial sepsis, extensive burns, the permeability of the vascular endothelium increases. This, in turn, results in leakage of albumin and a reduction in the effective circulating volume leading to hypotension.

- **Transcellular fluid:** Besides, there is an additional ECF compartment called transcellular fluid. It is small but physiologically important, amounting to 1–3% of body weight (Fig. 10.11).

  It includes the cerebrospinal fluid, aqueous humor, secretions of the gastrointestinal tract and associated organs (saliva, gastric juice, bile, pancreatic juice, intestinal juice, etc.), renal tubular fluid and bladder urine, synovial fluid and sweat. In these cases, the fluid is separated from the plasma by an epithelial cell layer in addition to a capillary endothelium. The epithelial layer modifies the electrolyte composition of the fluid so that transcellular fluids are not plasma ultrafiltrates (as are interstitial fluid and lymph). There is a constant turnover of transcellular fluids; they are continuously formed and absorbed or removed. Impaired formation, abnormal loss from the body or blockage of fluid passage can have serious consequences.

  The composition of ICF differs markedly from that of the ECF, as these compartments are separated from each other by a cell membrane. These differences in composition in the two compartments are a consequence of the Gibbs-Donnan equilibrium.

Sources of Water

Most of the foods, beverages, and many fruits and vegetables are good sources of water. Water is also available to the body as a result of metabolic breakdown of food for energy. The amount of water produced by the oxidation of nutrients, however, depends upon the type of the nutrient used in the body, e.g. 100 g of fats produce 107 ml, 100 g of carbohydrates produce 56 ml while 100 g of proteins produce 41 ml of water. On an average, the amount of endogenous water produced by an individual is nearly 300 ml per day.

RDA of Water

Daily need for water varies widely with variations in several characteristics of the person, e.g. body surface area, amount of body fat, metabolic rate, physical activity and environmental factors, as temperature, humidity, altitude, clothing, etc. ICMR-NIN (2020) Expert Group has suggested daily water requirement as 1.5 ml per Kcal ingested. Accordingly, total water requirement for sedentary adult male has been suggested as 2800 mL per day.

REGULATION OF BODY WATER

In a normal adult, the quantity of water intake is balanced by that which is eliminated from the body everyday, thus, maintaining a state of equilibrium (water homeostasis; Fig. 10.12).

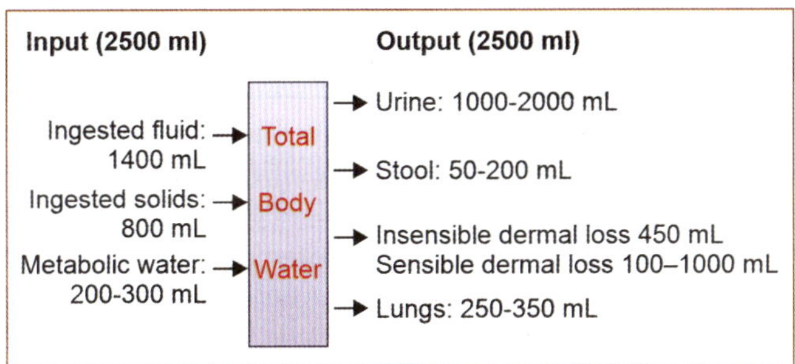

Fig. 10.12: Water homeostasis

Water balance is, thus, regulated by two mechanisms, i.e. by its intake as well as output.

- **Water intake**

  Main contributors of total water intake are the beverages (60–65%) and the foods (25–30%). Besides, daily metabolic water generation is 200–300 ml.

  Volume of the liquid ingested is regulated by thirst which is under the control of thirst center. Minimum requirement for water, however, is highly variable and depends upon several other factors such as:

  - **Obligatory losses:** There is an obligatory but variable loss of water in insensible perspiration, breath and feces. Sweating can greatly increase fluid loss and thus its demand.
  - **Disease conditions:** Fluid intake is also associated with physical condition and injury, e.g. fluid loss increases due to watery diarrhea or blood loss, etc. Human body has receptors in the right atrium, called baroreceptors which are sensitive to changes in osmotic pressure and blood volume. During certain pathological conditions, e.g. congestive heart failure, hepatic cirrhosis, nephrotic syndrome, etc. baroreceptors detect a decrease in blood volume despite an overall expansion of the ECF. This excess fluid in the ECF compartment gets collected in the tissues and cause edema.
  - **Dietary factors:** Sodium tends to hold water so extra sodium (salt) intake may increase water content of the body. Carbohydrate content of the diet affects both sodium and water balance. Increased amount of carbohydrate in the diet increases water retention while a low carbohydrate intake results in a loss of body fluid. Serum proteins influence water balance by their osmotic effect since proteins draw water from the interstitial fluid into the blood. If a low protein diet is consumed for a longer duration, serum albumin levels fall to such an extent that fluid accumulates between the cells and thus total body water is increased.

- **Water output**

  Water is removed from the body in the form of urine, feces, perspiration and expiration.

  - **Urine:** It is an important medium for the elimination of water presents in the body in excess of its requirement. Normally, about 1–2 L (60%) of water is excreted in the form of urine, daily. This is regulated by antidiuretic hormone (ADH), which promotes reabsorption of water from the distal renal tubules. In the absence of ADH (such as in diabetes insipidus) the urine is not concentrated and the urine output is highly increased, which may reach up to 15 L/day.
  - **Feces:** Normally, about 50–200 mL (4%) ml of water is excreted in the feces of an adult, daily. The value may increase considerably on a high vegetable diet, particularly in the presence of diarrhea.
  - **Perspiration:** The amount of water lost in the perspiration varies enormously. When the environmental temperature or humidity increases, sweat glands become active and thus in summer excessive water is lost via perspiration. Sweat removes a hypotonic solution which in addition to water also contains Na^+ and Cl^-. **Insensible perspiration** is the process whereby the body loses water continuously from the skin

surface and lungs. Contrary to the **visible perspiration** which removes hypotonic solution, insensible perspiration consists solely of water. Normally, from an adult human being about 600 ml (24%) of water is eliminated by this route, daily.

- **Expiration:** Nearly 250–350 ml (12%) of water is lost through exhalation from the lungs.

ELECTROLYTES

An electrolyte is a substance that ionizes when dissolved in suitable ionizing solvents such as water. This includes most soluble salts, acids and bases. Chemically, electrolytes are substances that become ions in solution and acquire the capacity to conduct electricity.

Electrolytes are present in the human body and the balance of the electrolytes in our body is essential for normal function of cells and organs. Common electrolytes that are measured in blood include sodium and potassium.

Biological functions of sodium and potassium are described in Table 10.3.

SODIUM

The adult human body contains ≈100 g of sodium, as sodium ions (Na^+). About half of this is found in the extracellular fluid while the remaining half in the cells and bone. Sodium is the **major cation in the ECF**. It exists in the body in association with several anions such as chloride, bicarbonate, phosphate, lactate and proteinate. High concentration of Na^+ along with low K^+ in the extracellular fluid is maintained by Na^+/K^+-ATPase (Na^+/K^+-pump).

Absorption and Excretion

Sodium is completely absorbed by the gastrointestinal tract. It is mainly excreted by the kidneys. Under normal physiological conditions, its daily urinary excretion is equal to its intake, since only less than 2% of the ingested sodium is eliminated in the feces. It is freely filtered by the glomerulus. About 70% of the filtered sodium is reabsorbed by the proximal tubules, 15% by the loop of Henle, 5% by the distal convoluted tubules and about 10% by the collecting ducts. Active reabsorption of Na^+ in the proximal tubule results in the passive reabsorption of Cl^- and HCO_3^- along with water. This helps to maintain electrical neutrality of the extracellular fluid while the reabsorption of water ensures normal osmotic pressure.

Sodium homeostasis is influenced by several general factors (Fig. 10.13).

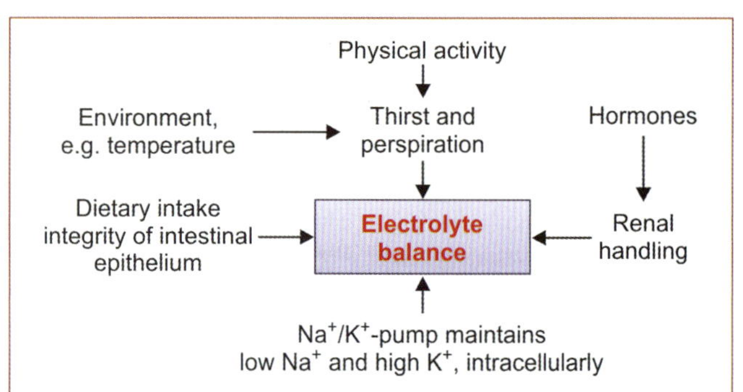

Fig. 10.13: Electrolyte balance. Aldosterone, secreted by the adrenal cortex, facilitates the retention of Na^+ and excretion of K^+ by the kidneys. Hypofunctioning of the adrenal cortex (Addison's disease) results in hyponatremia with hyperkalemia while hyperfunctioning of the adrenal cortex (Cushing's syndrome) results in hypernatremia with hypokalemia

Table 10.3: Biological functions of sodium and potassium in the body

Sodium	Potassium
1. Regulation of osmotic pressure of extracellular fluid	1. Regulation of intracellular osmotic pressure
2. Regulation of acid–base balance of extracellular fluid	2. Regulation of intracellular acid–base balance
3. GI and renal absorption of monosaccharides and amino acids	3. GI secretions
4. Maintenance of neuromuscular irritability and excitability	4. Maintenance of neuromuscular irritability and excitability
5. Maintenance of blood viscosity	5. Storage of proteins and glycogen
6. Cofactor for Na^+/K^+-ATPase	6. Cofactor for enzymes, e.g. Na^+/K^+-ATPase, pyruvate kinase, etc.

Sources of Sodium

The most important source of sodium is the common **table salt**, i.e. sodium chloride. Meat, seafoods, milk, cheese and bread are its good sources. Plant sources are usually low in sodium.

RDA of Sodium

Daily intake of sodium as sodium chloride varies from 5 to 15 g depending upon the climate.

POTASSIUM

Potassium is the **chief cation in the ICF**. Its functions are outlined in Table 10.3.

Potassium homeostasis is influenced by several general factors (Fig. 10.13).

Absorption and Excretion

Potassium is completely absorbed from the gastrointestinal tract. Less than 10% of the potassium is eliminated in feces. It is freely filtered at the glomerulus. Its active tubular reabsorption occurs throughout the nephron. Potassium is normally excreted almost entirely by the kidneys.

Sources of Potassium

Potassium is widely distributed in plants as well as animals, as the chloride, phosphate and carbonate salts of inorganic acids, organic acids and proteins. The good sources of potassium are coffee, cocoa, dried beans, wheat bran, most of the vegetables such as potato, tomato, dairy products, fish, eggs, meat and fruits like banana, peach and oranges.

RDA for Potassium

Normal intake of potassium has been recommended as about 4 g daily. However, its daily requirement has been suggested in relation of sodium in the ratio of 1:1, on a molar basis.

DISTRIBUTION OF ELECTROLYTES IN BODY FLUIDS

Electrolytes are distributed unevenly between ICF and ECF. Different concentrations of electrolytes in the two compartments are vital for the normal physiological processes. Since interstitial fluid and plasma are nearly similar in composition, they are considered together. Even though there are marked differences in the composition of ICF and ECF, their osmolarity is essentially the same.

Table 10.4 gives the differences in chemical composition of the ICF and plasma.

Table 10.4: Electrolyte distribution in various fluid compartments

Electrolyte	Concentration (mmol/L)	
	Intracellular fluid	Plasma
Total anions	**205**	**154**
Cl^-	2	103
HPO_4^{2-}	148	4
Others	55	47
Total cations	**205**	**154**
Na^+	10	142
K^+	160	4
Others	35	8

ELECTROLYTE BALANCE

Adequate hydration (water) and normal levels of electrolytes are important for proper functioning of the body.

Various mechanisms operate to maintain a normal electrolyte balance in body fluids (Fig. 10.13).

DERANGEMENTS ASSOCIATED WITH MAINTENANCE OF WATER AND ELECTROLYTE BALANCE

DERANGEMENTS ASSOCIATED WITH MAINTENANCE OF WATER BALANCE

Failure to regulate water balance results in dehydration (Chemistry to Clinics 10.2) and **edema** (Chemistry to Clinics 10.3).

Diet modifications, particularly reducing sodium intake often in conjunction with diuretic therapy is helpful in the treatment of conditions associated with excessive retention of sodium and water. However, when diuretic therapy is used along with sodium restriction, special attention should also be paid towards the need of potassium and other minerals whose excretion is also affected by the diuretics. For example, the use of diuretics such as furosemide and thiazides, may cause depletion of potassium, magnesium and zinc.

Any fluid intake below 2000 ml daily is considered to be a restriction. Sodium-restricted diet though is very helpful in preventing fluid accumulation; sometimes it is necessary to restrict both water as well as Na^+ intake. The restricted intake of water and Na^+ is termed

Chemistry to Clinics 10.2: Dehydration

Water deficit or volume depletion is referred to as dehydration. However, pure water deficit is rare and hence in clinical practice, the term 'dehydration' indicates water plus electrolyte deficit. Several conditions such as diarrhea, uncontrolled diabetes mellitus, diabetes insipidus, overdose of diuretics, heat stroke, etc. may lead to dehydration. Fluid and electrolyte status of these patients should be corrected at the earliest by employing suitable oral (oral rehydration solution) or intravenous (isotonic saline, dextrose-saline, Ringer lactate) fluids.

Chemistry to Clinics 10.3: Edema

Due to the retention of water along with sodium, both of these move from the blood to the interstitial fluid allowing maintenance of a relatively normal blood volume. When fluid retention is observable, the condition is called edema which takes the form of puffiness in the fingers and ankles or sometimes of the entire body (anasarca). Retention of sodium and water, as occurs in patients with congestive heart failure, increases workload on the heart and may precipitate an acute failure. A serious consequence of acute heart failure may be congestion in the lungs (pulmonary edema) and thus may lead to respiratory distress.

fluid restriction. In congestive heart failure, cirrhosis of the liver with ascites or any other disease in which intravascular volume is increased, fluid restriction may be employed to promote diuresis or to prevent life-threatening hyponatremia.

DERANGEMENTS ASSOCIATED WITH MAINTENANCE OF ELECTROLYTE BALANCE

Alterations in Sodium Homeostasis

Hyponatremia

It is defined as plasma Na^+ concentration **<135 mEq/L**. It is the most common disorder of body fluid and electrolyte balance. Most often it reflects a problem of too much water, not too little Na^+, in the plasma. Drinking large quantities of water rarely causes hyponatremia because of the large capacity of the kidneys to excrete dilute urine. If, however, plasma antidiuretic hormone (ADH) is not decreased when plasma osmolality is decreased or if the ability of the kidneys to dilute the urine is impaired, hyponatremia may develop even with a normal water intake.

Because Na^+ is the major solute in the plasma, it is not surprising that hyponatremia is usually associated with hypo-osmolality. However, hyponatremia may also occur with a normal or even elevated plasma osmolality.

- **Hyponatremia and hypoosmolality** can occur in the presence of a decreased, normal or even increased total body Na^+ (Chemistry to Clinics 10.4).

Chemistry to Clinics 10.4: Hyponatremia and Hypoosmolality

- **Hyponatremia and decreased total body Na^+:** It is seen with increased Na^+ loss such as with vomiting, diarrhea and diuretic therapy. The decrease in ECF volume stimulates thirst and ADH release. More water is ingested but the kidneys form osmotically concentrated urine, resulting in plasma hypo-osmolality and hyponatremia.
- **Syndrome of inappropriate ADH secretion (SIADH):** It occurs with neurological disease, severe pain, certain drugs (such as hypoglycemic agents) and with some tumors.
- **Hyponatremia and increased total body Na^+:** It is seen in edematous states such as congestive heart failure, hepatic cirrhosis and nephrotic syndrome. The decrease in effective arterial blood volume stimulates thirst and ADH release. The excretion of dilute urine may also be impaired because of decreased delivery of fluid to diluting sites along the nephron and collecting ducts. Although both Na^+ and water are retained by the kidneys in the edematous states, relatively more water is conserved leading to a dilutional hyponatremia.
- **General symptoms:** Muscle cramps, lethargy, fatigue, disorientation, headache, anorexia, nausea, agitation, hypothermia, seizures and coma. These symptoms, mainly neurological, are a consequence of the swelling of brain cells as plasma osmolality falls. Excessive brain swelling may be fatal or may cause permanent damage.
- **Treatment:** Identify and treat the underlying cause. If Na^+ loss is responsible for the hyponatremia, isotonic or hypertonic saline or NaCl by mouth is usually given. If the blood volume is normal or the patient is edematous, water restriction is recommended. Hyponatremia should be corrected slowly and with constant monitoring because too rapid correction can be harmful, resulting in central pontine myelinolysis.
- **Hyponatremia and increased plasma osmolality** is seen in hyperglycemic patients with uncontrolled diabetes mellitus. In this condition, the high blood glucose causes the osmotic withdrawal of water from cells and the extra water in the ECF space leads to hyponatremia. Plasma Na^+ falls by 1.6 mEq/L for each 100 mg/dl rise in blood glucose.
- **Hyponatremia and normal plasma osmolality** are seen in the so-called **pseudohyponatremia**. This occurs when plasma lipids or proteins are greatly elevated. These molecules do not significantly elevate plasma osmolality. However, they do occupy a significant volume of the plasma and because the Na^+ is dissolved only in the plasma water, the Na^+ measured in the entire plasma is low.

Hypernatremia

Hypernatremia is defined as plasma Na^+ concentration **>150 mEq/L**. It is **always hyperosmolar** and is characterized by edema, azotemia and anemia.

Accumulation of Na^+ in the body has been shown to result in a concomitant rise in blood pressure referred to as essential hypertension (Chemistry to Clinics 10.5).

Chemistry to Clinics 10.5: Salt Sensitive Hypertension

It is generally accepted that abnormal retention of salt (NaCl) by the kidneys is the major contributor to hypertension. Both the Na^+ and Cl^- in salt are critical; if chloride is replaced by bicarbonate or citrate ions in the diet then hypertension does not develop. Nonetheless, it is common to focus on Na^+ as the culprit because it is actively reabsorbed by the kidneys and the Cl^- usually just follows along. Salt retention leads to water retention and hence, higher volume and pressure in the vascular system. Dietary salt restriction and the use of diuretics, i.e. drugs that promote salt and water excretion, are highly effective in treating salt sensitive hypertension.

Multiple genes and environmental factors contribute to hypertension. Many of the implicated genes affect blood pressure by changing salt and water reabsorption by the kidneys. A good example is Liddle syndrome, an autosomal dominant disorder in which patients develop early and severe hypertension. In these patients, the renal epithelial Na^+ channel is constitutively activated, leading to excessive Na^+ and water reabsorption. They also develop hypokalemia caused by excessive renal loss of K^+. The hypertension can be effectively treated by a low-salt diet and the use of a diuretic drug, amiloride, which specifically blocks the overactive Na^+ channel.

Symptoms are primarily neurological which include tremors, irritability, confusion and coma.

Alterations in Potassium Homeostasis

Disorders of acid–base balance, water balance and administration of some drugs are often accompanied by alterations in potassium balance: Either potassium deficit (hypokalemia) or excess (hyperkalemia).

Hypokalemia

- Hypokalemia is defined as serum potassium concentration **<3.5 mEq/L**.
- It is seen in individuals taking potassium losing diuretics (carbonic anhydrase inhibitors, loop diuretics and thiazides), those with severe liver disease, gastrointestinal losses, and metabolic alkalosis. Hyperaldosteronism can cause excess excretion of potassium accompanied by increased retention of Na^+ which leads to depletion of plasma K^+. Prolonged hypokalemia, in turn, further causes damage to the kidneys.
- Both cardiac and skeletal muscles are affected by hypokalemia. Deficiency symptoms include muscular weakness, mental apathy, cardiac arrhythmias (irregular heartbeat), tachycardia (heartbeat more rapid than usual), hypotension, paralysis, bone fragility, etc.
- It can be corrected by oral KCl supplements and, if necessary, by suitable intravenous electrolytes.

Hyperkalemia

- Hyperkalemia is defined as serum potassium concentration **>5.5 mEq/L**.
- Hyperkalemia arises when K^+ excretion by the kidney is depressed such as in acute renal failure.
- Acidosis causes leakage of K^+ from the cell which may increase plasma K^+ while leaving the cells depleted of K^+.
- Potassium-sparing diuretics may lead to hyperkalemia.
- Early signs of cardiac damage include arrhythmia followed by a slowing of the heart rate, ventricular fibrillation and arrest in diastole.
- Hyperkalemia may lead to CNS depression, mental confusion, numbness or tingling of extremities and weakness of respiratory muscles resulting in difficulty in breathing and speech. High concentration of potassium is also toxic to the muscles and may cause paralysis.
- Under such situations, K^+ is excluded from the diet. Insulin and glucose promote the uptake of K^+ into the cells and this treatment is used for patients suffering from life-threatening hyperkalemia.

ARTERIAL BLOOD GAS (ABG) ANALYSIS

Arterial blood gas (ABG) analysis is important in the assessment of acid–base imbalance. The disturbances of acid–base balance are accompanied by characteristic changes in blood pH, pCO_2 and HCO_3^-, the normal values for which, in the arterial blood, are as follows:

pH	7.35–7.45
pCO_2	35–45 mm Hg
HCO_3^-	22–26 mmol/L

Besides, base excess and anion gap are also calculated.

Base Excess

Base excess is defined as the amount of acid required to titrate the blood to pH 7.4, at a pCO_2 of 40 mm Hg, at 37°C. If a blood sample is acidic, the base excess will be negative. The normal value is in the range of –2.0 to +3.0 mmol/L.

Anion Gap

Anion gap is the difference between the sum of Na^+ and K^+ (cations) from the sum of Cl^- and HCO_3^-

(anions). Anion gap thus represents plasma anions other than Cl^- and HCO_3^- which are not routinely measured such as lactate, citrate, ketone bodies (acetoacetate and β-hydroxybutyrate), etc.

$$\text{Anion gap} = (Na^+ + K^+) - (Cl^- + HCO_3^-)$$

Normal value for anion gap is in the range of 12–16 mmol/L. This is most commonly used to establish a differential diagnosis for metabolic acidosis.

As shown in Table 10.5, certain conditions resulting in metabolic acidosis are characterized by an increased anion gap while others do not lead to any change in the anion gap.

ARTERIAL BLOOD GAS (ABG) ANALYSIS IN VARIOUS DISORDERS

GENERAL CONCEPTS OF ABG

1. **Acidemia and alkalemia:** A blood pH below 7.35 (H^+ >45 nmol/L) indicates ***'acidemia'***, whereas a blood pH above 7.45 (H^+ <35 nmol/L) indicates ***'alkalemia'***. The range of pH values compatible with life is approximately 6.8 to 7.8 (H^+ = 160 to 16 nmol/L).
2. **Acidosis and alkalosis:** Four simple acid–base disturbances may lead to an abnormal blood pH: Respiratory acidosis, respiratory alkalosis, metabolic acidosis and metabolic alkalosis. The word 'simple' indicates a single primary cause for the disturbance. ***'Acidosis'*** is an abnormal process that tends to produce acidemia, whereas ***'alkalosis'*** is an abnormal process that tends to produce alkalemia.
3. **Identifying the primary disturbance:** If there is too much or too little CO_2, then a ***respiratory disturbance*** is present. If the problem is too much or too little HCO_3^-, then a ***metabolic disturbance*** (nonrespiratory disturbance) is present.

   Table 10.6 summarizes the various changes that occur in blood in each of the four simple acid–base disturbances.
4. **Compensatory mechanisms:** In considering acid–base disturbances, it is helpful to recall the Henderson-Hasselbalch equation discussed earlier. If the primary problem is a change in HCO_3^- or pCO_2, the pH can be brought closer to normal by changing the other member of the buffer pair in the same direction. For example, if pCO_2 is primarily decreased, a decrease in plasma HCO_3^- will minimize

Table 10.5: Clinical examples of anion gap

Condition	Explanation
High anion gap metabolic acidosis	
• Ketoacidosis	• Production of acetoacetic and β-hydroxybutyric acids
• Lactacidosis	• H^+ buffered by HCO_3^-, accumulation of lactate
• Uremia	• Sulfuric, phosphoric, uric and hippuric acids retained due to renal failure
• Salicylate intoxication	• Salicylate accumulation, lactacidosis, ketoacidosis
• Methanol intoxication	• Methanol metabolized to formic acid
• Ethylene glycol intoxication	• Ethylene glycol metabolized to glyoxylic, glycolic and oxalic acids
• Paraldehyde intoxication	• Paraldehyde metabolized to acetic and chloroacetic acids
Normal anion gap metabolic acidosis	
• Diarrhoea	• Loss of HCO_3^- in stool, renal conservation of Cl^-
• Renal tubular acidosis	• Loss of HCO_3^- in urine/decreased H^+ excretion, renal conservation of Cl^-

Table 10.6: Changes observed in major acid–base balance disorders

Acid–base disorder	Arterial blood			Compensatory response
	pCO_2	pH	HCO_3^-	
Respiratory acidosis	↑	↓	↑	↑ Renal H^+ excretion increases plasma HCO_3^- concentration
Respiratory alkalosis	↓	↑	↓	↑ Renal HCO_3^- excretion decreases plasma HCO_3^- concentration
Metabolic acidosis	↓	↓	↓	Hyperventilation decreases pCO_2
Metabolic alkalosis	↑	↑	↑	Hypoventilation increases pCO_2

the change in pH. In various acid–base disturbances, the lungs adjust the blood pCO_2 and the kidneys adjust the plasma HCO_3^- to reduce deviations of pH from normal; these adjustments are called ***'compensations'*** (Table 10.6).

Compensations, however, do not correct the underlying disorder and do not necessarily restore the normal blood pH.

DISORDERS OF ABG

Respiratory Acidosis

Respiratory acidosis is most often due to inadequate ventilation (hypoventilation) of the alveoli. This, in turn, results in the retention of CO_2 and a fall in blood pH. Alveolar hypoventilation occurs when the depth or rate of respiration is diminished, such as airway obstruction or a pulmonary disease. It will result in a rise in pCO_2. As pCO_2 rises, plasma pH drops and HCO_3^- concentration rises.

The kidneys compensate for the respiratory acidosis by increasing the output of H^+ in the urine. The filtered HCO_3^- is reabsorbed and the increased amounts of H^+ combine with the urinary buffers and are excreted in the urine. Thus, by excreting H^+ in the urine, kidneys increase plasma HCO_3^- concentration.

Respiratory Alkalosis

Respiratory alkalosis is produced by hyperventilation which results in the excessive removal of CO_2 from the blood. This, in turn, causes a fall in arterial blood pCO_2, a fall in plasma H^+ concentration, i.e. a rise in pH and a fall in plasma HCO_3^- concentration. Hyperventilation may be caused by anxiety, central nervous system injury involving the respiratory center, salicylate poisoning or fever. At high altitude also, due to decrease in total atmospheric pressure, alveolar pCO_2 falls and results in chronic respiratory alkalosis.

The kidneys compensate for the respiratory alkalosis by excreting HCO_3^- in the urine. A low pCO_2 leads to decreased H^+ secretion by the tubular epithelium. This, in turn, results in reduced reabsorption of the filtered bicarbonate and increases its excretion in the urine. This loss of HCO_3^- in the urine results in a further decrease in plasma HCO_3^- and plasma pH towards normal.

Metabolic Acidosis

Metabolic acidosis is characterized by the accumulation of nonvolatile acids (gain of fixed acids other than H_2CO_3) or loss of HCO_3^-. Gain of metabolically produced acid may be due to several reasons, such as:

1. Uncontrolled diabetes mellitus leading to the production of large quantities of ketone bodies (Chemistry to Clinics 10.6).

Chemistry to Clinics 10.6: Diabetic Ketoacidosis

Insulin deficiency leads to decreased glucose utilization, a diversion of metabolism towards the use of fatty acids and an overproduction of ketone bodies (acetoacetic acid and β-hydroxybutyric acid). Ketone bodies, sometimes called ketone body acids, are fairly strong acids (pKa 4–5). They are neutralized in the body by HCO_3^- and other buffers. Increased production of these acids leads to a fall in plasma HCO_3^-, an increase in plasma anion gap and a fall in blood pH (acidemia). This is diabetic ketoacidosis.

Complications: Severe acidemia, whatever its cause, has many adverse effects:

1. Impaired myocardial contractility, decrease in cardiac output, arteriolar dilation, fall in arterial blood pressure, cardiac arrhythmias.
2. Decreased hepatic and renal blood flow.
3. Respiratory muscle fatigue.
4. Activation of the sympathetic nervous system, increased metabolic demands, reduced ATP synthesis, hyperkalemia, protein catabolism.
5. Impaired neuronal metabolism and cell volume regulation leading to progressive obtundation and coma.

Respiratory compensation: Acidemia stimulates pulmonary ventilation resulting in a compensatory lowering of alveolar and arterial blood pCO_2. The consequent reduction in blood H_2CO_3 moves the blood pH back toward normal. The rapid, deep breathing that accompanies severe uncontrolled diabetes is called Kussmaul respiration and the breath gives the fruity smell of acetone, the volatile ketone body.

Renal compensation: The kidneys compensate for metabolic acidosis by reabsorbing all the filtered HCO_3^-. They also increase the excretion of titratable acid, part of which is composed of ketone bodies. But these acids can only be partially titrated to their acid form in the urine because the urine pH cannot go below 4.5. Thus, ketone bodies are excreted mostly in their anionic form; because of the requirement of electroneutrality in solutions, increased urinary excretion of Na^+ and K^+ results.

An important compensation for the acidosis is increased renal synthesis and excretion of ammonia. This adaptive response takes several days to develop fully but it allows the kidneys to dispose off large amounts of H^+ in the form NH_4^+. The NH_4^+ in the urine can replace Na^+ and K^+ ions thereby helping to conserve these valuable cations.

1. **Treatment:** The severe acidemia, electrolyte disturbances and volume depletion that accompany uncontrolled diabetes mellitus may be fatal. Correction of the acid–base disturbance is best achieved by addressing the underlying cause rather than just treating the symptoms. Therefore, the administration of a suitable dose of insulin by intravenous infusion is the key element of therapy. In some patients with marked acidemia (pH <7.10), $NaHCO_3$ solutions may be infused to speed recovery but this does not correct the underlying metabolic problem. Water and electrolyte corrections should be made.
2. Renal failure leading to reduced excretion of the metabolically produced acids.
3. Inadequate circulation due to cardiogenic or hemorrhagic shock which, in turn, promotes anaerobic glycolysis and increases the production of lactic acid.
4. Heavy exercise resulting in the production of lactic acid.
5. Ingestion of certain acidifying agents, such as ammonium chloride.

Metabolic acidosis may also be due to a loss of HCO_3^- from the body, such as due to diarrhea or abnormal excretion of HCO_3^- in the urine. Thus, an addition of strong organic or inorganic acid, or a loss of HCO_3^- results in a decrease in plasma HCO_3^- concentration in metabolic acidosis.

Two compensatory mechanisms are usually available to deal with the excess acid:

1. Due to the acidic pH, **respiratory system** is stimulated to hyperventilate. This, in turn, lowers the pCO_2 and hence the carbonic acid concentration in the blood. The respiratory compensation though is prompt but usually does not restore the blood pH to normal.
2. The other mechanism which begins almost instantly, is the **renal compensation**. The kidneys increase H^+ excretion. This however, takes time and is not adequate to return HCO_3^- concentration and the pH to normal.

Metabolic Alkalosis

10

Metabolic alkalosis is characterized by the intake of excess of alkali, i.e. by the gain of strong base or HCO_3^-, or abnormal loss of acid other than HCO_3^-. For example, the ingestion of excess sodium bicarbonate, used in treating gastric ulcer or the oxidation of organic anions, such as citrate, lactate and acetate. A common cause of abnormal loss of acid causing metabolic alkalosis, is prolonged vomiting or gastric lavage since loss of stomach contents results in net addition of HCO_3^- to the blood (Chemistry to Clinics 10.7).

It may also be a result of the rapid loss of body water, e.g. in diuresis, which in turn, may result in a temporary rise in HCO_3^- in plasma and extracellular fluid.

Characteristic arterial blood changes include a primary increase in plasma HCO_3^- concentration, a rise in pH, and a compensatory rise in pCO_2. Metabolic alkalosis is seldom long lasting. Chemical buffers in the body act to limit the alkaline shift in pH by liberating H^+. As the primary defect is an increase in plasma HCO_3^- concentration, the immediate physiological compensation is hypoventilation followed by increased renal excretion of HCO_3^-.

Chemistry to Clinics 10.7: Vomiting and Metabolic Alkalosis

Vomiting of acidic gastric juice results in metabolic alkalosis and fluid/electrolyte disturbances. The gastric parietal cells have H^+/K^+-ATPase in their luminal cell membrane and Cl^-/HCO_3^- exchanger in the basolateral cell membrane. When HCl is secreted into the stomach lumen and lost to the outside, there is a net gain of HCO_3^- in the blood and no change in the anion gap. The HCO_3^-, in effect, replaces lost plasma Cl^-.

Respiratory compensation: Ventilation is inhibited by the alkaline blood pH, resulting in a rise in pCO_2. This respiratory compensation, however, is limited because hypoventilation-induced hypoxemia stimulates breathing.

Renal compensation: The logical renal compensation for metabolic alkalosis is enhanced excretion of HCO_3^-. In people with persistent vomiting, however, the urine is sometimes acidic and renal HCO_3^- reabsorption is enhanced, thereby maintaining the elevated plasma HCO_3^-. This situation arises because vomiting is accompanied by losses of extracellular fluid (ECF) and K^+ that lead to a decrease in effective arterial blood volume, activation of the renin-angiotensin-aldosterone system and enhanced tubular H^+ secretion. With more H^+ secretion, more new HCO_3^- is added to the blood. The kidneys reabsorb filtered HCO_3^- completely even though the plasma HCO_3^- level is elevated and thus maintain the metabolic alkalosis.

Hypokalemia: Vomiting results in K^+ depletion because of a loss of K^+ in the vomitus, decreased food intake and most important quantitatively, enhanced renal K^+ excretion. Alkalosis results in a shift of K^+ into cells (including renal cells) and thereby promotes K^+

secretion and excretion. Elevated plasma aldosterone levels also favor K^+ loss in the urine.

Treatment: It primarily depends on eliminating the cause of vomiting. Correction of the alkalosis by administering an organic acid such as lactic acid does not make sense because this acid would simply be converted to CO_2 and H_2O; this approach also does not address the Cl^- deficit. The ECF volume depletion and the Cl^- and K^+ deficits can be corrected by administering isotonic saline and appropriate amounts of KCl. Because replacement of Cl^- is a key component of therapy, this type of metabolic alkalosis is said to be 'chloride-responsive'. After fluid and electrolyte replacement, the excess HCO_3^- (accompanied by surplus Na^+) will be excreted in the urine and the kidneys will return blood pH to normal.

RENAL TUBULAR ACIDOSIS (RTA)

It is a group of kidney disorders characterized by **chronic metabolic acidosis, a normal plasma anion gap and the absence of renal failure**. The kidneys show inadequate H^+ secretion by the distal nephrons, excessive excretion of HCO_3^-, or reduced excretion of NH_4^+. The following types are recognized:

- **Classic type 1 (*distal*) RTA:** The ability of the collecting ducts to lower urine pH is impaired. This condition can be caused by inadequate secretion of H^+ (defective H^+-ATPase or H^+/K^+-ATPase) or abnormal leakiness of the collecting duct epithelium so that the secreted H^+ diffuse back from the lumen into blood. Because the urine pH is inappropriately high, titratable acid excretion is diminished and trapping of ammonia in the urine (as NH_4^+) is decreased. Type 1 RTA may be the result of an inherited defect, autoimmune disease, treatment with lithium or the antibiotic amphotericin B, or diseases of the kidney medulla. The diagnosis is established by challenging the subject with a standard oral dose of NH_4Cl and measuring the urine pH over the next several hours. This results in a urine pH below 5.0 in healthy people. In subjects with type 1 RTA, however, urine pH will not decrease below 5.5. Treatment of type 1 RTA involves the daily administration of modest amounts of alkali (bicarbonate, citrate) sufficient to cover daily metabolic acid production.
- **Type 2 (*proximal*) RTA:** The HCO_3^- reabsorption by the proximal tubule is impaired leading to excessive losses of HCO_3^- in the urine. As a consequence, the plasma HCO_3^- falls and chronic metabolic acidosis ensues. In the new steady state, the tubules are able to reabsorb the filtered HCO_3^- load more completely, because the filtered load is reduced. The distal nephron is no longer overwhelmed by HCO_3^- and the urine pH is acidic. The NH_4Cl challenge results in a urine pH below 5.5. This disorder may be inherited (mutation in genes that code for carbonic anhydrase or Na^+/HCO_3^- cotransporters), may be associated with a number of acquired conditions that result in a generalized disorder of proximal tubule transport or may result from the inhibition of proximal tubule carbonic anhydrase by drugs such as acetazolamide. Treatment requires the daily administration of large amounts of alkali because when the plasma HCO_3^- is raised, excessive urinary excretion of filtered HCO_3^- occurs.
- **Type 3 RTA:** It is rare and shows ***mixed features*** of types 1 and 2.
- **Type 4 RTA:** It is also known as ***hyperkalemic distal RTA***. The collecting duct secretion of both K^+ and H^+ is reduced, explaining the hyperkalemia and metabolic acidosis. Hyperkalemia reduces renal ammonia synthesis resulting in reduced net acid excretion and a fall in plasma HCO_3^-. The urine pH can go below 5.5 after NH_4Cl challenge because there is a little ammonia in the urine to buffer secreted H^+. The underlying disorder is a result of inadequate production of aldosterone or impaired aldosterone action. Treatment of type 4 RTA requires lowering the plasma K^+ to normal; if this therapy is successful, alkali may not be needed.

Some Important Questions

1. **What are the important physiological functions of water in the body?**
2. **Discuss various factors responsible for the regulation of body water.**
3. **Describe physiological functions of sodium and its regulation.**
4. **Discuss important physiological functions of potassium and its regulation.**
5. **Define buffer. Name important buffers present in the body. Explain the role of various body buffers in the regulation of blood pH.**
6. **Explain:**
   i. Role of kidney in the regulation of blood pH
   ii. Various mechanisms of H^+ secretion
   iii. Disturbances of acid–base balance
   iv. Measures of acid–base imbalance
   v. Role of lungs in the regulation of blood pH
7. **Write notes on:**
   i. pH
   ii. Henderson-Hasselbalch equation
   iii. Chemical buffers in the body
   iv. Titratable acidity
   v. Respiratory acidosis
   vi. Respiratory alkalosis
   vii. Metabolic acidosis
   viii. Metabolic alkalosis
   ix. Base excess
   x. Anion gap
   xi. Diabetic ketoacidosis
   xii. Intracellular fluid
   xiii. Extracellular fluid
   xiv. Electrolytes
   xv. Na^+/K^+-ATPase
   xvi. Hyponatremia
   xvii. Hypernatremia
   xviii. Hypokalemia
   xix. Hyperkalemia
   xx. Anion gap
   xxi. Dehydration
   xxii. Edema

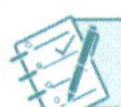

Multiple Choice Questions

1. **The following is a correct representation of pH:**
   A. $\log_{10}[H^+]$
   B. $\log_{10}[1/H^+]$
   C. $\log_e[H^+]$
   D. $\log_e[1/H^+]$
2. **The major buffer system in RBC is:**
   A. Bicarbonate
   B. Phosphate
   C. Hemoglobin
   D. Nonheme proteins
3. **The following is an 'open' buffer system:**
   A. Bicarbonate
   B. Phosphate
   C. Hemoglobin
   D. Plasma proteins

4. **The majority of titratable acid in the urine is:**
   A. Inorganic phosphate ($H_2PO_4^-$)
   B. Inorganic sulphate (H_2SO_4)
   C. Inorganic chloride (HCl)
   D. Carbonic acid (H_2CO_3)
5. **Alkalemia indicates the following H^+ concentration in blood:**
   A. <35 mmol/L
   B. <35 nmol/L
   C. <35 mol/L
   D. <35 pmol/L
6. **Salicylate poisoning is associated with:**
   A. Hyperventilation and respiratory alkalosis
   B. Hypoventilation and respiratory acidosis
   C. Hyperventilation and respiratory acidosis
   D. Hypoventilation and respiratory alkalosis

7. Increased renal HCO_3^- excretion is the main compensation observed in:

A. Metabolic acidosis
B. Metabolic alkalosis
C. Respiratory acidosis
D. Respiratory alkalosis

8. Increased anion gap is characteristic of:

A. Uncontrolled diabetes mellitus with metabolic acidosis
B. Salicylate poisoning with respiratory alkalosis
C. Status asthmaticus with respiratory acidosis
D. Prolonged gastric lavage with metabolic alkalosis

9. The sum of all buffering agents in blood is called:

A. Anion gap
B. Buffer base
C. Base excess
D. Buffering capacity

10. Water content is least in:

A. Adipose tissue
B. Bones
C. Muscles
D. Nervous tissue

CHAPTER 11

Minerals

Competency Achievement: The student should be able to:

BI6.9	Describe the functions of various minerals in the body, their metabolism and homeostasis
BI6.10	Enumerate and describe the disorders associated with mineral metabolism
PA14.1	Describe iron metabolism
PA16.1	Define and classify hemolytic anemia
PE13.1	Discuss the RDA, dietary sources of iron and their role in health and disease
PE13.2	Describe the causes, diagnosis and management of Fe deficiency
PE13.3	Identify the clinical features of dietary deficiency of iron and make a diagnosis
PE13.7	Discuss the RDA, dietary sources of iodine and their role in health and disease
PE13.8	Describe the causes, clinical features, diagnosis and management of deficiency of iodine
PE13.9	Identify the clinical features of iodine deficiency disorders
PE13.10	Discuss the National Goiter Control Program and their recommendations
PE13.11	Discuss the RDA, dietary sources of calcium and its role in health and disease
PE13.12	Describe the causes, clinical features, diagnosis and management of Ca deficiency
PE13.13	Discuss the RDA, dietary sources of magnesium and their role in health and disease
PE13.14	Describe the causes, clinical features, diagnosis and management of magnesium deficiency
DR17.4	Enumerate and describe the various changes in zinc deficiency

In addition to carbohydrates, lipids, proteins, vitamins and water, body also needs small amounts of a number of inorganic substances called minerals and trace elements. These are classified into 3 categories based on their daily requirements (Fig. 11.1).

CALCIUM

Amongst various minerals, calcium (Ca) is found in **highest concentration in the body** and is needed by all the cells. Adult human body contains nearly 1.0 to 1.2 kg

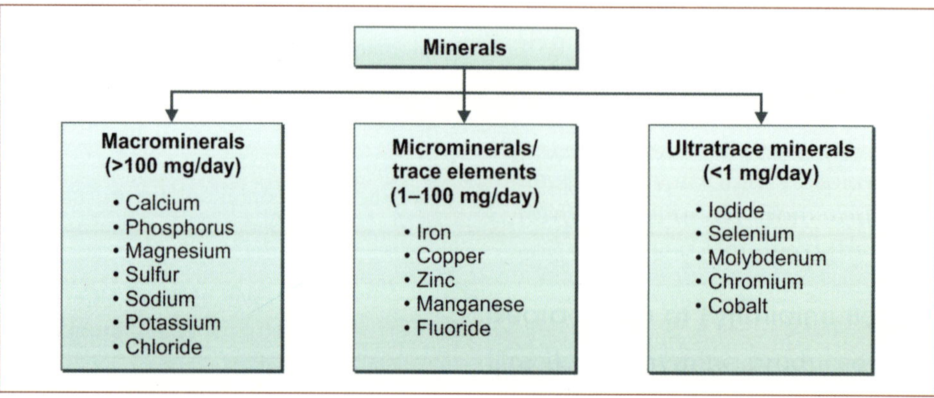

Fig. 11.1: Classification of minerals based on daily requirements

of calcium. About 99% of it is present in the skeletal tissue, i.e. in the bones and teeth while the remaining is found in the soft tissues, such as the muscle and the nervous tissue. Normal serum calcium level is 9–11 mg/100 mL. It is present in blood in three different forms:

1. About 45–50% of the total serum calcium is present in the **ionized form** as Ca^{2+} ions. It is freely exchangeable between the soft tissues, the extracellular fluid and the blood.
2. Nearly equal amount, i.e. 45–50% is **bound to proteins.**
3. The remaining 5–10% is present in the form of **salts,** with citrate, phosphate, etc.

Biological Functions of Calcium and its Role in Health and Disease

Calcium performs several roles in health and disease:

1. Calcification of the growing bones and teeth, and maintenance of the mature bones.
2. Activator of a number of enzymes, e.g. adenylate cyclase, ATPases, protein kinases, etc. Ca^{2+} activates phosphorylase kinase through its binding to calmodulin and thus increases the rate of glycogen breakdown. It activates pyruvate dehydrogenase phosphatase which, in turn, activates pyruvate dehydrogenase complex to produce acetyl-CoA. Ca^{2+} also regulates the enzymes of citric acid cycle, at several steps. For example, Ca^{2+} also activates isocitrate dehydrogenase and α-ketoglutarate dehydrogenase. Thus, Ca^{2+} stimulates the production of ATP.
3. Clotting of blood.
4. Contraction of muscles (excitation-contraction coupling).
5. Regulates the permeability of the capillary walls and excitability of the nerve fibers.
6. Secretion of various hormones and acts as a second messenger.
7. Decreases fluidity of the membranes.

Metabolism of Calcium

Only about 10–30% of the dietary calcium is normally **absorbed**. It is absorbed throughout the small intestine but mostly in the duodenum where pH is close to 7; as the pH increases towards the jejunum and ileum, absorption decreases. Both passive diffusion and calcitriol-mediated active transport are responsible for calcium uptake. Absorption depends upon several factors, such as calcium content of food, presence of interfering substances and the presence of vitamin D:

1. In vitamin D deficiency, calcium absorption is impaired.
2. Excess of phosphate lowers calcium absorption.
3. Phytic acid and related substances, present in unrefined cereals, interfere with the absorption of calcium.
4. Excessive amounts of fat, fiber and oxalate in the diet reduce calcium absorption, due to the formation of insoluble salts.
5. Higher amounts of dietary protein, lactose and acidic pH promote calcium absorption.

Calcium is excreted in the feces, urine and sweat

- Dietary calcium, which is not absorbed in the intestine, is excreted in the feces. Excretion in the feces continues even when its intake is low, thereby resulting in negative calcium balance.
- Depending upon its dietary absorption, amount of calcium excreted in the urine varies from 50 to 200 mg/day. Urinary excretion is increased (hypercalciuria) by ingestion of the excessive amount of protein in the diet, in acidosis, thyrotoxicosis, hypoparathyroidism and restricted physical activity.
- In tropical climate, calcium excretion is increased in sweat.

Calcium Homeostasis

Maintenance of serum calcium level within the normal limit is called calcium homeostasis. As mentioned above, nearly 45–50% of the serum calcium is present in the ionized form (Ca^{2+}). This form of calcium is freely exchangeable between the soft tissues, the extracellular fluid and the blood, and is called **diffusible calcium.** Most of the functions of calcium are performed by the ionized form (Ca^{2+}) only. Serum Ca^{2+} level is regulated in a complex manner by parathyroid hormone (PTH), vitamin D and calcitonin (Fig. 11.2).

- **Parathyroid hormone:** If serum Ca^{2+} concentration falls, secretion of PTH is increased. The hormone:
  - Acts directly on osteoclasts and increases dissolution of bone mineral. This process is called ***bone resorption.***
  - Increases reabsorption of Ca^{2+} from the kidney tubules. The overall effect of the two processes is to elevate serum Ca^{2+} level.
  - Stimulates 1-α-hydroxylase activity in the kidney which, in turn, activates vitamin D and converts it to 1,25-dihydroxycholecalciferol, also called ***calcitriol*** or ***active vitamin D.***

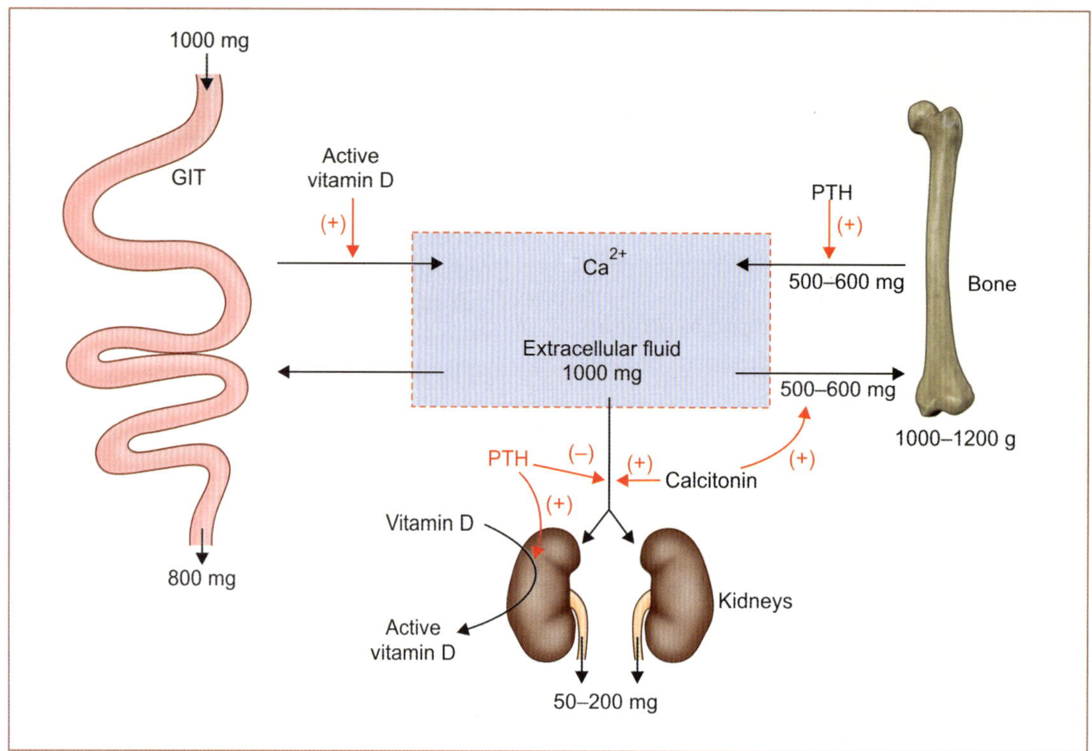

Fig. 11.2: Calcium homeostasis

- **Active vitamin D:** It increases serum Ca^{2+} concentration by promoting intestinal absorption of Ca^{2+} as well as its renal tubular reabsorption.
- **Calcitonin:** It is secreted when serum Ca^{2+} level rises. Its action is to lower serum Ca^{2+} level by promoting deposition of calcium, by the osteoblasts. It also promotes renal Ca^{2+} loss.
  Thus, PTH and calcitonin act in **opposite** directions in regulating serum calcium.

Calmodulin: It is a eukaryotic **Ca^{2+}-binding protein** that participates in numerous cellular regulatory processes. Calmodulin functions as a Ca^{2+} sensor and Ca^{2+} buffer in the cell, responding to changes in intracellular Ca^{2+} concentration which, in turn, affects the activities of a number of enzymes and acts as a second messenger for hormonal action.

RDA for Calcium

Daily requirement of calcium varies from individual to individual, due to the existence of several factors which affect availability of calcium. The RDA is 1000 mg for an adult. During pregnancy and lactation, its requirement is increased to about 1.2 g/day.

11

Dietary Sources of Calcium

Milk and milk products are rich sources of calcium. Besides milk, egg yolk, dry fruits, legumes, cabbage, cauliflower and leafy vegetables are good sources of calcium.

Deficiency Disorders of Calcium

A decrease in Ca^{2+} concentration in serum results in hypocalcemia. It may be due to increased pH, decreased intake or increased excretion of calcium. Hypocalcemia may also be caused by the deficiency of vitamin D or in hypoparathyroidism. Prolonged hypocalcemia may lead to faulty calcification of bone similar to that observed in rickets in children and osteomalacia in adults. Hypocalcemia may also contribute to osteoporosis.

Hypocalcemia affects motor nerves which become oversusceptible to stimuli, resulting in neuromuscular hyperexcitability and epileptiform convulsions. This is known as tetany (Chemistry to Clinics 11.1).

Chemistry to Clinics 11.1: Tetany

Causes: It may arise from various causes such as severe hypocalcemia (total serum calcium <7 mg/dl; ionized Ca^{2+} <2.5 mg/dl), hypoparathyroidism (may occur accidentally during thyroid surgery), hypomagnesemia, hyperphosphatemia, and alkalosis (at higher pH, more calcium is bound to albumin thus decreasing ionized calcium). Under these conditions, the membrane permeability for Na^{+} increases leading to rapid, successive, spontaneous depolarization.

Presentation: Neuromuscular excitability with painful muscle spasm is the chief symptom in adults and convulsive seizures in children.

Complication: Death may occur due to laryngospasm.

Emergency treatment: Intravenous calcium gluconate (preferred over calcium chloride because it causes less tissue necrosis, if extravasated), since it can correct low calcium and high potassium, and magnesium toxicity.

Osteoporosis: Decreased calcium intake, particularly during/after menopause leads to increased fragility and fractures of bones, mainly of the extremities and pelvis. This is due to **reduced bone density** (bone mass per unit volume) called osteoporosis. It is characterized by the loss of bone matrix and progressive demineralization. Thus, in contrast to osteomalacia where mineralization fails to occur on a normal osteoid matrix, in osteoporosis, **both the matrix formation and the subsequent calcification are at fault**. Increased supply of calcium in the food or oral supplementation of calcium along with the estrogen therapy in postmenopausal woman retards osteoporosis.

Besides calcium, vitamin C, vitamin K, magnesium, phosphorus, copper, zinc, manganese and boron are also important in bone formation. Vitamin D is also essential for the absorption and utilization of calcium. Therefore, an adequate diet sufficient in all the nutrients along with regular exercise is important for preventing osteoporosis.

Calcium Toxicity

Calcium toxicity may result in hypercalcemia, which may be due to increased intake of calcium, raised levels of plasma albumin or increased renal reabsorption of Ca^{2+} (Chemistry to Clinics 11.2).

Hypercalcemia may also by caused by hyperactivity of the parathyroid gland (hyperparathyroidism) or hypervitaminosis D. Hypercalcemia may lead to the formation of stones (calculi), loss of appetite, vomiting, constipation, weakness of muscles and sluggish reflexes.

Chemistry to Clinics 11.2: Milk-alkali Syndrome (Burnett's Syndrome)

In the past, excessive consumption of milk and antacids was a popular remedy among patients suffering from hyperacidity and indigestion. However, over a long period it results in hypercalcemia (calcium derived from milk and some calcium and magnesium containing antacids) and metabolic alkalosis. This is referred to as milk-alkali syndrome or Burnett's syndrome. Renal stones occur in extreme cases. The incidence has reduced considerably due to better treatment options for acid-peptic disease.

PHOSPHORUS

Phosphorus (P) is widely distributed in most of the tissues. A normal adult body contains nearly 600–800 g of phosphorus. About 75% of it is present in combination with calcium in the bones, teeth and skeletal tissues. The blood, muscle and the nerve tissue also contain fairly good amounts.

Biological Functions of Phosphorus and its Role in Health and Disease

Phosphorus is present in two forms, i.e. as inorganic phosphorus and organic phosphorus, both of which perform different functions.

A. Inorganic Phosphorus

1. It is essential with calcium, for the mineralization of bones and teeth. It is a part of the crystal, hydroxyapatite, which is laid down on collagen in the ossification process of bone formation.
2. Maintenance of acid–base balance. In the renal system, phosphate functions in the excretion of hydrogen ions. Filtered phosphate reacts with the secreted H^+ and releases Na^+ which gets reabsorbed through the renal tubules, under the influence of aldosterone.

B. Organic Phosphorus

It is the phosphorus found in the form of esters of various organic compounds, such as in phospholipids, nucleic acids, coenzymes, etc.

1. In the form of **phospholipids**, phosphorus is essential for the transport and metabolism of lipids and also forms an integral part of the cell membrane.
2. In the form of **nucleic acids**, it forms an important constituent of the cell nucleus and is essential for cell multiplication and protein synthesis.
3. **Organic esters** of phosphoric acid such as ADP, glucose-6-phosphate, etc. are necessary for metabolism and in the production of energy-rich compounds (ATP, creatine phosphate).
4. As a component of several coenzymes (TPP, $NADP^+$), it also participates in various enzyme catalyzed reactions.
5. It also acts as an activator for enzymes involved in phosphorylation/dephosphorylation processes.

Metabolism of Phosphorus

Depending upon the presence of other constituents, about 10–40% of the dietary phosphorus is **absorbed** as inorganic phosphate in the small intestine.

- Organic phosphate is hydrolyzed in the intestinal lumen and released as inorganic phosphate, through the action of pancreatic/intestinal phosphatases, e.g. alkaline phosphatase.
- Phosphorus present in animal foods, such as in milk and eggs, is absorbed to a greater extent than that is available from cereals and legumes, due to their high phytic acid (hexaphosphoinositol) content.
- Absorption of phosphorus also depends upon the dietary content of phosphorus (absorption of phosphorus is increased when its intake is low), as well as calcium and vitamin D.
- An increase in dietary magnesium also results in reduction in phosphate absorption.

Serum phosphorus: Absorbed phosphate exists in plasma in two forms, i.e. as phospholipids and in the inorganic form. The inorganic form, like calcium, can be either protein bound or free. In normal adult human beings, serum phosphorus (as inorganic phosphorus) varies from 2.5 to 4.5 mg/100 ml. Circulating phosphates are in equilibrium with the skeletal and cellular inorganic phosphates, as well as the organic phosphates. PTH and serum calcium regulate the level of phosphorus in the serum as well as its reabsorption by the renal tubules.

About two-thirds of the dietary phosphorus are **excreted** in the urine, while the remaining one-third is excreted in the feces. PTH increases excretion of phosphate by inhibiting its tubular reabsorption.

RDA for Phosphorus

Daily requirement of phosphorus is nearly similar to that of calcium. It varies from 1.0 to 1.2 g/day.

Dietary Sources of Phosphorus

Phosphorus is found in food containing phosphoproteins, nucleoproteins, phospholipids and glycerophosphates as well as inorganic phosphates chiefly of Ca and Na. Calcium-rich diets, e.g. milk, cheese and beans are also rich sources of phosphorus. Besides, eggs, cereals, fish and meat are also good sources of phosphorus.

Deficiency Disorders of Phosphorus

Deficiency of phosphorus may lead to several neuromuscular, skeletal and renal manifestations. Low serum phosphorus concentration may be a result of vitamin C deficiency and causes defective bone calcification. Similar to hypocalcemia, hypophosphatemia may also lead to rickets in children and osteomalacia in adults; in these conditions, the product of serum calcium and inorganic phosphorus which is normally 40 (10 mg calcium × 4 mg phosphorus), may decrease to <30.

MAGNESIUM

Adult human body contains nearly 20–25 g of magnesium (Mg). Nearly 75% of it is combined with calcium and phosphorus and is present in the bones. Bone magnesium is divided between the crystal lattice and the exchangeable surface pool. The remaining is present in the soft tissues, such as the muscle and the nervous tissue and in body fluids. In blood, most of the magnesium is intracellular.

Biological Functions of Magnesium and its Role in Health and Disease

1. Component of bone structure.
2. Nerve impulse transmission.
3. Magnesium ions (Mg^{2+}) act as activator for several enzymes, particularly those requiring ATP, such as glucokinase, hexokinase, acyl-CoA synthetase, alkaline phosphatase, DNA polymerase, RNA polymerase, etc.
4. Formation of cAMP and thus in mediating the effects of numerous hormones.
5. Electron transfer and stabilization of the redox centers.
6. Stabilizes the complex structures assumed by many RNAs.
7. Free nucleotides, which are anionic in nature, are usually associated with Mg^{2+} in the cells, e.g. Mg^{2+} provides stability to ATP.
8. Muscle contraction.

Metabolism of Magnesium

Nearly 50% of the dietary magnesium is absorbed from the small intestine. High intake of fat, calcium and phosphorus reduce magnesium absorption. An alkaline food also diminishes its absorption.

Magnesium is excreted both in the feces as well as in the urine. Intake of alkaline food reduces its intestinal absorption as well as urinary excretion.

RDA for Magnesium

Average daily requirement of magnesium is 370–440 mg.

Dietary Sources of Magnesium

It is widely distributed in several animal tissues and vegetables. Whole grain, cereals, potato, seafoods, coffee, tea and cocoa are good sources.

Deficiency Disorders of Magnesium

Magnesium deficiency (hypomagnesemia) is often observed in:

1. Alcoholics
2. Patients treated with certain types of diuretics
3. Metabolic acidosis
4. Uremia
5. Children suffering from kwashiorkor
6. Pregnancy (particularly during toxemia of pregnancy)
7. Rickets
8. Diarrhea and vomiting.

Deficiency symptoms include tremors, depression, hyperirritability, cardiac arrhythmias, muscular weakness and convulsions. Low levels of serum magnesium may also produce tetany (Chemistry to Clinics 11.1).

Magnesium Toxicity

Toxicity may be observed due to increased use of magnesium containing laxatives and antacids (Chemistry to Clinics 11.2).

Chief symptoms include drowsiness, lethargy and weakness.

IRON

The total quantity of iron (Fe) in normal adult human body is about 4 g. Most of it is present as a component of hemoglobin and myoglobin. Iron binds to different proteins either by its incorporation into a protoporphyrin ring or its interaction with other protein ligands. In the protoporphyrin ring, iron may be incorporated as Fe^{2+} or Fe^{3+} iron. The Fe^{2+}-protoporphyrin complex is called **heme** while Fe^{3+} proto porphyrin complex is designated as **hematin**.

Biological Functions of Iron and its Role in Health and Disease

Iron forms a component of several heme and nonheme proteins:

1. **Hemoproteins**
   - Hemoglobin is required for the transport of O_2 and CO_2.
   - Myoglobin is an oxygen-storage protein in muscles.
   - Cytochromes are required in the electron transport chain and oxidative phosphorylation.
   - Cytochrome P450 system is responsible for many biotransformation reactions.
   - Several enzymes contain heme iron, as a part of their prosthetic group, e.g. catalase, peroxidase, tryptophan pyrrolase, nitric oxide synthases, prostaglandin synthase, etc. As a component of the lysosomal enzyme myeloperoxidase, iron is required for phagocytosis and thus killing of bacteria by the neutrophils.
2. **Nonheme proteins:** Transferrin, ferritin and iron-sulfur proteins (ferridoxins).

Ferridoxins: These are nonheme iron proteins called **iron-sulfur centers** or iron-sulfur proteins. These consist of equal number of iron and sulfide ions and occur as prosthetic groups and are coordinated with cystine-sulfhydryl groups of proteins. Due to the presence of iron, Fe-S centers occur in the oxidized as well as the reduced state. Regardless of the number of Fe atoms present in them, the redox states of Fe-S clusters differ by one formal charge only.

Ferridoxins are involved in various enzymatic oxidation processes, such as in the mitochondrial electron transport chain. For example, complex I which passes electrons from NADH to CoQ, contains one molecule of FMN and 6 to 7 Fe-S clusters that participate in the electron transport.

Metabolism of Iron

Iron metabolism is unique in the sense that it operates largely as a closed system, i.e. it is regulated mainly at the absorption level. Whatever is absorbed is utilized by the body very efficiently and its losses are minimal. Thus, iron is called a **one-way substance** (Fig. 11.3).

Absorption of iron, mainly, occurs in the stomach, duodenum and upper part of the small intestine. Normally, only about 10% of the dietary iron is absorbed. Unabsorbed iron is excreted in the feces. Efficiency of absorption is increased up to 30% during severe iron deficiency.

Factor Affecting Iron Absorption

1. **Body iron status versus iron intake:** Absorption of dietary iron varies inversely with the iron stores of the body. Thus, iron absorption increases with its intake but up to a limit.
2. **Chemical form of dietary iron:** Heme iron is well absorbed. Iron in the ferrous form (Fe^{2+}) is more effectively absorbed than the ferric form (Fe^{3+}). The protein mucin in the duodenal lumen helps to solubilize and absorb Fe^{3+}.

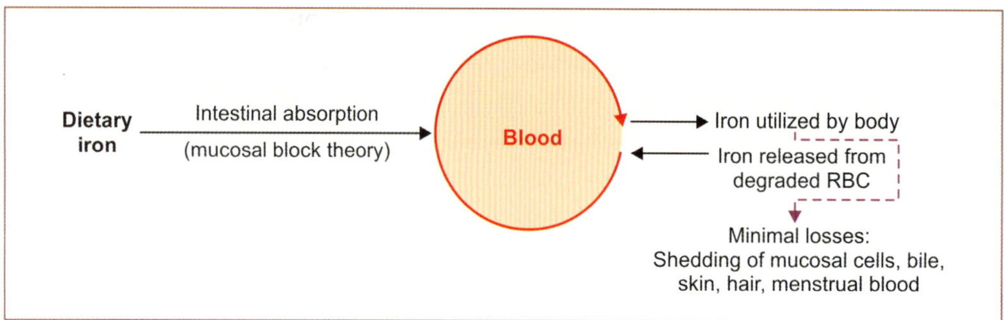

Fig. 11.3: Iron: A 'one-way substance'

3. **Reducing substances:** Amino acids, specially cysteine and the presence of various other reducing substances, such as vitamin C in the diet maintain the Fe^{2+} state of iron and thus promote its absorption.
4. **Complexing agents:** Iron from vegetables and cereals is poorly absorbed due to the presence of oxalates, phosphates, carbonates, phytates and fiber.
5. **Gastric hydrochloric acid:** It enhances iron absorption by stimulating pepsin-mediated digestion of dietary protein which, in turn, releases protein-bound iron.

Mucosal Block Theory of Iron Absorption

Mechanism: Iron may be absorbed as intact heme, Fe^{2+} and/or Fe^{3+}.

- Brush border of enterocytes contain a multi-protein complex called **paraferritin complex**. One of the proteins, called **divalent metal transporter 1** (DMT-1), transfers Fe^{2+} from the lumen to the cytosol (Fig. 11.4).
- On the other hand, **mucin** in the duodenal lumen helps to solubilize Fe^{3+} and makes it available for binding with a transmembrane protein called **integrin**, which interacts with another protein **mobilferrin** responsible for transferring iron from the luminal to the cytoplasmic surface of the cell accompanied by its reduction to Fe^{2+} by NADPH-dependent **ferrireductase**.
- In the mucosal cells, Fe^{2+} is again oxidized to Fe^{3+} form by a copper-containing protein called **ferroxidase I** or **ceruloplasmin**. The subsequent fate of iron depends on the total iron status of the body:
  - **If body iron stores are optimum or in excess:** Majority of the Fe^{3+} combines with **apoferritin** and is stored as mucosal **ferritin**. With the normal cell turnover, ferritin (and hence iron) is lost in the feces.
  - **When the body needs iron:** Majority of the mucosal iron is delivered across the cells to the blood (via a membrane protein called **ferroportin 1** which shuttles Fe^{2+} followed by its simultaneous oxidation to Fe^{3+} by another membrane protein called **hephaestin**) where it is trapped by **transferrin**, the iron-transport protein, to be delivered to the rest of the body. Importantly, ferroportin 1 is inhibited by a plasma protein called **hepcidin** (Chemistry to Clinics 11.3).

Chemistry to Clinics 11.3: Anemia of Chronic Disease

Hepcidin binds to ferroportin 1 and internalizes it within the enterocytes. This results in the retention of iron within cells, and a reduction in plasma iron levels. Hepcidin is thus the 'master regulator' of iron metabolism. It is partly responsible for the **anemia of chronic disease** (tuberculosis, rheumatoid arthritis, etc.), where hepcidin is released from the liver in response to inflammatory cytokines which results in an increased hepcidin concentration and a consequent decrease in plasma iron levels.

Ferritin: The Mucosal Iron Receptor

Ferritin is an iron containing protein involved in the **storage of iron**. The protein component is called **apoferritin,** which consists of 24 subunits of the H chains and the L chains that are arranged spherically. All the 24 units may be composed entirely of the H forms or the L forms or a mixture of the H and the L forms. In the heart apoferritin, the H form tends to predominate, whereas in the liver and spleen, apoferritins are composed mainly of the L form. The L form is also the main constituent of ferritin under conditions of iron overload. Their synthesis is regulated by the concentration of free intracellular iron. In a normal healthy adult, nearly 1500–2000 atoms of iron are bound in the whole ferritin complex. This ratio of iron to the polypeptide, however, is not constant since the apoprotein has the ability to gain and release iron, according to the physiological needs of the body:

- Uptake of iron is associated with the oxidation of Fe^{2+} to Fe^{3+}.

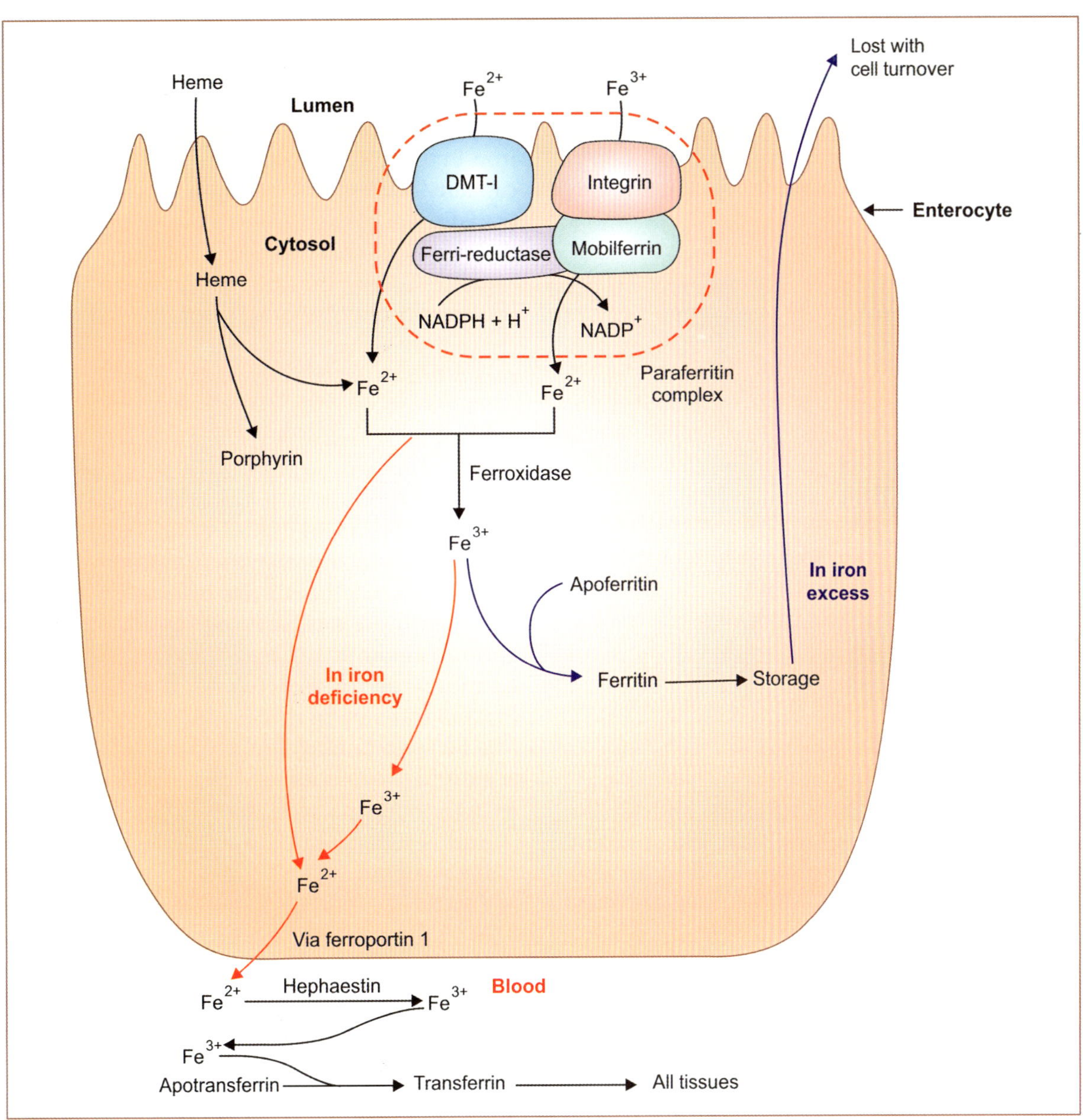

Fig. 11.4: Mechanism of iron absorption and mucosal block theory

- Intake of iron also regulates the rate of synthesis of apoferritin so that more protein is available for iron binding when the intake is high.

Therefore, ferritin acts both as a sink for iron during its excess intake as well as its source during iron deprivation. Apoferritin, also called **mucosal iron-receptor protein** in the upper small intestine, thus controls the absorption of iron as it has a very rapid turnover.

Ferroxidases (Multi-copper Oxidases)

The Fe^{2+} (reduced) and Fe^{3+} (oxidized) forms of iron are physiologically important since iron in hemoglobin is present in the Fe^{2+} state while it is transported in transferrin and stored in ferritin in the Fe^{3+} state. Oxidation requires copper-containing proteins designated as multi-copper oxidases or **ferroxidases**.

Ferroxidase I is identical with plasma **ceruloplasmin**, a copper-containing protein. Interconversion of Fe^{2+} to Fe^{3+} forms of iron is essential for its absorption and incorporation into various iron-containing proteins. The role of ferroxidases also points to the significance of copper in iron metabolism.

Table 11.1 summarizes various proteins involved in iron homeostasis.

Table 11.1: Key proteins participating in iron homeostasis

Paraferritin complex
• ***Divalent metal transporter 1*** (DMT-1): Transfers Fe^{2+} from the intestinal lumen to the cytosol of enterocytes. • ***Integrin***: Receives Fe^{3+} from lumen and transfers it to mobilferrin. • ***Mobilferrin***: Cytosolic shuttle for Fe^{3+}. • ***Ferrireductase***: Reduction of absorbed Fe^{3+} to Fe^{2+} in the cytosol.
Mucin: Solubilizes Fe^{3+} in the duodenal lumen and makes it available for binding with integrin.
Multi-copper oxidases (ferroxidases, e.g. ceruloplasmin, hephaestin): Oxidation of Fe^{2+} to Fe^{3+} in the cytosol/plasma.
Apoferritin: Intracellular iron storage as ferritin; 'mucosal iron receptor'.
Ferroportin 1: Exit of Fe^{2+} from enterocytes into blood.
Hephaestin: Oxidation of Fe^{2+} to Fe^{3+} during its exit (via ferro-portin 1) from enterocytes into blood.
Hepcidin: Inhibitor of ferroportin 1; 'master regulator' of iron absorption.
Apotransferrin: Transport of Fe^{3+} in plasma as transferrin.
Hemosiderin: Intracellular storage form of excess iron.

Iron Response Elements

The synthesis of receptors of transferrin and ferritin are reciprocally related to the cellular iron content. Specific untranslated sequences in the mRNA for both the proteins are designated as 'iron response elements' (**IRE**) which interact with the iron response element-binding protein (IRE-binding protein). Thus, when plasma iron levels are high, cells synthesize more ferritin while the mRNA for the transferrin receptor is degraded. On the other hand, when iron levels are low, mRNA for the transferrin receptors synthesizes more of the transferrin receptors while mRNA for the ferritin receptors becomes inactive.

From the mucosal cells Fe^{2+} passes into blood where it is oxidized to Fe^{3+} and is incorporated into **apoferritin**. Some of it is also incorporated into another serum protein called **apotransferrin,** which binds two Fe^{3+} atoms and is converted to transferrin (Fig. 11.4).

Transferrin and Total Iron-binding Capacity (TIBC)

Transferrin is a non-heme iron-containing serum glycoprotein (β_1-globulin) synthesized in the liver. It **transports iron** to the sites where it is required, such as in the bone marrow. The apoprotein part of transferrin is designated as apotransferrin. There are two iron-binding sites in an apotransferrin molecule. Though several metals can bind to apotransferrin, it has highest affinity for Fe^{3+}. **Iron is always transported in the Fe^{3+} form.** Although Fe^{2+} may be bound to apotransferrin, it rapidly gets oxidized to the Fe^{3+} form.

In a normal healthy adult, nearly one-third of the iron-binding sites is occupied. Thus, total iron-binding capacity (TIBC) of the serum is directly related to its transferrin concentration. TIBC is reduced in iron deficiency anemia but is increased in pernicious anemia and hemochromatosis. In iron overload, serum transferrin may be fully saturated. About 45% of the circulating transferrin is in the iron-free form and is called **unsaturated transferrin**.

There are specific receptors on the surface of many cells, for transferrin. **Transferrin receptor** is a transmembrane protein consisting of two subunits. Transferrin binds to its receptors and is internalized by the **receptor-mediated endocytosis**. The acid pH inside the lysosome causes iron to dissociate from the complex. After the release of iron, receptor-apotransferrin complex returns to the cell surface where apotransferrin is released for reutilization, i.e. to pick up more iron for its delivery to the site where needed. Plasma transferrin is in equilibrium with hemoglobin (the Fe^{2+}-containing hemoprotein) in the bone marrow erythroid precursors, as well as with ferritin in the liver.

- In the bone marrow, the Fe^{3+} is again reduced to Fe^{2+} and is incorporated into heme for the synthesis of hemoglobin.
- On the other hand, when there is a need for iron by the body, such as after hemorrhage, liver and spleen release their stores (ferritin). After ferritin reaches a low level, another iron storage protein, called **hemosiderin** releases iron.

Hemosiderin

Hemosiderin is an iron storage protein found as brownish granules in the cells. Excess of iron, such as during iron overload, stimulates the storage capacity of the newly synthesized apoferritin which may be partially degraded by proteolytic enzymes of the lysosomes. It is followed by the release of iron oxide micelles which form insoluble aggregates and get trapped in the secondary lysosomes. These insoluble aggregates of amorphous iron are designated as hemosiderin. In a normal healthy subject, very little hemosiderin is detectable. The quantity of hemosiderin **increases during iron overload**.

Only about 10% of dietary iron is absorbed but once absorbed, a very little of it is excreted. Nearly 1% of the red blood cells are continuously degraded in the reticuloendothelial system each day. In an adult human being, this results in the release of about 25 mg of iron, majority of which is conserved and reused.

- An adult male or a nonmenstruating female loses only about 1 mg of iron everyday.
- Nearly 50–60% of this is lost from the gastro-intestinal tract, either in the bile or by the shedding of the mucosal cells.
- The remaining is lost from the skin and the hair with practically no loss in the urine.
- In females, there is an additional loss of iron through menstruation, ranging from 1 to 3 mg/day.

RDA for Iron

Assuming about 10% efficiency of absorption, the recommended dietary allowance for iron is about 19 mg for normal adult males. The RDA is nearly 29 mg/day for nonpregnant females, during the reproductive stage of their life. This is on account of the increased loss during menstruation. According to ICMR-NIN (2020), iron requirement has been suggested as 27 mg/d during pregnancy and 23 mg/d during lactation.

Dietary Sources of Iron

Foods cooked in iron cookwares are the best sources of iron. Animal foods such as meat, fish and eggs are good sources of heme iron. Green leafy vegetables, cereals and legumes (whole grains) are good sources of non-heme iron. However, due to the presence of oxalates and phytates, iron from vegetable sources is poorly absorbed. Milk is a poor source of iron.

Deficiency Disorders of Iron

The commonest disorder is **iron deficiency anemia** (Chemistry to Clinics 11.4).

Chemistry to Clinics 11.4: Iron Deficiency Anemia

Causes

- ***Inadequate intake***: Malnutrition, pregnancy (increased fetal demand).
- ***Poor absorption***: Prolonged gastroenteritis, complete/partial gastrectomy.
- ***Increased losses***: Excessive blood loss during menstruation, gastrointestinal hemorrhage, hookworm infections.

Presentation: It is the commonest disorder of iron metabolism and the commonest form of nutritional anemia. It is a common feature in children, adolescent girls and females of the childbearing age, particularly in the developing countries.

- Children become dull, inactive, lose appetite and have poor growth.
- Deficiency of iron in females also reduces their work capacity. On exertion, such women get breathless and remain fatigued.
- Iron deficiency is also associated with decreased immunocompetence and susceptibility to infections.

Diagnosis: Low plasma iron and ferritin, increased plasma total iron-binding capacity (TIBC), low transferrin saturation (percent) and microcytic hypochromic blood picture (Fig. 11.5).

Treatment: Oral iron supplementation (parenteral iron in severe cases).

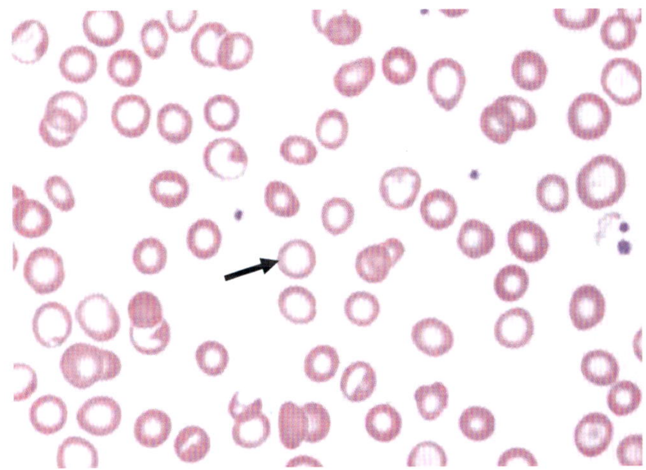

Fig. 11.5: Iron deficiency anemia morphologically characterized by variable degrees of microcytosis and hypochromia which results in widening of the central pallor accounting for greater than one-third of the total RBC diameter (arrow)

Anemia

Anemia is a condition which is characterized by a reduced number of circulating erythrocytes or reduced amount of hemoglobin in them, or both.

Types of Anemia: Based on the RBC size and the hemoglobin content, anemia is of three types:

1. **Microcytic hypochromic anemia:** The erythrocytes are much smaller in size and have reduced hemoglobin content. Their number may also be reduced but to a smaller extent. It is caused by iron deficiency (Fig. 11.5).
2. **Macrocytic hyperchromic/normochromic anemia:** The size of the erythrocytes is increased while their number is reduced, presenting the characteristic blood picture of megaloblastic anemia including pernicious anemia. It is caused by the deficiency of vitamin B_{12} and/or folic acid.

3. **Normocytic normochromic anemia:** The size as well as the hemoglobin content of the erythrocytes remains normal but number of the circulating erythrocytes is reduced. It is usually a result of internal or external hemorrhage.

Iron Toxicity

Iron toxicity may be a result of its overload (Chemistry to Clinics 11.5).

Chemistry to Clinics 11.5: Hemosiderosis and Hemochromatosis

Excess of iron, in the body, results in its deposition as hemosiderin in various tissues such as liver, spleen, skin and cardiac muscles. It is called **hemosiderosis**, which increases the risk of cardiovascular disease, besides hepatomegaly, pancreatitis and skin pigmentation (Fig. 11.6).

Repeated blood transfusions as required in thalassemia major, can lead to hemosiderosis. Other causes include alcoholic cirrhosis and chronic pancreatitis. A genetic susceptibility to iron overload is due to a failure of the regulation of iron absorption and leads to a condition called **hemochromatosis**, whose features are like hemosiderosis.

COPPER

The human body contains 100–150 mg of copper (Cu), out of which nearly 50% is found in the muscles and about 25% in bones.

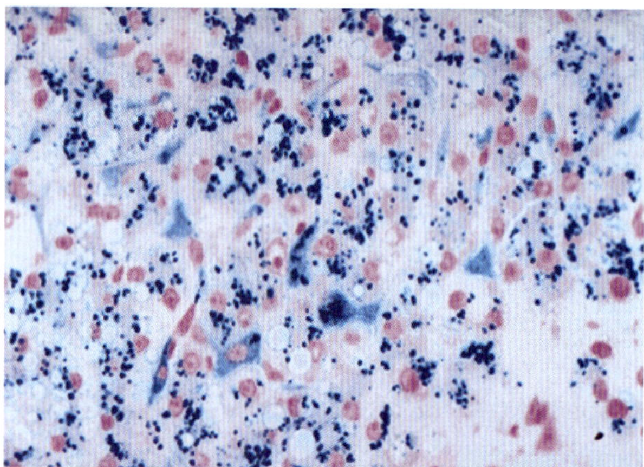

Fig. 11.6: Hemosiderosis: Prussian blue stain (for iron) of the liver to demonstrate large amounts of hemosiderin in the cytoplasm of hepatocytes and Kupffer cells

Biological Functions of Copper and its Role in Health and Disease

1. Copper is a component of many enzyme systems of metabolic importance (Table 11.2).
2. It is also an important constituent of several proteins, such as erythrocuprein, cerebrocuprein and hepatocuprein which are present in the bone marrow, brain and liver, respectively.

Metabolism of Copper

About one-third of the dietary copper is absorbed primarily from the duodenum. Phytate, zinc, ascorbic acid and certain amino acids inhibit copper absorption.

Table 11.2: Copper-containing enzymes and their metabolic importance

Enzymes	Metabolic importance
Multi-copper oxidases (ferroxidases)	Iron metabolism: Tissue-specific conversion of intracellular Fe^{2+} to Fe^{3+} to facilitate its storage or exit from cells, e.g. ferroxidase I (ceruloplasmin in enterocytes, liver, plasma), glycosylphosphatidylinositol-ceruloplasmin (brain), hephaestin (enterocytes), zyklopen (placental trophoblasts)
Cytochrome oxidase	Electron transport chain
δ-Aminolevulinate synthase	Synthesis of heme
Lysyl oxidase	Synthesis and maturation of collagen and elastin
Ascorbic acid oxidase	Interconversion of L-ascorbate (active vitamin C) and dehydroascorbate
Tyrosinase	Synthesis of melanin pigments
Dopamine β-oxidase	Synthesis of catecholamines
Superoxide dismutase (SOD)	Antioxidant
ATP7A	Intestinal copper absorption
ATP7B	Secretion of copper from hepatocytes into bile

- **ATP7A** (ATPase, Cu^{2+}-transporting α-polypeptide) is required for the intestinal uptake of dietary copper.
- Inside the intestinal mucosal cells, copper binds to another low molecular weight metal-binding protein called **metallothionein**. Copper absorption thus depends upon the availability of these proteins.
- In all tissues except the liver, another isoform of ATP7A is present in the Golgi complex where it regulates the availability of copper for its incorporation into copper-containing enzymes. However, if copper levels are elevated, this protein shuttles to the cell membrane and removes excess copper from the cell.
- After absorption, copper enters the plasma where almost all of it is present in the bound form. While some of it is loosely bound to albumin (called the direct reacting copper or the transport form of copper), most of it is bound to a specific copper-binding protein called **ceruloplasmin** (Fig. 11.7).

After absorption, copper is stored in the liver and is excreted via bile. The secretion of copper from the hepatocytes into the bile requires the enzyme **ATP7B** (ATPase, Cu^{2+}-transporting β-polypeptide). Very little copper is excreted in the urine.

Ceruloplasmin: It is a **copper containing α_2-globulin present in the plasma**. It is **synthesized in the liver** in the form of an apoprotein called **apoceruloplasmin**. After 6–8 atoms of copper are incorporated per molecule of apoprotein, it is converted into ceruloplasmin (Fig. 11.7).

Ceruloplasmin is also called **ferroxidase I** and is an example of multi-copper oxidase (Table 11.2).

Multi-copper oxidase helps in the oxidation of ferrous iron (Fe^{2+}) to the ferric iron (Fe^{3+}) for its incorporation into transferrin and ferritin. Thus, copper, through ceruloplasmin, **helps in iron metabolism**.

It should be remembered that plasma ceruloplasmin levels are raised nonspecifically during any ongoing acute inflammatory process in the body. Hence, ceruloplasmin is called an **acute phase reactant**.

RDA for Copper

A normal adult requires 1.5–1.7 mg of copper per day.

Dietary Sources of Copper

Copper is widely distributed in various types of foods. Nuts, leafy vegetables, dried legumes, egg yolk, fish and meat (liver) are good sources. Milk is a poor source of copper.

Deficiency Disorders of Copper

Some of the symptoms of copper deficiency include hypercholesterolemia, demineralization of bones, leukopenia, demyelination of the neural tissue and alopecia (loss of hair). There is also microcytic normochromic anemia which cannot be cured by iron supplementation alone, since copper, as ferroxidase, is essential for the intestinal absorption of iron and in its metabolism. Copper deficiency in infants has been found to be associated with a condition described as Menkes disease (Chemistry to Clinics 11.6).

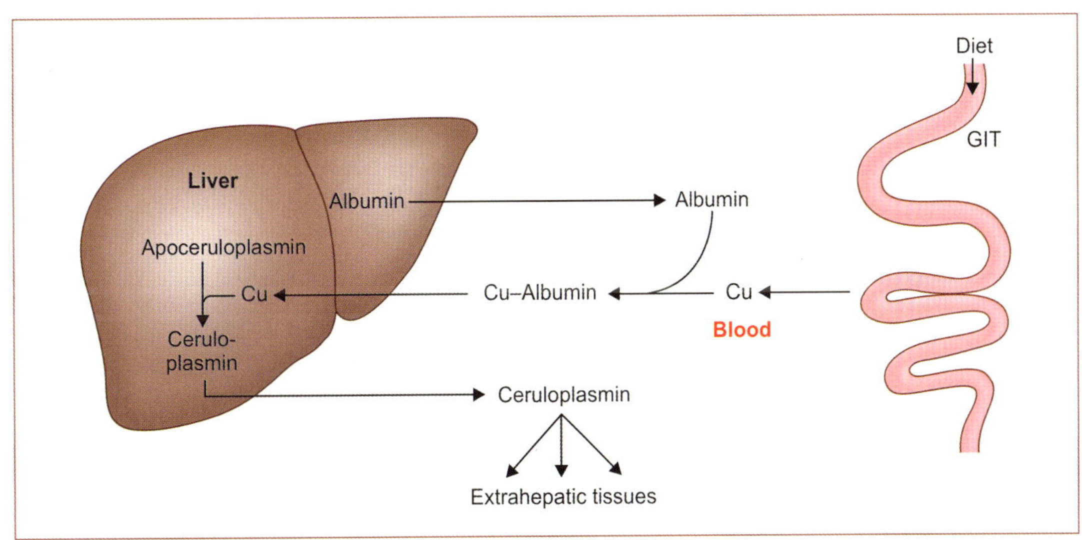

Fig. 11.7: Absorption and transport of copper

11

Chemistry to Clinics 11.6: Menkes Disease

It is an X-linked hereditary disease due to failure of copper absorption across the serosal membrane of intestinal mucosal cells. The molecular defect lies in the enterocyte membrane transport protein ATP7A. This, in turn, leads to low concentrations of copper in the plasma and the liver. Further, a defective ATP7A in other extrahepatic tissues results in deficiency of various copper containing oxidases (tyrosinase, lysyl oxidase, etc.) leading to various systemic manifestations such as skeletal malformation, mental retardation, defective thermoregulation and immunodeficiency. Menkes disease is also called **'kinky hair syndrome'** due to the failure to keratinize hair which become kinky and steel grey (Fig. 11.8).

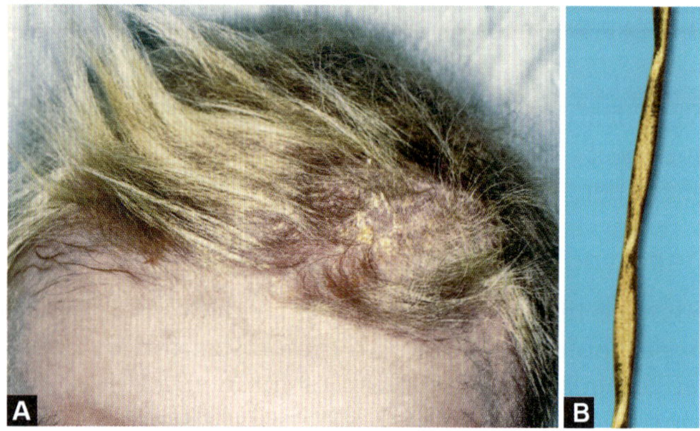

Fig. 11.8: Copper deficiency results in defective keratinization: (A) Menkes kinky hair which feels like steel wool (steely hair syndrome); (B) Pili torti: Twisting of the hair shaft on its own axis

Copper Toxicity

Copper toxicity may manifest as diarrhea, blue-green discoloration of the saliva, hemolysis, proteinuria and renal failure. Increased amount of copper is deposited in the liver and brain in **Wilson's disease** (Chemistry to Clinics 11.7).

Chemistry to Clinics 11.7: Wilson's Disease (Hepatolenticular Degeneration)

Causes: It is an autosomal recessive inherited disorder in which there is a positive copper balance due to deficient synthesis of ceruloplasmin in the liver. There is a defect in the incorporation of Cu^{2+} into newly synthesized apoceruloplasmin, to form ceruloplasmin. Besides, a defect in the ATP7B protein in the hepatocytes (responsible for copper-efflux into bile) is also a culprit. The net result is free Cu^{2+} accumulation to highly toxic levels mainly in the liver and the basal nuclei of the brain which promotes the generation of free radicals leading to extensive cell damage.

Presentation: Liver failure, neurological disturbances and characteristic Kayser-Fleischer rings in the cornea (Fig. 11.9).

Diagnosis

- Decreased plasma ceruloplasmin levels.
- Increased urinary excretion of copper which, in turn, causes renal tubular damage with hemoglobinuria and generalized aminoaciduria.
- Increased hepatic copper content on liver biopsy.
- Mutation analysis of *ATP7B* gene.

Treatment: Repeated administration of copper-chelating agents such as penicillamine.

IODINE

About 20–30 mg of iodine is present as iodide (I^-) in adult human body. Nearly two-thirds of it is present in the thyroid gland as free I^- as well as in the form of monoiodotyrosine, diiodotyrosine, T_3 and T_4.

Biological Functions of Iodine and its Role in Health and Disease

The important function of iodine is synthesis of the iodine-containing hormones, i.e. thyroxine (**T_4**) and triiodothyronine (**T_3**), the physiologically active substances that are formed by the thyroid gland.

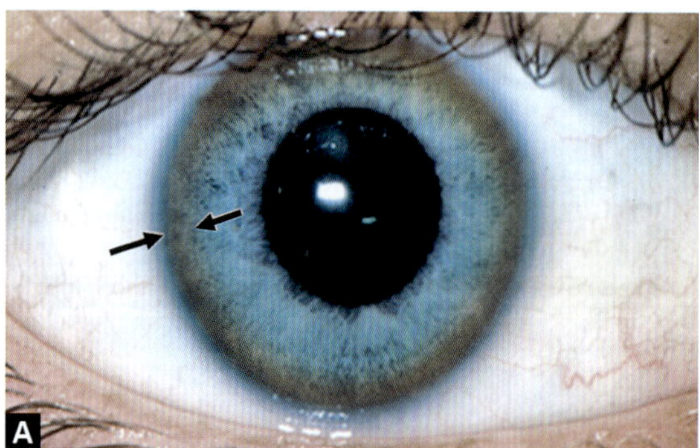

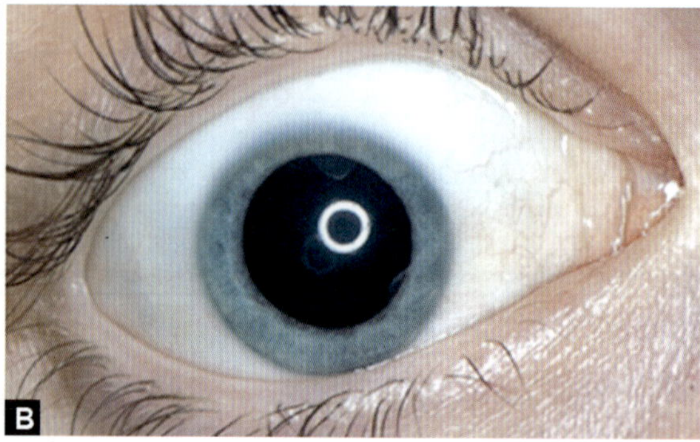

Fig. 11.9: Wilson's disease. (A) Kayser-Fleischer ring (arrows); (B) Complete resolution following copper-chelating (penicillamine) treatment

11

These hormones regulate basal metabolic rate throughout life, and during growth and development in children.

Metabolism of Iodine

Iodine is quickly absorbed from food and water as inorganic iodide (I^-) from the small intestine.

Depending upon the activity of the thyroid gland, a portion of the absorbed I^- is taken up by the gland (Chemistry to Clinics 11.8).

Chemistry to Clinics 11.8: Goitrogens

Some of the ingredients present in foodstuffs may prevent utilization of iodine by the thyroid gland. Such substances are called goitrogens, e.g. thiocyanate, perchlorate, goitrin, isoflavones, etc. and are abundant in cabbage, turnip, mustard-seeds, peanuts, sweet potatoes, soya beans, etc. Goitrogens are inactivated by heating/cooking. Hence, from a practical point of view, consumption of raw goitrogenic foods in large quantities over a long duration carries a risk of producing goiter.

In the epithelial cells of the thyroid gland, it is oxidized and gets conjugated with the thyroglobulin bound tyrosine residues, resulting in the formation of T_3 and T_4.

Nearly 90% of the plasma I^- is in the organic form, i.e. bound to protein and is called protein-bound iodine (PBI).

About 10% of the circulating organic iodine is excreted in the feces. Inorganic iodide is mostly excreted in the urine and partly through bile and saliva.

RDA for Iodine

Daily requirement of iodine is about 140µg

Dietary Sources of Iodine

To ensure adequate supply of dietary iodine, it is desirable to use iodized salt. Seafood, fruits, vegetables, cereals and meat are good sources. Iodine content of the food depends upon the iodine content of the soil in which these are grown.

Deficiency Disorders of Iodine

Iodine deficiency may lead to goiter. The term **goiter** simply refers to a diffuse enlargement of the thyroid gland due to any cause and it may be associated with overactivity or underactivity of the gland.

Endemic Goiter

Endemic goitrous belt: Iodine deficiency is common in some parts of the world. In India, certain sub-Himalayan regions contain less iodine in the soil. This part of the country is called the goitrous belt.

Mechanism of goiter: Dietary iodine deficiency causes depletion of thyroid iodine stores and therefore reduces output of the thyroid hormones. A decrease in serum T_4 stimulates release of pituitary thyroid stimulating hormone (TSH), resulting in hyperplasia of the thyroid gland. This, in turn, traps and processes the available iodine more efficiently. The gland returns to its normal size after sufficient amount of dietary iodine is available. This is called **simple goiter or colloid goiter**. Long-standing cases of simple goiter may lead to the development of nodules which are localized areas of cellular proliferation within the gland. This condition is called **nodular goiter**.

Presentation: The most characteristic feature is enlargement of the thyroid gland, to the extent that a large nodule can be visible in the neck (Fig. 11.10).

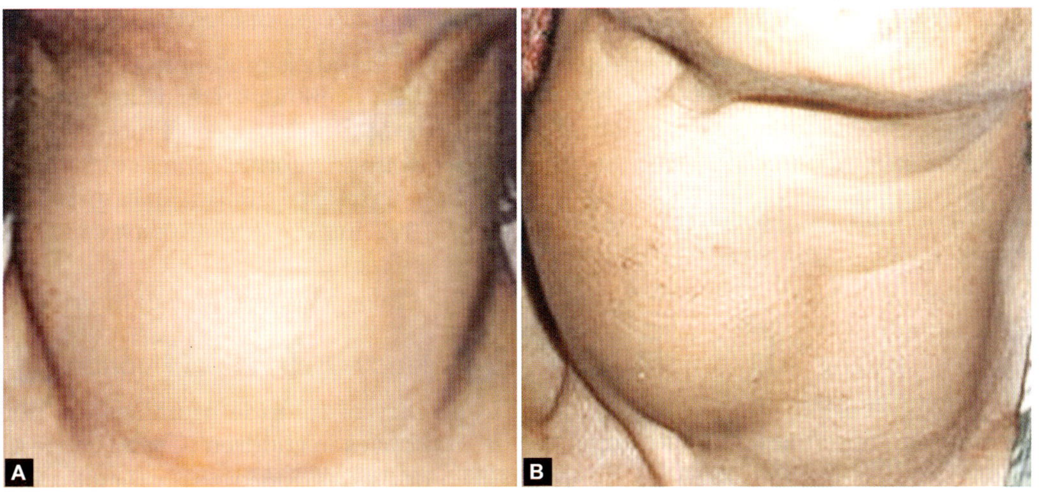

Fig. 11.10: (A) Simple colloid goiter; (B) Multinodular goiter

Complications: Severe deficiency of iodine in children may result in growth retardation, called cretinism, and myxedema in adults (Chemistry to Clinics 11.9).

Chemistry to Clinics 11.9: Cretinism and Myxedema

Cretinism: It is a condition of hypothyroidism in infants and children which, in turn, affects growth. A cretin child is a dwarf, has a thick tongue and skin, and is mentally retarded and sexually underdeveloped. The deficiency coincides with the critical perinatal period when thyroid hormones are required for neuronal development.

Myxedema: Severe hypothyroidism in adults leads to a condition called myxedema. The skin becomes thick and puffy, due to the deposition of mucous like slimy, viscous material (myxomatous material, mucopolysaccharides) in the skin of the face, hands and legs. Body weight is increased due to the retention of water and NaCl. There is mental dullness and hypersensitivity to cold. It is an emergency requiring intravenous thyroid hormone replacement and corticosteroids.

Prevention: Intake of sufficient iodine which may be accomplished by adding inorganic iodides to the source of drinking water or by the addition of iodides to the table salt.

Iodine Toxicity

Iodine toxicity may result in thyrotoxicosis.

National Goiter Control Program

Iodine deficiency disorders (IDD) are prevalent worldwide. In India, IDD was earlier thought to be a problem in the sub-Himalayan region, however, surveys, carried out subsequently, showed that no state in the country is completely free from IDD. Realizing the magnitude of the problem, Government of India launched **National Goiter Control Program (NGCP)** in 1962, and a policy decision of universal iodization of edible salt was taken in 1984. NGCP was renamed as **National Iodine Deficiency Disorders Control Program (NIDDCP)**, in August 1992, taking into consideration the control of wide-spectrum of IDD, like mental and physical retardation, deaf mutism, cretinism, stillbirth, abortion, etc.

Aim of the program

- Surveys to assess the magnitude of the IDD
- Universal iodization of salt and supply of iodized salt all over the country
- Resurvey after every 5 years to assess the extent of IDD and impact of iodized salt
- Laboratory monitoring of iodized salt and urinary iodine excretion
- Health education and publicity.

Services

- Replacement of common salt with iodized salt
- Use of iodized tablets to school children
- Use of iodized oil (1 ml injection of iodized oil to those suffering from IDD) for oral administration, as prophylaxis in IDD severe areas
- Mass communication for public awareness through mass media and public health programs.

FLUORIDE

Fluoride (F^-) is present in traces in human tissues, mainly in bones, teeth, thyroid gland and skin.

Biological Functions of Fluoride and its Role in Health and Disease

Fluoride promotes normal bone development, increases retention of calcium and phosphorus, and prevents osteoporosis during aging. It imparts stability to bones and enamel, due to formation of the highly insoluble **fluoroapatite** from hydroxyapatite. Hardening of dental enamel makes it resistant to acids.

Metabolism of Fluoride

Soluble fluorides are maximally (about 90%) absorbed through gastrointestinal tract. Absorption from drinking water is almost complete. After absorption, fluoride is distributed throughout the extracellular fluid. Only a small amount of it is deposited in dental enamel and the bones.

Fluoride is mainly excreted through urine.

RDA for Fluoride

Daily requirement has been defined as 2–3 mg.

Dietary Sources of Fluoride

Though fluoride is present in almost all foods in small quantities, drinking water is an important source of fluoride in a human diet. Fluoride content of water depends upon fluoride content of the soil. One part per million (1 ppm) of fluoride in drinking water supplies nearly 1–2 mg of fluoride/day which is sufficient to meet the requirement.

Tea is also a good source of fluoride.

Deficiency Disorders of Fluoride

Deficiency of fluoride promotes the development of **dental caries** in children (Chemistry to Clinics 11.10).

Fluoride deficiency also promotes **osteoporosis** in adults, particularly in postmenopausal women.

Chemistry to Clinics 11.10: Dental Caries

Dental caries is characterized by destruction of the tooth enamel as a result of the action of the microorganisms (normally present in the oral cavity) on carbohydrates, particularly during the formation of teeth (Fig. 11.11).

Breakdown of the enamel, in turn, exposes the dentine and leads to the development of dental caries (Fig. 11.12).

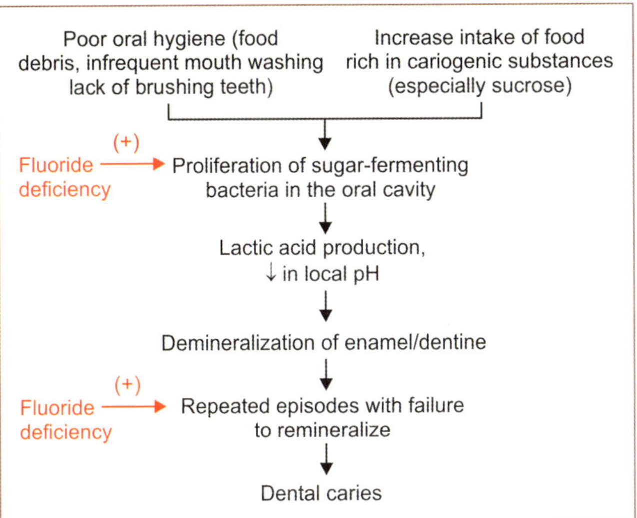

Fig. 11.11: Dental caries aggravated by fluoride deficiency

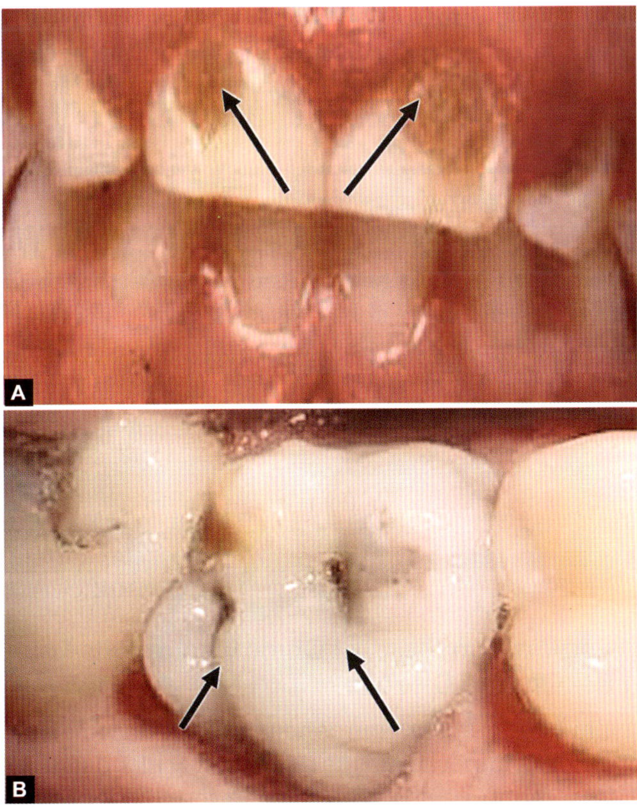

Fig. 11.12: Dental caries. (A) Characteristic lesions (arrows) on the enamel; (B) Cavities (arrows) in a neglected case of caries

Fluoride Toxicity

Large intake of fluoride results in **fluorosis** (Chemistry to Clinics 11.11).

Chemistry to Clinics 11.11: Endemic Fluorosis

Though some amount of fluoride is necessary for normal metabolism of the bones and teeth, large doses may be toxic and may lead to fluorosis which is an important public health problem in many parts of the world. High content of fluorosis in rocks may result in increased levels of fluoride in groundwater and its entry into the body.

Presentation: Muscle wasting (inhibition of protein biosynthesis) and impairment in energy metabolism (inhibition of enolase in glycolysis). Fluoride toxicity may manifest in two major forms, i.e. as dental fluorosis and skeletal fluorosis which together constitute endemic fluorosis:

- **Dental fluorosis:** It occurs mainly in children who are exposed to high fluoride intake before completion of mineralization of the tooth enamel. The teeth exhibit mottled enamel. Mottling is confined to permanent teeth and is characterized by multiple, minute white flecks and yellow/brown spots which are scattered irregularly over the tooth surface (Fig. 11.13).
- **Skeletal fluorosis:** The clinical features include pain, inflammation and restricted movement of the joints and stiffness of the spine. Further, significantly higher intake of fluoride (more than 3 mg/L, in drinking water) results in a variant of severe form of the skeletal fluorosis called genu valgum (knock-knee; Fig. 11.14).

Besides the features of dental and skeletal fluorosis, these individuals also exhibit extensive osteoporosis of the limb bones.

Prevention: Defluoridation of water and dietary interventions.

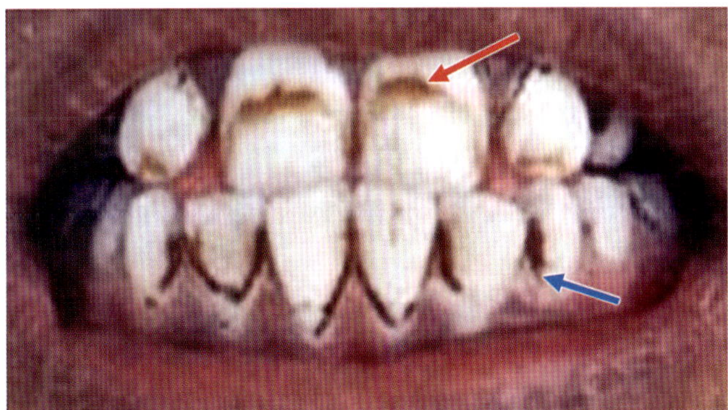

Fig. 11.13: Dental fluorosis. The teeth of the upper jaw (the two central incisors) show mottling and discoloration (red arrow) horizontally aligned on the enamel surface, away from the gums. It cannot be cleaned by a dentist. However, the teeth of the lower jaw show discoloration along the gums (blue arrow) due to dirty teeth (not fluorosis), which can be cleaned by a dentist

MANGANESE

Total body manganese (Mn) content of an adult human is about 10–12 mg. It is mainly concentrated in the bones,

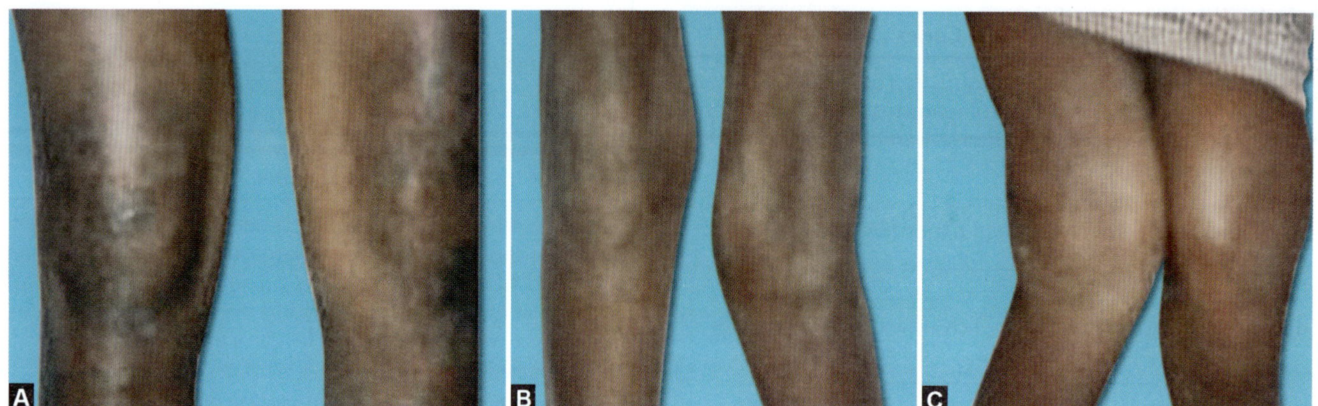

Fig. 11.14: Skeletal fluorosis. (A) Stage I: Swollen, painful and rigid knee joints; (B) Stage II: Deformed but mobile joints; (C) Stage III: Patient is crippled with severe restriction of movement

liver and kidney. Most of it is present in the mitochondria and plays an important role in biological oxidation.

Biological Functions of Manganese and its Role in Health and Disease

1. Cofactor for various enzymes such as hydrolases, decarboxylases and transferases, e.g. phosphorylases and phosphotransferases.
2. Synthesis of glycoproteins and proteoglycans, in the cartilages.
3. Stimulates biosynthesis of cholesterol and long chain fatty acids.
4. Prevents lipid peroxidation and exhibits lipotropic effects.

Metabolism of Manganese

Only about 5% of the dietary manganese is absorbed. Ethanol increases while dietary calcium, phosphorus and iron reduce its absorption.

Manganese is mainly excreted via bile, in the feces. Only a small fraction of it is excreted in the urine.

RDA for Manganese

Daily requirement is 4 mg.

Dietary Sources of Manganese

It is widely distributed in nuts, whole grain cereals, legumes and leafy vegetables. Tea is a rich source of manganese.

Deficiency Disorders of Manganese

Manganese deficiency leads to bone deformities, poor growth and ataxia in several animal species. Its deficiency has also been shown to decrease the synthesis of oligosaccharides, glycoproteins and proteoglycans.

Manganese Toxicity

Manganese is relatively nontoxic but toxicity can occur in manganese-ore mine workers. Inhalation poisoning produces severe psychotic symptoms and parkinsonism.

CHROMIUM

Total body chromium (Cr) content of adult humans is between 5 and 10 mg. It is present in two forms, i.e. in the trivalent form (Cr^{3+}) and the hexavalent form (Cr^{6+}). **The trivalent form of chromium is biologically active.** An organic compound of chromium is termed glucose tolerance factor (Chemistry to Clinics 11.12).

Chemistry to Clinics 11.12: Glucose Tolerance Factor

- It is a naturally occurring coordination complex between chromium (Cr^{3+}), nicotinic acid and glutathione (a tripeptide of three amino acids, i.e. glycine, glutamate and cysteine).
- It helps in the storage of insulin in the granules of the pancreatic β-cells as well as its secretion. It may also potentiate the effects of insulin by facilitating its interaction with the receptors and thus it is important in the removal of ingested glucose from the circulation.
- Chromium-picolinate is available commercially and is prescribed as an auxiliary drug to patients suffering from diabetes mellitus.

Biological Functions of Chromium and its Role in Health and Disease

1. Chromium, as a component of glucose tolerance factor, is important in the regulation of blood glucose.
2. Chromium is also important in the metabolism of lipoproteins and maintains normal level of cholesterol in the blood.

Metabolism of Chromium

Chromium is poorly absorbed. After its absorption, it combines with plasma β-globulin.

It is excreted in traces in the urine.

RDA for Chromium

Daily requirement for chromium has been suggested as 50 μg.

Dietary Sources of Chromium

Brewer's yeast, mushrooms, black pepper, meat (liver), cereals (whole grains), nuts and cheese are good sources.

Deficiency Disorder of Chromium

Chromium deficiency can impair glucose tolerance.

Chromium Toxicity

Chromium toxicity may be observed on occupational exposure to chromium dust which, in turn, may induce lung cancer.

SELENIUM

Selenium (Se) though is widely distributed in all the tissues but is present in higher amounts in the renal cortex, pancreas, pituitary and liver.

Selenoproteins

Selenoproteins are selenium containing proteins which have selenocysteine (**Se-C**) residues. The Se-C is incorporated into the peptide chain during its synthesis by the ribosomes, as the 21st amino acid, as a result of some variation in the standard translational machinary. The Se-C residues participate in redox reactions, such as those catalyzed by glutathione peroxidase which is a selenoprotein.

Biological Functions of Selenium and its Role in Health and Disease

1. An essential component of selenoproteins such as **glutathione peroxidase**, which protects the cells against the damage caused by H_2O_2. Thus, Se is an **antioxidant**. Further, it acts as a synergistic antioxidant with vitamin E and protects the cell membrane against free radicals.
2. Required in some of the immune mechanisms.
3. Biosynthesis of ubiquinone and thus essential for ATP biosynthesis in the mitochondria.

Metabolism of Selenium

Selenium is absorbed mainly in the duodenum.

It is excreted mainly in the feces and the expired air.

RDA for Selenium

The RDA for selenium has been suggested as 40 μg.

Dietary Sources of Selenium

Plant-foods, cereals, fish and meat are rich sources of selenium. Food content of selenium however, depends upon the selenium content of the soil.

Deficiency Disorders of Selenium

Selenium deficiency may be observed when its soil content is low. Deficiency may also be observed in protein energy malnutrition. Selenium deficiency may lead to liver necrosis, muscular dystrophy, cardiomyopathy and dilatation of the heart.

Selenium Toxicity

Very high intake of selenium may result in its toxicity and the condition is called **selenosis**. Its toxicity has been observed in workers in the paint, glass and ceramic industries. These individuals have difficulty in breathing due to inhalation of excessive selenium. High selenium intake may induce weight loss, hair loss, dermatitis, diarrhea, emotional disturbances (irritability) and garlic-like odor in breath.

Patients with primary neoplasms of the reticuloendothelial system show high levels of selenium in their sera. Excess of selenium as Se-C may replace sulfur in tissues and inhibits SH-containing enzymes.

ZINC

Total body content of zinc (Zn) in an adult is about 2.0 g. The choroid of the eye, liver, pancreas, prostate gland and prostatic fluid contain high concentrations of zinc.

Biological Functions of Zinc and its Role in Health and Disease

Zinc performs diverse biological functions (Table 11.3).

Metabolism of Zinc

Only about 20% of the dietary zinc is absorbed. Absorption of zinc occurs in the duodenum and the ileum. Phytate and dietary fiber decrease its absorption. They lower the availability of dietary zinc and thus increase its excretion in the feces. Zinc absorption is

Table 11.3: Functions of zinc

1. **Component of several enzymes**
   - Carbonic anhydrase
   - Lactate dehydrogenase
   - Alcohol dehydrogenase
   - Alkaline phosphatase
   - DNA and RNA polymerases
   - Retinene-retinal reductase
   - Cytosolic superoxide dismutase
2. **Blood glucose regulation:** Zinc forms a complex with insulin, helps in its storage and release from the β-cells of the pancreas.
3. **Maintains plasma vitamin A levels:** By stimulating the release of vitamin A from the liver into the blood.
4. **Taste sensation:** Zinc is a constituent of gustin, a salivary polypeptide necessary for the normal development of taste buds.
5. **Regulation of gene expression:** Essential component of zinc-finger motifs of various regulatory DNA binding proteins.
6. **Enhances immunity**
7. **Normal growth and reproduction.**

directly proportional to the levels of metallothionein in the intestinal mucosal cells.

Zinc is excreted through pancreatic juice.

Enteropancreatic circulation: Many digestive enzymes secreted from the pancreas contain zinc. Therefore, the gastrointestinal tract receives zinc from two sources during meal, i.e. sone from food and the other from the pancreatic secretions. The zinc circulates in the body from the pancreas to the small intestine and back to the pancreas via blood, thus completing the enteropancreatic circulation.

RDA for Zinc

Daily intake of about 13–17 mg is sufficient to meet zinc requirement.

Dietary Sources of Zinc

Good dietary sources are meat, seafoods, egg, legumes and milk. Colostrum is a very rich source of zinc.

Deficiency Disorders of Zinc

Since body stores of zinc are small, dietary deficiency can therefore produce symptoms promptly, particularly when its soil content is low (Chemistry to Clinics 11.13).

Chemistry to Clinics 11.13: Zinc Deficiency

Severe zinc deficiency is seen in alcoholics, chronic renal disease, severe gastroenteritis and malabsorption, and protein-energy malnutrition. Clinical manifestations include:

1. Poor wound healing, loss of appetite, poor growth and alopecia (loss of hair).
2. Impairment of sexual development in children.
3. Impairment in brain functions.
4. Certain fetal abnormalities during pregnancy besides hypogonadism, dwarfism (stunted growth) and gross skin lesions with severe acrodermatitis.
5. Delayed recovery from diarrhea.
6. Zinc deficiency affects spermatogenesis, parturition and lactation in experimental animals.

Zinc Toxicity

Zinc, when consumed in excessive amounts, produces toxic effects, such as acute gastrointestinal irritation, gastric ulcers, nausea and vomiting. It also interferes with the utilization and functions of copper, and may also cause anemia. Zinc-containing multivitamin cocktails are widely available commercially and need to be used with caution.

COBALT

Adult human body contains only 2–3 mg of cobalt (Co), mainly concentrated in the liver and the kidney.

Biological Functions of Cobalt and its Role in Health and Disease

1. Cobalt is an important constituent of **vitamin B_{12} (cobalamin)**, about 4% by weight. Vitamin B_{12} is the only compound of cobalt which is nutritionally effective in human beings and other monogastric animals.
2. Cobalt also acts as a cofactor for some enzymes, such as glycylglycine dipeptidase found in the intestinal juice.
3. Cobalt stimulates the production of erythropoietin which, in turn, promotes erythropoiesis.

Metabolism of Cobalt

Absorption and metabolism of cobalt is similar to that of vitamin B_{12}. It is stored in the liver and excreted via bile.

RDA for Cobalt

The RDA is 1–2 μg.

Dietary Sources of Cobalt

Its requirement can be met from dietary B_{12}. Foods from the animal origin are good sources of cobalt. Meat (liver) is a rich source.

Deficiency Disorders of Cobalt

Cobalt deficiency is not generally observed in human beings. Its deficiency may cause pernicious anemia, as seen due to the deficiency of vitamin B_{12}.

Cobalt Toxicity

Higher doses of cobalt may produce several toxic effects, such as polycythemia (increased erythrocytes in the blood), hypothyroidism, cardiomyopathy and heart failure.

MOLYBDENUM

An adult human body contains nearly 5 mg of molybdenum (Mo). Though it is present in all the tissues, liver and kidney contain large amounts.

Biological Functions of Molybdenum and its Role in Health and Disease

Molybdenum is an integral part of several flavoprotein containing oxidase systems, e.g. xanthine oxidase, aldehyde oxidase and sulfite oxidase. Thus, it helps in the transport of electrons. These enzymes contain a substituted pterin ring (molybdopterin) in which molybdenum is bound to two sulfur atoms.

Metabolism of Molybdenum

About 50% of dietary molybdenum is readily absorbed in the small intestine.

It is mainly excreted in the urine. Its excretion increases with high protein intake, particularly with a cysteine rich diet.

RDA for Molybdenum

Daily requirement for molybdenum is about 100–200 μg.

Dietary Sources of Molybdenum

Pulses, cereals, green leafy vegetables and meat are good sources. Dietary content of molybdenum depends upon molybdenum content of the soil.

Deficiency Disorders of Molybdenum

Molybdenum deficiency, due to the deficiency of molybdenum containing enzymes, may lead to reduced food consumption and mental retardation. Decreased xanthine oxidase activity may increase excretion of xanthine and decreases uric acid excretion.

Molybdenum Toxicity

Toxicity may occur on a high molybdenum diet. Molybdenum toxicity causes **molybdenosis** which is characterized by weight loss, anorexia, anemia, severe diarrhea and skeletal deformities. Very high amount of molybdenum also inhibits the absorption and utilization of copper.

Biological functions, dietary sources, RDA, deficiency disorders and toxicity symptoms of various minerals are shown in Table 11.4.

Table 11.4: Minerals and trace elements, their important biological functions, sources, daily requirements, deficiency disorders and toxicity symptoms

Mineral/trace elements	Biological functions	Sources	RDA*	Deficiency disorders	Toxicity
Calcium (Ca)	Calcification of teeth and bone, blood clotting, and cofactor for enzymes, such as adenylate cyclase, glycogen synthase, etc.	Milk and milk products, legumes, and dry fruits	1000–1200 mg	Tetany, osteoporosis	Renal stones
Phosphorus (P)	Calcification of teeth and bone, component of nucleic acids, regulation of blood pH and activator for enzymes involved in phosphorylation/dephosphorylation	Milk and milk products, eggs, meat, legumes, and cereals	1000–1200 mg	Neuromuscular, skeletal and renal manifestations	–

Contd.

Table 11.4: Minerals and trace elements, their important biological functions, sources, daily requirements, deficiency disorders and toxicity symptoms (Contd.)

Mineral/trace elements	Biological functions	Sources	RDA*	Deficiency disorders	Toxicity
Iron (Fe)	Component of heme and nonheme proteins, e.g. hemoglobin, catalase, cytochromes, etc.	Meat, green-leafy vegetables	19–29 mg	Anemia	Hemosiderosis
Copper (Cu)	Component of many enzymes, such as cytochrome oxidase, ceruloplasmin, tyrosinase, etc., also helps in iron metabolism	Meat, eggs, and legumes	1.5–1.7 mg	Menkes disease, anemia, neutropenia	Wilson's disease
Zinc (Zn)	Cofactor for various enzymes, such as carbonic anhydrase, DNA and RNA polymerases, alkaline phosphatase; also has role in insulin secretion and taste development	Meat, seafoods and legumes	13–17 mg	Poor wound healing, growth retardation	Gastrointestinal irritation
Iodine (I_2)	Synthesis of thyroid hormones	Iodized salt, seafoods	140 µg	Endemic goiter, myxedema, cretinism	Thyrotoxicosis
Fluoride (F^-)	Promotes normal bone and teeth development	Drinking water and tea	2–3 mg	Dental caries	Fluorosis
Magnesium (Mg)	Component of the bone structure, in nerve impulse transmission, also acts as cofactor for various ATP-dependent enzymes	Cereals, seafoods, tea and coffee	370–440 mg	Depression, muscle weakness, and tetany	Drowsiness and lethargy
Manganese (Mn)	Cofactor for various enzymes, such as hydrolases, decarboxylases, transferases, etc.	Nuts, whole grains, and tea	4 mg	Bone symptoms	Psychotic deformities
Chromium (Cr)	Regulation of blood glucose	Mushrooms, nuts and black pepper	50 µg	Glucose intolerance	Lung cancer
Selenium (Se)	Component of selenoproteins, such as glutathione peroxidase	Cereals, fish and meat	40 µg	Liver necrosis	Hair loss
Cobalt (Co)	Component of vitamin B_{12}	Liver	1–2 µg	Pernicious anemia	Polycythemia, hypothyroidism
Molybdenum (Mo)	Component of flavoprotein containing oxidases, such as xanthine oxidase	Pulses and cereals	100–200 µg	Affects growth, causes mental retardation	Anorexia and diarrhea

* ICMR-NIN (2020)

BIOCHEMICAL ASSESSMENT OF BODY STATUS OF MICRONUTRIENTS

Some biochemical parameters that can be used for assessment of the micronutrients (vitamins and minerals) status of the body are shown in Table 11.5.

Table 11.5: Biochemical assessment of micronutrient status

Lipid-soluble vitamins	Vitamin A	Serum retinol, serum retinol-binding protein
	Vitamin D	Serum vitamin D
	Vitamin E	Serum α-tocopherol, RBC hemolysis
	Vitamin K	Serum vitamin K, plasma prothrombin, prothrombin time
Water-soluble vitamins	Vitamin B_1	RBC transketolase, RBC thiamine pyrophosphate (TPP)
	Vitamin B_2	RBC glutathione reductase
	Niacin	Urinary N-methyl nicotinamide/2-pyridine ratio
	Vitamin B_6	Plasma B_6, RBC transaminase, urinary xanthurenic acid
	Biotin	Urinary biotin, urinary 3-hydroxyisovaleric acid
	Folic acid	RBC folate
	Vitamin B_{12}	Serum vitamin B_{12}, urinary methylmalonic acid
	Vitamin C	Plasma and leukocyte vitamin C
Minerals	Sodium	Serum Na^+
	Potassium	Serum K^+
	Chloride	Serum Cl^-
	Magnesium	Serum Mg^{2+}
	Calcium	Serum Ca^{2+}
	Phosphorus	Serum PO_3^-
	Copper	Serum copper and ceruloplasmin, RBC superoxide dismutase
	Zinc	Plasma and hair zinc
	Iodine	Urinary iodine, serum thyroxin, serum TSH
	Selenium	RBC selenium, RBC glutathione peroxidase
	Iron	Hb, hematocrit, serum ferritin, serum total iron-binding capacity, serum iron, serum transferring saturation, RBC protoporphyrin

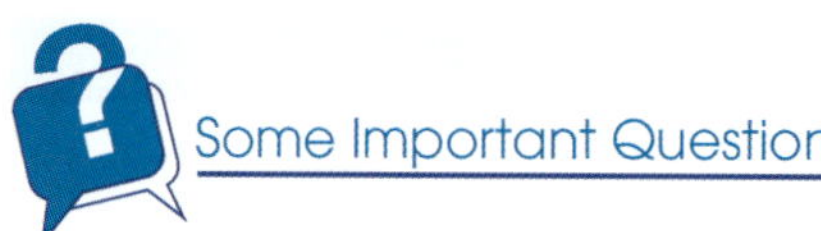

1. **Describe dietary sources, daily requirement and functions of calcium in the human body.**
2. **Describe the role of calcium and phosphorus metabolism in relation to calcitonin, parathyroid hormone and 1,25-dihydroxycholecalciferol.**
3. **Name iron containing proteins and explain their functions. How iron metabolism is regulated? Mention disorders related to iron metabolism.**
4. **Describe in brief:**
   - i. Absorption and transport of iron
   - ii. Osteoporosis
   - iii. Calcium homeostasis
   - iv. Fluoride as a nutrient
   - v. Role of copper in iron metabolism
   - vi. Significance of zinc-containing proteins in the body
5. **Write notes on:**
   - i. Copper toxicity
   - ii. Biological functions of selenium
   - iii. Wilson's disease
   - iv. Fluorosis
   - v. Dental caries
   - vi. Biochemical role of calcium
   - vii. Calmodulin
   - viii. Tetany
   - ix. Ferredoxins
   - x. Ferritin
   - xi. Ferroxidases
   - xii. Transferrin
   - xiii. Anemia
   - xiv. Hemochromatosis
   - xv. Ceruloplasmin
   - xvi. Menkes disease
   - xvii. Cretinism
   - xviii. Myxedema
   - xix. Selenoproteins
   - xx. Molybdenosis
6. **Discuss**
   - i. Biochemical role of magnesium
   - ii. Mucosal block theory of iron absorption
   - iii. Endemic goiter
   - iv. Biochemical role of manganese
   - v. Glucose tolerance factor
   - vi. Biochemical significance of zinc
   - vii. Biochemical role of cobalt
   - viii. Biochemical assessment of micronutrient status.

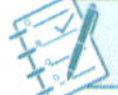

Multiple Choice Questions

1. Calcium absorption is decreased by all of the following *except*:

A. Acidic pH B. Phosphates
C. Oxalates D. Alkaline pH

2. Tetany may occur in all of the following *except*:

A. Hypocalcemia
B. Hypomagnesemia
C. Acidosis
D. Alkalosis

3. The normal serum 'Ca × P' product (each expressed in mg/dl) is:

A. 10–20
B. 20–30
C. 30–40
D. 40–50

4. Magnesium toxicity may occur with:

A. Excessive use of Mg-containing antacids
B. Treatment with diuretics
C. Metabolic acidosis
D. Uremia

5. In iron deficiency anemia, TIBC:

A. Increases
B. Decreases
C. Remains unchanged
D. Cannot be calculated

6. Hemosiderosis may be observed in:

A. Multiple blood transfusions for thalassemia major
B. Chronic pancreatitis
C. Alcoholic cirrhosis
D. All of the above

7. 'Kinky hair syndrome' is due to a genetic deficiency of:

A. Keratin
B. Collagen
C. Elastin
D. ATP7A

8. Goitrogens include:

A. Thiocyanate and perchlorate only
B. Goitrin and isoflavones only
C. Perchlorate and goitrin only
D. All of the above

9. Glucose tolerance factor consists of:

A. Cr^{3+}, nicotinic acid, GSH
B. Zn^{2+}, nicotinic acid, GSH
C. Cr^{3+}, pyridoxine, GSH
D. Zn^{2+}, pyridoxine, GSH

10. Insulin storage and release requires:

A. Zn
B. Ca
C. Fe
D. Mn

CHAPTER 12

Metabolism of Hemoglobin

Competency Achievement: The student should be able to:

BI6.11 Describe the functions of heme in the body and describe the processes involved in its metabolism and describe porphyrin metabolism

BI6.12 Describe the major types of hemoglobin and its derivatives found in the body and their physiological/ pathological relevance

BI5.2 Describe and discuss functions of proteins and structure-function relationships in relevant areas, e.g. hemoglobin and selected hemoglobinopathies

PY2.3 Describe and discuss the synthesis and functions of hemoglobin and explain its breakdown. Describe variants of hemoglobin

PA16.1 Define and classify hemolytic anemia

PA16.3 Describe the pathogenesis, features, hematologic indices and peripheral blood picture of sickle cell anemia and thalassemia

PA16.4 Describe the etiology, pathogenesis, hematologic indices and peripheral blood picture of acquired hemolytic anemia

Heme is an organic, ring-shaped molecule that forms a prosthetic group of hemoproteins. In fact, heme is named for the Greek derivative for **blood**, which is where it was first identified. **The red color of blood is produced by the heme**. It, though, is **synthesized in** all mammalian tissues, its synthesis, however, is most pronounced in the **bone marrow** and **the liver**, because of the requirement for its incorporation into hemoglobin and cytochromes, respectively.

Heme is made from **4 *pyrroles***, which are small pentagon-shaped molecules. Each pyrrole ring contains 4 carbons and 1 nitrogen (Fig. 12.1).

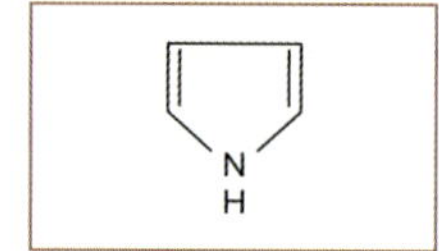

Fig. 12.1: A pyrrole ring

Four pyrroles together form a ***tetrapyrrole***. If the tetrapyrrole has substitutions on the side chains which allow it to hold a metal ion, it is called a **porphyrin**. **Heme consists of one atom of ferrous ion** (Fe^{2+}) and a tetrapyrrole ring, called **protoporphyrin IX** (Fig. 12.2).

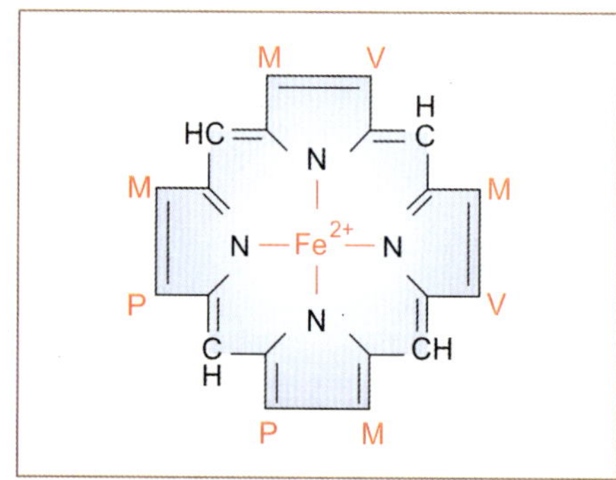

Fig. 12.2: Heme

HEME-CONTAINING PROTEINS

Heme-containing proteins, also referred to as **hemoproteins**, are among the most versatile of **metalloproteins**. They have one or several characteristic iron porphyrins operating as cofactors in the protein matrices, i.e. include those proteins that contain heme as a prosthetic group. For example:

- **Hemoglobin:** It transports oxygen.
- **Myoglobin:** It stores oxygen.
- **Cytochromes:** They participate in the electron transport chain.
- **Catalase:** It detoxifies hydrogen peroxide.

- **Peroxidases:** They detoxify hydrogen peroxide and organic peroxides.
- **Tryptophan pyrrolase:** It catalyzes the first step in tryptophan catabolism.
- **Nitric oxide synthases:** They catalyze the synthesis of nitric oxide.
- **Prostaglandin synthase:** It catalyzes the synthesis of prostaglandins.

TYPES OF HEME

In nature, there are a number of different iron porphyrin variants, which correspond to the many functions it must serve in an organism. Specific proteins use the varying side chains to attach to, and change the properties of the heme. However, the base structure (tetrapyrrole) is always the same, e.g. **heme A, heme B, heme C, heme D,** etc.

Heme A

Heme A is a bimolecular heme that is made up of macrocyclic ligand, called porphyrin, chelating an iron atom. It contains a methyl side chain at a ring position that is oxidized to **a formyl group** and **hydroxy-ethylfarnesyl group**. Moreover, the iron tetrapyrrole heme is attached to **a vinyl side** and **an isoprenoid chain**. It is known to be relatively comparable to heme O, since both include farnesyl.

It works in the **electron transport chain** as part of ***cytochrome** c*, and is involved in transporting proteins and catalyzing reactions.

Heme B

Heme B prosthetic group consists of **an iron atom** which is **able to bind to one oxygen molecule** in the center of a protoporphyrin. The **protoporphyrin is composed of four pyrrole rings** that are **linked together by a methene bridge, four methylene groups, two vinyl groups** and **two propinoic acid side chains**. Thus, each pyrrole ring consists of one methyl group. Two of the pyrrole rings have a vinyl group side chain, while the other two rings have a propionate group, independently. The prosthetic group is, usually, bound within the protein matrix in an area known as the **heme pocket**.

Several well-known hemoproteins such as myoglobin, hemoglobin, horseradish peroxidise (HRP), cytochrome b_5 and cytochrome P450 have heme B in the heme pocket.

Heme B carries oxygen and the proteins, it is attached to help it release the oxygen at the appropriate time. Typically, heme B is bound to apoprotein with a single coordination bond between the heme iron and the amino acid side chain. The biological function of the group is for delivering oxygen to body tissues, such that bonding of ligand of gas molecules to the iron atom of the protein group changes the structure of the protein by amino acid group of histidine residue around the heme molecule. The iron contained in heme B is bounded to four nitrogens of the porphyrin and one electron donating atom of the protein, which puts it in a pentacoordinate state. The iron turns into a hexa-coordinate when carbon monoxide is bounded.

The heme group gives myoglobin and hemoglobin the ability to bind oxygen because of the presence of iron atom. It also contributes to the red color found in muscles and blood. Each heme group contains an iron atom that is able to bind to one oxygen (O_2) molecule. Each hemoglobin protein can bind four oxygen molecules. The iron atom, usually in the ferrous oxidation state (Fe^{2+}), lies between four pyrrole rings but slightly bends away (0.4 Å) from the plane. The iron ion has two extra binding sites, called the fifth and sixth coordination sites on each side of the pro-toporphyrin plane. Usually, the fifth coordination binds with proximal histidine, whereas the sixth coordination binds to an oxygen. When oxygen binds to iron, the iron becomes slightly smaller allowing it to move into the plane of the porphyrin ring. A distal histidine binds to oxygen to make sure reactive oxygen is not released. The distal histidine will not allow the release of oxygen when the iron is in the Fe^{3+} state.

Heme C

Heme C differs from heme B in that the two vinyl sides from the heme B are substituted with a **covalently thioether linkage with the apoprotein**. Because of this connection, heme C has difficulty in dissociating from holoprotein and cytochrome *c*.

Heme C functions a **crucial role in apoptosis**, because some molecules of cytoplasmic cytochrome *c* must contain heme C. As a consequence, **this leads to cell destruction**.

Heme D

Heme D is another form of heme B. Instead, the **hydroxylated propionic acid side chain forms a gamma-spirolactone**.

Heme D reduces oxygen in water of bacteria with a low oxygen tension.

Heme O

Heme O contains **four methylene groups**, while the rest of the structure is similar between heme O and heme A.

FUNCTIONS OF HEME IN THE BODY

Hemes are used for two known reasons, i.e. **to carry oxygen** and **to transport**, or **store, electrons**. Organisms use the heme molecule, **in complex with specially-shaped proteins**, like ***hemoglobin*** and ***myoglobin***, which are made to help the heme complex hold, or release, oxygen at the appropriate times.

Heme has two important functions:

1. Transport of Gases

Heme binds oxygen and CO_2, and transports them throughout an organism. Special proteins, like **hemoglobin** and **myoglobin**, then force the heme to release its oxygen at the appropriate time.

- **Hemoglobin:** Hemoglobin is a globular protein, present in high concentration in **RBC**. It **binds oxygen in the lungs** and **transports it to the cells**. It **also transports CO_2 and H^+ from the tissues to the lungs**. Hemoglobin **also carries and releases NO in the blood vessels of the tissues**. When the blood cells pass through the lungs, they bind up as much oxygen as the iron in the heme can handle. The blood cells then travel to various parts of the body, such as the muscles. These cells are actively using up oxygen and releasing carbon dioxide as a by-product. Carbon dioxide forms an acid in the blood plasma, lowering the pH of the blood. Like all proteins, hemoglobin reacts to change in pH, by changing shape. This change in shape forces the oxygen off the heme complex, releasing the oxygen into the blood plasma. The oxygen diffuses into the muscle cells, where it is bound by myoglobin and transported to the mitochondria and is used.
- **Myoglobin:** Myoglobin also has a heme group, but it operates in a different way so that oxygen remains tightly bound, until reaching the mitochondria. It is the hemoprotein found in **muscles** and is made up of a **single polypeptide chain** that binds and protects the heme prosthetic group. It acts as a **reservoir of oxygen** and releases the same only when the muscle pO_2 falls to very low levels, such as during strenuous exercise.

Hemoglobin Versus Myoglobin

Although both myoglobin and hemoglobin are oxygen-binding proteins, there are distinct structural and functional differences between the two, as highlighted in Table 12.1.

Table 12.1: Comparison between myoglobin and hemoglobin

Parameters	Myoglobin	Hemoglobin (HbA_1)
Structural aspects		
Primary structure		
Number of amino acids	153	α-chain: 141, β-chain: 146
Molecular weight	17,000	64,500
Secondary structure		
α-helices	8 (A to H)	7 in each chain (A to G)
Proximal His F8	Present	Present
Distal His E7	Present	Present
Tertiary structure		
Shape	Globular	Globular
Size	4.5 × 3.5 × 2.5 nm	4 times larger
Surface	Polar	Polar
Interior	Nonpolar, binds heme	Nonpolar, each chain binds heme
Quaternary structure	Absent (single polypeptide chain)	Present ($\alpha_2\beta_2$)
Functional aspects		
Allosteric modulation	No	Yes, mainly by 2,3-BPG
P50	5 mm Hg	26 mm Hg
Positive cooperativity	No	Yes
Kinetics	Rectangular hyperbola	Sigmoid
O_2-affinity	Higher	Lower
Function and location	To store oxygen and release it during exercise, hence located in myocytes	To transport oxygen from lungs to all tissues, hence located in RBC

Presence of free myoglobin or hemoglobin in the urine is called myoglobinuria and hemoglobinuria, respectively (Chemistry to Clinics 12.1).

Chemistry to Clinics 12.1: Myoglobinuria and Hemoglobinuria

Myoglobinuria refers to the presence of myoglobin in the urine; the latter turns brown ('tea colored'). Causes include extensive muscle breakdown (rhabdomyolysis), malignant hyperthermia and certain drugs such as HMG-CoA reductase inhibitors (statins) and gemfibrozil used to lower serum cholesterol and triglycerides, respectively. Patients who are prescribed the above drugs should be instructed to immediately report to the physician in case of unexplained shoulder pain (suggestive of rhabdomyolysis), alteration in urine color and oliguria (impending renal shutdown due to deposition of excess myoglobin in the renal tubules).

Myoglobinuria, however, cannot be differentiated from hemoglobinuria on the basis of urine color and dipstick test for blood (both give a positive test due to the presence of heme). However, serum is not discolored in case of myoglobinuria whereas it is pink-brown in case of hemoglobinuria (as compared to hemoglobin, myoglobin is cleared very rapidly from plasma). Further, serum CK-MM may be raised in case of myoglobinuria due to rhabdomyolysis.

2. Holding of Electrons

The second important function of heme is holding electrons and facilitating reactions in the electron transport chain. During oxidative **phosphorylation** in the mitochondrial membrane, electrons are passed down a series of reactions, which slowly extract their energy before depositing them in water and carbon dioxide. The energy gained is stored in the bonds of the molecule of *ATP*, which most organisms use as a primary source of energy (*see* Chapter 9).

The heme groups in the cytochromes are different than those in hemoglobin, for they have different functions and bind to different proteins.

METABOLISM OF HEME

BIOSYNTHESIS OF HEME

In the biosynthesis of heme, firstly, the **four pyrrole rings are formed**. The organic portion of heme is derived from eight residues each of glycine and succinyl CoA. Some of the reactions occur in the mitochondria while others (the intermediate steps) take place in the cytosol (Fig. 12.3).

1. In the first step, **succinyl-CoA** (an intermediate of the Krebs cycle) condenses with **glycine** and forms **δ-aminolevulinic acid (ALA)** in the mitochondria. The reaction is catalyzed by **δ-aminolevulinic acid synthase** (**ALA synthase**, i.e. enzyme 1 or **E1**), which requires pyridoxal phosphate (PLP) as a coenzyme. This is the rate-limiting step of heme synthesis. The enzyme is synthesized in the cytosol and is incorporated into matrix of the mitochondria.
2. In the next step, **two molecules of ALA** condense asymmetrically and **form porphobilinogen**. This reaction is catalyzed by aminolevulinic acid dehydratase (**ALA dehydratase, E2**), a zinc containing enzyme present in the cytosol. It consists of eight subunits, four of which interact with the substrate.

   ALA dehydratase is sensitive to heavy metals, particularly lead. **ALA levels are elevated in lead poisoning**.
3. Porphobilinogen undergoes deamination by porphobilinogen deaminase (**hydroxymethylbilane synthase** or uroporphyrinogen I synthase, **E3**) and forms a linear tetrapyrrole, called hydroxymethylbilane.
4. With the ring closure catalyzed by **uroporphyrinogen I cosynthase** (**E4**), hydroxymethylbilane is converted to uroporphyrinogen I.

   Alternatively, **uroporphyrinogen III cosynthase** converts hydroxymethylbilane to **uroporphyrinogen III**. Only types I and III are found in nature. **Porphyrins with symmetric arrangement of the substituent groups** on its four rings are classified as **type I porphyrins**, while those **with asymmetric substitutions** are classified as **type III porphyrins** (Fig. 12.4).

   Under normal conditions, the uroporphyrinogen formed is almost exclusively the type III isomer. **Heme is** also a **type III porphyrin**.
5. **Uroporphyrinogen** I or III **is converted to** the respective **coproporphyrinogen** by **uroporphyrinogen decarboxylase** (**E5**). The enzyme is inhibited by iron salts.
6. **Coproporphyrinogen III** enters mitochondria and is **converted to protoporphyrinogen IX**. The reaction is catalyzed by **coproporphyrinogen oxidase** (**E6**) and requires molecular oxygen. The enzyme does not act on coproporphyrinogen I.

   These porphyrins are identified as belonging to series IX, since they were designated ninth in a series of the postulated isomers.
7. **Protoporphyrinogen oxidase** (**E7**) acts on **protoporphyrinogen IX** and **converts it to protoporphyrin IX**, in the mitochondria. Protoporphyrin IX is water insoluble. Its excessive amounts are excreted by the biliary system into the intestinal tract.

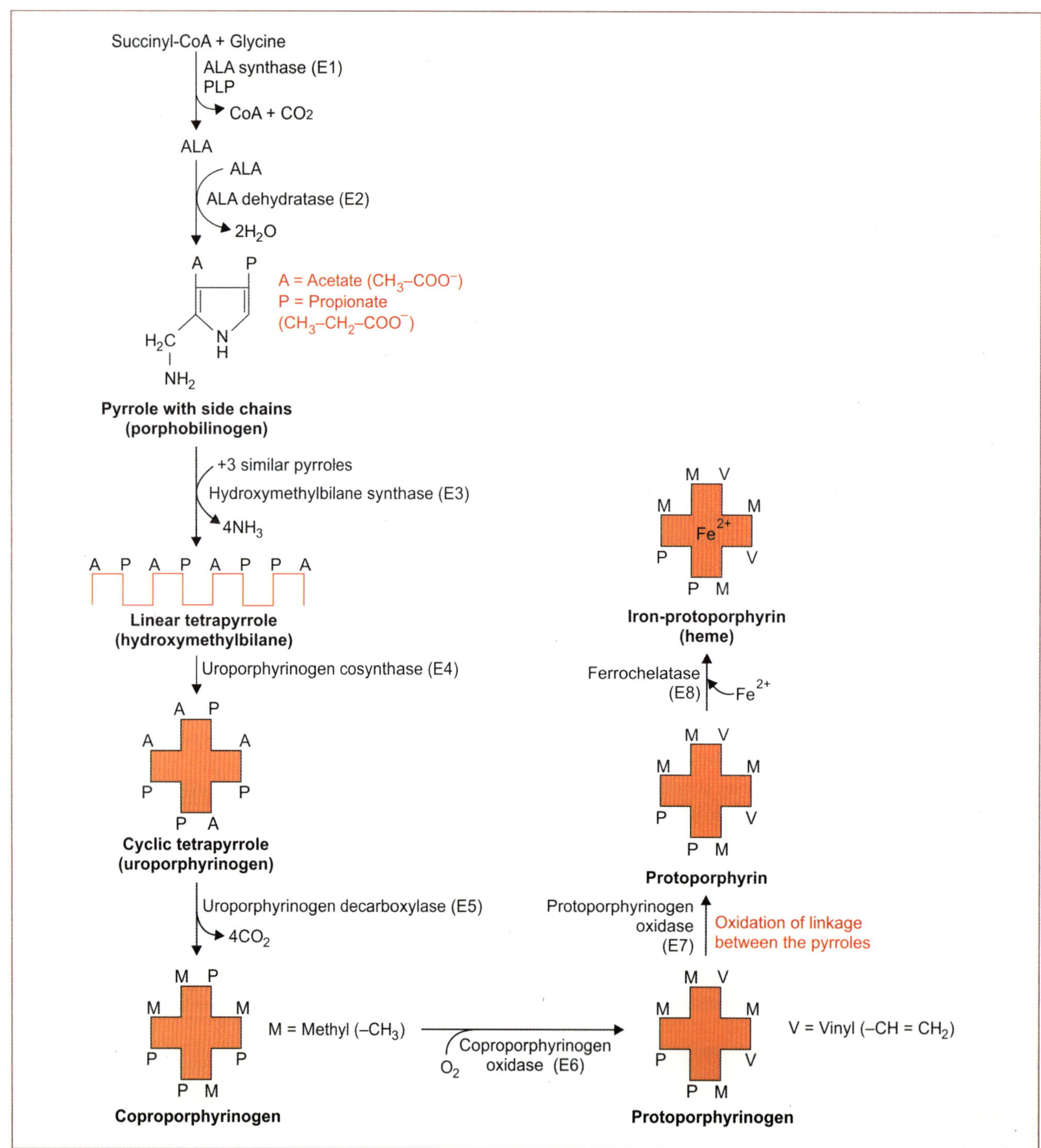

Fig. 12.3: Heme biosynthesis

8. In the final step of **heme synthesis, ferrous iron (Fe^{2+}) is inserted into the protoporphyrin IX**. The reaction is catalyzed by **ferrochelatase (E8)**, which requires reducing substances. The **enzyme is sensitive to** heavy metals, especially, **lead**. It is also sensitive to **iron deprivation**. Thus, **heme** is an **iron-centered cyclic tetrapyrrole** (Fig. 12.2).

Regulation of Heme Biosynthesis

ALA synthase occurs in two forms, called **hepatic-ALA (ALA-S1)** and **erythrocytic-ALA (ALA-S2)**. ALA-S1 controls the rate-limiting step of heme synthesis. Further, heme acts, both, as a repressor of synthesis of the enzyme as well as an inhibitor of its activity.

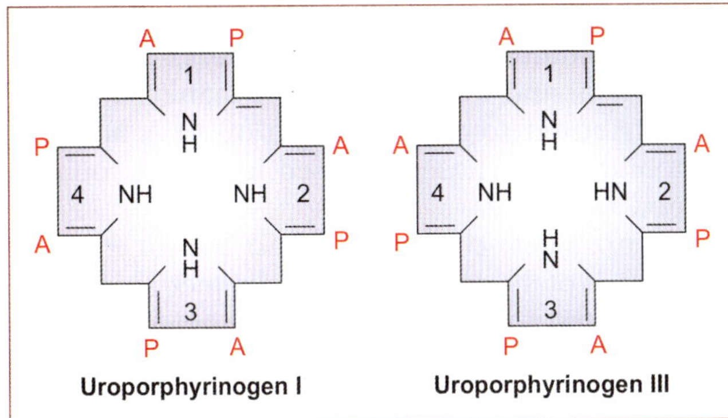

Fig. 12.4: Type I and type III porphyrinogen

Many drugs, which are metabolized by hemoprotein cytochrome P450, result in diminished intracellular heme concentration that, in turn, causes increased synthesis of hepatic ALA synthase. Decreased heme concentration causes derepression of ALA synthase with a corresponding increased rate of heme synthesis. Various factors, like administration of glucose or hematin (oxidized form of heme), can affect drug-mediated derepression of ALA synthase. They may repress ALA synthase resulting in diminished production of harmful heme precursors.

SALIENT FEATURES OF PORPHYRIN BIOSYNTHESIS

- **Rule of 8:** Porphyrin biosynthesis requires **eight molecules** each of succinyl CoA and glycine are required to synthesize one heme molecule. Further, eight enzymes, i.e. E1–E8, participate in the process. Hence, eight different porphyrias can occur.
- Out of the eight enzymes, E1, E6, E7 and E8 are mitochondrial, while the other four enzymes (E2, E3, E4 and E5) are cytosolic.
- E1 catalyzes the rate-limiting step. It is repressed by heme (autoregulation) and induced by barbiturates (sedatives), griseofulvin (antifungal) and alcohol.
- E2 and E8 are sulfhydryl enzymes, which can be inhibited by inorganic lead (Chemistry to Clinics 12.2).
- Humans synthesize porphyrins with asymmetric side chains, i.e. the type III porphyrin.
- **Porphyrinogens** are unstable and are easily **auto-oxidized** in the presence of light into the corresponding stable **porphyrins**. However, E7 catalyzes the only known enzymatic conversion of a porphyrinogen to a porphyrin.
- Porphyrinogens are colorless, whereas porphyrins are colored. The double bonds joining the pyrrole rings in porphyrins are responsible for the characteristic absorption and fluorescence of these compounds. Double bonds are absent in porphyrinogens.
- Porphyrins exhibit characteristic absorption spectra with maximum absorbance (**Soret band**) at 400 nm.
- Porphyrins emit purple-red fluorescence upon UV exposure so that small amounts can be detected easily in biological samples.
- Synthetic porphyrins are of clinical interest (Chemistry to Clinics 12.3).

Chemistry to Clinics 12.2: Lead Poisoning

- **Inorganic lead poisoning** is an occupational hazard to workers employed in the battery and paint manufacturing industries. Further, children who are in the habit of scraping and eating wall-paints are also at risk. Inorganic lead binds to sulfhydryl proteins including ALA-dehydratase and ferrochelatase participating in heme biosynthesis, resulting in symptoms of porphyrias (an example of acquired porphyria) as well as anemia. In addition, inorganic lead displaces calcium from its various binding proteins leading to neuromuscular manifestations.
- On the other hand, **organic lead**, i.e. lead tetraethyl is added to petrol where it serves as an 'anti-knock' and protects the automobile engine. The automobile exhaust is thus rich in organic lead and is a health hazard to workers in the automobile industry. Organic lead does not result in porphyria; rather, because of its high affinity for membrane lipids it produces CNS toxicity.

Chemistry to Clinics 12.3: Photodynamic Therapy

Synthetic porphyrins can be administered to cancer patients whereby they get deposited in the tumor and exert cytotoxicity upon laser exposure (cancer photodynamic therapy), e.g. porfimer used in lung cancer and esophageal cancer.

PORPHYRIAS

Porphyrias are a group of disorders due to abnormalities in the pathway of heme biosynthesis.

These can be genetic or acquired. Based on the site of overproduction, porphyrias are either **hepatic** or **erythropoietic,** or sometimes **mixed** (Table 12.2).

Clinical Manifestations and Laboratory Diagnosis of Porphyrias

- Deficiency of an enzyme in the heme biosynthetic pathway blocks the distal part of the pathway, resulting in reduced heme synthesis. This leads to **derepression** of **ALA synthase** (except when this enzyme itself is missing) and the accumulation of proximal metabolites. In fact, clinical manifestations

Table 12.2: Types of porphyrias (deficient enzyme is given in parentheses)

Hepatic porphyrias	Erythropoietic porphyrias
• ALA dehydratase deficiency (E2)	• X-linked sideroblastic anemia (E1)
• Acute intermittent porphyria (E3)	• Congenital erythropoietic porphyria (E4)
• Porphyria cutanea tarda (E5)	• Erythropoietic protoporphyria (E8)
• Hereditary coproporphyria (E6)	
• Variegate porphyria (E7)	

may be triggered by intake of substances that induce ALA synthase, such as alcohol and barbiturates. In general, the clinical and laboratory features depend on whether the defect lies before the cyclization of the tetrapyrrole or after it (the cyclization is catalyzed by E4, i.e. uroporphyrinogen III cosynthase).

- In case of a **pre-cyclization defect**, there are predominantly **neurovisceral** (e.g. acute pain abdomen) and **neuropsychiatric** manifestations. It is attributed to accumulation of ALA and porphobilinogen whose increased levels are found in blood and urine.
- In case of a **post-cyclization defect**, there is enhanced synthesis of the corresponding symmetric as well as asymmetric porphyrinogens. These get converted to their respective porphyrins, which can be detected in the urine/feces. Deposition of excess porphyrins is responsible for **cutaneous reactions** (porphyrins deposited in the skin get excited on UV light exposure) and **red-purple fluorescence in tissues**/body fluids (Greek *'porphyria'* = purple; Fig. 12.5).

Management of Porphyrias

- Avoidance of inducers of ALA synthase
- Administration of intravenous dextrose or hematin to suppress ALA synthase
- Administration of β-carotene to suppress skin reactions.

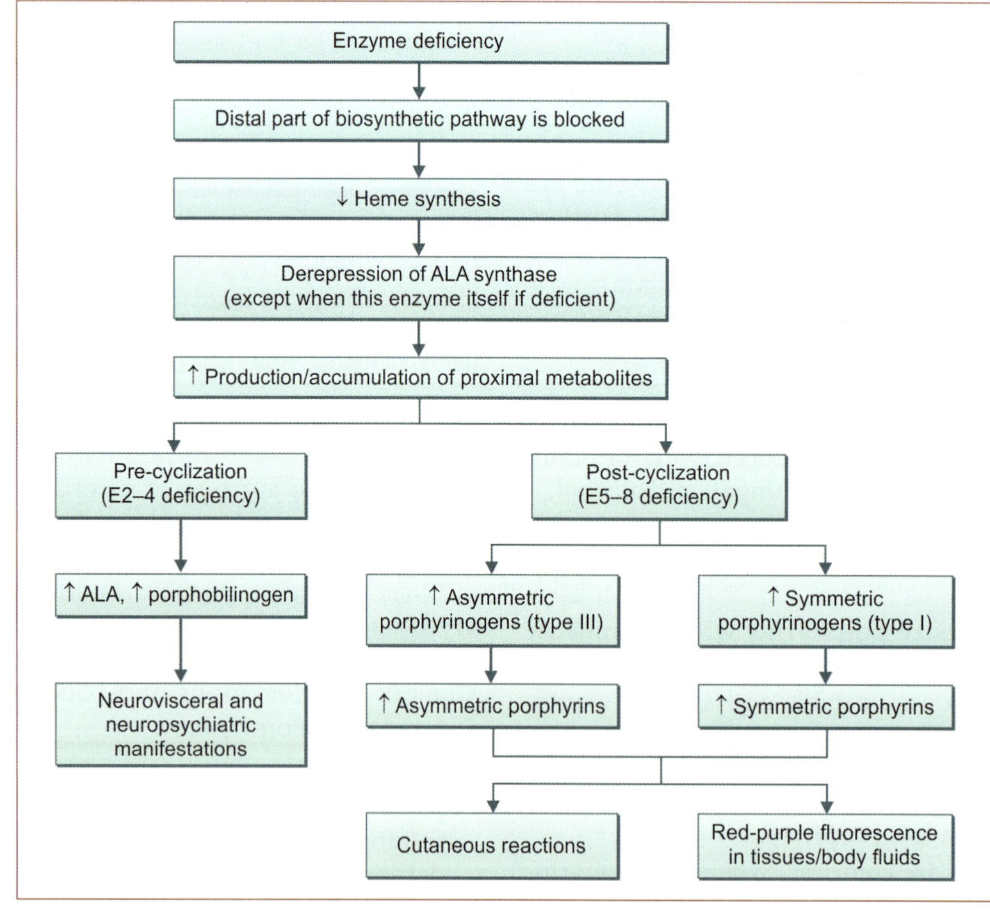

Fig. 12.5: Porphyrias: Biochemical-clinical correlations

DEGRADATION OF HEME

As we know, red blood cells (RBCs) have a limited lifespan of, approximately, 100–120 days, the senescent cells are recognized by their membrane changes, removed and engulfed by the reticuloendothelial system at the extravascular sites.

Degradation of the RBC occurs mainly in the **spleen, bone marrow, liver and lymph glands**. Complete degradation of heme, from hemoglobin, occurs mainly in the liver. If degradation of the RBC occurs in the tissues other than liver, hemoglobin is transported to the liver by means of the haptoglobin. After an aged RBC is recognized by a macrophage, it is rapidly engulfed to form a phagosome. This, in turn, fuses with a primary lysosome and forms a secondary lysosome where cathepsins result in complete degradation of cellular proteins including globin of hemoglobin, to the constituent amino acids which are utilized for general metabolic needs. Heme is released and converted to bile pigments in the endoplasmic reticulum of the cell.

Degradation of heme leads to the synthesis of bilirubin (Fig. 12.6):

Decreased lifespan of circulating erythrocytes results in **hemolytic anemia** (Chemistry to Clinics 12.4).

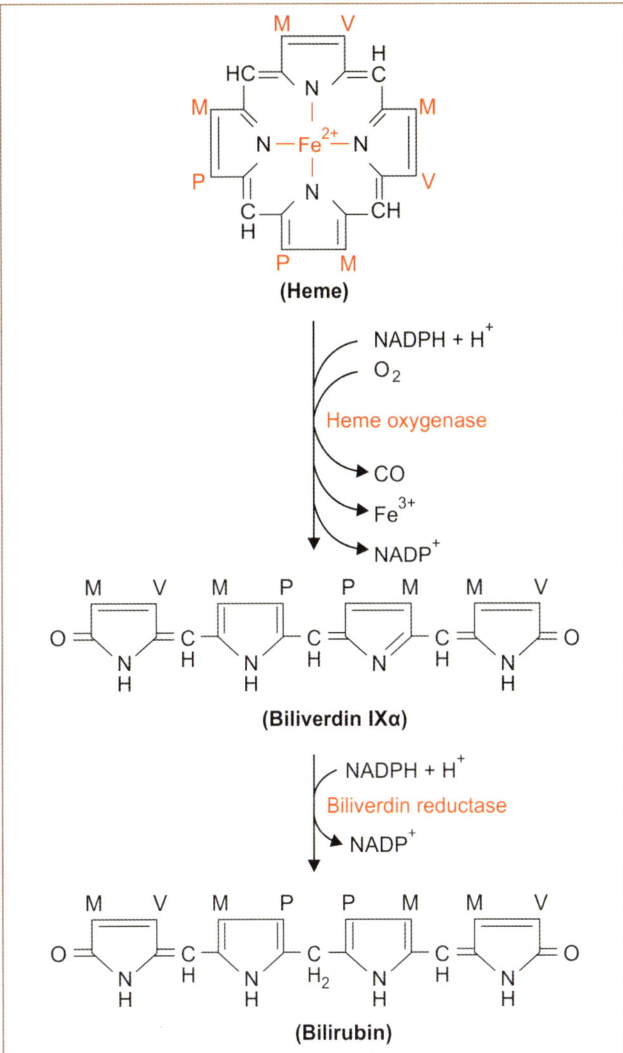

Fig. 12.6: Formation of bilirubin from heme

Chemistry to Clinics 12.4: Hemolytic Anemias

Hemolytic anemias refer to **decreased lifespan of circulating erythrocytes**. These are often accompanied by a regenerative response manifested by erythroid hyperplasia of the bone marrow and increased circulating reticulocytes. The peripheral blood smear may show morphologic evidence of erythrocyte destruction, including spherocytes, and occasionally Heinz bodies, and other forms of poikilocytosis, depending on the pathogenesis of the anemia (Fig. 12.7).

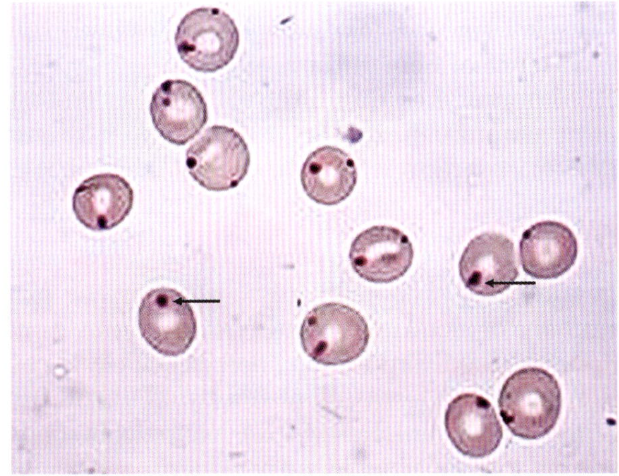

Fig. 12.7: Heinz bodies (arrows) are inclusions in the RBC composed of denatured or precipitated hemoglobin, revealed in a peripheral blood smear stained with methyl violet. They decrease cell membrane flexibility

Symptoms of hemolytic anemia may include abnormal paleness or lack of color of the skin, yellowish skin, eyes and mouth (jaundice); dark-colored urine; fever, weakness, dizziness, confusion, enlarged spleen and liver; increased heart rate (tachycardia) and heart murmur.

Types of hemolytic anemia

There are two main types of hemolytic anemia, i.e. inherited and acquired.

- **Inherited:** With the inherited type, parents pass the genes for the condition onto their children. Two common causes of this type of anemia are sickle cell anemia and thalassemia. These conditions produce red blood cells that do not live as long as normal red blood cells.

- **Acquired:** With this type of anemia, one is not born with a certain condition. Our body makes normal red blood cells, but they are later destroyed.

ACQUIRED HEMOLYTIC ANEMIA

Acquired hemolytic anemias may develop as the result of **immunological reactions** consequent on the **administration of certain drugs**.

Types of Acquired Hemolytic Anemia

The acquired hemolytic anemia can be divided into two main groups as **immune hemolytic anemias** (where the production of antibodies mediates red cell destruction) and **nonimmune hemolytic anemias** (which are of numerous diverse causes).

- **Autoimmune hemolytic anemia (AIHA):** It is the most common type of acquired hemolytic anemia and is caused by the destruction of RBCs by autoantibodies directed against erythrocytes. AIHA can result in intravascular or extravascular hemolysis:
  - **Intravascular hemolysis** is complement mediated and caused by IgM or complement-fixing IgG directed against RBC antigens, resulting in lysis of RBCs directly in the plasma and leading to jaundice or hyperbilirubinemia, elevated LDH and low haptoglobin.
  - In contrast, **extravascular hemolysis** is typically mediated by IgG without complement-fixing characteristics. Extravascular hemolysis may result in little or **no increase in LDH** and **bilirubin**, presumably, because RBCs are destroyed in the phagocytic cells of the reticuloendothelial system rather than in the plasma itself. Urinalysis may show **hemoglobinuria** in the **absence of hematuria**.
- **Nonimmune hemolytic anemias:** The main causes of nonimmune hemolysis are infections, traumatic and microangiopathic disorders, chemical and physical agents, and acquired disorders of the red cell membrane.

Laboratory tests: Laboratory tests that are useful for the diagnosis of acquired hemolytic anemia include peripheral blood film examination, reticulocyte count, direct antiglobin test (Coombs' test), LDH, bilirubin, aspartate aminotransferase (AST), haptoglobin, hemoglobinemia, methemalbumin and hemopexin, and hemoglobinuria and hemosiderinuria. Bone marrow examination may be useful to uncover an underlying cause.

Treatment: In treating drug-induced hemolytic anemia, the implicated drug should be discontinued immediately.

Hemolytic Disease of the Newborn

Hemolytic disease of the newborn is the result of interaction of maternal IgG antibodies that have crossed placenta, and incompatible fetal red blood cells in fetal circulation. ABO and Rh incompatibilities are the first and second most common causes, respectively. The ABO type is less severe and occurs predominantly in group A or B infants, and group O mothers. Rh-related hemolysis is more severe and may lead to intrauterine death or hydrops fetalis.

METABOLISM OF BILIRUBIN

1. **Synthesis of bilirubin:** Heme is degraded in the reticuloendothelial cells to a linear tetrapyrrole, **biliverdin IXa** by a microsomal enzyme system designated as **heme oxygenase system.** The enzyme system requires molecular oxygen and NADPH, and is induced by heme.
   - Heme oxygenase system catalyzes the **cleavage of the α-methenyl bridge**, releasing carbon monoxide (CO), which may be trapped by hemoglobin and, eventually, exhaled.
   - **Biliverdin** is, thereafter, reduced to **bilirubin** (also called **unconjugated bilirubin**) by biliverdin reductase (Fig. 12.6).
   - Iron released from the porphyrin ring is transferred from the cells by an iron transport protein called transferrin and is made available for the resynthesis of new hemoglobin.

   Besides the senescent RBCs, bilirubin is also derived from the turnover of other heme-containing proteins, such as cytochromes.
2. **Transport of unconjugated bilirubin:** At physiological pH, bilirubin is poorly soluble in an aqueous solution. If RBCs are degraded in the liver, further metabolism of bilirubin occurs ***in situ***, but bilirubin formed in other tissues is transported to the liver from where it is taken up at the sinusoidal surface of the hepatocytes by a carrier-mediated saturable system. Bilirubin, normally, present in the blood, is bound to **albumin** and is transported to the liver. Fatty acids, thyroxine and certain drugs (such as aspirin or sulfonamide) **compete** with bilirubin for binding sites on albumin.
3. **Conjugation of bilirubin in the liver:** Hepatocytes trap bilirubin by means of a specific binding protein called **protein Y or ligandin** (a family of glutathione-S-transferases). Once in the hepatocytes, the propionyl side chains of bilirubin are conjugated with **UDP-glucuronate,** which is derived from the oxidation of UDP-glucose. This reaction is catalyzed by **UDP-glucuronyl transferase** and results in the formation of **conjugated bilirubin** (Fig. 12.8).

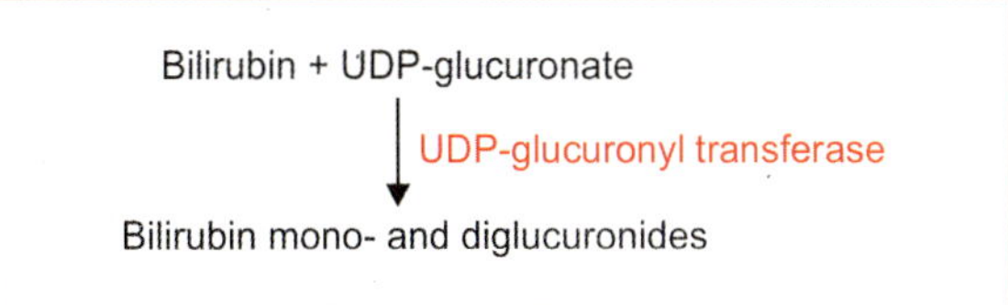

Fig. 12.8: Conjugation of bilirubin in the liver

4. **Biliary secretion of conjugated bilirubin:** In the normal bile, **bilirubin diglucuronide** is the major form of excreted bilirubin with only a small amount of the **bilirubin monoglucuronide**. As bilirubin diglucuronide is much more water soluble than free bilirubin, transferase, thus, facilitates excretion of bilirubin via bile duct into the intestine.
5. **Synthesis of urobilinogens:** As bilirubin diglucuronide is poorly absorbed by the intestinal mucosa, glucuronide residues are released in the terminal ileum and large intestine by intestinal **β-glucuronidases** and by the enzymes produced by anaerobic bacteria. The released bilirubin is reduced to colorless linear tetrapyrroles called stercobilinogen, mesobilinogen and urobilinogen. These compounds are **collectively referred to as urobilinogens**. A large portion of the urobilinogens is excreted in the feces.
6. **Enterohepatic circulation of urobilinogen:** Some of the urobilinogens (up to 2%) are also reabsorbed passively from the intestine and return to the liver via the portal venous blood. A majority of these recirculating pigments are taken up the liver and **re-excreted** in the bile, thereby completing the enterohepatic circulation of urobilinogen.
7. **Formation of urobilin:** Most of the reabsorbed urobilinogen is taken up by the liver and is re-excreted in the bile. A small portion of the urobilinogens (2–5%), however, escapes hepatic extraction, reaches the peripheral circulation and is excreted in urine. The fecal and urinary urobilinogens are **auto-oxidized** to form orange-yellow colored compounds called **urobilins** or **stercobilins** (Fig. 12.9).

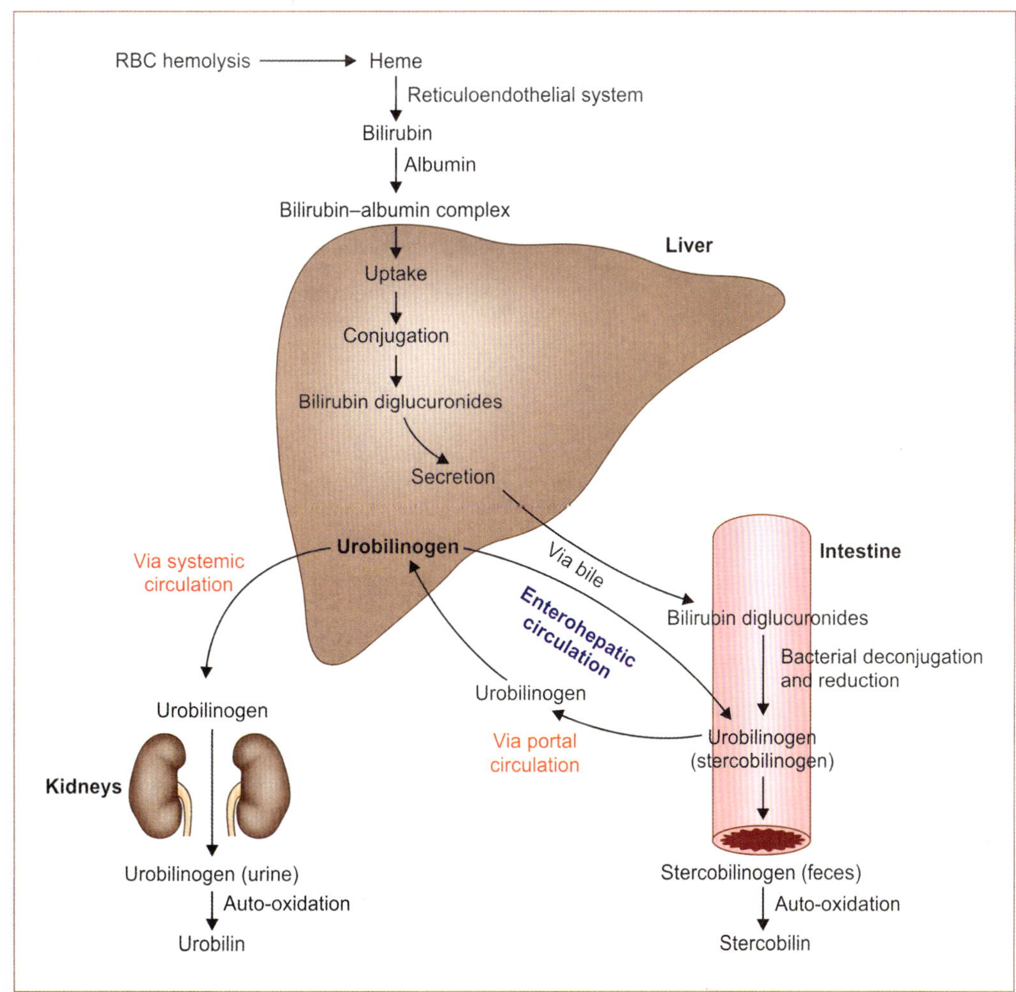

Fig. 12.9: Bilirubin metabolism

Plasma Bilirubin and van den Bergh Reaction

In the normal state, plasma bilirubin concentration is 0.3–1.0 mg/dl. Almost all of this is **unconjugated bilirubin** bound noncovalently to albumin and does not react until it is released by the addition of an organic solvent, such as methanol. The reaction with diazonium salt yields azo dye after the addition of methanol and is called **indirect van den Bergh reaction**. Unconjugated bilirubin binds so tightly to serum albumin and lipid that it does not diffuse freely in plasma, and therefore, does not lead to an elevation of bilirubin in the urine.

In contrast, **conjugated bilirubin** is relatively water soluble and elevation of conjugated bilirubin leads to its high urinary excretion with the characteristic deep yellow-brown color to the urine. The conjugated bilirubin is also referred to as direct bilirubin because it can be coupled readily with diazonium salt to yield azo dye. This is called the **direct van den Bergh reaction**.

HYPERBILIRUBINEMIA

A raised concentration of bilirubin in plasma is described as hyperbilirubinemia. It may be due to excessively high concentration of either free bilirubin or conjugated bilirubin. The skin, eyes and urine of the patient gradually become pigmented with a yellow to yellow-green coloration and the clinical condition is described as **jaundice** (Chapter 13).

TYPES OF HEMOGLOBIN AND THEIR PHYSIOLOGICAL/PATHOLOGICAL RELEVANCE

STRUCTURE–FUNCTION RELATIONSHIP OF HEMOGLOBIN

Structure of Hemoglobin

Hemoglobin is a metalloprotein that has heme as a prosthetic group that is attached to globin protein chains. It has a **quaternary structure**, i.e. it is a tetramer having four protein subunits (globin chains).

Normal adult hemoglobin, i.e. hemoglobin found in normal adult human beings, has **two alpha chains** and **two beta chains** ($\alpha_2\beta_2$).

Heme pocket: Each polypeptide of the globin subunit contains a heme prosthetic group, which is positioned within a hydrophobic pocket of the globin subunit, referred to as heme pocket. Since hemoglobin has a quaternary structure with four monomeric subunits, it has **four heme-binding sites for O_2**. Hemoglobin has a P50 (partial pressure of oxygen, pO_2) at which a hemoprotein is 50% saturated) of 26 mm Hg and shows sigmoidal oxygen-binding kinetics which makes it favorable for loading O_2 at a high partial pressure in the lungs, transporting it and unloading it at the low partial pressure prevailing in the metabolizing tissues (Fig. 12.10).

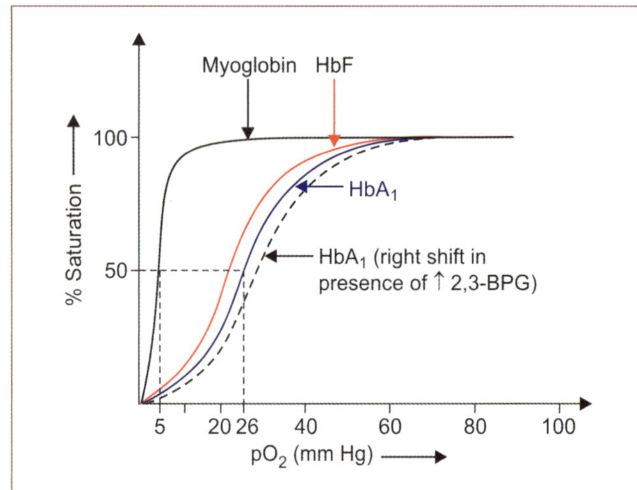

Fig. 12.10: Oxygen binding kinetics of myoglobin and hemoglobin

NORMAL ADULT HEMOGLOBIN AND ITS PHYSIOLOGICAL RELEVANCE

FUNCTIONS OF NORMAL ADULT HEMOGLOBIN

The main physiological function of hemoglobin is to transport gases, i.e:

- It **binds oxygen in the lungs** (oxygenation) and **transports it to the cells** (deoxygenation).
- Further, it **also transports CO_2 and H^+ from the tissues to the lungs**.

TRANSPORT OF O_2 FROM LUNGS TO THE EXTRAPULMONARY TISSUES

Hemoglobin binds oxygen in the lungs (**oxygenation**) and transports it to the cells (**deoxygenation**).

Oxygenation and deoxygenation of hemoglobin: Ferrous ion (Fe^{2+}), in heme, can form **five** or **six ligand bonds**, depending upon whether or not the O_2 is bound to the molecule.

- **Fe^{2+} is linked to the four nitrogen atoms of the pyrrole rings** of the porphyrin.
- It is **also linked** through a coordinate bond **to** the imidazole nitrogen of a histidine, designated as the **proximal histidine** (**His F8**; Fig. 12.11).

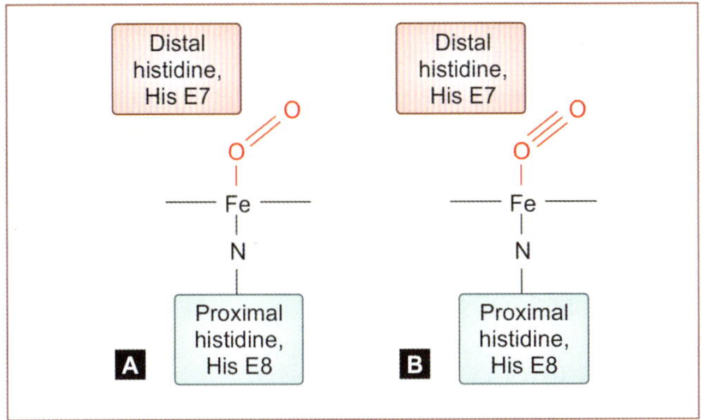

Fig. 12.11: In oxyhemoglobin (A), **oxygen** binds to the heme plane at an angle due to steric hindrance imposed by His E7. **Carbon monoxide** binds in the same stereochemical orientation (B) but with a much **higher affinity**

- The O_2, when bound to hemoglobin, i.e. **in oxyhemoglobin**, forms a **sixth coordinate bond with Fe^{2+}**. The O_2 gets placed between the Fe^{2+} and the nitrogen of the imidazole ring of another histidine molecule, designated as the **distal histidine (His E7)**. The binding of oxygen is affected by **allosteric modulators** such as 2,3-bisphosphoglycerate, H^+, CO_2, Cl^- and temperature; an increase in any of these modulators shifts the curve to the right.
- **In deoxyhemoglobin, this sixth coordinated position of Fe^{2+} is unoccupied.**

T and R Conformation: Ferrous ion in deoxyhemoglobin has a slightly larger radius and gets placed in the center of porphyrin with a conformational constraint on His F8. This, in turn, results in some distortion of the porphyrin ring and the deoxy conformation of hemoglobin is, thus, referred to as the **T** (Tense) **conformational state**. With the binding of O_2 to the Fe^{2+}, the favorable free energy of bond formation overcomes the repulsive interaction between His F8 and porphyrin, the Fe^{2+} moves into the plane of the porphyrin ring and triggers a conformational change in the hemoglobin molecule from **T** to the **R** (Relaxed) **conformational state** (Fig. 12.12).

It is important to note that binding of the one molecule of oxygen to a polypeptide chain in hemoglobin facilitates sequential binding of more oxygen molecules, a phenomenon called **positive cooperativity**.

The T and R conformational equilibrium of hemoglobin **controls delivery of the O_2 and the NO to the tissues, and transport of the CO_2 away from the tissues**. The **equilibrium** between the T and the R state **is regulated by the H^+ ions concentration**, which are released as the T conformation is converted to the R conformation. The imidazole group of His 146 (β) is a major contributor for proton dissociation during the transition from T to R conformation.

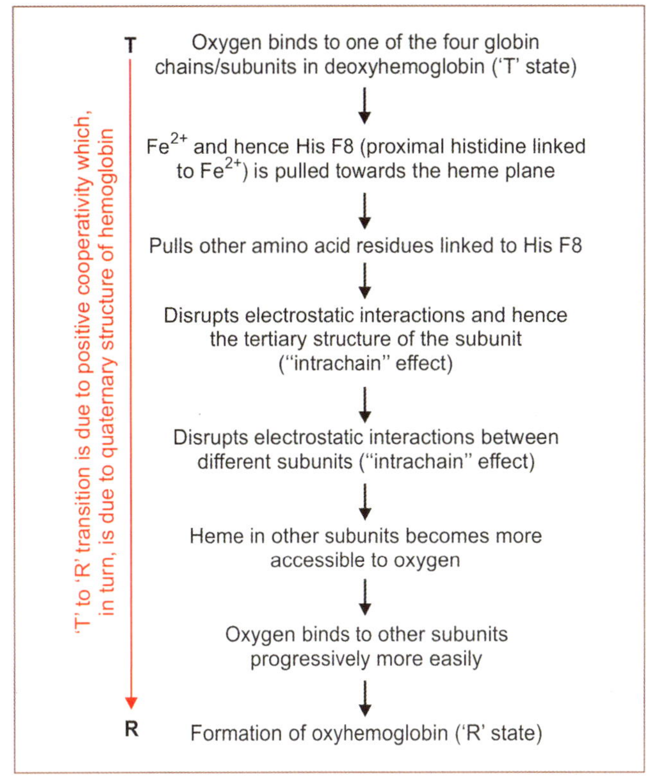

Fig. 12.12: Mechanism of oxygenation of hemoglobin in the lungs. In the peripheral tissues, the phenomenon is reversed

The 2,3-bisphosphoglycerate (2,3-BPG) is an intermediate synthesized in an **off-shoot of glycolysis**. It is present in small amounts in all the cells with large concentration in **RBC**. It is the **most important allosteric modulator of hemoglobin**, with high affinity to the T conformation (deoxyhemoglobin) and not to the R conformation (oxyhemoglobin). It forms salt bridges through its negatively charged phosphate groups to the positively charged residues in the hemoglobin chains. As BPG **binds tightly to T conformation**, it forces the curve to the right and, thus, the delivery of O_2 (Chemistry to Clinics 12.5).

Bohr effect: The affinity of oxygen for hemoglobin is also affected by **pH**. The affinity of oxygen for hemoglobin decreases as the pH becomes more acidic. This is known as Bohr effect. In other words, there is an increase in acidity of hemoglobin as it binds O_2 or increase in basicity of hemoglobin as it releases oxygen.

Bohr effect suggests that an **increase in H^+ concentration favors the release of oxygen from oxyhemoglobin**. Conversely, oxygenation of hemoglobin accompanies lowering of pH of the solution.

Chemistry to Clinics 12.5: Importance of 2,3-BPG

- Since the binding-affinity of 2,3-BPG for heme is less in case of fetal hemoglobin (P50 = 20 mm Hg), the oxygen-dissociation curve of fetal hemoglobin is towards the left of adult hemoglobin (Fig. 12.10). This, in turn, helps in the transfer of oxygen from the mother to the fetus.
- In conditions that cause hypoxia (lack of O_2, such as anemia, smoking and high altitude), the metabolism of the RBC switches over to produce more BPG.
- Prior to transfusion, blood is preserved in ACD (acid-citrate-dextrose) and with the passage of time the BPG levels fall. The blood thus fails to deliver adequate oxygen to the recipient. Hence, inosine is added to blood at the time of storage, which acts as a precursor of BPG and maintains its levels.

Under conditions of lack of O_2, anaerobic glycolysis occurs, which, in turn, produces more lactic acid and, thus, lowers the tissue pH. This causes more release of O_2. Thus, the combined effect of 2,3-BPG and increased acidity leads to a marked reduction in oxygen binding capacity of hemoglobin and, therefore, promotes oxygen release.

TRANSPORT OF CO_2 FROM EXTRAPULMONARY TISSUES TO LUNGS

Transport of CO_2 from tissues to the lungs (for its removal) along with the transport of O_2 from lungs to the tissues is linked with the protons, generated by the Bohr effect, is achieved by two different mechanisms:

- **Isohydric transport:** The metabolizing cells utilize O_2 and produce CO_2, which diffuses from the cells and enters RBCs, in capillaries of the tissues.
  - **In the RBCs:** Within the RBCs, CO_2 is dissolved in water, and is rapidly converted to H_2CO_3 by the enzyme **carbonic anhydrase**. Spontaneously, carbonic acid is dissociated to HCO_3^- and H^+. The H^+ binds to deoxyhemoglobin, forcing the $O_2{\cdot}Hb$ equilibrium from oxyhemoglobin to deoxy-hemoglobin with the dissociation of O_2, which then diffuses out of the RBCs to the cells of tissues. The HCO_3^-, in turn, diffuses out of the RBCs, and is transported (in plasma) to the lungs (Fig. 12.13A).
  - **In the lungs:** In the lungs, high O_2 pressure forces the reaction in the opposite direction, i.e. it promotes the conversion of **deoxyhemoglobin to oxyhemoglobin**. During this process, H^+ ions are dissociated and combine with HCO_3^- to reform carbonic acid. The carbonic anhydrase now catalyzes the conversion of H_2CO_3 to CO_2 and H_2O. The CO_2 diffuses out of the blood, into the lungs alveoli, and is expired into the air (Fig. 12.13B).

  About 80% of the cellular CO_2 is transported from tissues to the lungs by this mechanism, i.e. as HCO_3^-, referred to as **isohydric transport of CO_2**.
- **Carbaminohemoglobin:** Hemoglobin also transports, nearly, 15–20% of the CO_2 by a second mechanism, i.e. via formation of the carbamino-hemoglobin.
  - **From cells of the tissues**, CO_2 diffuses into the RBCs, in capillaries, reacts with the **NH_2-terminal groups of hemoglobin** polypeptide chains and forms carbaminohemoglobin. This

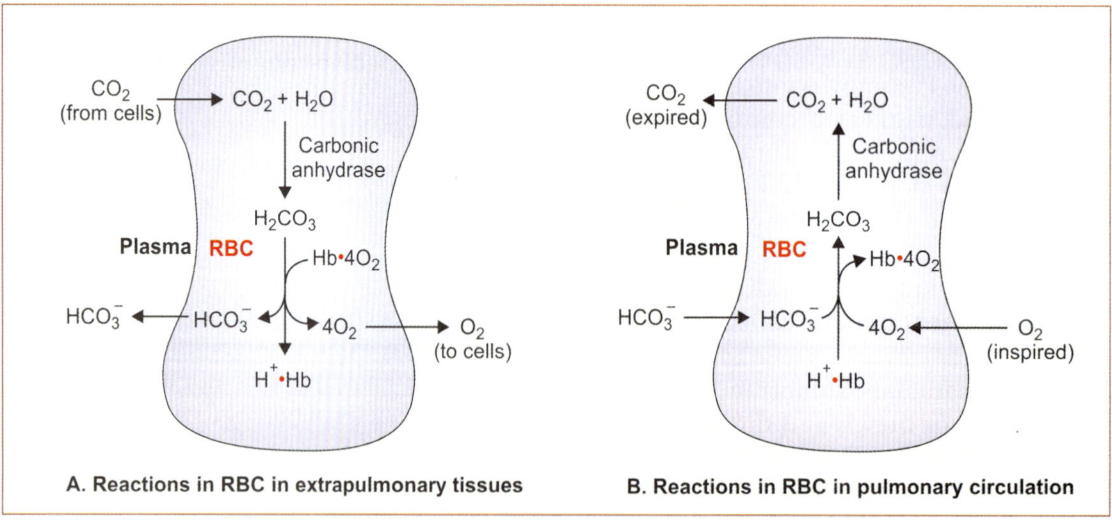

Fig. 12.13A and B: Isohydric transport of CO_2 as bicarbonate

12

reaction also produces H^+, which promotes dissociation of O_2 from hemoglobin. Accordingly, O_2 diffuses out of the RBCs to the tissues (Fig. 12.14A).

- **In the lungs**, high O_2 pressure forces the reaction in the opposite direction. This, in turn, leads to expiration of CO_2 from the lungs. Free H^+ thus promotes dissociation of the carbamino group, from Hb to reform CO_2, which is expired from the lungs (Fig. 12.14B).

Transport of Nitric Oxide

Nitric oxide (NO) is a potent **vasodilator**. It has a very short lifetime in the blood but is prevented from rapid destruction by hemoglobin. Hemoglobin reversibly binds NO. As hemoglobin changes from the oxy (R) conformation to the deoxy (T) conformation, it dissociates the bound NO to glutathione (GSH). NO is thus released as glutathione–nitric oxide complex (GS-NO). Glutathione not only stabilizes NO against its rapid degradation but also efficiently delivers it to the cells of the blood vessel wall and promotes relaxation of the vascular wall. This, in turn, facilitates the transfer of gases between the blood and the cells of the tissues.

STRUCTURE–FUNCTION RELATIONSHIPS OF HEMOGLOBIN AND HEMOGLOBINOPATHIES

As discussed above, hemoglobin has a quaternary structure and that the normal adult hemoglobin has two alpha chains and two beta chains ($\alpha_2\beta_2$). Any change in its structure, i.e. the type of the globin chain and/or its size, results in a variant of normal adult hemoglobin, which in turn, results in a group of pathological disorders referred to as hemoglobinopathies.

HEMOGLOBIN VARIANTS AND THEIR PATHOLOGICAL RELEVANCE

Several variants of normal adult hemoglobin are known to occur at different developmental stages in human beings (Table 12.3).

Table 12.3: Different types of human hemoglobins

Hemoglobin	Chain composition	Developmental stage
HbA_1	$\alpha_2\beta_2$	Adult
HbA_2	$\alpha_2\delta_2$	Adult
HbF	$\alpha_2\gamma_2$	Fetus
Hb·Gower-1	$\zeta_2\varepsilon_2$	Embryo
Hb·Portland	$\zeta_2\gamma_2$	Embryo

- **Embryonic hemoglobin:** Embryonic hemoglobin contains two zeta chains along with either two epsilon ($\zeta_2\varepsilon_2$) or two gamma chains ($\zeta_2\Upsilon_2$). Accordingly, these are referred to as **Hb Gower-1** and **Hb Portland**, respectively. Embryonic hemoglobin is found in the embryonic stage, i.e. in the **first month after conception**.
- **Fetal hemoglobin:** Fetal hemoglobin (HbF) predominates in the blood of the human fetus. HbF contains two α chains along with two γ chains ($\alpha_2\gamma_2$). After birth, fetal hemoglobin is rapidly replaced with the adult hemoglobin (HbA_1), whose synthesis

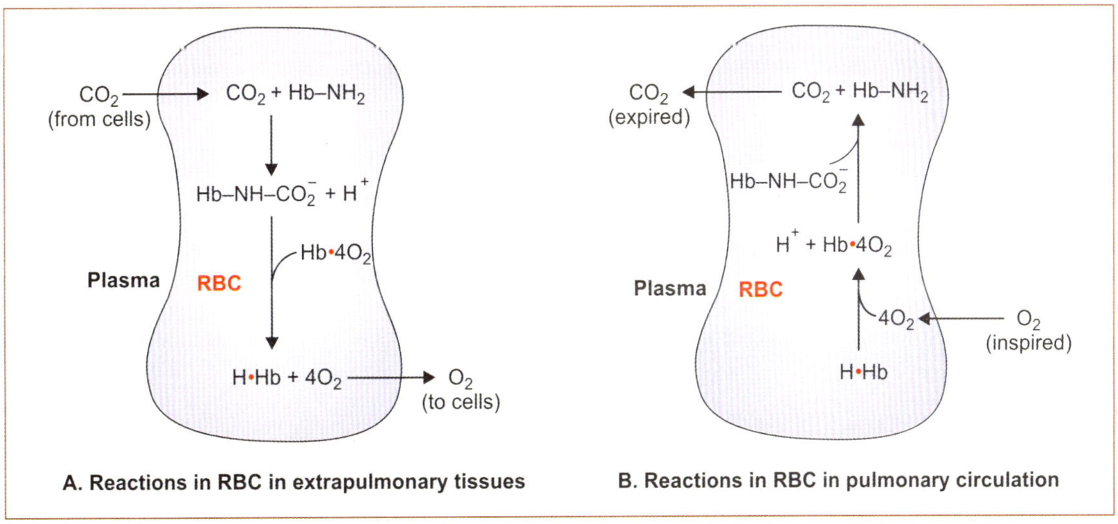

Fig. 12.14A and B: Transport of CO_2 as carbaminohemoglobin

actually starts in the late fetal life. HbF comprises only about 0.5% of the total hemoglobin in adults.

- **Minor adult hemoglobin:** Minor adult hemoglobin, also referred to as HbA_2, comprises only about 2.5% of the normal adult hemoglobin (HbA_1). It consists of two α chains and two δ chains ($\alpha_2\delta_2$). HbA_2 has a reduced efficiency to transport oxygen compared to HbA_1.
- **Glycated hemoglobin:** It results from a covalent linkage between hemoglobin and carbohydrates (Chapter 3).

HEMOGLOBINOPATHIES

Hemoglobinopathies refers to a group of pathological conditions (such as methemoglobinemia, sickle cell anemia, etc.) that may be a result of **structurally and/or functionally abnormal hemoglobin** (**hemoglobin variant**). The pathological relevance may be due to **genetic** or **acquired** defect, in **heme** (hemopathy) or **globin** structure (globinopathy; Table 12.4).

- The variant hemoglobins denature easily and precipitate within the RBCs, forming **Heinz bodies**, which, in turn, can damage the cell membrane (Fig. 12.7).
- In some cases, the change may be clinically insignificant; while in others it may cause different types of anemias or some serious disease.

Table 12.4: Hemoglobinopathies

1. Hemopathies
A. Defective heme synthesis: Porphyrias, iron deficiency anemia
B. Defective heme function: Methemoglobinemia, CO poisoning
2. Globinopathies
A. Qualitative defect (globin mutated but synthesized in normal quantities): Sickle cell anemia, hemoglobin C
B. Quantitative defect (globin normal but synthesized in reduced quantities): Thalassemia, protein energy malnutrition

Methemoglobinemia

Methemoglobin (Met-Hb) is nonfunctional hemoglobin with $\mathbf{Fe^{3+}}$ instead of Fe^{2+}. Normally, Met-Hb levels are <1%. Spontaneously formed Met-Hb is reduced (regenerating normal hemoglobin) by protective enzyme systems, e.g. NADH-methemoglobin reductase (cytochrome *b*5 reductase, major pathway) and NADPH-methemoglobin reductase (minor pathway; Fig. 12.15).

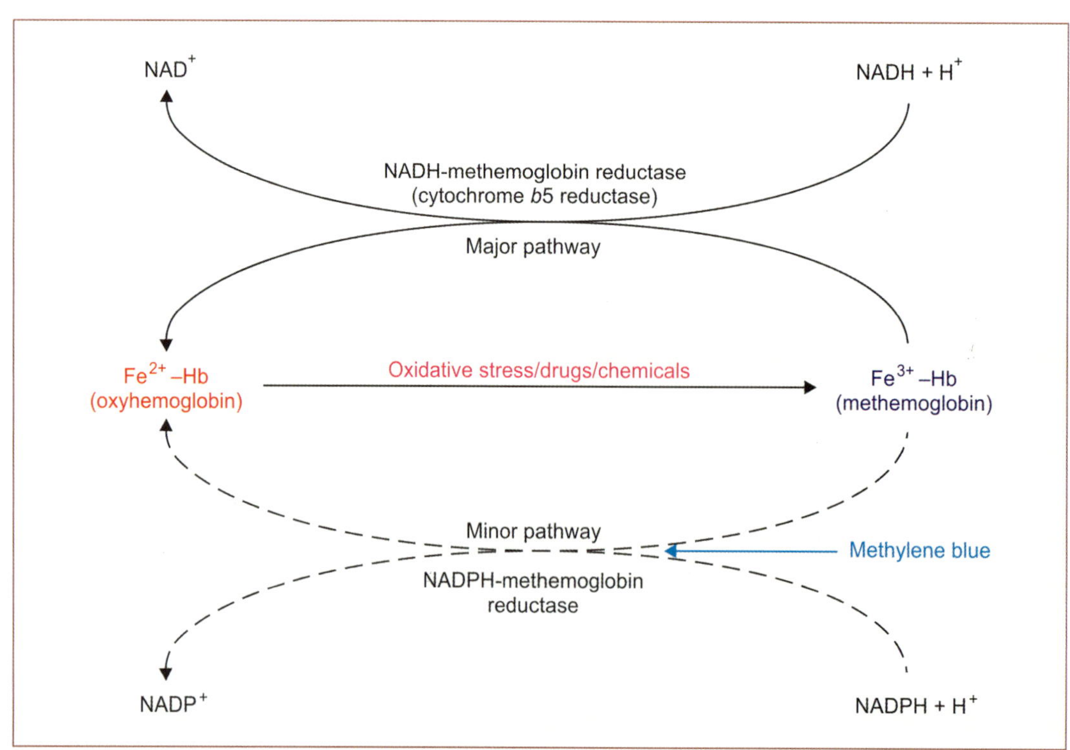

Fig. 12.15: Interconversion of oxyhemoglobin and methemoglobin

12

Cause and types of methemoglobinemia: Elevated Met-Hb occurs when the mechanisms that defend against oxidative stress within the RBC are overwhelmed along with failure to reconvert Met-Hb back to oxyhemoglobin:

- **Congenital:** Either due to deficiency of Met-Hb reductase or due to mutated hemoglobin (termed HbM) which exists in the ferric state and cannot be reduced by Met-Hb reductase.
- **Acquired:** Exposure to certain drugs/chemicals (Table 12.5).

Table 12.5: Common drugs/chemicals causing acquired methemoglobinemia

- Benzocaine: Anesthetic
- Sulfonamides: Antibiotics
- Dapsone: Treatment of leprosy
- Organic nitrates (e.g. nitroglycerin): Treatment of angina pectoris
- Inorganic nitrates: Preservatives

Outcome of methemoglobinemia: It reduces the ability of RBC to release oxygen to tissues, with the oxyhemoglobin dissociation **curve shifted to the left**. Hypoxia occurs due to the decreased oxygen-binding capacity of Met-Hb as well as the increased oxygen-binding affinity of other subunits in the same hemoglobin molecule which prevents them from releasing oxygen at the partial pressure of oxygen in tissues. Patients with high concentration of Met-Hb show **cyanosis** (bluish color of the skin; Fig. 12.16).

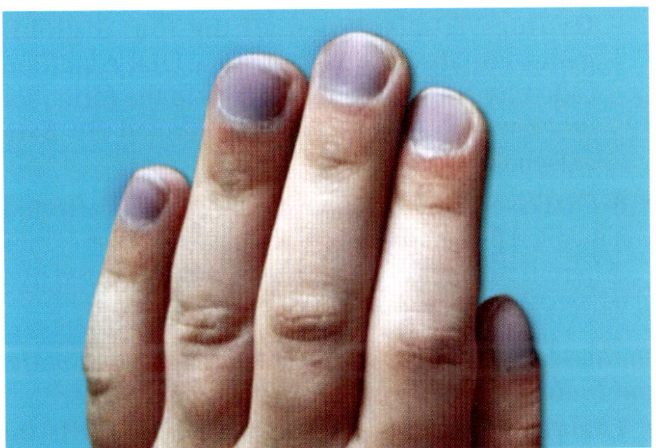

Fig. 12.16: Cyanosis of nail beds in **methemoglobinemia**

Treatment of methemoglobinemia: Intravenous **methylene blue**, which is reduced to leukomethylene blue by erythrocyte Met-Hb reductase in the presence of NADPH. Leukomethylene blue then reduces Met-Hb to oxyhemoglobin. Later, the patient may be switched over to oral methylene blue.

Carbon Monoxide Poisoning

Carbon monoxide (CO) has 200-fold **higher affinity** for binding isolated heme (free from globin) as compared to oxygen. However, due to steric constraints imposed by His E7 (distal histidine), this affinity is reduced substantially in the presence of globin (Fig. 12.11).

CO-poisoning is an industrial hazard, e.g. **automobile** industry. It causes **cherry-red** discoloration of skin and **hypoxia** (Fig. 12.17).

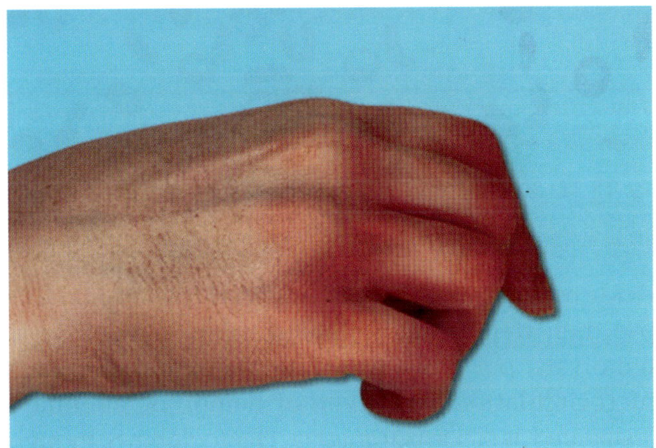

Fig. 12.17: Cherry-red discoloration of skin in **carbon monoxide poisoning**

CO-poisoning can be rapidly **fatal** and requires the prompt administration of **hyperbaric oxygen**.

Sickle Cell Disease

The most common of all hemoglobinopathies is sickle cell disease, which is characterized by the presence of **sickle cell hemoglobin (hemoglobin S or HbS)**.

Molecular defect in HbS: It is a variant form of the normal adult hemoglobin (HbA_1), in which a substitution occurs in the sixth position of the β-globin chain. Whereas in HbA_1, this position is occupied by a glutamic acid residue, in HbS, it is substituted by valine (**β_6 Glu → Val**). The molecular basis for this is a point mutation, i.e. a change in a single nucleotide within the codon from GAA or GAG which codes for glutamic acid to GUA or GUG which codes for valine.

Outcome of HbS: Due to the presence of valine in place of glutamic acid, sickle cell hemoglobin has a lower negative charge than normal hemoglobin. As a result, HbS gets polymerized and precipitate within the RBCs, particularly, **in the deoxygenated state**. This, in turn, makes the red blood cells assume a **sickle-shape,** instead of the normal biconcave shape (Fig. 12.18).

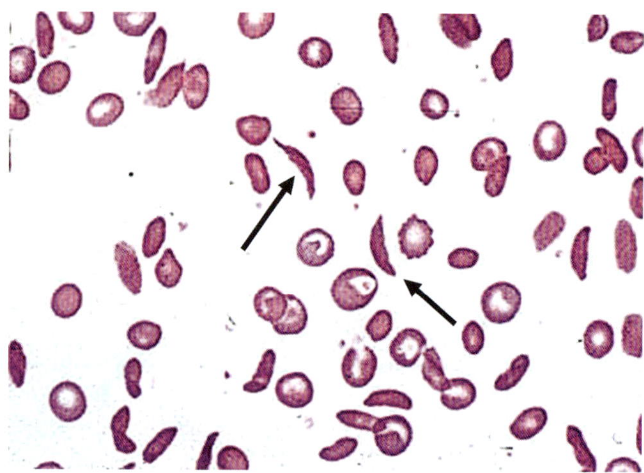

Fig. 12.18: Sickled red blood cells (arrows) in a peripheral blood smear

Sickle cell anemia: The sickle-shaped (distorted) RBCs lose their deformability, resulting in higher rate of hemolysis, particularly, while negotiating through microcirculation. This type of hemolytic anemia is designated as sickle cell anemia. Hemoglobin S, though, binds and releases oxygen, but abnormally. During any illness such as dehydration, infection, etc., these patients are at risk of occlusion of capillaries by the sickle-shaped RBCs, leading to gross tissue hypoxia and damage. These irregular blood cells die prematurely, resulting in a chronic shortage of red blood cells. This can cause painful swelling in the feet and hands, as well as fatigue and **jaundice** (Chapter 13).

Sickle cell trait: Only **homozygous individuals for HbS exhibit the disease**. Those who are heterozygous for HbS do not exhibit symptoms of sickle cell anemia, except under extreme conditions of hypoxia. This is due to the reason that such individuals have 50% HbA_1 and 50% HbS in their RBCs. This is called sickle cell trait.

Diagnosis of the sickle cell disease: Diagnosis can be made by:

1. **Hemoglobin electrophoresis.**
2. **Sickling test:** Sickling of the RBCs, on a blood film, can be induced by the addition of reducing agents such as sodium metabisulfite or sodium dithionite, and confirmed microscopically.
3. **Genetic tests** (mutation analysis).

12

Treatment of Sickle Cell Disease

1. Always **maintain adequate hydration.**
2. **Blood transfusions** during acute attacks (sickle crisis).
3. **Bone marrow transplantation.**

Thalassemias

Thalassemias are a family of related genetic disorders due to defective synthesis of the globin chain(s).

Molecular defect: Thalassemias arise due to the **deletion of one or more globin-like genes** in either the **globin gene clusters** or due to a **defect in transcription** and/or **processing of mRNA** of the globin gene (α-globin gene: Chromosome 16; β-globin gene: Chromosome 11).

Types of Thalassemias

- **α-Thalassemia:** If there is a reduced synthesis or total lack of synthesis of α-globin mRNA, the disease is classified as **α-thalassemia**. The **α-thalassemia** patients may be missing one to four α-globin genes and have **different subtypes**:
  - **α-Thalassemia-1:** If **one α-globin gene is missing**, the condition is called **α-thalassemia-1 (α-thal-1)**.
  - **α-Thalassemia-2:** When **two α-globin genes are missing**, it is called **(α-thal-2)**.

    Both, these conditions are associated with mild to moderate anemia.
  - **HbH disease:** If **three α-globin genes are missing**, it results in the formation of a tetramer of four β-globins. This condition is called **HbH disease**.
  - **Hydrops fetalis:** When **all the four α-globin genes are absent**, it results in a fatal condition, called **hydrops fetalis.** It results in the formation of a tetramer of four ϒ-chains, termed **Hb Barts** (4ϒ-chains).
- **β-Thalassemia:** If β-globin mRNA level is affected, it is called **β-thalassemia**. β-Thalassemias also exhibit different degrees of severity and can be caused by a variety of defects or deletions.

Thalassemias are also grouped as thalassemia major and thalassemia minor

- **Thalassemia minor:** When the **child inherits the defective gene from one parent**, there are usually minor symptoms and is called **thalassemia minor** or trait (whether α or β).
- **Thalassemia major:** On the other hand, if **inheritance of the defective genes is from both the**

parents and results in a symptomatic disease requiring treatment, it is called **thalassemia major** (α or β).

Diagnosis of Thalassemias

1. **Hemoglobin electrophoresis**.
2. **Genetic tests** (mutation analysis).

Treatment of Thalassemias

1. Children require **repeated blood transfusions** for survival, which, unfortunately, results in iron overload, hemosiderosis and organ damage. Hence, **iron chelation** is required and is achieved by injections of **desferoxamine** or **oral deferasirox**.
2. **Bone marrow transplantation.**

Hemoglobin C

Hemoglobin C is another variant of HbA_1 where β_6 Glu is replaced by lysine. This, in turn, results in the formation of aggregates and reduces survival time for the red blood cells. This form of hemoglobinopathy exhibits more limited pathological effects and is commonly found among certain Black African population.

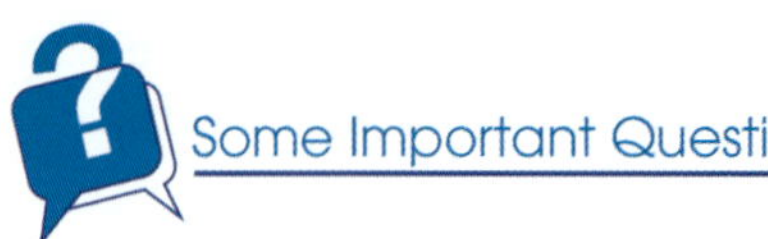

Some Important Questions

1. **Describe the biosynthesis of heme. How heme biosynthesis is regulated?**
2. **What is porphyria? Describe various types of porphyrias.**
3. **Describe how heme is degraded? Discuss the metabolic fate of bilirubin.**
4. **Describe:**
   i. Oxygenation and deoxygenation of hemoglobin.
   ii. Isohydric transport of CO_2.
5. **Compare:**
   i. Myoglobin and hemoglobin.
   ii. Myoglobinuria and hemoglobinuria.
6. **Write notes on:**
   i. Acute intermittent porphyria
   ii. Hyperbilirubinemia
   iii. Heme-containing proteins
   iv. Different types of hemoglobin
   v. Hemoglobinopathies
   vi. Sickle cell anemia
   vii. Thalassemias
   viii. Bohr effect
   ix. Carbaminohemoglobin
   x. Carbon monoxide poisoning
   xi. Methemoglobinemia

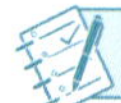

Multiple Choice Questions

1. **In the plasma, conjugated bilirubin is bound to:**
   A. α_2-Globulin
   B. α_1-Globulin
   C. β-Globulin
   D. None of the above
2. **In hydrops fetalis, the number of missing α-globin gene is/are:**
   A. 1 B. 2
   C. 3 D. 4
3. **The following has the highest oxygen affinity:**
   A. HbF B. HbA_1
   C. HbA_1C D. Myoglobin
4. **Acidemia may have the following effect:**
   A. Stimulates oxygen release from oxy-Hb
   B. Inhibits oxygen release from oxy-Hb
   C. No effect
   D. Inactivates oxy-Hb
5. **Organic lead poisoning is an occupational hazard in:**
   A. Paint industry
   B. Battery industry
   C. Automobile industry
   D. All of the above

CHAPTER 13

Organ Function Tests

Competency Achievement: **The student should be able to:**

BI6.13 Describe the functions of the kidney, liver, thyroid and adrenal glands

BI6.14 Describe the tests that are commonly done in clinical practice to assess the functions of these organs (kidney, liver, thyroid and adrenal glands)

BI6.15 Describe the abnormalities of kidney, liver, thyroid and adrenal glands

PY2.5 Describe different types of anaemias and Jaundice

PY4.8 Describe and discuss gastric function tests, pancreatic exocrine function tests and liver function tests

PY7.8 Describe and discuss renal function tests

PY8.4 Describe function tests: Thyroid gland; adrenal cortex, adrenal medulla and pancreas

PA25.1 Describe bilirubin metabolism, enumerate the etiology and pathogenesis of jaundice, distinguish between direct and indirect hyperbilirubinemia

KIDNEY (RENAL) FUNCTION TESTS

Kidneys form a paired organ system. The functional unit of the kidney is called **nephron**. Each kidney has nearly one million nephrons. Each nephron consists of a renal corpuscle and its attached renal tubule.

- **The renal corpuscle** consists of a tuft of capillaries called ***glomerulus*** surrounded by the ***Bowman's capsule***. The glomerulus of the nephron is formed from a specialized capillary network. The resulting structure is relatively impermeable to most proteins >60 kD.
- **The tubule** comprises proximal convoluted tubule, loop of Henle, distal convoluted tubule and collecting ducts. ***The proximal tubule*** is the most active part of the nephron. It facilitates the reabsorption of 60–80% of the glomerular filtrate volume, ≈70% of the filtered load of Na^+ and Cl^-, most of K^+, glucose, bicarbonate, phosphate and sulfate. Proximal tubules secrete 90% of the H^+ excreted by the kidneys. The main function of the ***loop of Henle*** is to generate concentrated urine. The distal convoluted tubule actively reabsorbs sodium and chloride ions. It is relatively impermeable to water but in presence of ADH, its permeability to water increases making urine concentrated. It secretes ammonium and hydrogen ions.

The collecting duct is the final segment of renal tubule which is involved in sodium reabsorption and potassium excretion mainly due to the action of aldosterone. ADH further enhances the water reabsorption resulting in low volume concentrated urine.

BIOCHEMICAL FUNCTIONS OF THE KIDNEY

Primary function of the kidneys is the filtration and excretion of waste products, both exogenous and endogenous. Besides, kidneys play a central role in the homeostatic mechanisms of the human body, synthetic and hormonal functions (Fig. 13.1).

- **Reabsorption of vital substances:** Substances that are vital to the body are reabsorbed, e.g. glucose. Glucose is, normally, completely reabsorbed by the proximal tubule. Amino acids are also reabsorbed in the proximal tubule by several specific transport mechanisms. Most of the filtered phosphate is also reabsorbed in the proximal tubule by the processes that are linked to the reabsorption of sodium and water. Reabsorption of phosphate, however, is inhibited by parathyroid hormone and increased by vitamin D.
- **Excretion of waste products:** The excretory function of the kidneys serves to get the body rid of most of

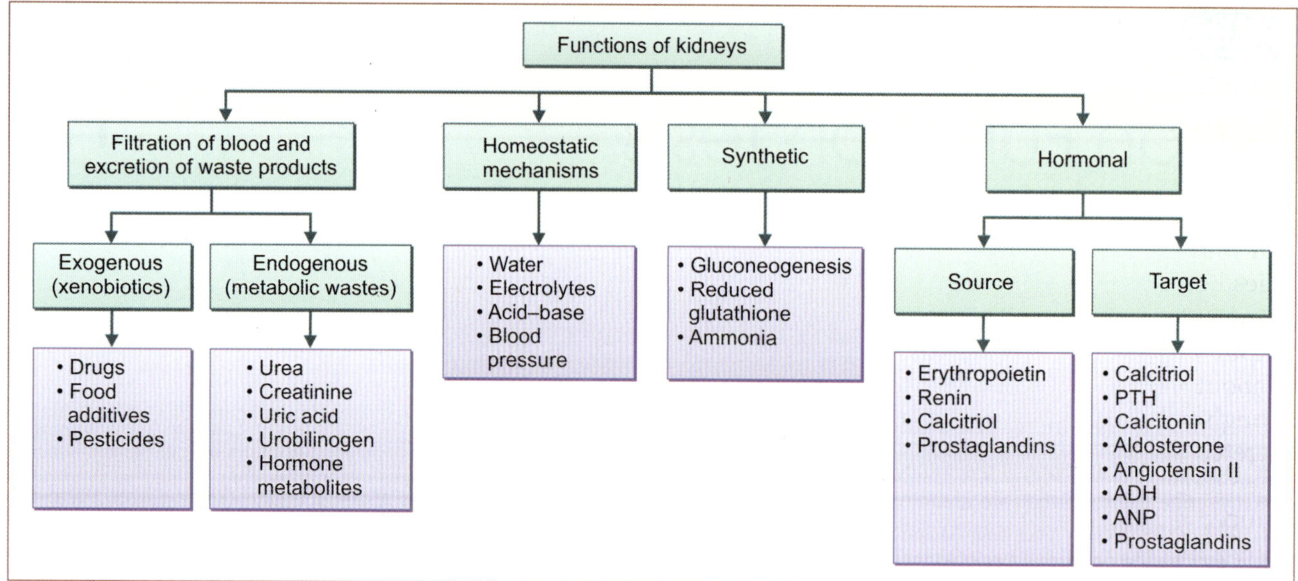

Fig. 13.1: Overview of functions of the kidneys

the undesirable end products of metabolism including various organic and inorganic substances along with water in the urine. Only a small amount of protein is normally excreted in the urine. But the **end products of metabolism**, e.g. urea, creatinine, uric acid, etc. **are largely excreted in the urine**.

Urine

Urine is defined as the fluid excreted by the kidneys, passed through the ureters, stored in the urinary bladder and discharged through the urethra. In a healthy individual, it is a sterile and clear solution which has amber color, a characteristic odor, pH of about 5.0 to 6.0 and specific gravity of about 1.024. The volume of the urine excreted (about 1.5 L/day or nearly 1 ml/min) is the net effect of two opposing processes, i.e. ultrafiltration of nearly 180 L of fluid per day (nearly 125 ml/min) across glomerular capillaries and the reabsorption of more than 99% of this ultrafiltrate by transport processes operating in the renal tubules.

Glomerular filtration rate: Urine formation begins with the elaboration of a protein free ultrafiltrate of plasma across the walls of the glomerular capillaries. The rate of ultrafiltration is referred to as glomerular filtration rate (**GFR**, Chemistry to Clinics 13.1).

GFR is defined as the **volume of plasma cleared of a particular substance by both the kidneys in one minute**. GFR is determined by three factors:

1. The balance of pressures acting across the capillary wall.
2. The rate at which plasma flows through the glomeruli.
3. The permeability and the total surface area of the filtering capillaries.

Chemistry to Clinics 13.1: Decrease in GFR

A decrease in GFR is expected when:

- Glomerular hydrostatic pressure is reduced: Hypotensive shock.
- Tubule hydrostatic pressure is increased: Ureteral or bladder neck obstruction.
- Plasma oncotic pressure rises to unusually high levels: Hemoconcentration due to dehydration, multiple myeloma.
- Renal blood flow is decreased: Circulatory collapse, heart failure.
- Permeability and/or total filtering surface area is reduced: Acute or chronic glomerulonephritis.

Endocrine Functions

The endocrine functions of the kidney may be regarded as either primary or secondary. In its **primary** endocrine function, kidney **produces** erythropoietin, renin, active vitamin D (calcitriol) and prostaglandins (PGE_2 and PGI_2), both of which are concerned with the control of renal circulation. In the **secondary** endocrine function, kidney is a **target** for the hormones produced either within the kidney itself (e.g. calcitriol) or elsewhere (e.g. aldosterone, ADH, angiotensin II, ANP, PTH, etc.).

TESTS THAT ARE COMMONLY DONE IN CLINICAL PRACTICE TO ASSESS FUNCTIONS OF THE KIDNEY

EXAMINATION OF URINE

Clinical features of renal disease commonly arise from alterations in the chemical composition of the body which may be suspected after detection of abnormalities in the urine:

- **Urine volume:** In temperate climate, 24 hours urine output varies from 800 to 2500 ml with an average of about 1500 ml. **Oliguria** is the failure to produce enough urine (<500 ml/day) to enable solutes to be excreted in adequate amounts. Oliguria develops when renal blood flow and/or GFR are reduced, e.g. reduced blood volume, septicemia, cardiac failure, acute glomerulonephritis and acute tubular necrosis. If untreated, it results in complete lack of urine output or **anuria**. **Polyuria** is a persistent increase in urinary output (>3000 ml/day) which may be due to an increased osmotic load (diabetes mellitus), disturbances in the concentration mechanism (diabetes insipidus), certain drugs or excessive water intake.
- **Urine pH:** In a healthy individual, urine pH ranges from 4.3 to 8.0. pH >8.0 indicates urinary tract infection with an organism which splits urea and forms ammonia. In certain circumstances, the ability to excrete H^+ is suppressed.
- **Urine proteins:** Routine side-room testing of urine for the presence of protein is a part of the clinical examination of a patient. Routine testing for protein is usually carried out on an early morning specimen, as this is normally the most concentrated sample of the urine (Chemistry to Clinics 13.2).

  Microalbuminuria is a useful index of early, preclinical renal impairment (Chemistry to Clinics 13.3).

Chemistry to Clinics 13.2: Proteinuria

Proteinuria may be observed in:

1. Individuals with a benign cause, e.g. postural or exercise proteinuria. Physiological proteinuria may also be seen during pregnancy.
2. Patients with conditions that cause transient proteinuria, e.g. fever, congestive cardiac failure.
3. In patients with an organic renal disease, proteinuria may be classified as:
   i. Minimal proteinuria (<1 g/24 h) as in chronic pyelonephritis.
   ii. Moderate proteinuria (1.0–3.5 g/24 h) as in diabetic and hypertensive nephropathy.
   iii. Heavy proteinuria (>3.5 g/24 h) as in nephrotic syndrome.
4. Overflow proteinuria may be found in multiple myeloma where Bence Jones proteins are excreted.

Chemistry to Clinics 13.3: Microalbuminuria

It was previously thought that plasma albumin is not filtered at the glomerulus. However, the fact is that albumin does cross the filtration barrier but the majority is reabsorbed by the proximal tubules with the help of transport proteins called cubilin and megalin. Values below the lower limit refer to normoalbuminuria while values above the upper limit refer to **macroalbuminuria** (or simply 'albuminuria'). A repeat measurement is suggested after 2–3 months to confirm the diagnosis. **Microalbuminuria** refers to urinary albumin excretion with respect to any one of the following criteria:

1. 30–300 mg/24 h (for 24 h urine sample).
2. 30–300 mg/L (for spot urine sample).
3. 30–300 mg albumin/mg creatinine (called albumin/creatinine ratio [ACR] for spot urine sample).

Microalbuminuria is an indicator of

1. Glomerular endothelial dysfunction.
2. Pre-clinical renal impairment in diabetic nephropathy and hypertensive nephropathy.
3. The need to implement rigorous control of blood glucose and blood pressure.

ANALYSIS OF BLOOD COMPONENTS

Blood Urea

Blood urea level in a normal individual may vary between 15 and 35 mg/dl. Urea is the **major** nitrogen containing metabolic product of protein catabolism in humans, accounting for >75% of the nonprotein nitrogen (NPN) which is eventually excreted. Urea is filtered freely by the glomeruli, moderately reabsorbed and secreted by the tubules. In a normal kidney, 40–70% of the highly diffusible urea moves passively out of the renal tubule into the interstitium. Measurement of blood urea is widely used as a test of renal function although it may be raised due to renal or nonrenal factors (Chemistry to Clinics 13.4).

Chemistry to Clinics 13.4: Increased Blood Urea

Pre-renal factors: High protein diet, protein catabolic states, gastrointestinal hemorrhage, treatment with cortisol, some cases of chronic liver disease, decreased renal perfusion due to dehydration (severe diarrhea, vomiting and burns).

Renal factors: Acute and chronic glomerulonephritis, acute and chronic renal failure.

Post-renal factors: Ureteric stones, stricture urethra, ureteric fibrosis, carcinoma of ureters/urinary bladder/prostate.

Serum Creatinine

Normal serum creatinine concentration varies between 0.7 and 1.5 mg/dl. Creatine is synthesized in the kidney, liver and muscles. A portion of free creatine in muscle is spontaneously and irreversibly converted to its anhydride, i.e. creatinine. Free creatinine thus is a waste product of creatine. Its daily production is related to **muscle mass** and does not vary greatly from day to day. The level of creatinine in the blood remains fairly constant. Serum creatinine values are lower in children than in adults, in women than in men (due to lower muscle mass), and during pregnancy. Meal containing meat may slightly increase serum creatinine concentration.

Creatinine is freely filtered by the glomerulus. Although it is not reabsorbed to any great extent by renal tubules, a small amount of creatinine is secreted. Its secretion is increased with the increasing levels of plasma creatinine. In patients with acute renal failure, value may reach 4–6 mg/dl while values >10 mg/dl are seen in untreated chronic renal failure. Determination of serum creatinine thus gives a useful indication of the **degree of renal failure** (Chemistry to Clinics 13.5).

Chemistry to Clinics 13.5: Increased Serum Creatinine

An increase in serum creatinine is observed in:

1. Any condition in which there is decreased renal perfusion, e.g. reduced blood pressure, fluid deprivation or renal artery stenosis.
2. Most diseases in which there is loss of functioning nephrons, e.g. in acute and chronic glomerulonephritis, acute and chronic renal failure.
3. Diseases where pressure is increased on the tubular side of the nephron, e.g. in urinary tract obstruction due to prostatic enlargement.

Serum Cystatin C

Cystatin C is a 13 kD protein constitutively produced by all nucleated cells. Its plasma levels are **independent** of diet, muscle mass or inflammatory conditions. It is freely filtered at the glomerulus, completely reabsorbed and degraded by cells lining the proximal convoluted tubules. It is not secreted by the tubules. Thus, its plasma levels are determined by GFR. It is a **sensitive biomarker to detect kidney disease much earlier** than that possible with the determination of serum creatinine (Chemistry to Clinics 13.6).

Blood pH, Gases and Electrolytes

Diminished capacity to excrete H^+ results in metabolic acidosis, the severity of which may be estimated by the measurement of arterial H^+ concentration, HCO_3^- content and pCO_2. Estimations of serum sodium, potassium, calcium and phosphate are also of value in certain conditions, e.g. in chronic renal failure or in metabolic acidosis accompanied by hyponatremia, hyperkalemia, hypocalcemia and hyperphosphatemia.

Chemistry to Clinics 13.6: Creatinine-blind GFR and Cystatin C

Though creatinine is filtered at the glomerulus, serum creatinine does not rise appreciably until the GFR drops below 60 ml/min. This is because creatinine undergoes tubular secretion and partly compensates for a declining GFR so that serum creatinine rises only when the secretory capacity is saturated. Thus, many patients with mild-moderate decrease in GFR are missed if serum creatinine is used as the sole diagnostic criterion for renal disease. The critical range of GFR, 50–70 ml/min, is called the **'creatinine-blind GFR'**. However, elevation in serum cystatin C occurs in this range as it does not undergo tubular secretion. Therefore, cystatin C provides a superior assessment of renal function.

TESTS FOR THE ASSESSMENT OF GLOMERULAR FUNCTIONS

Tests that are done to assess glomerular functions include kidney (renal) clearance test, renal plasma flow and filtration fraction test.

Renal Clearance

Clearance is defined as the volume of plasma from which the substance whose clearance is to be estimated is completely cleared-off by the two kidneys per minute. The clearance of a substance can be calculated by the mathematical relationship (formula),

$$C_s = \frac{U_s \times V}{P_s}$$

where

C_s = Clearance of substance (ml/min, i.e. ml of plasma cleared of a substance in 1 min)

U_s = Urine concentration of the substance (mg/dl)

V = Volumetric flow rate of urine (ml/min)

P_s = Plasma (blood or serum) concentration of the substance (mg/dl).

Measurement of clearance thus requires measurement of plasma and urine concentrations of the marker plus a reliable urine collection. A substance, which can be considered as a suitable marker of glomerular filtration should meet several criteria (Table 13.1).

Table 13.1: Desirable characteristics of a substance for determining its clearance and hence glomerular filtration rate (GFR)

Desirable characteristics	Urea	Creatinine	Cystatin C
Blood level independent of diet	No	No	Yes
Blood level independent of muscle mass	Yes	No	Yes
Day-to-day blood level within narrow limits	More variable (15–35 mg/dl)	Less variable (0.7–1.5 mg/dl)	Least variable (0.52–0.95 mg/L)
Freely filtered at the glomerulus	Yes	Yes	Yes
No tubular reabsorption	≈50% reabsorption by passive diffusion	Yes	Yes
No tubular secretion	Moderate secretion	Mild-moderate secretion	Yes
Day-to-day urinary excretion within narrow limits	More variable (25–30 g/day)	Less variable (1–2 g/day)	Yes (minimal excretion)
Blood level or clearance value representative of GFR	≈60%	≈80–90%	≈95%

Clearly, in the long-term monitoring of renal function, the **choice is: Cystatin C > Creatinine > Urea**.

- **Inulin clearance:** Inulin is a polymer of fructose. It is filtered by the glomeruli but is neither reabsorbed nor secreted by the tubules. Inulin clearance is nearly equal to GFR. Normal value for GFR as per inulin clearance found in adults is about 125 ml/min. Although inulin meets most of the above criteria for measuring GFR, it is not suitable for routine use as it is not an endogenous substance and has to be administered intravenously.
- **Urea clearance:** Urea clearance depends upon the volume of urine excreted in one min. Urea clearance may be calculated as standard urea clearance or maximum urea clearance.
  - **Standard urea clearance:** It is calculated when the urine volume is <2 ml/min. Standard urea clearance is calculated by taking square root of V, i.e. $\sqrt{V}$:

    Standard urea clearance (ml/min) = $U/P \times \sqrt{V}$

    where U and P are the concentrations of urea in urine and blood (mg/100 ml) respectively, while $\sqrt{V}$ is the square root of the volume of urine excreted (ml/min). The mean value for standard urea clearance is 54 ml/min.
  - **Maximum urea clearance:** When the volume of urine excreted is ≥2 ml/min, urea clearance is calculated as the maximum urea clearance, calculated by putting the actual value of V in the above equation, instead of $\sqrt{V}$. The mean value for maximum urea clearance is 75 ml/min.

    Since urea clearance depends on urine flow rate and also because urea is affected by dietary protein, urea clearance is not preferred to estimate GFR.
  - **Creatinine clearance:** Creatinine, as mentioned above, is generated spontaneously from creatine and gains access to the urine by glomerular filtration. Moreover, creatinine clearance is not affected by the volume of urine excreted or by dietary protein intake. It is, therefore, preferred as a measure of GFR.

    Creatinine clearance per 1.73 m^2 surface area is low at birth (35–40 ml/min) but reaches normal adult levels (80–120 ml/min) by 6 months of age. Creatinine clearance declines with age. However, it is increased by 20% during pregnancy.

Plasma Flow

Measurement of renal plasma flow can be done by renal excretion rate of a substance undergoing both glomerular filtration as well as tubular secretion, e.g. ρ-aminohippuric acid (PAH). At low blood levels, PAH clearance is used as a measure of renal plasma flow. Renal plasma flow as determined with PAH in normal adults is about 700 ± 130 ml/min.

Filtration Fraction

Filtration fraction is the fraction of plasma passing through the kidney which is filtered at the glomerulus. It is obtained by dividing the value of inulin clearance by the value of PAH clearance.

TESTS FOR THE ASSESSMENT OF TUBULAR FUNCTIONS

Tests that are done to assess tubular functions include urine concentration test, urine dilution test and urine acidification test.

Urine Concentration Test

Urine concentration (water deprivation) test can be done by measuring the osmolality of a specimen of the urine which is obtained after water deprivation or after the administration of vasopressin (ADH). Urine osmolality (Osm) is determined by the number of particles of solute per kg water. In normal subjects, restriction of water intake for 8 hours results in maximal stimulation of ADH secretion. Since ADH acts on the collecting tubules and promotes reabsorption of water, it results in concentrated urine.

For water deprivation test, the subject should not take water, coffee or tea and should not smoke but can have light breakfast until the start of the test. No fluids should be given for 8 hours. Thereafter, osmolality of the urine (after 8 hours) should be measured and the value should reach 800 mOsm/kg (or specific gravity of 1.022). If the urine sample has less osmolality or specific gravity, it indicates impaired renal concentrating power either due to tubular defect or due to decreased ADH secretion.

The patient should, however, be weighed at the start and after 5 and 8 hours. The test should be stopped if weight loss is >3% of body weight. The water deprivation test procedure is potentially dangerous when renal concentrating ability is impaired, e.g. in diabetes insipidus.

Urine Dilution Test

Urine dilution (water excretion) test is done to assess the ability of the kidneys to eliminate water. This function is tested by measuring urinary output after ingesting a large volume of water. In normal subjects, at least 750 ml of water is excreted within 4 hours.

After an overnight fast, the subject is asked to empty the bladder. The person is then given 1000 ml of water to drink within 20 minutes. Urine samples are collected at hourly intervals during the next 4 hours. The specific gravity of one of these specimens should fall to at least 1.003, while its osmolality should be <100 mOsm/kg. If renal function is impaired, the quantity eliminated in 4 hours will be less, depending on the degree of impairment. Specific gravity of the urine is often 1.010 or higher in conditions of oliguria.

The test is not advisable in patients with adrenal insufficiency.

Urine Acidification Test

The ability of the kidneys to produce acidic urine is also a function of the tubules. Hence, this test is called urine acidification test and is carried out without any restriction.

The person is asked to empty the bladder. Thereafter, ammonium chloride (0.1 g/kg body weight) is given in a gelatin capsule. Urine samples are collected one hourly for 8 hours. During the test, the patient may eat normally and should drink about 200 ml of water per hour. The pH of the urine is measured. It should be between 4.6 and 5.0. In patients with renal tubular acidosis, pH of the urine does not fall below 5.3 even after a dose of ammonium chloride.

Various renal function tests are summarized in Fig. 13.2.

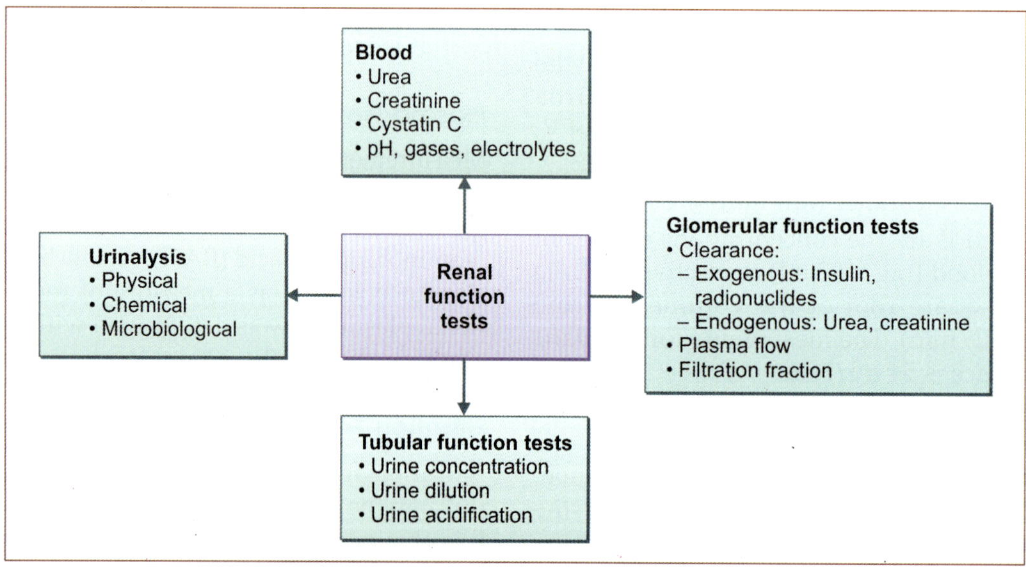

Fig. 13.2: Renal function tests

ABNORMALITIES OF KIDNEYS

CHRONIC KIDNEY DISEASE

Chronic kidney disease (CKD), usually, means that kidneys do not work in the normal way. The kidneys then cannot remove waste products from the body. Damage to the filter system can also allow blood and protein to leak into the urine.

CKD can exist on its own or in combination with other long-term conditions such as high blood pressure, diabetes or diseases that affect the blood vessels (vascular disease).

The major risk with CKD is that of developing problems affecting the heart and blood vessels such as heart attacks and strokes.

There are various stages of chronic kidney disease (CKD), ranging from mild loss of kidney function to complete kidney failure, but not all CKD conditions progress to the most serious stage.

Kidney disease is measured and categorised using a blood test which gauges the estimated glomerular filtration rate and a urine test which shows the urine albumin:creatinine ratio.

The definition of CKD includes all individuals with an eGFR of less than 60 ml/min/1.73 m^2 on at least 2 occasions 90 days apart (with or without markers of kidney damage).

Biochemical markers of kidney disease include: albuminuria (ACR >3 mg/mmol), **hematuria** (or presumed or confirmed renal origin) and **electrolyte abnormalities** due to tubular disorders.

Around 10% of people with CKD may reach a stage that is known as established renal failure when the kidneys can no longer work well enough to keep us healthy and alive, and support from dialysis treatment or a kidney transplant is considered.

ANEMIA

Anemia is common in people with kidney disease and one of its most important complications. Healthy kidneys produce erythropoietin (EPO), a hormone that stimulates the bone marrow to produce red blood cells. Diseased kidneys, however, often do not make enough EPO. As a result, the bone marrow makes fewer red blood cells (Chapter 11).

CHRONIC PYELONEPHRITIS

Chronic pyelonephritis (CP) is the long-term damage done by recurrent urine infection to the drainage system of the kidney. The cause of CP is unclear, partly, because the condition may exist with no evidence of infection. It can be caused by reflux nephropathy, in which the kidneys are damaged by the backward flow of urine into the kidney, due to a leaky valve between the bladder and the ureter.

NEPHROTIC SYNDROME

Nephrotic syndrome is a kidney condition characterized by:

- Very high levels of protein in the urine (proteinuria)
- Low levels of protein in the blood
- Swelling, especially around the eyes, feet and hands.

Other indicators include a high cholesterol level in the blood and sticky blood, which can cause blood clots in the legs (deep vein thrombosis) or lungs (pulmonary embolus). Urinary loss of albumin leads to compensatory increase in synthesis of globulins and apoproteins. This enhances lipoprotein synthesis and a corresponding increase in cholesterol.

LIVER FUNCTION TESTS

Liver is the **largest organ** of the body, weighing about 1200–1500 g in adults. Traditionally, it is divided into two lobes, i.e. the right lobe and the left lobe. The functional unit of the liver is acinus which comprises the group of hepatic parenchymal cells called hepatocytes.

BIOCHEMICAL FUNCTIONS OF THE LIVER

Liver may be called the **chemical workshop** of the body. It performs a variety of functions, which are shown in Fig. 13.3.

TESTS THAT ARE COMMONLY DONE IN CLINICAL PRACTICE TO ASSESS FUNCTIONS OF THE LIVER

Various biochemical tests to assess liver functions for the diagnosis and follow-up of liver disease are briefly described here.

Serum Bilirubin

Bilirubin is an orange-yellow pigment derived from the senescent red blood cells in the liver, spleen and bone marrow. Daily bilirubin production in adults averages 250–300 mg. Approximately, 85% of this is derived from the heme moiety of hemoglobin which is released from the erythrocytes that are destroyed in the reticulo-endothelial cells. The rest of it is formed from

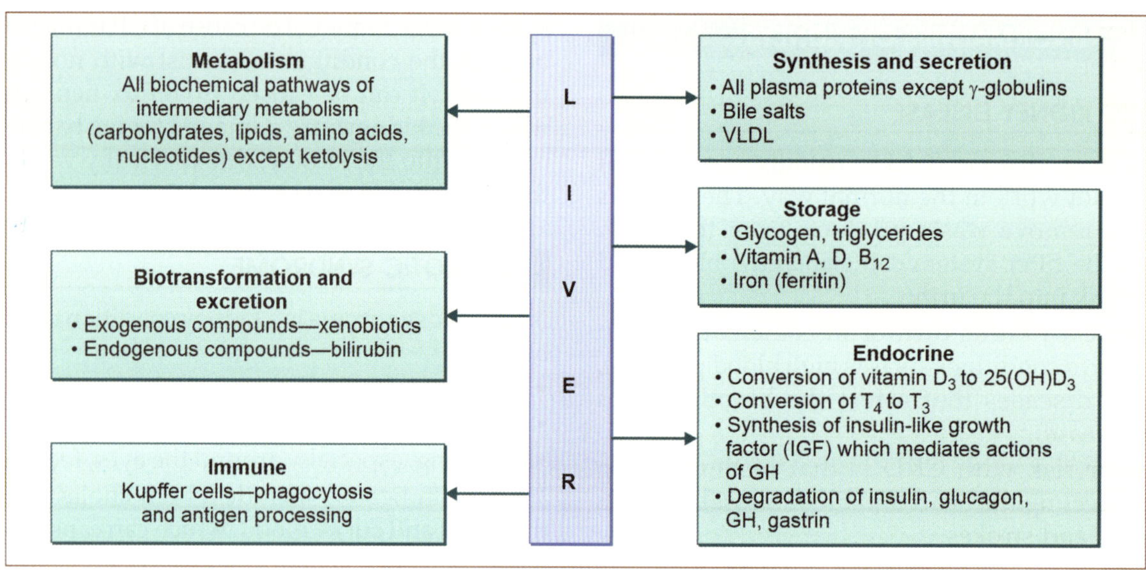

Fig. 13.3: Functions of liver

catabolism of other hemoproteins such as myoglobin, cytochromes and heme-containing enzymes.

Serum contains two different forms of bilirubin, i.e. the **unconjugated (lipid soluble)** form which is bound to albumin and is transported from the reticulo-endothelial system to the liver, and the **conjugated (water soluble)** form which has been regurgitated from the liver into the plasma. Majority of the bilirubin in plasma is unconjugated (Chemistry to Clinics 13.7).

Disorders of bilirubin metabolism lead to **hyperbilirubinemia** and serial measurement of bilirubin is helpful in knowing severity of liver disease. Bilirubin fractionation is helpful in the differential diagnosis of **jaundice**.

Chemistry to Clinics 13.7: Delta Bilirubin

Normally, only traces of conjugated bilirubin are non-enzymatically, irreversibly and covalently bound to albumin. Since it is not filtered at the glomerulus, its half-life reflects that of albumin (14 days, i.e. longer than that of the conventional conjugated bilirubin which is easily filtered out at the glomerulus). This is delta bilirubin, which is not measured separately in the laboratory. This fraction increases with the duration of biliary outflow obstruction of any cause, i.e. cholestasis. Thus, some patients recovering from cholestatic jaundice continue to have clinical jaundice for about 2 weeks despite biochemical recovery (apparently normal serum conjugated bilirubin and absence of urinary bile pigments.

13

Urinary Urobilinogen

Normally, 0.5–4.0 mg of urobilinogen is excreted in the urine in 24 hours. Increased excretion of urobilinogen occurs when hepatocellular function is impaired. Urobilinogen may also increase in the urine if there is an excess of urobilinogen in the gastrointestinal tract that exceeds the capacity of the liver to re-excrete it, e.g. in hemolysis, viral hepatitis and cirrhosis. In contrast, when biliary excretion of bilirubin is impaired, e.g. in cholestasis, urinary excretion of urobilinogen is decreased due to limited delivery of bilirubin to the gut and due to low rate of urobilinogen production. This also results in clay-colored or chalky white stool of patients with cholestatic jaundice.

Fecal Stercobilinogen

Stercobilinogen content of feces of patients with stone obstruction is closer to the lower limit of normal while it is low or absent in those with malignant obstruction. It may thus be of value to distinguish between obstruction due to stone in the bile duct or that due to neoplasm.

Serum Enzymes

In liver diseases, serum levels of several enzymes are elevated. These include:

- **Transaminases (aminotransferases):** These constitute a group of enzymes that catalyze interconversion of amino acids and α-keto acids by the transfer of an amino group. **ALT (SGPT) and AST (SGOT)** are the two such enzymes which are liberated into the blood whenever liver cells are damaged. Increased plasma activities of these enzymes are a sensitive index of hepatic damage. In viral hepatitis and other forms of the liver disease associated with hepatic necrosis, serum SGPT and

SGOT levels are **elevated even before clinical signs and symptoms of the disease** appear. Peak values occur between day seven and day twelve. Activities thereafter gradually decrease reaching towards normal levels by the third to fifth week of recovery. Increased levels may also be observed in extra-hepatic cholestasis, the increase being comparatively higher with more chronic obstruction. Five to ten folds elevation of both the enzymes occur in patients with primary or metastatic carcinoma of the liver. Although serum levels of both GPT and GOT become elevated whenever a disease process affects the liver, **GPT however, is more liver specific**.

- **Alkaline phosphatase (ALP):** It catalyzes hydrolysis of a variety of substrates at a pH of about 10. The enzyme is present in all tissues of the body, particularly at high levels in intestinal epithelium, kidney tubules, bone (osteoblasts), liver and placenta. Serum ALP measurements are of particular interest in the investigation of hepatobiliary diseases and bone disease associated with increased osteoblastic activity. The response of the liver to any form of **biliary tree obstruction** is to synthesize more ALP, by way of its **induction**. Elevation tends to be **more marked in extrahepatic obstruction** than in intrahepatic obstruction. **Increased ALP in children is a normal finding** due to ongoing bone growth associated with enhanced osteoblastic activity.
- **Glutamate dehydrogenase (GDH):** It is found mainly in the liver, heart, muscle and kidney. GDH is present in normal serum only in traces but increased activities are observed in hepatocellular damage.
- **5′-Nucleotidase (5′-NT):** It is a phosphatase that acts only on nucleoside-5′-phosphate such as AMP and releases inorganic phosphate. Serum 5′-NT activity is increased two to six folds in hepatobiliary diseases. This may be due to extrahepatic causes (such as stone/tumor/fibrosis obstructing the bile duct) or may arise from intrahepatic conditions (such as cholestasis caused by chlorpromazine, malignant infiltration of the liver, or biliary cirrhosis).
- **Gamma-glutamyl transferase (γ-GT):** It is also called γ-glutamyl transpeptidase. It transfers γ-glutamyl group from peptides and other compounds, to some acceptor. Even though renal tissue has its highest level, the enzyme present in the serum originates primarily from the hepatobiliary system. It is highest in cases of intrahepatic or post-hepatic biliary obstruction. Further, elevated levels of γ-GT occur in sera from people who are heavy alcoholics. Thus, γ-GT is of significance in detecting **alcohol-induced liver disease**.

Prothrombin Time (PT)

Increased PT observed in hepatocellular disease (e.g. cirrhosis) is not correctable by vitamin K injections whereas that due to cholestasis is correctable. Thus, serial measurements of PT can be used to **differentiate between cholestasis and severe hepatocellular disease**.

ABNORMALITIES OF THE LIVER

JAUNDICE

Jaundice is a **physical sign** characterized by yellow appearance of the patient resulting from the deposition of bile pigment (bilirubin) in the skin, mucous membranes and sclera (Fig. 13.4).

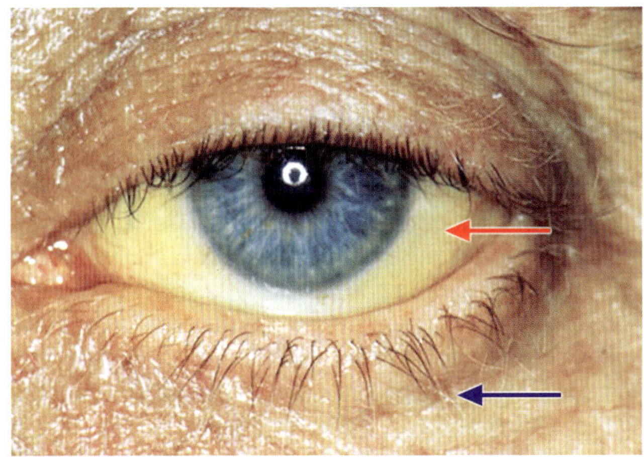

Fig. 13.4: Jaundice: Yellow discoloration of skin (blue arrow) and sclera (red arrow)

These tissues are rich in **elastin** which has a high affinity for bilirubin. Jaundice is the most characteristic clinical manifestation of hyperbilirubinemia.

Types of Jaundice

Depending on serum bilirubin levels, jaundice is either clinical or latent. Jaundice is apparent clinically (**clinical jaundice**) when serum bilirubin concentration is >2 mg/dl. If serum bilirubin concentration is <2 mg/dl it is called **latent jaundice (subclinical jaundice)** since at this stage it is not yet detectable, clinically.

Depending on the cause of jaundice, it may be of three types, i.e. **pre-hepatic, hepatic and post-hepatic jaundice**. In this classification, the liver is taken as the reference organ because the key reaction in bilirubin metabolism, i.e. conjugation of bilirubin, occurs in the liver. Biochemical differentiation of three types of jaundice is given in Table 13.2.

Table 13.2: Biochemical differentiation of three types of jaundice

Sample	Biochemical parameter	Types of jaundice		
		Pre-hepatic	Hepatic	Post-hepatic
Blood	Serum bilirubin	↑	↑↑	↑↑↑
	Type of bilirubin	Unconjugated	Mixed	Conjugated
	Serum transaminases, especially ALT (SGPT)	N	↑↑↑	↑
	Serum alkaline phosphatase	N	↑	↑↑↑
	Serum-5′-nucleotidase	N	↑	↑↑↑
	Prothrombin time (PT)	N	↑	↑
	Effect of parental vitamin K on PT	–	Remains ↑	↓ (normalizes)
Urine	Urobilinogen	↑↑	N/↑	↓/–
	Bilirubin	–	–	↑↑
	Bile salts	–	–	↑
Stool	Stercobilinogen	↑	↓	↓/–

- **Pre-hepatic jaundice:** It is also called **hemolytic jaundice** since it results from excessive hemolysis of RBC as observed in hemolytic anemia. It is characterized by increased serum unconjugated bilirubin which may be due to increased hemolysis, decreased uptake of unconjugated bilirubin across hepatocyte membrane (as in Gilbert syndrome) or decreased biotransformation (as in neonatal jaundice or Crigler-Najjar syndrome).
  - **Hemolysis:** In disorders associated with hemolysis, most commonly hemolytic anemia, the rate of bilirubin production is increased which may exceed the amount that can be removed by the liver. This, in turn, results in unconjugated hyperbilirubinemia (Chemistry to Clinics 13.8).

Chemistry to Clinics 13.8: Hemolytic Jaundice

Common causes are sickle cell anemia, thalassemia major, malaria, snake bite, mismatched blood transfusion and drug induced in case of patients suffering from G6PD deficiency.

  - **Gilbert's syndrome:** This is a heterogeneous group of disorders which is inherited as an autosomal recessive trait. Several defects including the deficiency of bilirubin glucuronyl-transferase, defective hepatic uptake of bilirubin and decreased red cell survival have been described. There is a mild unconjugated hyper-bilirubinemia.
  - **Neonatal jaundice:** It is also called **physiological jaundice of the newborn**. Every infant exhibits some transient unconjugated hyperbilirubinemia between the second and the fifth day of life. Since at this stage the **liver is still immature,** the activity of the hepatic enzyme glucuronyl transferase may be inadequate to completely conjugate the bilirubin. Hence, unconjugated bilirubin level remains at ≈5 mg/dl. The activity of glucuronyl transferase increases within 2 weeks after birth and serum bilirubin returns to normal. Naturally, in a premature infant, physiological jaundice is more pronounced (Chemistry to Clinics 13.9).

Chemistry to Clinics 13.9: Kernicterus

In neonates, serum unconjugated bilirubin >18 mg/dl may lead to deposition of bilirubin in the lipid-rich basal ganglia resulting in kernicterus (Fig. 13.5).

It is a life-threatening condition because bilirubin exerts neuro-toxicity by multiple mechanisms:

1. Damage to membrane transport systems such as Na^+/K^+-ATPase.
2. Uncoupling of oxidative phosphorylation.
3. Impaired synthesis and/or function of DNA and proteins (including enzymes).
4. Impaired synthesis of neurotransmitters and/or synaptic transmission.

Treatment requires UV phototherapy, which degrades bilirubin into water soluble forms that are readily excreted. Phenobarbitone is also useful.

  - **Crigler-Najjar syndrome:** This disorder is known to exist in two forms. **Type I** is the clinically severe form and is due to complete absence of glucuronyl transferase. **Type II** has moderate clinical findings and is due to partial deficiency of the enzyme. In

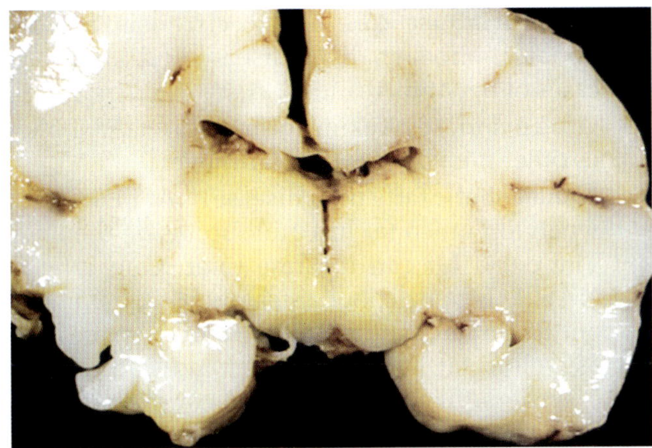

Fig. 13.5: Kernicterus: Cut-section of brain showing permanent yellow staining of basal ganglia due to deposition of unconjugated bilirubin

both the conditions, unconjugated bilirubin is significantly raised.

- **Hepatic jaundice:** In jaundice due to primary liver disease, the serum, usually, exhibits elevated levels of both conjugated and unconjugated bilirubin. **Hepatitis and cirrhosis** constitute the most common disorders associated with conjugated and unconjugated hyperbilirubinemia.
  - In most instances of **viral hepatitis**, besides a rise in serum conjugated and unconjugated bilirubin, there is also a variable increase in alanine aminotransferase (ALT, also called serum glutamate pyruvate transaminase or SGPT) and aspartate aminotransferase (AST, also called serum glutamate oxaloacetate transaminase or SGOT).
  - Besides, inhalation, ingestion or parenteral administration of a number of pharmacological and **chemical agents** such as carbon tetrachloride, acetaminophen, isoniazid and chlorpromazine may also result in liver injury (called **toxic or drug-induced hepatitis**) leading to hepatic jaundice.

    Some other conditions include Dubin-Johnson syndrome and Rotor syndrome.
  - **Dubin-Johnson syndrome:** It is a benign, autosomal recessive condition characterized by elevated levels of conjugated as well as unconjugated bilirubin along with dark-brown pigmentation in the liver cells (Fig. 13.6).

    The defect lies in the secretion of conjugated bilirubin into the bile canaliculi.
  - **Rotor syndrome:** Its features are the same as that of Dubin-Johnson syndrome except that no abnormal pigmentation occurs.

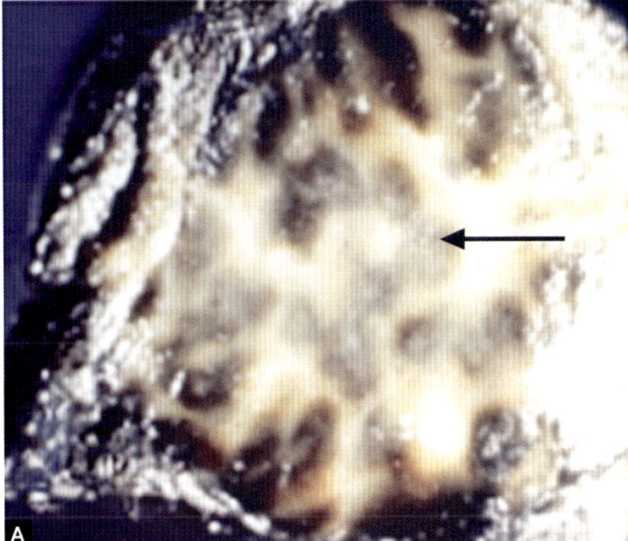

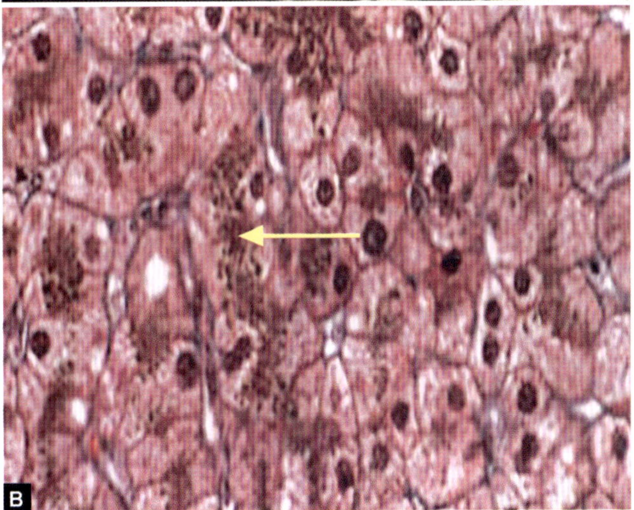

Fig. 13.6: Dubin-Johnson syndrome. (A) Gross liver specimen showing multiple areas of dark pigmentation (black arrow); (B) Light micrograph of a section through liver showing accumulation of large coarse granules of a brown pigment (yellow arrow). The pigment contains a complex association of melanin-like compound, lipofuscin and unidentified bilirubin degradation products. The defect lies in the secretion of conjugated bilirubin from hepatocytes into bile canaliculi and accumulation of the pigment in lysosomes

- **Post-hepatic jaundice:** It refers to post-hepatic cholestasis caused by **obstruction** of the bile duct outside the liver. Obstructive jaundice, most often, may be due to stones in the common bile duct/hepatic duct (choledocholithiasis), carcinoma of the head of pancreas or carcinoma of the bile duct (cholangiocarcinoma). Serum of such a patient contains excessive amount of the **conjugated bilirubin**. It is also characterized by the presence of excessive amount of bilirubin in the urine.

Since unconjugated bilirubin is not soluble in water, it is not excreted in the urine. Only conjugated bilirubin is excreted in the urine of patients with obstructive jaundice. It is an indirect test for the increased concentration of conjugated bilirubin in the serum.

Due to obstruction to the flow of bile, free cholesterol excretion as well as bile acid excretion decreases. Both will eventually lead to hypercholesterolemia in such patients.

OTHER KINDS OF LIVER DISEASES

Besides jaundice, there are many other kinds of liver diseases:

- **Diseases caused by viruses:** Diseases caused by viruses, such as hepatitis A, hepatitis B and hepatitis C:
  - **Hepatis A is a result of** eating or drinking something that is tainted by fecal matter.
  - **Hepatitis B** through unprotected sex or taking drugs with shared needles.
  - **Hepatitis C** comes from infected blood with shared needles or in connection with HIV.
- **Immune system problems**
  - **Autoimmune hepatitis** inflames liver. It can lead to other disorders and even liver failure. It strikes girls and women more often than boys or men.
  - **Primary biliary cholangitis** attacks tiny tubes in the liver called bile ducts. Primary sclerosing cholangitis scars bile ducts, and it can eventually block them. The bile builds up inside the liver and that makes it harder for the liver to work. It may lead to liver cancer.
- **Liver cancer and tumors**
  - **Liver cancer (hepatocellular carcinoma)** affects women more often than men and African-Americans more often than whites. It is more likely if one has hepatitis or drinks too much alcohol.
  - **Bile duct cancer** strikes the tubes that run from liver to small intestine to carry bile. This kind of cancer mainly affects people over age 50.
  - **Liver cell adenoma** is a tumor that does not have cancer. Women who take birth control pills for a long time are more prone than other people to develop it.
- **Diseases caused by drugs:** Diseases caused by drugs, poisons or too much alcohol, e.g. fatty liver disease and cirrhosis:
  - **Alcohol abuse** can lead to cirrhosis. So, can nonalcoholic fatty liver disease and long term cases of hepatitis B and C.
  - **Drug overdoses:** Taking too much acetaminophen or other medications can harm liver.
  - **Nonalcoholic fatty liver disease** (NAFLD) is there when too much fat has built up inside the liver. The extra fat can inflame liver. One type of NAFLD is nonalcoholic steatohepatitis. It means one has inflammation and cell damage in the liver, as well as fat. It can scar liver and lead to other disorders, like cirrhosis. Dire complications of liver disease include:
    - **Acute liver failure:** This happens when one does not have a long-term liver disease but liver quits working within a very short time, may be days or weeks. That may happen because of an overdose of acetaminophen, infections or because of prescriptions drugs.
    - **Cirrhosis** is a build up of scars in the liver. The more scars replace the healthy parts of the liver, the harder it is for the liver to do its job. Over time, it may not work like it should.
- **Inherited disorders:** Inherited disorders include conditions such as hemochromatosis and Wilson's disease.
  - **Hemochromatosis** makes the body store up too much of the iron from food. The extra iron builds up in liver, heart or other organs. It can lead to life-threatening conditions such as liver diseases, heart disease or diabetes.
  - **Wilson's disease** makes copper build up in liver and other organs. Its first symptoms usually show up when one is between the age of 6 and 35, most often in teens. It not only affects liver, but it can also cause nerve and psychiatric problems.

THYROID FUNCTION TESTS

Main function of the thyroid gland is to **synthesize and secrete thyroid hormones**, i.e. T_3 and T_4.

TESTS THAT ARE COMMONLY DONE IN CLINICAL PRACTICE TO ASSESS FUNCTIONS OF THE THYROID GLAND

Biochemical tests to establish, if there is any thyroid dysfunction, include the measurements of the thyroid hormones (T_3 and T_4) and TSH in serum. Other tests include radioactive iodine uptake, protein bound iodine, serum cholesterol, etc. (Table 13.3).

Table 13.3: Biochemical assessment of thyroid status

Parameter	Hyperthyroidism	Hypothyroidism
Serum T_4	↑	↓
Serum T_3	↑	↓
Serum TSH	↓ (primary) ↑ (secondary)	↑ (primary) ↓ (secondary)
TRH-stimulation response	Not performed	↑ (primary) ↓/Delayed (secondary)
Serum PBI	↑	↓
RAI uptake	↑	↓ (↑ in endemic goiter)
Thyroid-stimulating antibodies	↑ (Graves' disease)	–
BMR	↑	↓
Serum cholesterol	↓	↑

SERUM LEVELS OF THYROID HORMONES

Measurement of the concentration of T_4 and T_3 in the serum is used in confirming the diagnosis of hyperthyroidism or hypothyroidism.

- **Thyroxine (T_4)**

  Serum thyroxine or $\mathbf{T_4}$ value in a normal person ranges from 5 to 12 mg/dl. In hyperthyroidism, serum T_4 concentration is increased to >12 mg/dl whereas in hypothyroidism the value is <5 mg/dl (Chemistry to Clinics 13.10).

Chemistry to Clinics 13.10: Low Serum T_4

Serum total T_4 concentration is low in hypoproteinemia such as in chronic liver disease, nephrotic syndrome and euthyroid patients who are on drugs that block T_4 binding to thyroxine-binding globulin (TBG), e.g. salicylates. Treatment with androgens, cortisol and some anticonvulsants, e.g. phenytoin, may produce spuriously low serum total T_4 concentration.

Free thyroxine (**FT_4**), however, provides more reliable information than does total T_4.

- **Tri-iodothyronine (T_3)**

  Normal value for serum T_3 varies between 70 and 190 ng/dl. Serum T_3 concentration is low at birth. The value rises to near adult level in early childhood and then is maintained up to 30 years of age, after which it again falls (Chemistry to Clinics 13.11).

Chemistry to Clinics 13.11: Serum T_3 versus T_4

In some conditions, serum T_3 concentration is disproportionally high relative to serum T_4, e.g. in all types of hyperthyroidism and early thyroid failure in which the gland is exposed to enhanced stimulation by TSH. Serum T_3 thus is a superior indicator of hyperthyroidism because thyroidal T_3 production is often increased early, such as in Graves' disease where serum T_3 becomes abnormal before serum T_4. Serum T_3 measurement however, is not of diagnostic value in hypothyroidism but is a useful test to monitor the adequacy of therapy. In early hypothyroidism, serum T_3 concentration may be normal despite subnormal value for T_4.

Measurement of reverse T_3 (rT_3, a catabolic product of T_4) may also be helpful in some cases, e.g. in low T_3 syndrome where rT_3 concentration is increased.

- **Thyroid-stimulating hormone (TSH)**

  Reference value for serum TSH concentration is in the range of 0.3–5.0 mU/L (Chemistry to Clinics 13.12).

Chemistry to Clinics 13.12: Significance of Serum TSH

Serum TSH measurements are useful:

1. To differentiate between pituitary and hypothalamic cause of hypothyroidism (Table 13.4).

   Measurement of TSH is most useful and sensitive for primary hypothyroidism. When feedback suppression of the pituitary is reduced by a deficient production of thyroid hormones, TSH rises in an attempt to increase the production of these hormones. Rise in TSH occurs while the patient is still asymptomatic. It is thus an early and sensitive indicator of hypothyroidism. In a hypothyroid patient, the finding of low TSH indicates deficient pituitary secretion of TSH or deficient hypothalamic secretion of TRH.
2. In determining the response to exogenous TRH in the investigation of hypo- and hyperthyroidism
3. To monitor the response to therapy with antithyroid drugs (in patients with hyperthyroidism) or thyroid hormone replacement (in patients with hypothyroidism).
4. For the follow-up of patients who have undergone thyroid surgery or developed hypothyroidism following radiation.
5. In the assessment of hyperthyroidism: Serum TSH is subnormal in all patients with hyperthyroidism as a result of feedback suppression except in pituitary TSH secreting adenoma and tertiary hyperthyroidism (Table 13.5).

STIMULATION/SUPPRESSION TESTS

- **TRH stimulation test:** Thyrotropin-releasing hormone (TRH) stimulation test is used to assess the functional state of the TSH secretory mechanism. Serum TSH is assayed before and 20, 30 and 60

Table 13.4: Classification of hypothyroidism based on the primary site of defect

Hypothyroidism	Primary site of defect	Causes
Primary	Thyroid gland	Endemic goiter (iodine deficiency), autoimmune thyroiditis (Hashimoto's disease), following radioiodine therapy for treating thyrotoxicosis
Secondary	Pituitary gland	Pituitary tumor (except TSH-secreting adenoma), radiation or surgery
Tertiary	Hypothalamus	Hypothalamic tumor, radiation or surgery

Table 13.5: Classification of hyperthyroidism based on the primary site of defect

Hyperthyroidism	Primary site of defect	Causes
Primary	Thyroid gland	Autoimmune overstimulation (Graves' disease)
Secondary	Pituitary gland	TSH-secreting pituitary adenoma
Tertiary	Hypothalamus	TRH-secreting hypothalamic tumor

minutes after a standard dose of TRH. In normal individuals, serum TSH peaks are observed in 30 minutes and values generally range between 5 and 30 mU/L. A normal response excludes the possibility of thyrotoxicosis. In hyperthyroidism, no significant rise in TSH occurs because elevated thyroid hormones inhibit TSH production. In primary hypothyroidism, TSH response to TRH is exaggerated and is of diagnostic significance. It is often useful in differentiating between pituitary and hypothalamic lesion as the cause of secondary hypothyroidism.

- **Thyroid suppression test:** Normally, exogenous thyroid hormone suppresses pituitary TSH secretion, resulting in a decrease in RAIU. An abnormal suppression test is observed in hyperthyroidism, irrespective of the underlying cause. A normal suppression test excludes the diagnosis of hyperthyroidism.

AUTOIMMUNE PROFILE

Antibodies against thyroid peroxidase (**anti-TPO antibodies**) may be detected in the serum of some hypothyroid patients. In Graves' disease, long-acting thyroid stimulator (LATS) is detectable in serum.

OTHER TESTS

- **Radioactive iodine uptake:** As iodine plays an important role in the metabolism of the thyroid gland, radioactive iodine uptake (RAIU) is used for thyroid function studies. Usually 10 μCi (microcuries) of sodium or potassium iodide is administered orally (^{125}I delivers low radiation dose, hence it is preferred over ^{131}I). The radioactivity mixes uniformly with the endogenous iodide in the extracellular fluid. Percentage of the iodide entering and leaving the extracellular space per unit time, which is accumulated by the thyroid in the steady state, is assessed. RAIU is usually measured 24 hours after the administration of the isotope. Normally, 24 hours RAIU uptake is 5–30% of the administered dose. Values above the normal range indicate hyperfunctioning of the gland and are useful in the diagnosis of hyperthyroidism. RAIU is also used as a part of thyroid suppression test.
- **Protein-bound iodine:** Serum protein-bound iodine (PBI) is an indirect measure for assessing thyroid function since about 90% of the iodine in serum is bound to thyroxine. PBI value in a normal subject ranges from 4 to 8 mg/100 ml. In hypothyroidism, PBI value varies from 0.2 to 2.5 mg/100 ml whereas in hyperthyroidism PBI value ranges from 9 to 18 mg/100 ml.
- **Basal metabolic rate (BMR):** It is a measurement of oxygen consumption in the basal state. BMR is raised in hyperthyroidism and is reduced in hypothyroidism.
- **Serum cholesterol:** Increase in serum cholesterol is observed in hypothyroidism whereas it is decreased in hyperthyroidism or thyrotoxicosis. Hypercholesterolemia is due to decreased 7-α-hydroxylase activity. This is normally induced by thyroid hormones which enhance the conversion of cholesterol into bile acids which is then excreted by bile, thereby decreasing the cholesterol levels.

- **Serum calcium:** Hyperthyroidism may result in increased plasma calcium along with increased plasma alkaline phosphatase activity.
- **Glucose tolerance test (GTT):** It is sometimes abnormal in patients with hyperthyroidism who may show a diabetic type of response.

ABNORMALITIES OF THE THYROID GLAND

HYPERTHYROIDISM

Hyperthyroidism is a clinical syndrome, which results from exposure of body tissues to excess circulating levels of free thyroid hormones. Females are more affected than males. Main causes include **Graves' disease**, **multinodular goiter** and **toxic adenoma**.

HYPOTHYROIDISM

Hypothyroidism is a deficiency of thyroid activity such as in **myxedema** and **cretinism:**

- **Myxedema:** Myxedema is a form of hypothyroidism in which there is accumulation of mucopolysaccharides in the skin and other tissues in adults.

  In severe hypothyroidism, a slimy, myxomatous substance, consisting of hyaluronic acid and chondroitin sulfate complexed with protein, is deposited in the extracellular matrix of the skin, causing water to accumulate osmotically. This produces a puffy appearance of the face, hands, legs and feet, called myxedema (Fig. 13.7).

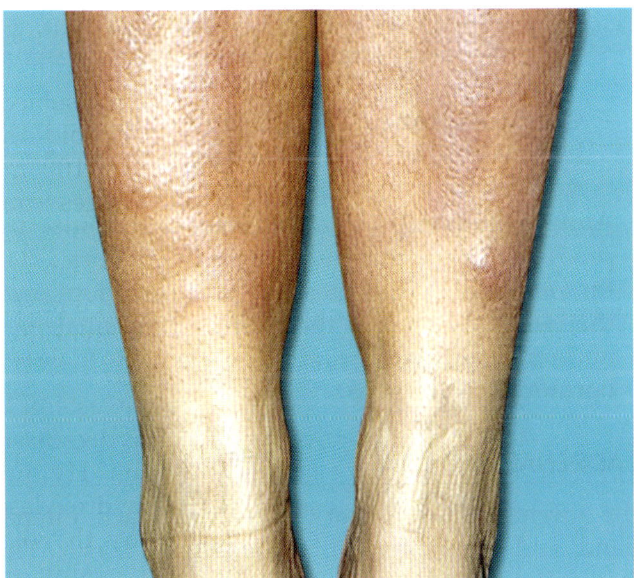

Fig. 13.7: Myxedema

- **Cretinism:** Cretinism is the term used to describe **hypothyroidism in children** (Chemistry to Clinics 13.13).

Chemistry to Clinics 13.13: Cretinism

Deficiency of thyroid hormones in the perinatal period during which the differentiation of neurons, development of neuronal circuits and myelination occurs, leads to mental retardation. Thyroid hormone replacement must be made in the first few months of postnatal life to prevent permanent mental retardation. If treatment is initiated after behavioral deficits have occurred, the retardation cannot be reversed. In addition, the physical growth of the child is also impaired. The features are collectively known as cretinism.

On the other hand, thyroid hormone deficiency later in life also influences the functions of the nervous system. Cognitive functions including speech and memory are impaired and body movements are slow and clumsy. These changes, however, can be reversed with thyroid hormone therapy.

AUTOIMMUNE THYROID DISEASES

- **Hashimoto's disease:** The thyroid gland is infiltrated by lymphocytes and elevated levels of antibodies against several components of thyroid tissue (e.g. antithyroid peroxidase [anti-TPO] and antithyroglobulin antibodies) are found in the serum. The thyroid gland is partly or completely destroyed, resulting in **hypothyroidism**.
- **Graves' disease:** Stimulatory antibodies to the thyroid-stimulating hormone (TSH) receptor activate thyroid hormone synthesis, resulting in **hyperthyroidism**. Bulging of eyes (exophthalmos) is a characteristic feature due to increase in retro-ocular fibro-adipose tissue and inflammatory edema of extraocular muscles (Fig. 13.8).
- **Postpartum thyroiditis:** It, usually, occurs within 3 to 12 months after delivery. The disease is characterized by a transient destruction-induced thyrotoxicosis (**hyperthyroidism**), often followed by a period of **hypothyroidism** lasting several months. Many patients, eventually, return to the euthyroid state. The postpartum occurrence of the disorder is likely a result of increased immune system function following the suppression of its activity during pregnancy. Since 5–10% of women develop postpartum thyroiditis, it is recommended that thyroid function (serum T_4, T_3 and TSH levels) be monitored postpartum at 2, 4, 6 and 12 months in all women with thyroid peroxidase antibodies or symptoms suggestive of thyroid dysfunction.

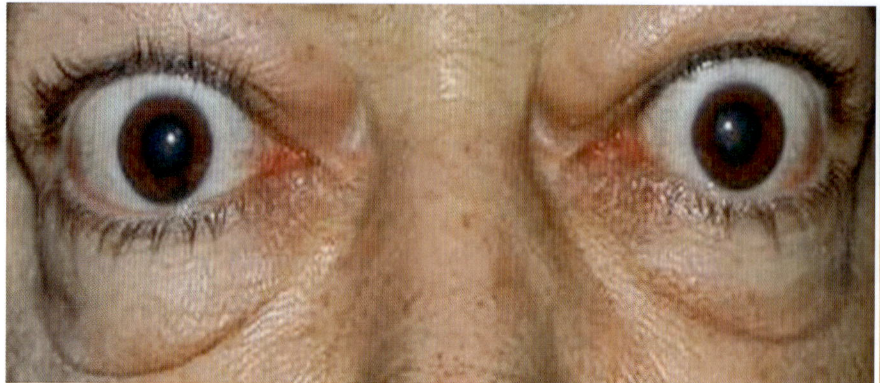
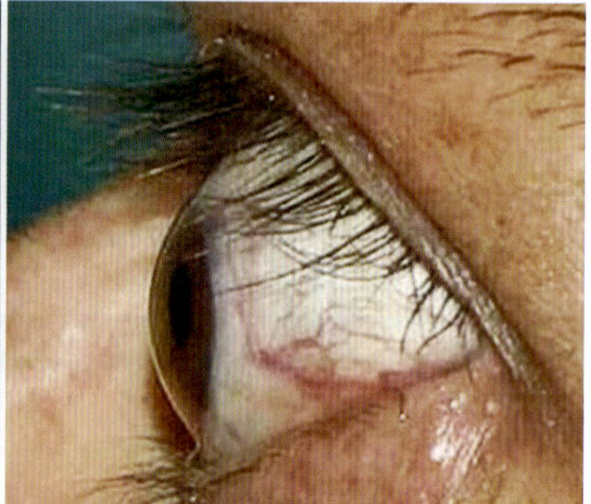

Fig. 13.8: Exophthalmos in Graves' disease

ADRENAL GLAND FUNCTION TESTS

The **adrenal glands** (also known as **suprarenal glands**) are endocrine glands found above the kidneys that produce a variety of hormones including adrenaline and the steroids, aldosterone and cortisol.

FUNCTIONS OF THE ADRENAL GLAND

An adrenal gland is made of two main parts, i.e. outer cortex (called **adrenal cortex**, which produces **steroid hormones)** and an inner medulla (called adrenal medulla, which produces catecholamines). **Both have very different functions.**

ADRENAL CORTEX

The **adrenal cortex** is the outer region and also the largest part of an adrenal gland. It is divided into three separate zones, i.e. **the zona glomerulosa**, **the zona fascilulata** and **the zona reticularis**.

Each zone is responsible for producing specific hormones:

13

- **Mineralocorticoids** are produced in the **zona glomerulosa**. The principle mineralocorticoid is **aldosterone** that plays a central role in regulating blood pressure and certain electrolytes (sodium and potassium). Aldosterone sends signals to the kidneys, resulting in the kidneys absorbing more sodium into the bloodstream and releasing potassium into the urine. This means that aldosterone also helps regulate the blood pH by controlling the levels of electrolytes in the blood.
- **The glucocorticoids** are synthesized in the **zona fasciculata**. Glucocorticoids released by the adrenal cortex include:
  - **Cortisol:** Also referred to as **hydrocortisone** regulates how the body converts fats, proteins and carbohydrates to energy. It also helps regulate blood pressure and cardiovascular function.
    - One of the primary activities of cortisol is to **increase available glucose to the nervous system** by breaking down protein and fat to glucose in the liver. It helps block glucose uptake into tissues other than the central nervous system.
    - Cortisol also has powerful **anti-inflammatory** and **antiallergy actions**. It decreases the activities of the immune system to reduce inflammation conditions. Because of this, it is used to treat dermatitis, insect bites, inflammation from arthritis and ulcerative colitis.
    - Cortisol reduces the capacity of osteoblasts to produce new bone tissue and decreases the absorption of calcium in the gastrointestinal tract.
  - **Corticosterone:** This hormone works with hydrocortisone to regulate immune response and suppress inflammatory reactions.
- **Androgens** (**DHEA** and **androgenic steroids)** are produced in the innermost layer of the cortex, i.e. the **zona reticularis**. These are precursor hormones that are converted in the ovaries into female sex hormones (**estrogens**) and in the testes into male sex hormones (**androgens**).

ADRENAL MEDULLA

The adrenal medulla is at the center of each adrenal gland, and is surrounded by the adrenal cortex. The chromaffin cells of the medulla are the body's main source of the catecholamines (adrenaline and noradrenaline) released by the medulla, hormones that initiate the flight or fight response. Approximately, 20% noradrenaline (norepinephrine) and 80% adrenaline (epinephrine) are secreted here. The adrenal medulla releases its secretions directly into the blood.

- **Epinephrine:** Epinephrine, most commonly known as **adrenaline**, rapidly responds to stress, by increasing heart rate and rushing blood to the muscles and brain. It also spikes blood sugar level by helping convert glycogen to glucose in the liver.
- **Norepinephrine:** Norepinephrine, also known as **noradrenaline**, works with epinephrine in responding to stress. However, it can cause vasoconstriction (the narrowing of blood vessels). This results in high blood pressure.

TESTS THAT ARE COMMONLY DONE IN CLINICAL PRACTICE TO ASSESS FUNCTIONS OF THE ADRENAL GLAND

BLOOD AND URINE LEVELS OF ADRENAL HORMONES

Measuring blood and urine levels of adrenal hormones, is often the first step in diagnosing a variety of disorders associated with adrenal gland dysfunction.

- **Aldosterone:** Both blood levels and urinary excretion of aldosterone may be measured. Overproduction (hyperaldosteronism) or underproduction (hypoaldosteronism) of aldosterone may be caused by tumors or other abnormalities within the adrenal glands (primary, e.g. adrenal cancer) or may result from problems outside the adrenals (secondary).
- **Cortisol:** Cortisol levels can be tested through **blood, urine** or **saliva**. Usually, both, blood levels and urine levels (known as free cortisol) are measured.

  Oversecretion of cortisol, most often, caused by a benign adrenal tumor, results in Cushing's syndrome. Undersecretion may indicate a form of adrenal insufficiency known as Addison's disease. The test is used in the diagnosis of these diseases and as a way to assess the functioning of the adrenal and pituitary glands.

  - **Blood cortisol** levels, naturally, rise and fall throughout the day. They are, usually, highest in the morning and lowest around midnight, but there are also variations that depend on the person. Normal results for a blood sample taken at 8 a.m. range between 6 and 23 micrograms per deciliter (μg/dl).

    Higher than normal cortisol levels may indicate that:

    - Pituitary gland is releasing too much ACTH due to a tumor or excess growth of the pituitary gland,
    - A tumor in the adrenal gland resulting in excess cortisol production, or
    - One may have tumor elsewhere in the body that is involved in cortisol production.

    Lower than normal cortisol levels may indicate that:

    - One has Addison's disease, which occurs when production of cortisol by adrenal glands is too low, or
    - Hypopituitarism, which occurs when production of cortisol by the adrenal glands is too low because the pituitary gland is not sending proper signals.
  - **The urine test** is done over a period of 24 hours.
    - The cortisol urine test tends to be more comprehensive than the other types of cortisol tests.
    - A normal adult range for cortisol levels in urine is, usually, between 3.5 and 45 micrograms per 24 hours.
- **18-Hydroxycortisol:** It is a product of cortisol metabolism. It is produced in excessive amounts in patients with primary hyperaldosteronism. Measuring blood levels of this hormone can help to determine whether primary hyperaldosteronism is caused by a tumor called adrenal adenoma, or by overgrowth (hyperplasia) of adrenal tissue; levels are significantly higher in people with an adenoma.
- **DHEA-S:** DHEA-S (dehydroepiandrosterone-sulfate) is a sex hormone (androgen) synthesized by the adrenal gland. It is a precursor to testosterone. In women, the adrenal glands are the major, and sometimes only, source of androgens. Elevated DHEA-S levels are associated with virilism (male body characteristics), hirsutism (excessive hair growth), amenorrhea (absence of menstruation) and infertility. Adrenal abnormalities such as tumors may lead to abnormally high DHEA-S levels.

OTHER TESTS

- **Dexamethasone-suppression test:** Dexamethasone suppression test measures the response of the adrenal glands to ACTH. Dexamethasone is given and levels of cortisol are measured. Cortisol levels should decrease in response to the administration of dexamethasone.

There are two different types of dexamethasone suppression tests, the low-dose test and the high-dose test. Each type can either be done in an overnight or standard (3 days) way. For the low-dose overnight method, 1 mg of dexamethasone is given at 11 p.m. and the blood is drawn at 8 a.m. for a cortisol measurement.

In the standard **low-dose method**, urine is collected over 3 days (stored in 24-hour collection containers) for measurement of cortisol. On day 2, a low dose (0.5 mg) of dexamethasone is given by mouth every 6 hours for 48 hours.

For the **high-dose** overnight method, a baseline cortisol is measured on the morning of the test and then 8 mg of dexamethasone is given at 11 p.m. Blood is drawn at 8 a.m. for cortisol measurement. For the standard high-dose test, urine is collected over 3 days (stored in 24-hour collection containers) for measurement of cortisol. On day 2, a high dose (2 mg) of dexamethasone is given by mouth every 6 hours for 48 hours.

- **ACTH stimulation test:** The ACTH stimulation test measures how well the adrenal glands respond to adrenocorticotropic hormone (ACTH), a hormone produced in the pituitary gland that stimulates the adrenal glands to release cortisol.

  This is the most specific test for diagnosing adrenal insufficiency. Blood cortisol levels are measured before and after a synthetic form of ACTH is given by injection.
- **Insulin-induced hypoglycemia test:** The insulin-induced hypoglycemia test is used to determine how the hypothalamus, pituitary and adrenal glands respond to stress. During this test, blood is drawn to measure the blood glucose and cortisol levels, followed by an injection of fast-acting insulin. Blood glucose and cortisol levels are measured again 30, 45 and 90 minutes after the insulin injection. The normal response is for blood glucose levels to fall (this represents the stress) and cortisol levels to rise.

ABNORMALITIES OF THE ADRENAL GLAND

ABNORMALITIES OF THE ADRENAL CORTEX

- **Hyperfunctioning of the adrenal cortex** can result in
  - **Cushing's syndrome** (Chemistry to Clinics 13.14)

Chemistry to Clinics 13.14: Cushing's Syndrome

Cause: It is due to increased production of cortisol by the adrenal cortex. However, prolonged use of corticosteroids for the treatment of some diseases also result in Cushing's-like features (iatrogenic Cushing's syndrome).

Presentation: Most of the features can be explained from the known biochemical functions of cortisol (Table 13.6).

- Hypercortisolism promotes deposition of adipose tissue in characteristic sites, notably the upper face (producing typical moon-like face), the interscapular area (producing buffalo-hump) and the mesenteric bed (producing truncal obesity) (Fig. 13.9A).

  The skin is thinned and weakened so that weight gain results in stretching and sometimes hemorrhages, giving the appearance of stretch marks or striae (Fig. 13.9B).
- It is also accompanied by increased hepatic gluconeogenesis and insulin resistance which, in turn, can cause impaired glucose tolerance or secondary diabetes mellitus.
- Other features include osteoporosis, diastolic hypertension, central adiposity, hirsutism and amenorrhea. Plasma and urine cortisol levels are variably elevated.
- Occasionally, hypokalemia, hypochloremia and metabolic alkalosis are present, particularly with ectopic production of ACTH.

Diagnosis: Plasma cortisol at 8 AM is >140 nmol/L (>5 μg/dl) after 1 mg dexamethasone challenge at midnight.

  - **Hyperaldosteronism** (Chemistry to Clinics 13.15)
- On the other hand, **hypofunctioning of the adrenal cortex** may cause **Addison's disease** (Chemistry to Clinics 13.16).

Table 13.6: Salient features of Cushing's syndrome

Normal biochemical function of glucocorticoids	Result of excess secretion of glucocorticoids (Cushing's syndrome) or prolonged use as a drug (iatrogenic Cushing's syndrome)
Anti-insulin action	Impaired glucose tolerance, diabetes mellitus
Protein catabolism	Muscle weakness
Lipogenesis in adipose tissue of selected body parts	Moon-like face, buffalo hump, truncal obesity
Immunosuppression	Susceptibility to infections
Weak mineralocorticoid-like activity	Water retention, edema, diastolic hypertension

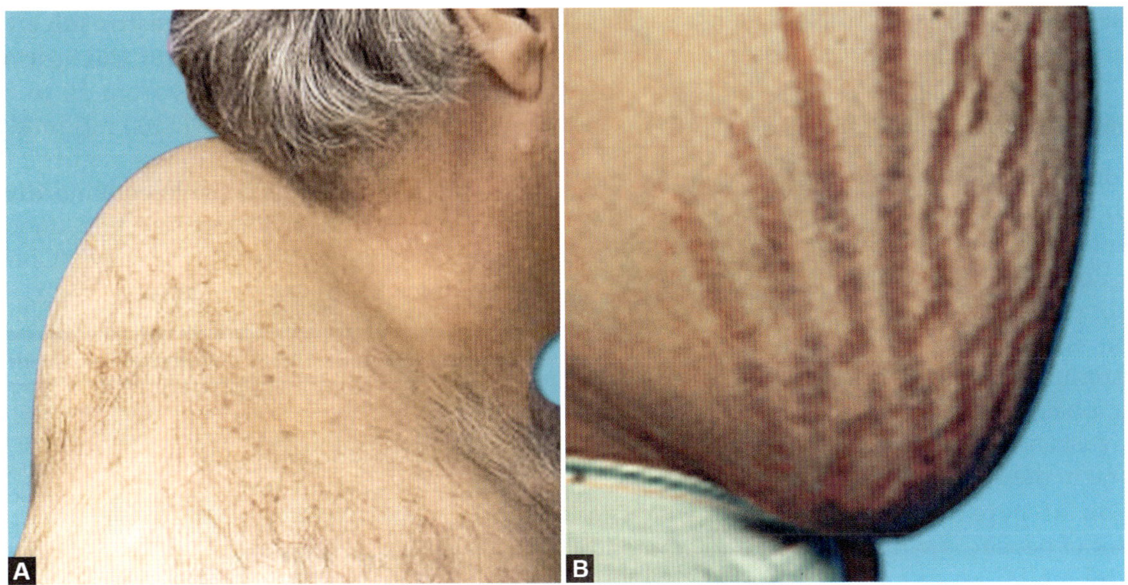

Fig. 13.9: Cushing's syndrome. (A) Buffalo hump; (B) Striae

Chemistry to Clinics 13.15: Hyperaldosteronism

It is a syndrome associated with hypersecretion of aldosterone (mineralocorticoids). In **primary hyperaldosteronism**, cause for excessive aldosterone production is an adenoma within the adrenal gland **(Conn's syndrome)**. The disease is characterized by hypokalemia, diastolic hypertension and muscle weakness. **Secondary hyperaldosteronism** refers to increased production of aldosterone in response to activation of the renin-angiotensin-aldosterone system. Secondary hyperaldosteronism in patients with accelerated hypertension is due to elevated plasma renin levels. In contrast, patients with primary hyperaldosteronism have suppressed plasma renin levels.

Chemistry to Clinics 13.16: Addison's Disease

It results from progressive destruction of adrenal glands. Half of the patients have circulating adrenal antibodies. Adrenal tuberculosis is a common cause in India. The disease is characterized by weakness, anorexia, nausea and vomiting, weight loss, cutaneous and mucosal pigmentation, hypotension and hypoglycemia. Serum sodium, chloride and bicarbonate levels are reduced while serum potassium is elevated. There may also be mild-to-moderate hypercalcemia.

ABNORMALITIES OF THE ADRENAL MEDULLA

Increased production of the hormones of the adrenal medulla may result in a condition designated as **pheochromocytoma** (Chemistry to Clinics 13.17).

Chemistry to Clinics 13.17: Pheochromocytoma

It is a tumor of the adrenal medulla. It is called the **'10% tumor'** because nearly 10% are bilateral, 10% are multiple, 10% are extra-adrenal, 10% are malignant, 10% are familial and 10% occur in children. Patients with pheochromocytoma produce, store and secrete increased amounts of catecholamines. Hypertension is the most common sign. Most of the patients secrete greater amount of norepinephrine. There is impaired glucose tolerance, elevated hematocrit and hypercalcemia in majority of the patients. Diagnosis is established by the increased urinary excretion of catecholamines or catecholamine metabolites, particularly **vanillylmandelic acid (VMA)**.

GASTRIC FUNCTION TESTS

The stomach functions as a temporary storage organ for food. It secretes about 2–3 liters of gastric juice every day. Most of this juice is produced by exocrine glands located in the body and fundus of the stomach. These exocrine secretory glands contain three types of secretory cells, i.e. the chief cells, the parietal cells and the mucous cells.

- **The chief cells**, located in the basal regions of these glands and also in the glands of the antrum, secrete **pepsinogen** (the inactive precursor of pepsin).
- **The parietal cells** secrete **HCl**. In addition to converting pepsinogen to pepsin, HCl provides optimum pH for the activity of this enzyme. The parietal cells also secrete **intrinsic factor** necessary for the intestinal absorption of vitamin B_{12} which is required for formation of normal RBCs.
- **The mucous cells** are located at the necks of these glands, in the glands of the antrum and scattered throughout the gastric epithelial lining. These cells secrete **alkaline mucous containing fluid** which

coats the gastric wall and protects against various forms of damage to the gastric mucosa.

BIOCHEMICAL FUNCTIONS OF THE STOMACH

- **Secretion of HCl:** The important function of the stomach is that parietal cells secrete an iso-osmotic solution of HCl with a hydrogen ion concentration ≈150 mEq/L (pH 0.9–1.0). Both excitatory and inhibitory mechanisms regulate gastric HCl secretion. The gastric mucosa is rich in histamine, a potent stimulus of parietal cell secretion. During the cephalic phase, there is release of acetylcholine as well as gastrin, both of which cause the release of histamine in the vicinity of the parietal cells.
- **Secretion of pepsin:** Pepsinogen, the inactive precursor of pepsin, is synthesized by and stored in the chief cells as zymogen granules. Once pepsinogen enters the gastric lumen, HCl and pre-existing pepsin convert it to pepsin. Both acetylcholine and peptides stimulate secretion of HCl by the parietal cells and thus, in turn, play an important role in the activation of pepsin as well as in the maintenance of the highly acidic environment required for its optimal activity (Fig. 13.10).

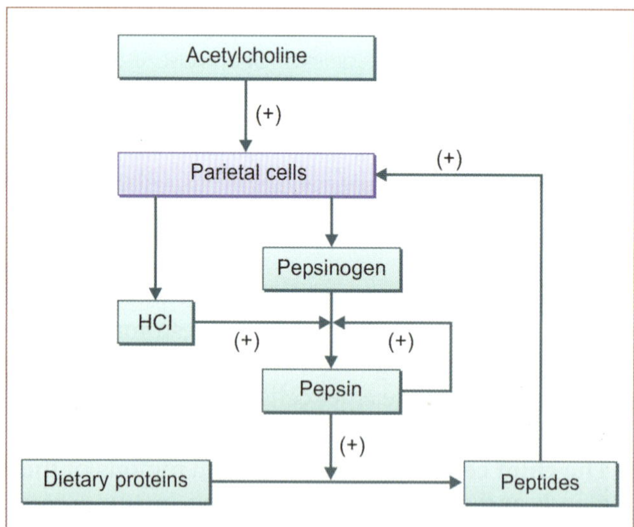

Fig. 13.10: Secretion and activation of pepsinogen

TESTS THAT ARE COMMONLY DONE IN CLINICAL PRACTICE TO ASSESS FUNCTIONS OF THE STOMACH

13

The content of the stomach after nearly 12 hours of fast is defined as **gastric residue (residuum)**. It is obtained by aspiration through a gastric tube (**Ryle's tube**) and examined for the following:

- **Physical characteristics of gastric juice**
  - **Volume:** Total volume of the resting gastric residue normally varies from 20 to 50 ml. An increase in the volume (>100 ml) may be due to hypersecretion, retention or regurgitation from duodenum and is considered abnormal. Various causes include pyloric obstruction, duodenal ulcer or Zollinger-Ellison syndrome (Chemistry to Clinics 13.18).

Chemistry to Clinics 13.18: Zollinger-Ellison Syndrome

It is due to a gastrin-secreting tumor of the endocrine pancreas. Excess gastrin overstimulates gastric acid secretion resulting in abdominal pain, mucosal ulceration and diarrhea. It is suspected in patients of acid-peptic disease who fail to respond to conventional treatment with H2-receptor blockers and proton pump inhibitors.

  - **Consistency:** The resting gastric juice is fluid in consistency. It may be viscous in the presence of mucus. Food particles may be present in carcinoma of the stomach.
  - **Color:** The resting gastric content is usually colorless. It may be slightly yellow or green due to regurgitation of bile, or red/brown due to the presence of blood.
- **Chemical constituents of gastric juice**
  - **Bile:** It may be found in gastric residuum as a result of intestinal obstruction or ileal stasis.
  - **Mucus:** Small amount of mucus is found normally. Increased amounts may be seen in gastritis and gastric carcinoma.
  - **Blood:** Accidental trauma to the gastric mucous membrane during the passage of Ryle's tube may result in traces of blood in the gastric juice. Increased amounts of blood may be present due to gastric carcinoma, erosive gastritis or bleeding peptic ulcer.
  - **Organic acids:** Lactic and butyric acids may be present in large amounts in hypoacidity, achlorhydria and carcinoma of the stomach. In the absence of free HCl, these organic acids are formed in increased amounts by bacterial fermentation of food, as food is retained in the stomach for longer periods (usually more than 6 hours) at neutral or alkaline pH.
  - **Pepsin:** Absence of pepsin is seen in a condition called achylia gastrica. Decreased pepsin levels are seen in diseases associated with chief cell mass, atrophic gastritis and gastric carcinoma. Increased pepsin activity may be observed in disease

associated with increased gastric output as in patients with Zollinger-Ellison syndrome, duodenal ulcer, gastritis and after the administration of proton pump inhibitors such as omeprazole.

- **Estimation of free acidity**

  The main acid in the gastric juice is HCl which is a strong mineral acid. It accounts for free acidity. HCl is secreted by the parietal cells at a concentration of about 150 mEq/L with pH <1.0. As the parietal secretion gets mixed with other gastric constituents, the concentration of hydrogen ions usually reaches <40 mEq/L with a pH of 1.5–3.5.

  Concentration of free acidity in gastric residue in normal individuals varies from 0 to 40 mEq/L (Chemistry to Clinics 13.19).

Chemistry to Clinics 13.19: Gastric Acidity

- **Hyperchlorhydria: When free acidity is increased**, the condition is called hyperchlorhydria. It occurs in duodenal and gastric ulcers, and in diseases of the gallbladder.
- **Hypochlorhydria: Decreased secretion of HCl** is called hypochlorhydria. It is observed in gastric carcinoma, chronic gastritis, constipation and anemias.
- **Achlorhydria: Complete absence of HCl** in the gastric juice is called achlorhydria. It occurs in pernicious anemia. Absence of free HCl in gastric residue is considered abnormal only if the condition persists after maximal stimulation with pentagastrin. In the absence of HCl, bacterial fermentation of food is increased which leads to the formation of lactic acid. A small percentage of the healthy individuals (about 4% of the young ones and 25% at age 60 years) may have no free HCl in the fasting stomach.

- **Estimation of total acidity**

  Total acidity in gastric residue includes hydrogen ions occurring as free HCl, mucoproteins, acid salts and organic acids, such as lactic and butyric acids. The total acid concentration in a normal state is usually 10–50 mEq/L.

STIMULATION OF GASTRIC SECRETION

Many compounds or processes such as test meal, alcohol, caffeine, gastrin, pentagastrin or insulin stimulate gastric secretion and, in turn, the secretion of HCl.

- **Test meals:** Stimulation of gastric secretion by administration of a test meal such as toast with water or tea (Ewald's meal) was practiced in the past. This test however, is not used these days.
- **Alcohol:** 50–100 ml of 7% ethyl alcohol (3.5 ml ethanol in 50 ml water) may be administered through the syringe attached to the tube as a stimulant for HCl secretion.
- **Caffeine:** Caffeine sodium benzoate, 500 mg in about 200 ml of water, may be administered into the stomach through a gastric tube as a stimulant of gastric secretion.
- **Histamine:** Histamine is a powerful stimulant for the secretion of gastric juice. It causes secretion of an increased volume of highly acidic gastric juice with low pepsin content. Two types of histamine tests may be carried out.
  - **Standard histamine test:** In the standard histamine test, subcutaneous injection of histamine (0.01 mg/kg body weight) is given and the gastric contents are removed. Absence of free HCl in gastric secretion after histamine indicates achylia gastrica.
  - **Augmented histamine test:** A large dose of histamine (0.04 mg/kg body weight) is given for the augmented histamine test. In pernicious anemia no free HCl is secreted but in other forms of achlorhydria some amount of free HCl may be secreted, after augmented histamine stimulation test is performed (Chemistry to Clinics 13.20).

Chemistry to Clinics 13.20: Antihistaminics

Sometimes a high dose of histamine may cause a severe reaction mediated through H1 receptors. Under such a condition, an injection of H1 antihistamine may be given intramuscularly. This does not interfere in gastric stimulation because the gastric effects of histamine are mediated through H2 receptors.

- **Insulin:** Intravenous injection of 0.1–0.2 U/kg body weight of soluble insulin may also be given for the stimulation of gastric secretion and gastric samples are withdrawn after every 15 min. This is called **Hollander test**. Insulin stimulation is helpful to ascertain the effectiveness of vagotomy in patients with duodenal ulcer. In these patients, concentration of free HCl may be as high as 1200 mEq/L. After successful vagotomy, since there is no response to insulin, gastric acidity remains at a low level of 15–20 mEq/L before as well as after insulin administration.

  As insulin may cause hypoglycemia the test is not preferred.
- **Gastrin and pentagastrin:**
  - **Gastrin** is the most powerful stimulus for gastric HCl secretion. Gastrin is administered in a single subcutaneous dose of 2 mg/kg body weight.

- **Pentagastrin**, a synthetic pentapeptide with a physiologically active part of the gastrin molecule, is also a potent stimulus for gastric HCl secretion and is commonly used these days.

Basal acid output: The fasting content of the stomach is aspirated and its volume is measured. This is termed as the basal acid output (**BAO**). The secretions are collected at 15 minute intervals for 1 hour.

Maximal acid output: Pentagastrin is then given at a dose of 6 mg/kg body weight subcutaneously and post-stimulation secretions are again collected at 15 min intervals for the next 1 hour. This acid output is termed as the maximal acid output (**MAO**).

This test is useful in differentiating the diagnosis of achlorhydria and hyperchlorhydria. In normal persons, the BAO ranges from 0–10 mEq/h. After stimulation with pentagastrin, MAO varies from 0–35 mEq/h. A large volume of fasting juice indicates obstruction of gastric outlet. A very high BAO suggests that the patient has Zollinger-Ellison syndrome.

PANCREATIC EXOCRINE FUNCTION TESTS

The pancreas serves two functions which are carried out by different groups of cells within the organ. These two groups of cells are designated as the endocrine and the exocrine portions of the pancreas.

Endocrine Pancreas

The endocrine pancreas consists of group of cells known as the **islets of Langerhans**, which are embedded in the exocrine portion of the gland. Islets are composed of four major cell types, each of which synthesize and secrete a different hormone. These include glucagon producing alpha cells, insulin producing beta cells, somatostatin producing delta cells and a pancreatic polypeptide producing F cells.

Exocrine Pancreas

The exocrine secretory cells are called acinar cells arranged in sac-like clusters called acini. These cells secrete a small volume of juice containing the digestive enzymes of the pancreas. The acini are connected by small intercalated ducts to larger ducts that converge into one duct which delivers the exocrine secretion of the pancreas into the duodenum. The epithelial cells lining the intercalated ducts secrete a relatively large volume of juice with a high concentration of the alkaline salt sodium bicarbonate.

13

BIOCHEMICAL FUNCTIONS OF THE EXOCRINE PANCREAS

Production and secretion of pancreatic juice: Exocrine functions of the pancreas, as described above, include the production and secretion of pancreatic juice, which is rich in several enzymes and bicarbonate.

Total volume of pancreatic juice secreted in a normal human is 500–800 ml/24 hours. It is **strongly alkaline** with a pH of about 8.0. Its alkalinity is **due to the presence of bicarbonate** (HCO_3^-), since pancreatic juice contains nearly 70–100 mEq/L of HCO_3^-.

Bicarbonate neutralizes acid that arrives in the duodenum from the stomach and **performs two functions:**

1. It protects the delicate lining of the upper small intestine from damage by acid.
2. It ensures optimal pH for activity of the pancreatic digestive enzymes (Chemistry to Clinics 13.21).

Chemistry to Clinics 13.21: Acute Pancreatitis

Acute pancreatitis is a condition in which activated proteolytic enzymes are liberated from the pancreatic acinar cells, and in turn, attack the pancreas itself. This self-digestion process often results in reduced output of both pancreatic digestive enzymes as well as bicarbonate.

The pancreas also secretes several digestive enzymes (Table 13.7).

Regulation of exocrine pancreatic secretion

Secretion of the pancreatic juice is controlled by two mechanisms, i.e. by **hormonal control** and the **nervous control** (via vagus nerve).

- Two **hormones**, secretin and cholecystokinin, which are released from the duodenal mucosa during the intestinal phase of digestion regulate bicarbonate and enzyme secretion by the pancreas.
  - **Secretin** is released into the blood in response to HCl. After its release, the hormone stimulates the intercalated duct cells of the pancreas to secrete bicarbonate-rich juice. The secretion, in turn, neutralizes the acid that causes secretin to be released and so reduces the stimulus for additional secretin release until more acid enters the duodenum from the stomach.
  - **Cholecystokinin** is released from duodenal mucosa in response to protein and lipid digestion products. The hormone stimulates the pancreatic acinar cells to secrete digestive enzymes. As a result, more digestion products are produced which further stimulate the pancreas to secrete more enzymes. The process continues as long as food remains in the small intestine to be digested (Fig. 13.11).

Table 13.7: Digestive enzymes of the pancreatic juice

Enzyme	Substrate	Digestion products
Trypsin	Proteins and peptides	Small peptides
Chymotrypsin	Proteins and peptides	Small peptides
Carboxypeptidase A and B	Proteins and peptides	Peptides and amino acids
Amylase	Starch	Oligosaccharides, maltose
Lipase	Triacylglycerols	Monoacylglycerols and free fatty acids
Phospholipase A_2	Lecithin	Lysolecithin and free fatty acid
Cholesterol esterase	Cholesterol esters	Cholesterol and free fatty acids
RNase	RNA	Ribonucleotides
DNase	DNA	Deoxyribonucleotides

- Vagus stimulation also **helps in the secretion of enzymes**.

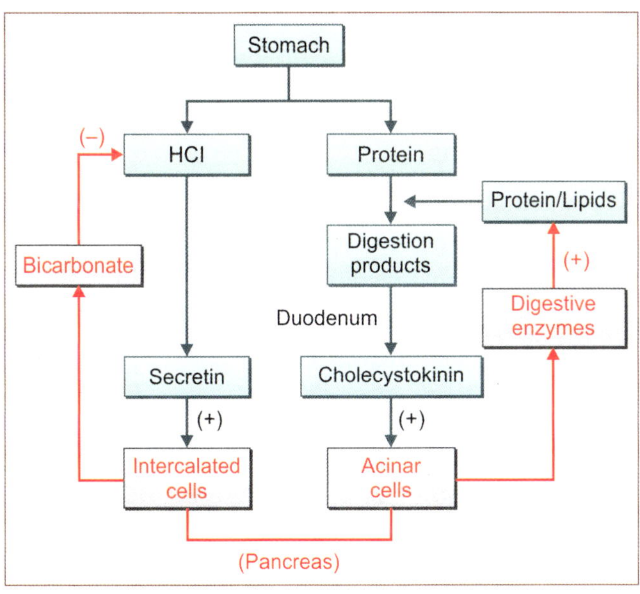

Fig. 13.11: Regulation of exocrine pancreatic secretion

TESTS THAT ARE COMMONLY DONE IN CLINICAL PRACTICE TO ASSESS EXOCRINE FUNCTIONS OF THE PANCREAS

Volume and Bicarbonate Concentration of the Pancreatic Juice

The exocrine secretory capacity of the pancreas is assessed by intubating the duodenum and subjecting the pancreas to stimulation with a test meal, secretin or pancreozymin. After the duodenal contents are aspirated, the patient is given secretin (1 unit/kg body weight) intravenously and the aspirate is examined for volume, bicarbonate content and amylase activity.

In pancreatitis, there is usually a reduction in the volume of pancreatic juice as well as its bicarbonate output. In the milder form of pancreatitis, volume of the pancreatic juice and its bicarbonate contents are fairly normal but enzyme activities particularly the activity of amylase is reduced. Patients with chronic pancreatitis are unable to secrete juice of high bicarbonate content (<90 mEq/L). Carcinoma of the head of pancreas obstructs the overall volume flow.

Estimation of Enzymes in Serum/Urine

- **Serum and urinary amylase:** Serum and urine amylase activities are increased in acute pancreatitis. In early stages of the disease, determination of serum amylase is of great diagnostic importance. Rise starts within 2–12 hours of the onset of pain and usually returns to normal within 3–5 days. There is also an increase in urinary amylase.
- **Serum lipase:** Serum lipase activity rises slower than that of amylase, within 4–8 hours and normalizes by 7–14 days. Thus, it remains elevated for a longer duration than serum amylase. Further, serum lipase as compared to serum amylase is elevated more often in patients with pancreatic carcinoma.
- **Serum elastase:** Elastase I is a pancreatic proteolytic enzyme that hydrolyzes scleroproteins, a basic ingredient of the connective tissue. It is produced in the acinar portion of the pancreas and appears in the exocrine pancreatic secretion as zymogen (pro-elastase). This, in turn, is activated by trypsin. Serum elastase I is of significance in the later stages of acute pancreatitis or in patients with relapse or cystic complications of chronic pancreatitis. Elastase I remains abnormally elevated longer than amylase.

Some Important Questions

1. Briefly discuss:

i. Thyroid function tests
ii. Kidney function tests
iii. Renal clearance tests
iv. Gastric function tests
v. Differential biochemical diagnosis of jaundice
vi. Pancreatic function tests
vii. Liver function tests

2. Write notes on:

i. Neonatal jaundice
ii. GFR
iii. Tubular function tests
iv. Cystatin C
v. Zollinger-Ellison syndrome
vi. Delta bilirubin

Multiple Choice Questions

1. The following proteins are not synthesized in the liver:

A. α_1-Globulins
B. α_2-Globulins
C. γ-Globulins
D. β-Globulins

2. Highest concentration of γ-GT normally occurs in:

A. Liver
B. Kidneys
C. Small intestine
D. Lungs

3. The maximum urea clearance is:

A. 54 ml/min
B. 75 ml/min
C. 100 ml/min
D. 125 ml/min

4. The normal inulin clearance is:

A. 54 ml/min
B. 75 ml/min
C. 100 ml/min
D. 125 ml/min

5. A useful index of renal plasma flow is:

A. Inulin clearance
B. PAH clearance
C. Creatinine clearance
D. Urea clearance

6. LATS antibodies are seen in:

A. Graves' disease
B. Hashimoto's disease
C. Postpartum thyroiditis
D. Myxedema

7. All are autoimmune in nature, *except*:

A. Endemic goiter
B. Hashimoto's disease
C. Graves' disease
D. Postpartum thyroiditis

8. What is not associated with Cushing's syndrome

A. Hypokalemia
B. Hypochloremia
C. Metabolic alkalosis
D. Respiratory alkalosis

9. Achylia gastric is associated with:

A. Loss of HCl secretion
B. Loss of enzymes
C. Loss of both HCl secretion and enzymes
D. None of the above

10. Exocrine function of pancreas cannot be assessed by:

A. Serum lipase level
B. Serum elastase level
C. Serum insulin level
D. Serum amylase level

CHAPTER

14

Structure and Functions of Nucleic Acids

Competency Achievement: The student should be able to:

BI7.2 Describe the structure and functions of DNA and RNA and outline the cell cycle

Nucleic acids are the macromolecules constituted by the repeated monomeric units called nucleotides (*see* Chapter 7).

Nucleic acids include **DNA (deoxyribonucleic acid)** and **RNA (ribonucleic acid)**. They are strongly acidic in nature and, thus, are negatively charged at physiological pH. Nucleic acids occur in association with basic proteins, such as histones and protamines. They store information and make it available to the cell.

DEOXYRIBONUCLEIC ACID

DNA (deoxyribonucleic acid) stores genetic information and is called the chemical basis of heredity. DNA is a double-stranded polymer of deoxyribonucleotides, which are linked by phosphodiester bonds.

Various features of DNA structure were first described by Watson-Crick; therefore, it is called the Watson-Crick model or Watson-Crick structure of DNA. Watson-Crick described that:

- DNA is a **polynucleotide** of deoxyadenylate (dAMP), deoxyguanylate (dGMP), deoxycytidylate (dCMP) and thymidylate (TMP).
- The information content of a DNA molecule resides in the **sequence** in which these monomers (purine and pyrimidine deoxyribonucleotides) are ordered.
- The polymer possesses a **polarity** where one of its ends has a 5′-hydroxyl or phosphate terminus while the other end has a 3′-phosphate moiety or a hydroxyl group.
- DNA molecule is **double-stranded**.
- The two chains run **antiparallel** to each other, i.e. one strand runs in the 5′→3′ direction while the other in the 3′→5′ direction (Fig. 14.1).
- Both the polynucleotide chains are wound around a common axis so as to form a **right-handed helix**. The double helix so formed is nearly 2 nm in diameter.
- A base occupies the core of the helix while sugar-phosphate chains run along the periphery and form two grooves of unequal width. These are called the **major groove** and the **minor groove** (Fig. 14.2).
- The helix has a **pitch** (rise/turn) of 3.4 nm and has 10 base pairs within each turn.
- The two strands of the double-stranded molecule are held together by **hydrogen bonds** between a purine base and a pyrimidine base of the respective polynucleotide chain.

```
5′—— A — G — C — C — G — T — T — A — A — A — G — C — G — T — A ———— 3′
     |   |   |   |   |   |   |   |   |   |   |   |   |   |   |
3′—— T — C — G — G — C — A — A — T — T — T — C — G — C — A — T ———— 5′
```

Fig. 14.1: A double-stranded nucleic acid molecule

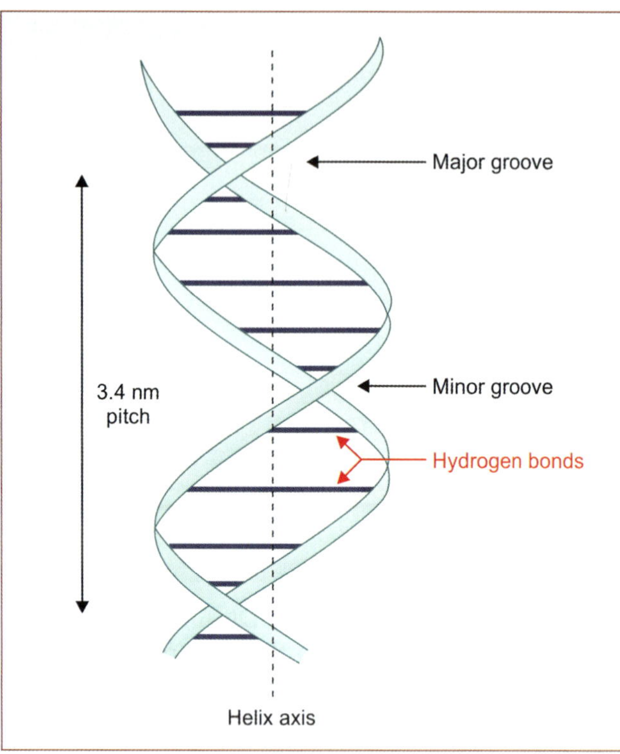

Fig. 14.2: DNA double-helix

- **Chargaff's rule:** The base-pairing is very specific, as A is linked to T with two hydrogen bonds and G is linked to C with three hydrogen bonds (Fig. 14.3).

DNA molecule thus has equal number of adenine and thymine residues (A=T) as well as guanine and cytosine residues (G≡C). This relationship is known as Chargaff's rule.

The hydrogen-binding interaction, a phenomenon known as **complementary base pairing**, results in specific association of the two chains of a double helix. It finds application in DNA denaturation/renaturation.

Denaturation and Renaturation (Melting and Annealing) of DNA

Two strands of the DNA double helix get separated (referred to as **melting**) when a solution of duplex DNA is heated above certain temperature. This process of complete separation (or unwinding) of the two strands *in vitro* is called **denaturation**.

- It results in breakage of hydrogen bonds between the bases causing separation of the base pairs.
- Denaturation of DNA also results in qualitative changes in physical properties of the DNA such as decrease in viscosity or increase in ultraviolet absorbance, called **hyperchromicity**, at 260 nm.

The temperature at which DNA is half denatured is called **melting temperature** or **Tm** of DNA. At Tm, absorbance of UV light is 50% between the maximum and minimum. The Tm depends on nature of the solvent, concentration of ions in the solution and pH, and base composition of the DNA.

When the melted sample of DNA is slowly cooled to temperature below Tm, it results in reformation of complementary base pairs, as per Chargaff's rule, and form DNA double helix. This is referred to as **renaturation** or **annealing** (Fig. 14.4).

Denaturation/renaturation cycle is used in the polymerase chain reaction.

The process of the formation of RNA–DNA (hybrid) double helix, from the complementary strands of RNA and DNA, is called **hybridization**.

Short stretches of RNA–DNA hybrids are known to occur during initiation of DNA replication, by small fragments of RNA.

T=A

C≡G

Fig. 14.3: Hydrogen bonds in DNA

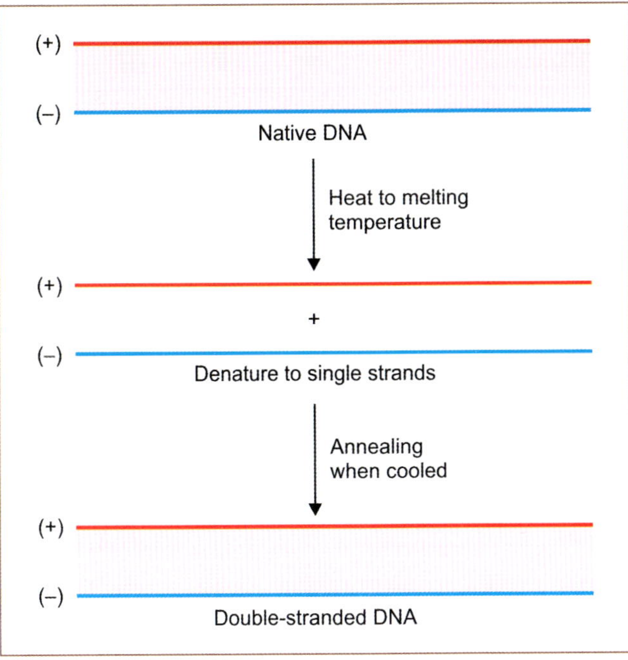

Fig. 14.4: Denaturation and annealing of DNA

STRUCTURAL FORMS OF DOUBLE HELIX DNA

A double helix DNA can assume various distinct structures, depending upon base sequence and composition of the solvent. There are 3 major structural forms of DNA, described as B-DNA (described by Watson and Crick), A-DNA and Z-DNA (Table 14.1).

Plasmids

Plasmids are small, circular, **extrachromosomal DNA** molecules, 1–200 kb in size, which are found in most species of bacteria. Plasmid DNA carries genetic information and undergoes replication.

Plasmids facilitate the transfer of genetic information from one bacterium to another, and are used as vectors in recombinant DNA technology, e.g. *E. coli* plasmid pBR322. These small circular DNA molecules automatically replicate in a bacteria or yeast cell and provide resistance to antibiotics (Fig. 14.5).

Plasmids that contain DNA sequences, called cos sites, required for packaging DNA into the phage particle are designated as **cosmids**. Cosmids can accept very large DNA fragments (35–40 kb).

Mitochondrial DNA

Mitochondria contain circular molecules of DNA, referred to as mtDNA, each one of which codes for various polypeptides required for the process of oxidative phosphorylation. The mtDNA is maternally inherited and has a high rate of mutation (*see* Chapter 1).

Functions of DNA

DNA controls every aspect of cellular function, i.e.

- It makes copies of itself as a cell divides and thus transfers genetic information from one generation to the next. This process is known as replication.
- DNA also determines the properties of a living cell and regulates biological information by controlling protein synthesis.
- The biological information passes from one class of nucleic acid to another, i.e. from DNA to RNA. This is known as transcription.

Table 14.1: Comparison of different types of DNA

Parameter	B-DNA	A-DNA	Z-DNA
Formation	Commonest form	Formed from B-DNA under dehydrating conditions	Transiently formed from B-DNA during transcription; may relieve torsional strain
Overall proportions	Long, thin	Short, broad	Elongated, slim, zig-zag [due to complementary polynucleotides with alternating purines and pyrimidines, such as poly d(CG) • poly d(GC) or poly d(AC) • poly d(TG)]
Helix rotation sense	Right-handed	Right-handed	Left-handed
Base pairs per turn	10	11	12
Pitch	3.4 nm	2.8 nm	4.5 nm
Helix axis location	Through base pairs	Major groove	Minor groove
Major groove	Wide, intermediate depth	Very narrow and deep	Flattened out
Minor groove	Narrow, intermediate depth	Very broad and shallow	Very narrow and deep

14

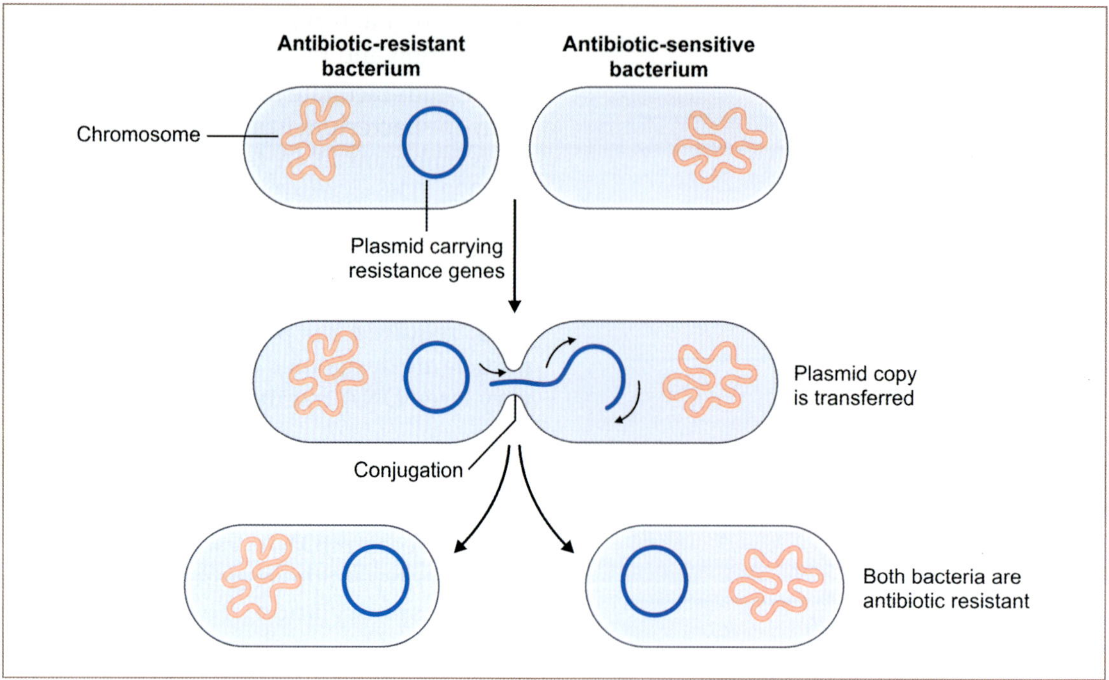

Fig. 14.5: Plasmid-mediated transfer of antibiotic resistance

- The sequence of bases in RNA is then translated into the sequence of amino acids and forms a protein. This is called translation.

DNA molecule thus serves as a template both for the transcription of information into RNA as well as for the replication of information into daughter DNA (Fig. 14.6).

RIBONUCLEIC ACIDS

Ribonucleic acids (RNA) also have purine and pyrimidine bases, and 3′,5′-phosphodiester linkages but RNAs have several specific structural differences from DNA.

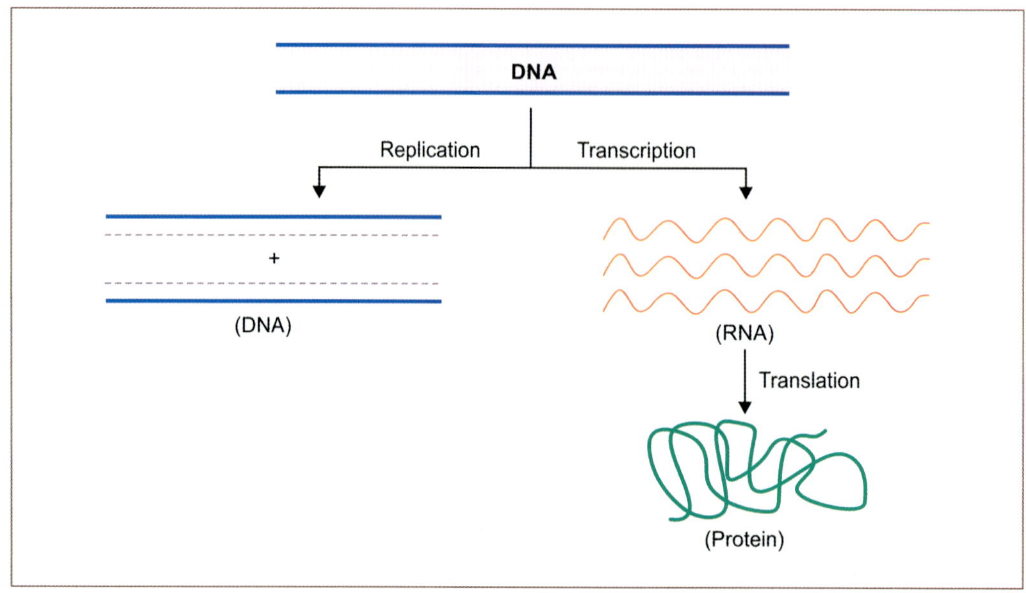

Fig. 14.6: Cellular functions of DNA

DIFFERENCES BETWEEN DNA AND RNA

1. As the name suggests, the sugar moiety in RNA is ribose instead of deoxyribose in DNA.
2. RNA does not contain thymine (which is present in DNA); instead, it has uracil.

   RNA is a polymer of ribonucleotides of adenine, guanine, cytosine and uracil.
3. Unlike DNA, RNA is generally a single-stranded molecule. Therefore, in RNA, guanine content may not necessarily be equal to its cytosine content. Similarly, the adenine content need not to be equal to the uracil content.
4. RNA is alkali labile because of the presence of 2′-hydroxyl groups.

TYPES OF RNA

Three main classes of RNA, i.e. messenger RNA, ribosomal RNA and transfer RNA are found in all eukaryotic as well as prokaryotic cells. Although all three types of RNA are involved in protein biosynthesis, they differ from each other with respect to their size, composition, location within the cell, and functions.

Messenger RNA

Messenger RNAs (mRNAs) are most heterogeneous, highly elongated and short-lived molecules. These are synthesized within the nucleus as a result of the transcription of a DNA molecule. Their features include:

- The mRNA transcript has 5′→3′ polarity which is complementary to the coding strand of its gene (DNA molecule) but there occurs a difference in the pyrimidine base, as mRNA contains uracil in place of thymine present in the DNA strand (Fig. 14.7).
- The mRNA conveys message (information) from the gene to the protein synthesizing machinery. This information is present in the mRNA molecule in the form of codons (the sequence of nucleotides as triplets). Each mRNA serves as a template on which specific sequence of amino acids is polymerized to form a specific protein, the ultimate product of a gene.
- The mRNA is, generally, stable in eukaryotes but quite unstable in prokaryotes.

  In mammalian cells, the primary transcription product of DNA is a larger molecule called heterogeneous nuclear RNA (**hnRNA**). The hnRNA molecules undergo post-transcriptional changes and form mRNA which are released into the cytoplasm where they serve as templates for protein biosynthesis.

Transfer RNA

Transfer RNAs (tRNAs) are much smaller in size, and consist of nearly 75 to 90 ribonucleotides. tRNA molecules comprise about 15% of the total cellular RNA. tRNA is also known as soluble RNA (sRNA) because it is found in the soluble fraction of the cell.

There are about 40 different tRNAs, each one of which fulfills the role of an adaptor molecule and has a sequence called anticodon. Thus, each tRNA, bearing an amino acid, has a unique property of locating itself at the correct codon for translation of information (present in the sequence of nucleotides of mRNA) into specific amino acids in the protein chain.

Specific tRNAs although differ from each other in their nucleotide sequence, as a class they have many common features:

- The nucleotide sequence (the primary structure) allows extensive folding and intramolecular base-pairing to form a secondary structure, giving the clover leaf-like appearance (Fig. 14.8).

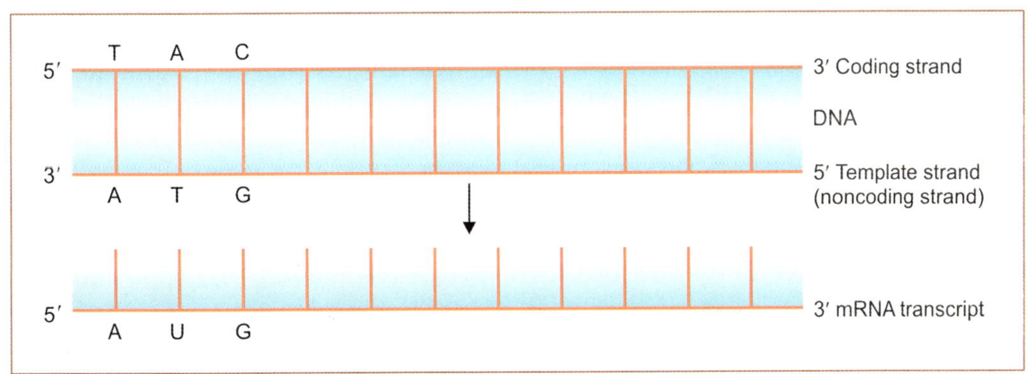

Fig. 14.7: mRNA transcript from a DNA molecule

14

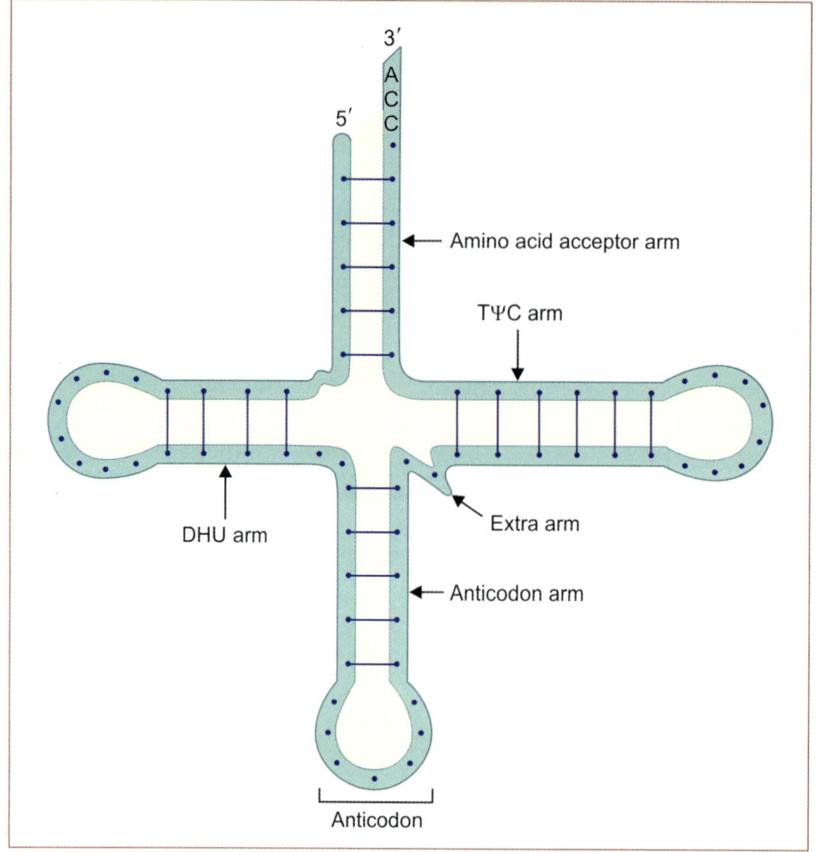

Fig. 14.8: tRNA

- All tRNAs, in addition to the 4 usual bases (A, G, C and U), also have several unusual (modified) bases, e.g. 7-methylguanine, thymine, dihydrouracil, pseudouracil, hypoxanthine, etc.
- All tRNA molecules have 4 main arms, which are designated as the amino acid acceptor arm, the anticodon arm, DHU arm and TΨC arm. In addition, there is also a small loop, designated as extra arm.

Amino acid acceptor arm: The amino acid acceptor arm has a 7 base-paired stem which terminates in CCA (5′→3′ sequence) whose A (the adenosyl moiety) accepts an amino acid. The carboxyl group of the amino acid forms an ester linkage with 3′-hydroxyl group of the adenosyl moiety.

Anticodon arm: The anticodon arm has 5 base pairs and a loop which has a triplet nucleotide sequence (the anticodon), complementary to the codon. This anti-codon is responsible for the specificity of a tRNA molecule.

14

The other two arms have unusual bases and are named accordingly as the DHU arm and the TΨC arm.

DHU arm: The DHU arm has dihydrouracil (DHU) in its loop and 3 or 4 base-paired stem.

TΨC arm: The TΨC arm has a sequence of thymine (T), pseudouracil (Ψ) and cytosine (C) in the loop, and a stem having 5 base pairs.

Extra arm: An extra arm may have 3–5 base pairs.

Ribosomal RNA

Ribosomal RNAs (rRNAs) are present in the ribosomes, in association with a number of polypeptides. Ribosomes are found in the cytoplasm and contain nearly 80% of the total cellular RNA. Ribosomes combine to form polyribosomes which are the active units in protein biosynthesis.

Both mRNA and tRNA interact on ribosomes to translate the information transcribed from the gene into the specific protein molecule. Mammalian ribosomes are very complex with a sedimentation velocity of 80S. Each ribosome has 2 subunits, i.e. a large subunit (60S) and a small subunit (40S). The large subunit contains 3 different rRNAs, i.e. 5S, 5.8S and 28S along with more than 50 specific polypeptides. The small subunit has an 18S rRNA and nearly 30 polypeptides (Fig. 14.9).

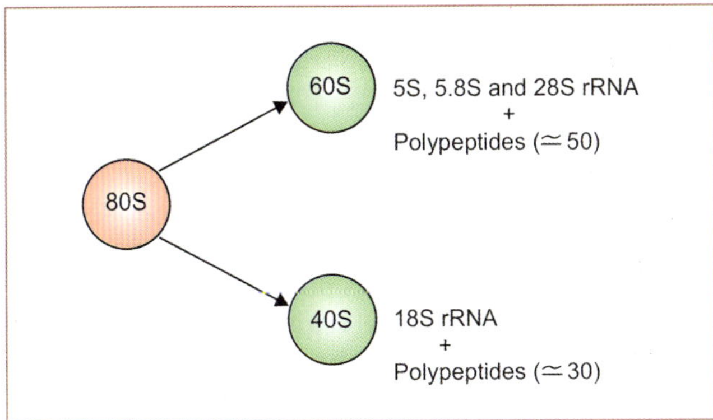

Fig. 14.9: Mammalian ribosomes

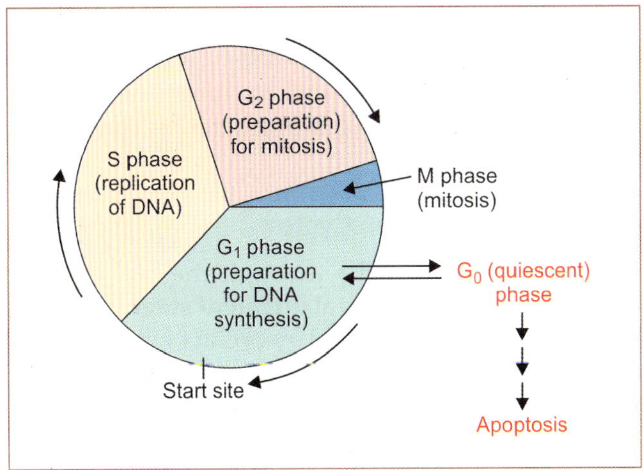

Fig. 14.10: Cell cycle

CELL CYCLE

The **cell cycle**, or **cell-division cycle**, is the series of events that take place in a cell that cause it to divide into two daughter cells. These events include the duplication of its DNA (DNA replication) and some of its organelles and subsequently, the partitioning of its cytoplasm and other components into two daughter cells in a process called cell division. This cyclic process results in cell proliferation and is called **proliferative cell cycle.**

In cells with nuclei, i.e. in eukaryotes, the cell cycle is divided into two main stages referred to as interphase and the mitotic (M) phase (including mitosis and cytokinesis). **During interphase**, the cell grows; accumulating nutrients needed for mitosis, and replicates its DNA and some of its organelles. **During the mitotic phase**, the replicated chromosomes, organelles, and cytoplasm separate into two new daughter cells.

Phases of the Cell Cycle

The eukaryotic cell cycle consists of four distinct phases referred to as **G_1 phase**, **S phase** (synthesis), **G_2 phase** and **M phase** (mitosis and cytokinesis; Fig. 14.10).

The stages in the cell cycle between one mitosis and the next (which include G_1, S and G_2) are known, collectively, as the **interphase**.

M phase is itself composed of two tightly coupled processes, called **mitosis** (in which the cell's nucleus divides) and **cytokinesis** (in which the cell's cytoplasm divides forming two daughter cells).

Activation of each phase is dependent on the proper progression and completion of the previous one. While some cells are constantly dividing, some cell types are at rest. These cells may exit G_1 and enter a **resting state called G_0**.

- **G_1 phase**
  - Cell increases in size
  - Cellular contents duplicated
- **S phase**
  - DNA replication
  - Each of the 46 chromosomes (23 pairs) is replicated by the cell
- **G_2 phase**
  - Cell grows more
  - Organelles and proteins develop in preparation for cell division
- **M phase**
  - Mitosis, followed by cytokinesis (cell separation)
  - Formation of two identical daughter cells
- **G_0 phase**

  After completing mitosis, some cells, e.g. hepatocytes enter a prolonged phase, out of the cell cycle, called the **quiescent phase** (G_0). Concentration of the various regulatory molecules, such as growth factors, can divert the cell into G_0, or stimulate quiescent cells to active cycling.
  - **Nonproliferative** (nondividing) **cells in multicellular eukaryotes**, generally, enter the quiescent G_0 phase from G_1 and **may remain quiescent for long periods of time, possibly indefinitely** (as is often the case for **neurons**). This is very common for cells that are fully differentiated.
  - **Some cells enter the G_0 phase semipermanently** and are considered post-mitotic, e.g. **liver, kidney** and **stomach cells.**

- Many cells **do not enter G_0** and continue to divide throughout an organism's life, e.g. **epithelial cells**.

Quiescence can be followed by **apoptosis** if it lasts too long while uncontrolled proliferation can lead to **neoplasm/tumor**.

Regulation of the Cell Cycle

The progression of cells through the cell cycle is controlled by **checkpoints at different stages**. This cell cycle is also closely regulated by **cyclins which control cell progression** by activating **cyclin-dependent kinase (CDK) enzymes**.

- **The checkpoints:** To ensure the proper replication of cellular components and division, there are control mechanisms known as **cell cycle checkpoints** after each of the key steps of the cycle that determine if the cell can progress to the next phase. The checkpoints detect if a cell contains damaged DNA, and ensure those cells do not replicate. The **restriction point (R)** is **located at G_1** and **is a key checkpoint**. The vast majority of cells that pass through the R point will end up completing the entire cell cycle. **Other checkpoints** are located at the **transitions between G_1 and S**, and **G_2 and M**.

  If damaged DNA is detected at any checkpoint, **activation of the checkpoint results in increased protein *p53* production**. The p53 is a **tumor suppressor gene** that **stops the progression of the cell cycle** and **starts repair mechanisms** for the damaged DNA. **If** this DNA **cannot be repaired**, then it ensures the **cell undergoes apoptosis** and can no longer replicate.
- **Cyclins and Cyclin-dependent Kinases:** Two key classes of regulatory molecules called **cyclins** (the proteins, whose concentration increase or decrease throughout the cycle) and **cyclin-dependent kinases (CDKs)**, determine a cell's progress through the cell cycle. **Cyclins form the regulatory subunits** and **CDKs the catalytic subunits** of an activated heterodimer. Cyclins have no catalytic activity and CDKs are inactive in the absence of cyclin. **When activated by a bound cyclin, CDKs phosphorylate substrates**, which are essential **for progression through the cell cycle**. **CDKs are constitutively expressed in cells**, whereas **cyclins are synthesized at specific stages of the cell cycle**, in response to various molecular signals.

  An example of a **tumor suppressor protein** is **retinoblastoma protein (*Rb*)**. The *Rb* restricts the ability of a cell to progress from G_1 to S phase in the cell cycle. CDK phosphorylates ***Rb*** to ***pRb***, making it unable to restrict cell proliferation. This allows cells to divide normally in the cell cycle.

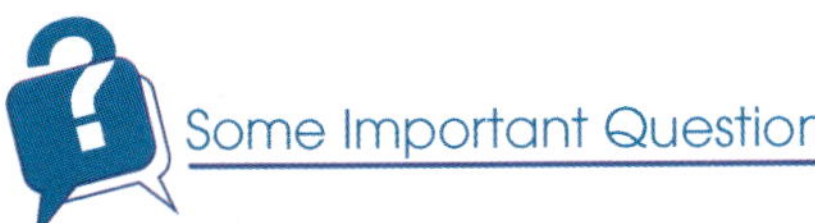

Some Important Questions

1. Describe various special features of the Watson-Crick model of DNA.

2. What are various types of RNAs? Describe their functions.

3. Explain:

i. Structure and function of tRNA
ii. Differences between DNA and RNA

4. Write notes on:

i. Ribosomes
ii. B-DNA
iii. A-DNA
iv. Z-DNA
v. Plasmid
vi. Mitochondrial DNA
vii. hnRNA
viii. Cell cycle
ix. Cyclins
x. Cyclin-dependent kinases

Multiple Choice Questions

1. At physiological pH, nucleic acids are:

A. Negatively charged
B. Positively charged
C. Uncharged
D. Uncharged zwitterions

2. Proliferative cell cycle consists of:

A. Synthetic phase, mitosis, the interphase and the gap 2 phase
B. Synthetic phase, mitosis, the quiescent phase and the gap 2 phase
C. Mitosis, the interphase, the quiescent phase and the gap 2 phase
D. Synthetic phase, mitosis, the interphase and the gap 1 phase

3. In the Watson-Crick DNA model, the number of hydrogen bond(s) between G and C is/are:

A. 1 B. 2
C. 3 D. 4

4. During DNA denaturation, the following bond(s) is/are broken:

A. Phosphodiester
B. Hydrogen
C. Glycosidic
D. All of the above

5. The Watson-Crick model originally described the following:

A. Z-DNA B. B-DNA
C. A-DNA D. Denatured DNA

6. The biologically commonest form of DNA is:

A. B-DNA B. A-DNA
C. Z-DNA D. None of these

7. The diameter of Watson-Crick B-DNA double helix is:

A. 0.2 nm B. 2.0 nm
C. 0.34 nm D. 3.4 nm

8. hnRNA is found in the:

A. Nucleus
B. Cytoplasm
C. Ribosomes
D. Smooth endoplasmic reticulum

9. The specificity of a tRNA molecule lies in the:

A. Amino acid acceptor arm
B. Anticodon arm
C. TΨC arm
D. DHU arm

10. 80% of total cellular RNA is present in the:

A. Cytosol B. Ribosomes
C. Nucleoplasm D. Nucleolus

CHAPTER 15

Processes of Replication, Transcription and Translation

Competency Achievement: **The student should be able to:**

BI7.2 Describe the processes involved in replication and repair of DNA and the transcription and translation mechanisms

REPLICATION

The **process of DNA synthesis** is called **replication**. It is a semiconservative process.

Semiconservative Process

During replication, each strand of the double-stranded DNA serves as a **template** for the synthesis of a new strand, in a very accurate manner. Since both the strands of the parental DNA double helix can serve as template and produce two daughter DNA molecules, therefore, after a round of replication, each of the two newly formed double-stranded DNA molecules contain one strand from the parental double-stranded DNA while the other one is a newly synthesized complementary strand.

This process of DNA replication where after each round of replication, one strand in a double helix is maintained intact (parental strand) and combines with the other one which is a newly synthesized daughter strand, is called **semiconservative** replication (Fig. 15.1).

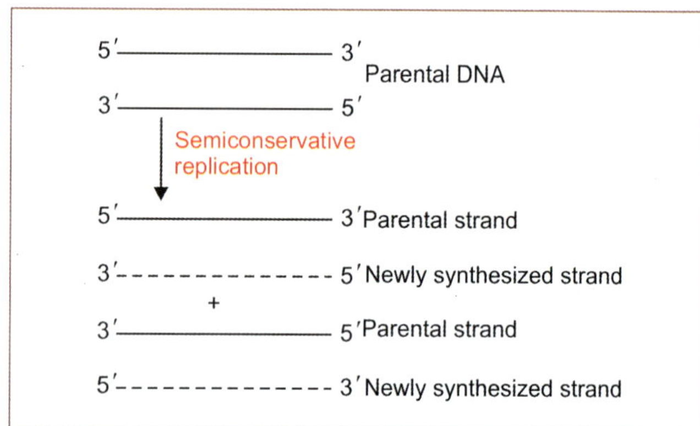

Fig. 15.1: Semiconservative replication

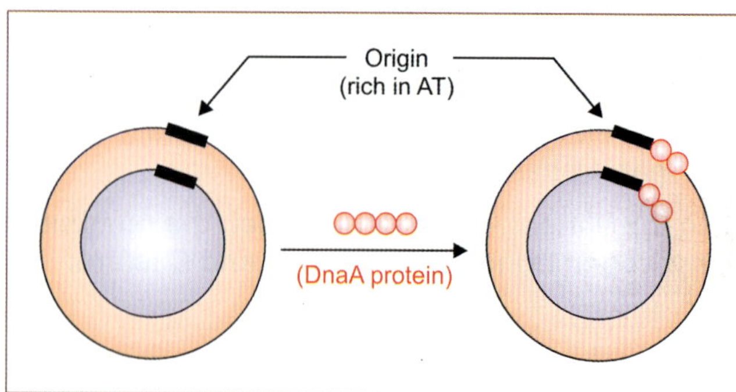

Fig. 15.2: Binding of DnaA at origin of replication

Cellular Requirements for DNA Replication

The following proteins/enzymes are required by the cell for the process of replication:

- **DnaA protein:** DnaA is a protein that binds at the origin of replication. It is also called the **origin-binding protein.**

  Nearly, **20–50 monomers of DnaA bind** at the specific **nucleotide consensus sequence that** is present at the origin of replication. This binding in turn requires ATP and results in **separation (melting) of two strands of the DNA** (Fig. 15.2).

- **Single strand DNA-binding protein:** Single strand DNA-binding (SSB) protein binds to the single-stranded DNA and prevents the two strands from rejoining. They are stripped-off the SSB-protein, before the replication begins.

  In eukaryotes, the two strands of DNA, after their separation, are covered with another protein, which is referred to as **replication protein A,** also called

replication factor A. It is functionally similar to the SSB-protein, which occurs in prokaryotes.

- **Helicases:** Helicase is the enzyme that separates two strands of the DNA. This enzyme initiates the unwinding of the double helix, at the single-stranded region, adjacent to the duplex and functions in a particular polarity only.
  In eukaryotes, helicase activity is associated with the enzyme **DNA polymerase δ.**
- **Topoisomerases:** As we know, chromosomes of many bacteria and viruses are the circular molecules of the double helix DNA and have a peculiar twisted appearance. This is referred as **supercoiling** or **superhelicity** (Fig. 15.3).

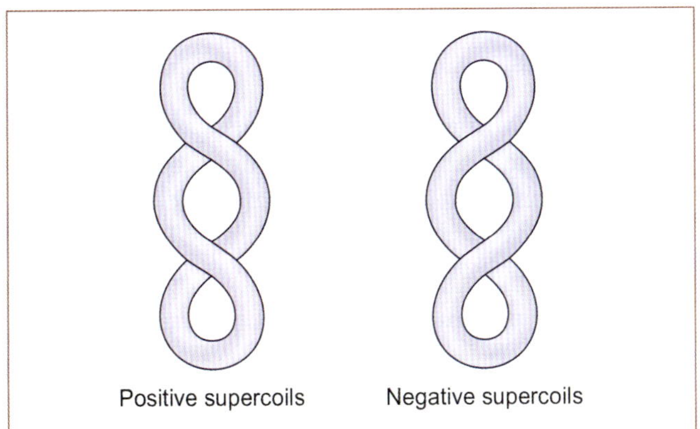

Fig. 15.3: The coiling of duplex DNA around its own axis is called supercoiling. Positive supercoils twist the DNA in the same direction as the turns of the right-handed double helix. Positively supercoiled DNA is overwound (wound more tightly). Negative supercoils twist the DNA about its axis in the opposite direction from the clockwise turns of the right-handed double helix. Negatively, supercoiled DNA is underwound (and thus favors unwinding of duplex)

The group of enzymes, called topoisomerases overcomes supercoiling. They are endonucleases, which **alter topological coiling of the circular DNA.** They introduce nicks in one or both the strands, remove supercoils, and reseal the ends. There are several types of topoisomerases (Table 15.1).

Topoisomerase II inhibitors are in common clinical use (Chemistry to Clinics 15.1).

Chemistry to Clinics 15.1: Topoisomerase II Inhibitors

Antimicrobials of the quinolone category such as norfloxacin, ciprofloxacin, ofloxacin, etc. and some anticancer agents such as doxorubicin and etoposide, block topoisomerase II activity. These compounds thus arrest DNA replication as well as RNA transcription, which explains the high clinical potency of these drugs. On the other hand, drugs like camptothecin, anthracycline, etc., interfere only with the enzyme catalyzed resealing of the DNA strands. They do not affect the overall activity of the enzyme but convert these topoisomerases into the DNA-breaking agents. Since DNA degradation leads to cell death, these drugs are used in the treatment of certain hematological neoplasms, e.g. leukemias and lymphomas.

If the topological problems are not corrected, it may stop unwinding of the parent DNA and hence, DNA replication.

- **DNA polymerases:** DNA polymerases (DNA-dependent DNA polymerases) are the enzymes that catalyze the synthesis of the complementary strand, on the single-stranded DNA template. They add nucleotides at the free 3′-OH group and extend the chain in 5′→3′ direction (Fig. 15.4).
  Different types of the DNA polymerases are found in prokaryotes and eukaryotes.

Table 15.1: Topoisomerases: Salient features

Type	Target DNA	Activity		ATP	Effects in	
		Endonuclease	Ligase	required	Prokaryotes	Eukaryotes
I	One strand	Yes	Yes	No	Relax negative supercoils	Relax both negative and positive supercoils
II	Both strands	Yes	Yes	Yes	Relax both negative and positive supercoils. Introduce negative supercoils into relaxed DNA (gyrases)	–
III	One strand	Yes	Yes	No	Remove circular DNA products called catenates which are generated just prior to the completion of DNA replication	–
Reverse gyrase	Both strands	Yes	Yes	Yes	Found in archaebacteria: Introduce positive supercoils into DNA and prevent denaturation from high temperature and acidity	–

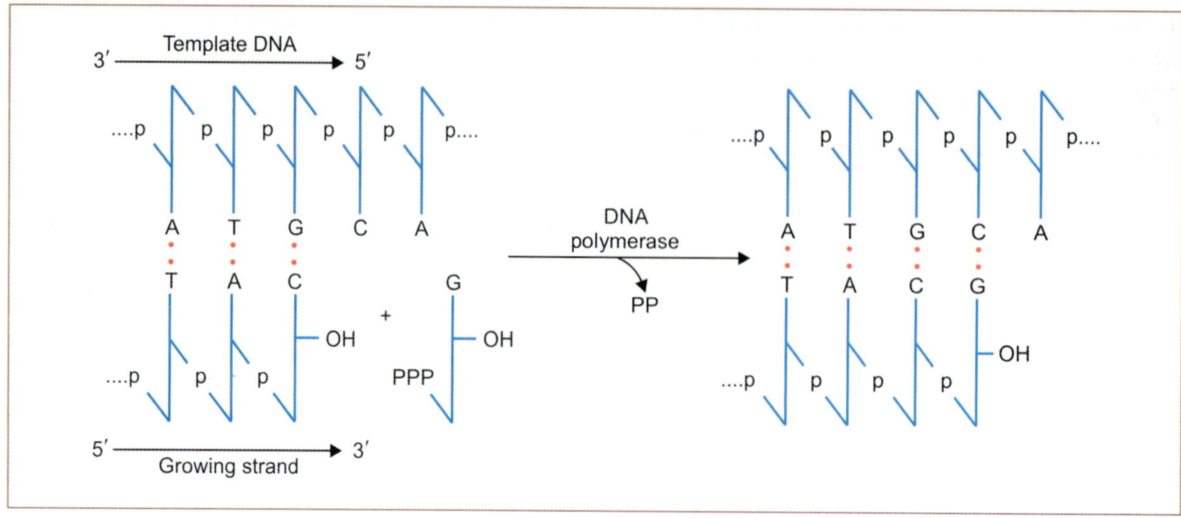

Fig. 15.4: Action of DNA polymerase

– *DNA polymerases in prokaryotes*

Three distinct forms of the enzyme are found in prokaryotes. These are designated as DNA polymerase I, II, and III.

- **DNA polymerase I: DNA polymerase I (pol I)** has **three distinct activities,** i.e. it has 5′→3′ **polymerase (synthetic) activity** and both, 3′→5′ and 5′→3′ **exonuclease (hydrolytic) activity.** **The enzyme has two fragments,** which are referred to as the large fragment and the small fragment:
  - **The large fragment** is designated as **Klenow fragment**. It has 5′→3′ **polymerase** and 3′→5′ **exonuclease activities.**
  - The **small fragment** has 5′→3′ **exonuclease activity.**

  DNA polymerase I also **edits mistakes** and its **proofreading action** suggests that the enzyme has high fidelity in DNA replication. It is also important in the repair of the damaged DNA.
- **DNA polymerase II: DNA polymerase II (pol II)** has 5′→3′ **polymerase** activity along with the 3′→5′ **exonuclease activity** but lacks 5′→3′ exonuclease activity. It mainly participates in the process of DNA repair.
- **DNA polymerase III: DNA polymerase III (pol III)** is a more complex enzyme, as it consists of at least **ten different subunits. All the subunits** together form a labile multisubunit enzyme, known as **pol III holoenzyme**. It **polymerizes** DNA and **edits mistakes** but lacks nick-translation.

15

– *DNA polymerases in eukaryotes*

Five different types of DNA polymerases are found in eukaryotes. These are designated as DNA polymerase α, β, γ, δ and ε. **All** have **5′→3′ synthetic activities**. With the exception of the polymerase γ, which occurs in mitochondria, they are involved in the chromosomal DNA synthesis as well as its repair.

- **DNA polymerase α: DNA polymerase α (pol α)** has 5′→3′ **polymerase activity** but lacks proofreading (exonuclease) activity. Thus, **it can replicate DNA** but **cannot correct its mistakes**. It also has tightly **associated primase activity,** which is concerned with the priming (initiation) of replication. It is also called the **lagging strand replicase.**
- **DNA polymerase δ: DNA polymerase δ (pol δ) has,** 5′→3′ **polymerase activity** and 3′→5′ **exonuclease (proofreading) activity. Pol δ** has a very **high processivity when associated with a protein** called **proliferating cell nuclear antigen** (PCNA). The **pol δ-PCNA complex** is designated as the **leading strand replicase** (Chemistry to Clinics 15.2).

Chemistry to Clinics 15.2: Proliferating Cell Nuclear Antigen (PCNA)

PCNA is a protein (**cyclin**) which forms a trimer ring around a DNA double helix. It binds to a variety of other nuclear proteins and organizes biochemical processes at the DNA replication fork. It functions in DNA synthesis, repair, chromatin remodeling, regulation of cell cycle and apoptosis. It is a cell proliferation marker hence, a tumor with higher number of PCNA-positive cells is likely to be more aggressive and better respond to anticancer drugs. Anti-PCNA antibodies occur in many cancers as well as autoimmune diseases, e.g. systemic lupus erythematosus.

- **DNA polymerase ε: DNA polymerase ε (pol ε),** though resembles pol δ, but is **highly processive even in the absence of the factor, PCNA.** It also has 3′→5′ **exonuclease activity** and is involved in repairing of the damaged nuclear DNA.
- **DNA polymerase β: DNA polymerase β (pol β)** is a small polypeptide. Its biological function is not yet known.
- **DNA polymerase γ: DNA polymerase γ (pol γ) occurs exclusively in mitochondria** and is involved in the mitochondrial DNA replication only.

Reverse Transcriptase

RNA-dependent DNA polymerase, designated as **reverse transcriptase**, is also a member of the **polymerase family of enzymes**. It is found in **retroviruses** (RNA-containing eukaryotic viruses), such as **human immunodeficiency virus (HIV)**, which is the causative agent of the **acquired immunodeficiency syndrome (AIDS).**

Reverse transcriptase **catalyzes synthesis of the double-stranded DNA, from the single-stranded RNA template.**

PROCESS OF REPLICATION IN PROKARYOTES

DNA replication is a complex process, which involves initiation, elongation and termination.

Initiation of DNA Replication

Initiation of DNA replication involves formation of the replication fork and synthesis of the RNA primer.

Formation of Replication Fork

- **Replication starts at** the site referred to as **origin of replication**. It is designated as ori C, in *E. coli*. The sequence of nucleotides at the origin is **rich in AT**.
- The **DnaA protein binds at the origin**.
- Binding of DnaA at the AT-rich region **promotes unwinding of the two strands of the parent DNA.**
- After the two strands get separated, the **circular chromosome exhibits a bubble-like structure**, called **replication bubble (replication eye).** The branch point in the replication bubble, at which DNA synthesis begins, is called **replication fork.** Formation of the replication fork initiates stepwise assembly of various proteins and enzymes that are required for DNA replication (Fig. 15.5).
- With the movement of the enzyme helicase **two single-stranded regions of the parent DNA are generated.**
- Subsequently, the SSB-protein covers the two strands and keeps them apart from each other.

Synthesis of RNA Primer

- Synthesis of RNA primer begins with the **formation of prepriming complex** (prepriming assembly),

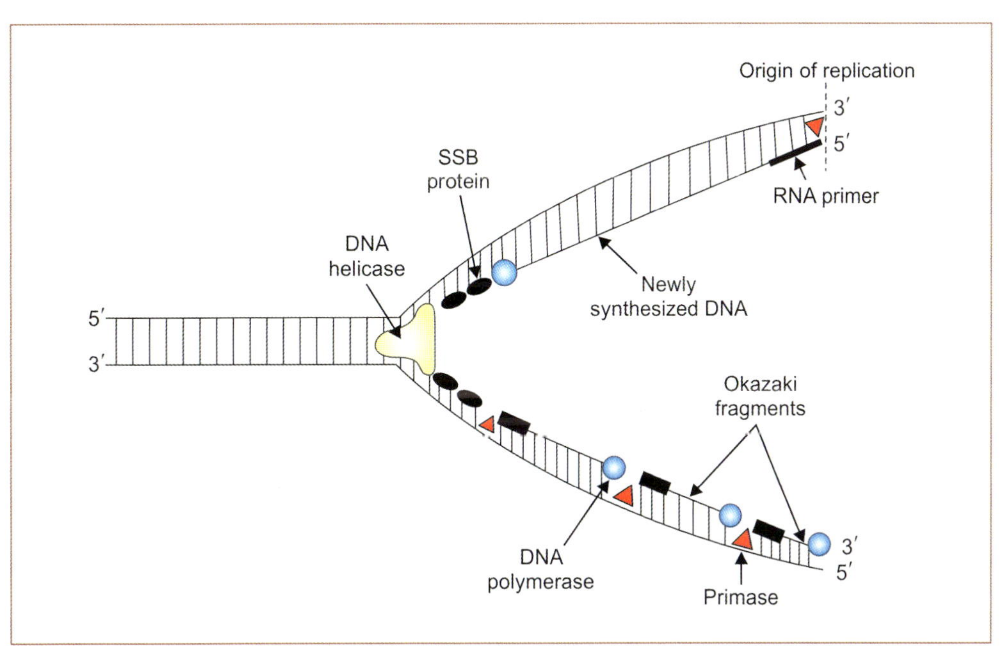

Fig. 15.5: A replication fork

15

which consists of **DnaB**, **DnaC** and four other proteins referred to as **n, n′, n″** and **i**.

- The pre-priming complex **associates with the enzyme primase** (called RNA polymerase) and **forms primosome (the priming complex)**.
- The **primosome interacts with the template** (at the replication fork) and **begins the synthesis of the RNA primer**. Whereas, only one priming complex is required to initiate the synthesis of the leading strand, multiple copies of the complex are required for the synthesis of the lagging strand.
- After the site of the primer, initiation has been recognized, SSB-proteins are displaced and the primase lays down the primer.

  Note: During the process of replication, two antiparallel DNA strands are simultaneously replicated at the two advancing replication forks in the 5′→3′ direction, but differently. One of its strands is **synthesized continuously** (in the direction of the movement of the replication fork). This is called the **leading strand**. On the other hand, the **other strand** is synthesized **discontinuously**, i.e. in small fragments (though it is also synthesized in the 5′→3′ direction only). This strand is called the **lagging strand**. These **fragments** are called **Okazaki fragments**. Okazaki fragments vary in size from about 100–200 deoxyribonucleotides, in eukaryotes, to nearly 1000–2000 deoxyribonucleotides, in prokaryotes.

Elongation of Replication

Elongation of replication is carried out by an assembly referred to as **replisome (replicase system).** Various components of the replisome are shown in Table 15.2.

Table 15.2: Components of a replisome

Component protein/ enzyme	Functions
DnaA	Unwinding of two strands of DNA at the origin of replication
DnaB	Helicase activity, unwinds DNA for creation of the initiation bubble
Topoisomerase II	Removal of supercoils
SSB-protein	Binds to single strands of the DNA, to keep two strands apart from each other.
DnaC	Binding with the SSB-protein at the origin of replication
Primase	Synthesis of the RNA primer
n, n′, n″ and i proteins	Primosome assembly
DNA polymerase III	Chain elongation on the 3′-OH group of the primer
DNA polymerase I	Excision of the primer and gap-filling
DNA ligase	Ligation of the polynucleotide fragments

A replisome exists only as a protein complex, which is associated with the particular structure that DNA takes at the replication fork.

- The replisome (which contains two polymerase III holoenzymes) synthesizes the leading strand as well as the lagging strand.
- It moves, as a single unit, in the 5′→3′ direction along the leading strand, whereas the lagging strand template loops around to permit the holoenzyme to extend the primed lagging strand. After completing the synthesis of an Okazaki fragment, holoenzyme (on the lagging strand) is relocated to the new primer, near the replication fork, and extends the RNA primer to form a new Okazaki fragment. At each location, DNA polymerase uses RNA primer, for the synthesis of DNA. After the polymerase reaches the end of the single-stranded template, it takes over the next primer that is annealed to the template, as DNA–RNA hybrid.
- In eukaryotes, the primers may be formed at several locations, which are determined by nucleosome spacing. This, in turn, results in **continuous synthesis of the leading strand** and **several RNA primed Okazaki fragments** (which are separated from each other by the single-stranded nicks) **on the lagging strand**. In this process, synthesis of the leading strand is always ahead of the synthesis of the lagging strand.
- Thereafter, **DNA polymerase I replaces ribonucleotides** (from RNA primer) **with the deoxyribonucleotides** and finally, the **nicks are sealed by DNA ligase.**

Termination of the Process of DNA Replication

A protein designated as the **Tus protein** (terminator utilization substance), arrests the movement of the replication fork and **terminates DNA replication**.

- The Tus protein acts as a contra-helicase and **binds** to a region called **ter site,** which has **GT rich termination sequence.** This in turn **prevents advancement of the replication fork**, by arresting the action of **DnaB.** Finally, **delinking of the parent strands,** from the daughter strands, is catalyzed by the enzyme topoisomerase.

DIFFERENCES IN PROCESSES OF REPLICATION IN PROKARYOTES AND EUKARYOTES

As shown in Table 15.3, DNA replication in **eukaryotes differs from** the process in **prokaryotes** in several ways.

Table 15.3: Differences in DNA replication between prokaryotes and eukaryotes

Prokaryotes	Eukaryotes
Replication begins at the origin	Replication begins at multiple sites, simultaneously
SSB-protein keeps two strands separate	Replication protein A keeps two strands separate
Only negative supercoils are relaxed	Both negative and positive supercoils are relaxed
There are three types of DNA polymerases, called polymerase I, II and III	There are three types of DNA polymerases, called polymerase α, β, γ, δ and ε.
Helicase is a specific enzyme	Helicase activity is associated with DNA polymerase α
Primase is a specific RNA polymerase	Primase activity is present in DNA polymerase α
Both the DNA strands are synthesized by DNA polymerase III	Leading strand is synthesized by DNA polymerase δ while lagging strand is synthesized by DNA polymerase α
Very long Okazaki fragments are synthesized	Small size Okazaki fragments are synthesized
The process is simple, rapid and error-prone	The process is complex, slow but accurate

1. The amount of DNA present in the eukaryotic cell is much more than the prokaryotic cell.
2. **Eukaryotic cell contains large number of the DNA polymerase molecules** (often more than 20,000) as compared to the small number (a few dozen), that occur in a prokaryotic cell.
3. **Origin of replication** in eukaryotes has specific sequences, termed **autonomous replicating sequences (ARSs)**. Each such sequence is 100–200 base-pair (bp) in size and has **AT-rich central region**. It is the 11-bp element and is designated as **ARS-ACS (autonomous consensus sequence).**
4. Initiation of the **DNA replication occurs at several origins of replication,** simultaneously, in eukaryotes. DNA segment between the two origins of replication is termed as **replicon**. An average human chromosome may contain about 100 replicons, hence, replication may proceed at nearly 200 forks, simultaneously.
5. **Eukaryotic DNA synthesis requires a protein,** called **replication protein A** (replication factor A), which is functionally as the SSB-protein in prokaryotes.
6. In eukaryotes, **helicase** activity is associated with the DNA **polymerase δ.**
7. **Eukaryotic DNA is packed** along with the histones, **as chromatin, in the nucleosomes.** The DNA gets separated from histones, prior to its replication, just ahead of the replication fork.

   After replication, histones again **get associated** with the upcoming daughter duplexes and form nucleosomes.
8. Cyclins and cyclin-dependent kinases regulate initiation of DNA synthesis in eukaryotes.

   Moreover, DNA synthesis in eukaryotes is confined to the synthetic phase (**S phase)** only. This is followed by the gap period (G_1). Thereafter, cell division occurs during mitosis (M phase), which again follows a gap period (G_2).

   On the other hand, DNA is replicated through most of the cell cycle in prokaryotes and the cell division occurs immediately after the DNA synthesis has ceased.
9. In eukaryotes, **synthesis of the leading strand** and the **lagging strand** is carried out **by different enzymes.**

   In prokaryotes, DNA synthesis is catalyzed by two similar but distinct subunits of the same enzyme, i.e. DNA polymerase III.
10. **Ends of the eukaryotic chromosomes have unusual structures,** called **telomeres,** which are also replicated.

TELOMERES

- Telomeres are 1000 or more nucleotides long **tandem repeats** (copies of short **G- and T-rich** oligonucleotide sequences) present at the **3′-end** of the strand (at the end of each chromosome).
- A telomere also has a 12–16 nucleotides long single strand **overhang**, which serves as a template for the primer that initiates the synthesis of the final Okazaki fragment on the lagging strand (Fig. 15.6).
- In drosophila, the lengthening of these chromosomal ends is carried out by the transposition of DNA segments known as transposons.

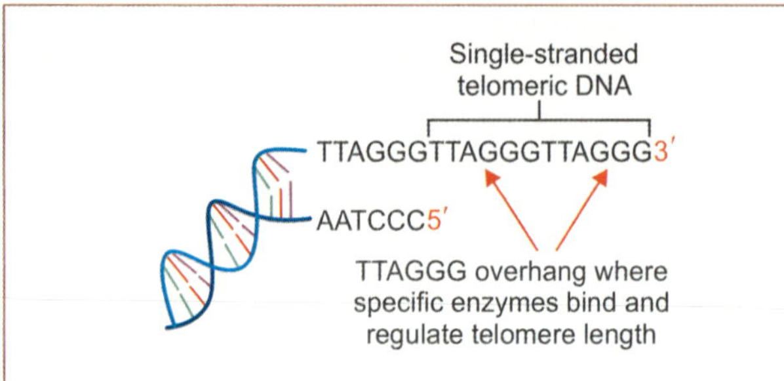

Fig. 15.6: Telomere

- In most of the eukaryotes, telomere replication is carried out by a specialized reverse transcriptase, designated as **telomerase**.

Telomerases: These are ribonucleoproteins whose **RNA** components have enzyme activity. Such a component contains a segment that is complementary to the repeating telomeric sequence and acts as an internal template. Its function, therefore, is similar to that of reverse transcriptase.

Absence of the telomerase shortens the chromosome with each round of replication and contributes to **normal senescence** of the cell. Maintenance of the chromosomal length thus depends on the action of telomerase.

Importance of Telomeres

- Required for the **complete replication** of the chromosomes.
- To form **caps that protect** the chromosomes from nucleases and other destabilizing forces.
- **Prevent the ends** of chromosomes from **fusing** with one another.
- Unlike somatic cells, **germ cells of the gonads retain telomerase activity** and telomeres of the chromosomes do not shrink after cell division. Consequently, each offspring begins life as a zygote that contains telomeres of maximum length.
- Telomere repeats gradually decrease with aging and serve as a **mitotic clock.**
- Telomere shortening plays a key role in **protecting from cancer**. Unlike normal somatic cells that lack detectable telomerase activity, majority of cancer cells contain active telomerase activity and are 'immortalized'.

DNA REPLICATION IN MITOCHONDRIA

15

Mitochondrial chromosome of the mammals is a 15 kb segment. It is **circular** and contains 500–600 nucleotides long **D-loop** that undergoes frequent cycles of degradation and resynthesis.

- During replication of the mitochondrial DNA (mtDNA), the D-loop is extended.
- Replication of the mtDNA is carried out by the process in which synthesis of the leading strand precedes the synthesis of the lagging strand.
- The leading strand, in turn, displaces the lagging strand template to form a displacement loop (D-loop).
- When the D-loop has reached more than half the way around the chromosome, the lagging strand origin is exposed and its synthesis proceeds in the opposite direction around the chromosome. The synthesis of the lagging strand is thus only less than half complete by the time the synthesis of the leading strand is terminated (Fig. 15.7).

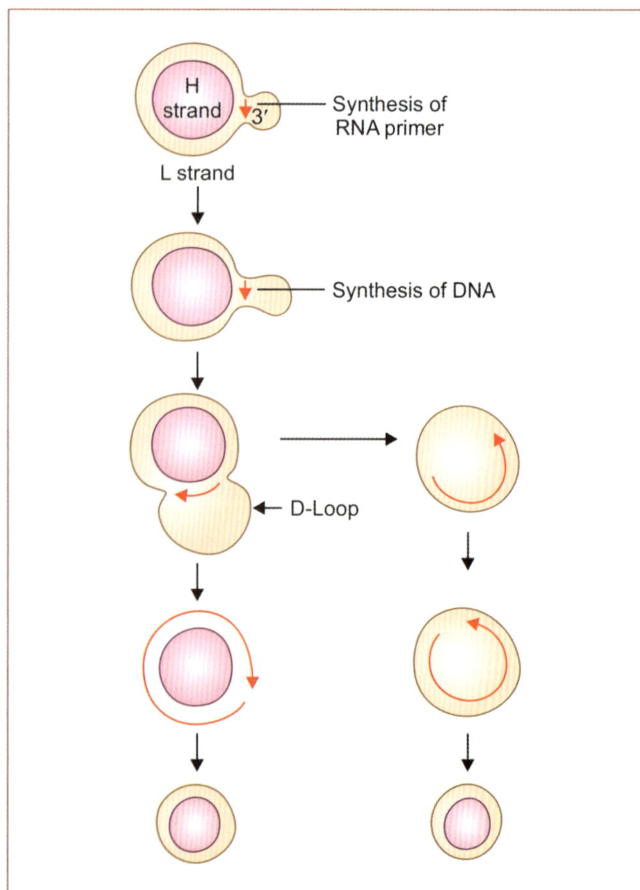

Fig. 15.7: DNA replication in mitochondria

NUCLEOSOMES

Nucleosomes are the **lowest level of chromosome organization**.

- Eukaryotic DNA being large is **packed** in chromatin in association with the basic proteins called **histones**, which are rich in lysine and arginine. These are positively charged molecules and form ionic bonds with the DNA which is negatively charged.

- There are five classes of histones, designated as **H1, H2A, H2B, H3 and H4**.
- Two molecules each of H2A, H2B, H3 and H4 form an **octamer-structured core** of the individual nucleosome around which a segment of the DNA double helix is wound twice, forming a negatively supertwisted helix. These DNA segments are small (approximately, 50 nucleotides), and are called **linker DNA** (Fig. 15.8).

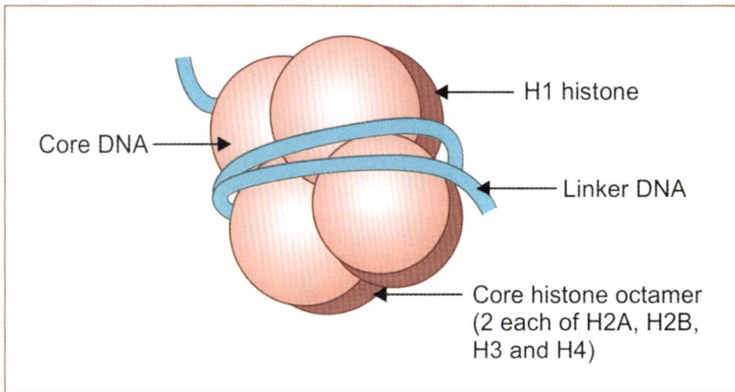

Fig. 15.8: Nucleosome/chromatosome

- Histones-octamer joined by the linker DNA, forms a nucleosome (nucleofilament).
- Thereafter, H1 binds to the DNA chain, between the nucleosome beads, and helps in packaging of the nucleosome into a more compact structure. Strictly speaking, a **nucleosome** consists of **1¾ turns of DNA (≈146 bp)** around the histone-octamer, whereas when the DNA makes **two full turns (≈166 bp)**, the resulting structure is called a **chromatosome**.
- Synthesis of the new histones occurs mainly during the **S phase**, simultaneously with the replication of DNA.
- Newly synthesized DNA inherits some parental histones which combine with an equal amount of the new histones, to complete the structure of the nascent nucleosomes that are formed behind the moving replication fork.

REPAIR OF DNA

DNA is the **only macromolecule** that is repaired rather than degraded. DNA repair is a high-priority process for the maintenance of **integrity of the genetic information** and other cellular functions. It is a **very efficient** process with less than 1 out of 1000 accidental changes which may result in a **mutation**. There are several processes for DNA repair, each one of which can repair a certain type of the damage.

REPLACEMENT OF THE DAMAGED DNA SEGMENT

A segment of the damaged DNA is repaired by the process called **excision repair**. The process is catalyzed by different enzymatic systems, each one of which is specific for the repair of a specific type of damage. These repair systems are capable of recognizing and excising damaged DNA, replacing the same with newly synthesized, properly base-paired segment. The process includes incision at the site of damage, excision of the damaged segment, resynthesis of the new strand at the site of damage and ligation of the two ends. Such systems exist both in eukaryotes and prokaryotes.

Excision Repair in Prokaryotes

Excision repair is carried out by the replacement of the damaged DNA, depending upon the extent of the damage in the two strands. It includes base excision repair and nucleotide excision repair.

Base Excision Repair

It eliminates modified bases like those that have been deaminated, methylated or modified chemically.

- The modified bases are hydrolytically removed by the enzymes termed **DNA glycosylases**, e.g. deaminated cytosine (uracil) is removed by uracil DNA glycosylase. DNA glycosylases remove the damaged base by hydrolyzing the glycosidic bond.
- This, in turn, produces a deoxyribosephosphate residue, i.e. having only the sugar moiety which is linked with a phosphate but is without a base. Such a site is designated as an **apurinic-apyrimidinic site (AP site)**. Such a site may also be generated by spontaneous hydrolysis of a purine or pyrimidine. It may be called **depurination** or **depyrimidination**.
- After an AP site has been created, AP endonuclease nicks phosphodiester backbone at the AP site and excises the sugar-phosphate residue, creating a gap of one nucleotide.
- This gap is filled by the action of DNA polymerase I.
- Finally, DNA ligase seals the ends (Fig. 15.9).

Nucleotide Excision Repair

It is activated when a **bulky lesion** has been produced, such as due to the interaction of DNA with a polycyclic aromatic hydrocarbon, like benzo(a)pyrene (generated by tobacco smoke). Chemotherapeutic drugs, like **cisplatin,** may also result in the formation of thymine-cisplatin adducts. The dimerization of the adjacent pyrimidines, induced by **UV light**, may also result in generation of a bulky lesion.

15

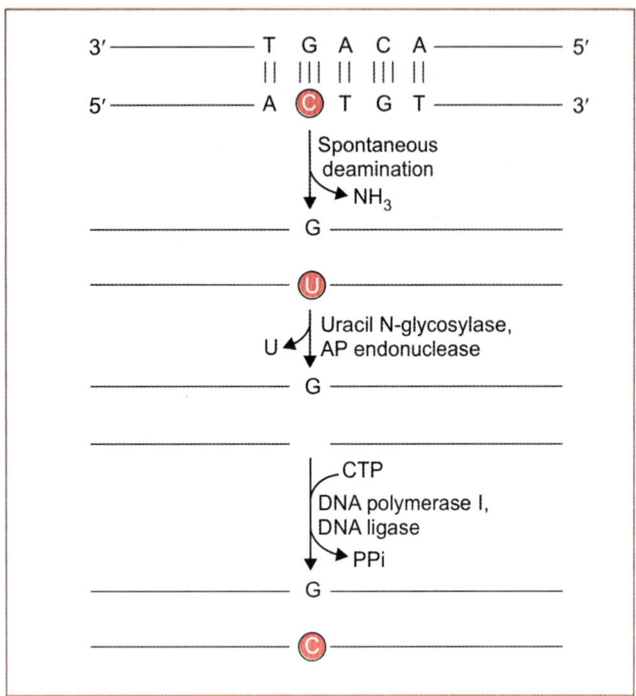

Fig. 15.9: Base excision repair in prokaryotes

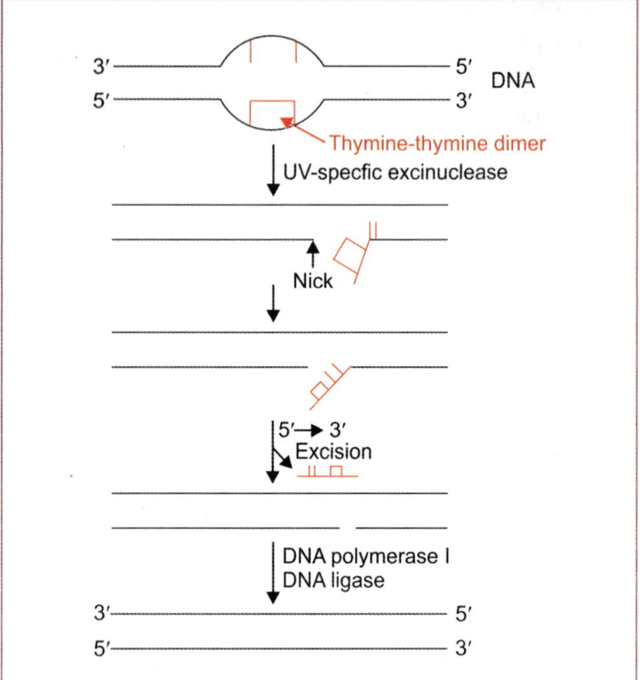

Fig. 15.10: Nucleotide excision repair in prokaryotes

In *E. coli,* such a repair is initiated by recognition of the distortion of DNA by an endonuclease system which is a product of three genes, i.e. UvrA, UvrB and UvrC. This endonuclease system is designated as excision nuclease or **excinuclease**. In this process:

- A tetramer, consisting of two UvrA and two UvrB proteins, is formed. This, in turn, causes local melting of DNA (at the expense of ATP) and locates the bulky lesion.
- UvrB makes 3′ incision, followed by a 5′ incision by UvrC.
- It leads to the release of an oligonucleotide including the bulky lesion, e.g. the pyrimidine dimer.
- Thereafter, UvrD (a helicase) unwinds DNA and releases the above excised oligonucleotide.
- DNA polymerase then displaces UvrB and fills the gap.
- The repair is completed by DNA ligase (Fig. 15.10).

Excision Repair in Eukaryotes

In eukaryotes, the process is similar to that in prokaryotes except that the endonuclease activity of human cells consists of 16–17 different polypeptides compared to only four proteins of *E. coli.*

- Nucleotide excision repair of human DNA begins with the binding of a protein designated as xeroderma pigmentosum A (**XP-A**) to a dimer which consists of two other proteins, i.e. XP-F and ERCC-1 (excision repair component). XP-A binds to the dimer between XP-F and ERCC-1 and forms a complex, XP F-XP A-ERCC-1. Its XP-A component recognizes the damaged site and binds to it.
- Thereafter, a replication protein (HSSB) also binds to XP-A and gets associated to the damaged site.
- There is also involvement of an additional enzyme complex known as general transcription factor **TFIIH**, essential for transcription initiation as well as for nucleotide excision repair. Two of its subunits, i.e. XP-B and XP-D are helicases and are involved in kinking and unwinding of DNA at the damaged site. The TFIIH interacts with XP-C and the whole complex gets associated to the damaged site through XP-A.
- Subsequently, XP-G also gets associated with this complex to complete the excinuclease system.
- The 3′ nick is introduced by XP-G while XP-F in association with ERCC-1 makes the 5′ nick.
- This, in turn, results in excision of an oligonucleotide.
- The gap is filled by polymerases γ and ε.
- Finally, DNA ligase seals the nick.

Defects in nucleotide excision repair have been shown to result in various hereditary disorders, such as xeroderma pigmentosum, Cockayne's syndrome and trichothiodystrophy (Chemistry to Clinics 15.3).

15

Chemistry to Clinics 15.3: Disorders Associated with Defects in the Process of Nucleotide Excision Repair in Eukaryotes

- **Xeroderma pigmentosum:** This is a condition characterized by varying levels of UV sensitivity and corresponding deficiencies in DNA repair system, such as a mutation in XPV gene. These patients exhibit sunlight-induced **photodermatosis** characterized by severe skin reactions that range from skin ulceration to the development of skin cancer (Fig. 15.11).

  Some of its forms are also accompanied by neurological abnormalities due to abnormal gene expression and DNA deterioration caused by the accumulation of the damaged DNA.
- **Cockayne's syndrome:** This condition is associated with mutations in XP-D and XP-B genes. It is characterized by growth and mental retardation, neurological deficiencies and photosensitivity but not increased rate of cancer or skeletal abnormalities.
- **Trichothiodystrophy:** This is caused by mutations in XP-B, XP-G and TFIIH-associated excision repair subunits. These patients have scaly skin, brittle hair, and short stature and neuroskeletal abnormalities.

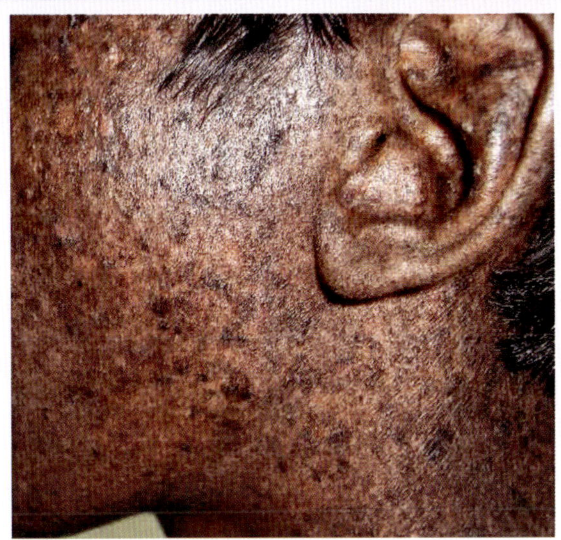

Fig. 15.11: Xeroderma pigmentosum: An inherited disease characterized by photosensitivity, epithelial atrophy and hyperpigmentation

TRANSCRIPTION

Transcription refers to the **process of RNA synthesis,** by which a DNA sequence is transcribed into the RNA transcript.

The process of RNA synthesis requires an appropriate sequence of **DNA as a template,** and the enzymes called **RNA polymerases.**

Promoter Regions

Each cycle of the transcription process begins as well as ends with the recognition of some **specific sites in the DNA template.** The site, where **RNA polymerase binds** is called **promoter.**

The **nucleotide in the promoter region is assigned a negative number if, it is present towards the 5′-site,** i.e. **prior to the transcription start site.** This position is also referred as the **upstream.**

A nucleotide is assigned a **positive number if** it is present **towards the 3′-site,** i.e. **after the transcription start site.** This position is called the **downstream.**

The **first nucleotide at the transcription start site is** referred to as **+1.**

Certain conserved sequences have been shown to **occur in the promoter region** both in prokaryotes and eukaryotes.

In Prokaryotes

The RNA polymerase binds at the site, which is extending nearly **45 base pair** (bp) **upstream** and **10 bp downstream,** of the transcription start site. Within this region, **there are two highly conserved short (oligonucleotide) sequences,** called **pribnow box** or **–10 sequence** and **–35 sequence** (Fig. 15.12).

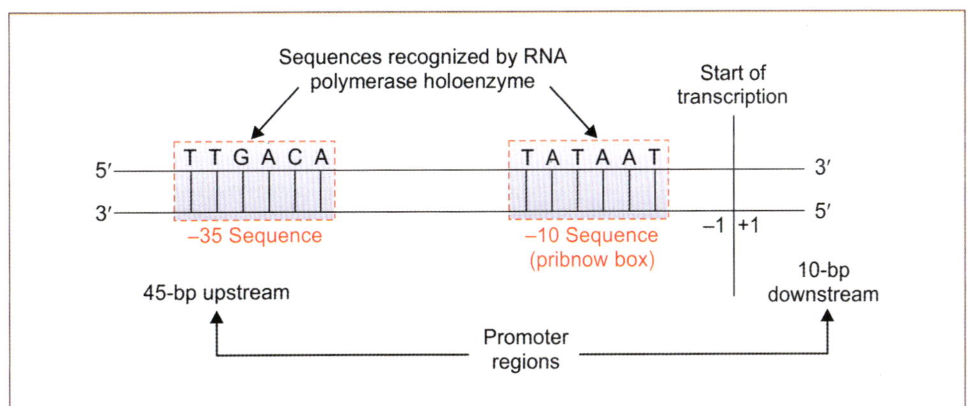

Fig. 15.12: Promoter regions in prokaryotes

15

In Eukaryotes

The promoters region, in eukaryotes, has three different highly conserved sequences, which are referred to as the **TATA box, the GC box and the CAAT box**. In addition to them, transcription in eukaryotes is also affected by certain **other promoter elements, called enhancers.**

RNA Polymerases

RNA polymerases synthesize RNA in the 5′→3′ direction, using a DNA template. They initiate polymerization of the ribonucleotides at the consequence sequence, on a promoter site, and do not need a primer.

Different types of RNA polymerases are found in prokaryotes and eukaryotes.

In Prokaryotes

A single type of the **RNA polymerase** synthesizes all types of RNAs in bacteria. It is a **multienzyme complex**. The core enzyme **consists of** four peptides, i.e. it has **two a, one b,** and **one b′** subunits. It cannot recognize the promoter region on the DNA template without the addition of another protein, i.e. the fifth subunit, which is designated as the sigma (σ) factor. The binding of the σ factor with the core enzyme results in the formation of the holoenzyme, which in turn initiates the synthesis of RNA.

In Eukaryotes

Three different **types of the RNA polymerases** have been identified in eukaryotes. These are referred to as RNA polymerase I, II and III.

RNA polymerase I transcribes **ribosomal RNA (rRNA)**, genes for which are located within the nucleolus.

RNA polymerase II transcribes **mRNA**. It synthesizes large RNA particle, which is the precursor of the mRNA and the small nuclear RNAs (snRNAs).

RNA polymerase III produces small RNA molecules, which are processed to give various types of tRNA, and some snRNAs.

In addition to the above three types of RNA polymerases, eukaryotes also have another type of RNA polymerase, called mitochondrial RNA polymerase (mtRNA polymerase), which is responsible for the synthesis of mRNA, tRNA and rRNA within the mitochondria.

PROCESS OF TRANSCRIPTION IN PROKARYOTES

The process of RNA synthesis occurs in 3 steps, which are referred to as initiation, elongation, and termination.

Initiation of Transcription

RNA polymerase holoenzyme binds to the DNA template and locates a promoter. After the holoenzyme (RNA polymerase with the sigma factor) has recognized the promoter, it binds there and forms a complex. This in turn results in unwinding of nearly 10 nucleotide base pairs of the DNA double helix. The unwound DNA then binds to the initiating ribonucleotide triphosphate, usually a purine ribonucleotide (GTP or ATP), and the holoenzyme forms the first phosphodiester bond.

Elongation of the RNA Transcript

After the initiation of the process, RNA polymerase translocates to the next position and continues the synthesis. After the enzyme has begun to synthesize the RNA transcript, its σ subunit is released and the core enzyme continues the process.

The template strand gets attached to the growing RNA chain, by base pairing. The enzyme topoisomerase, which is a component of the transcription complex, helps in the process of unwinding and restoring the DNA double helix (Fig. 15.13).

Termination of the Transcription Process

RNA polymerase complex also recognizes the termination sequence, which is present at the end of the gene, and terminates the process.

Termination of the transcription process can occur in either of the two modes. Either, the enzyme itself recognizes the termination region on the DNA template, by the process which is referred to as **rho (ρ) independent termination.** Alternatively, termination of the process may require an additional protein, which is designated as ρ factor, for the release of the RNA transcript. This is termed as the **ρ-dependent termination.**

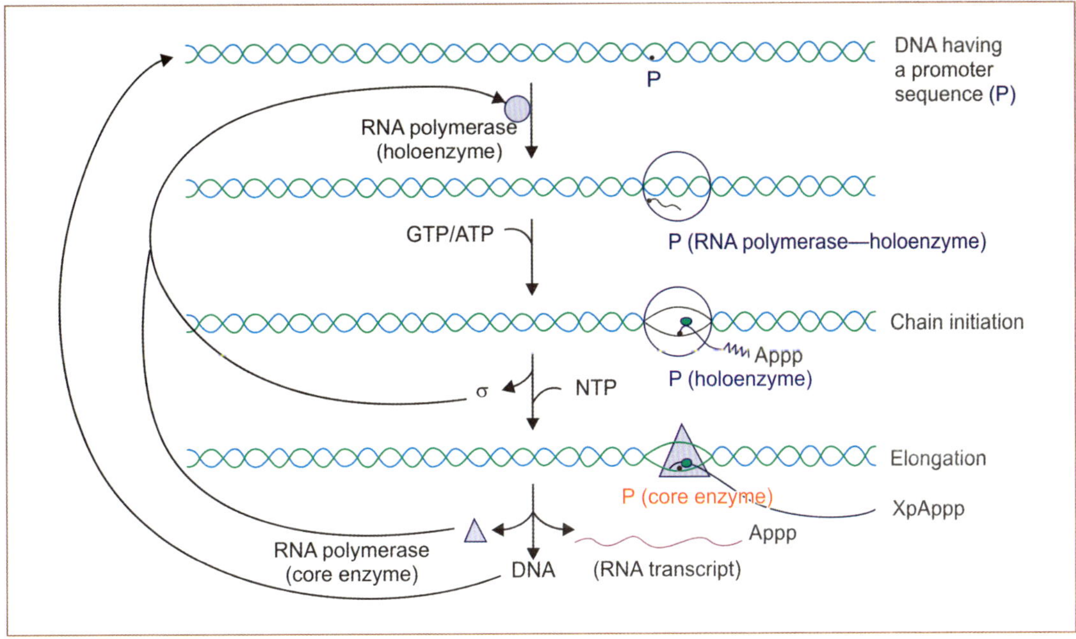

Fig. 15.13: Process of RNA transcription

DIFFERENCES IN THE PROCESS OF TRANSCRIPTION IN PROKARYOTES AND EUKARYOTES

Transcription in eukaryotes is more complex than prokaryotes. Whereas, transcription in prokaryotes requires only an appropriate sequence of the DNA as a template, the enzyme RNA polymerase (holoenzyme) and ribonucleoside triphosphates as the substrates, initiation of the process in **eukaryotes requires several additional molecular events:**

1. Chromatin, though is organized in the nucleosomes however, some of its part, which is containing the promoter sequences, is not well organized and is not accessible to the transcription machinery. Such a nucleosomal organization requires **DNase activity** for proper access by the transcription machinery.
2. Certain gene-specific sequences, referred to as **enhancers,** are also needed. These sequences stimulate transcription as well as binding of various transcription factors.
3. Besides RNA polymerases, certain additional proteins, called **transcription factors,** are required. They bind to some sequences in the promoter region, for the initiation of the process. These transcription factors also facilitate binding of the RNA polymerase.
4. Eukaryotes have **three distinct types of RNA polymerases**, each one of which is specific for the particular class of RNA.

Differences in the process of transcription between prokaryotes and eukaryotes are shown in Table 15.4.

Table 15.4: Differences in the process of transcription between prokaryotes and eukaryotes

Prokaryotes	Eukaryotes
No nucleosomal organization is required as chromatin is easily accessible to the transcription machinery	Nucleosomal organization is required, which is done by the enzyme DNase. This is essential for proper access by the transcription machinery
Promoter region, for the binding of the RNA polymerase, is simple	Promoter region is complex, and binds RNA polymerase with other transcription factors
There is only one type of RNA polymerase	There are three distinct forms of the enzyme RNA polymerase, one for each class of the RNA. These are referred to as RNA polymerase I, II and III
Introns are rarely found in the primary transcript	Introns very commonly occur in the primary transcript
Post-transcriptional modifications are restricted to tRNA and rRNA only	Post-transcriptional modifications take place in all the three types of RNAs

POST-TRANSCRIPTIONAL MODIFICATIONS OF THE RNA TRANSCRIPT

Primary transcripts of **tRNA and rRNA are processed** post-transcriptionally **both in prokaryotes and eukaryotes. In prokaryotes**, mRNA is generally, identical to its primary transcript and does not require modifications, whereas **in eukaryotes, mRNA** genes are transcribed as pre-mRNA primary transcripts which are extensively **modified, post-transcriptionally.**

- **Post-transcriptional modifications of the mRNA transcript in eukaryotes**
  The mRNA transcript undergoes following modifications:
  - **Addition of poly(A) tail:** The poly(A) tail of 40–200 adenine nucleotides is added to the free 3′-end of the mRNA primary transcript by a polymerase. This polyadenylation does not require a template.
    This poly(A) tail helps in the stabilization of the mRNA and facilitates its exit from the nucleus (Fig. 15.14).
  - **Splicing:** The primary mRNAs transcript, called pre-mRNA or **heterogenous nuclear RNA (hnRNA),** contains two types of sequences called **introns** and **exons**.
    Introns, also called **intervening sequences,** are the noncoding sequences that are present in pre-mRNA but not in mature **mRNA.** The other sequences, which are expressed or retained, are called **exons**.
    As **pre-mRNA is** extruded from the RNA polymerase complex, it is rapidly **bound by small nuclear ribonucleoproteins** (snRNPs or **snrnps**). Different snrnps bind to the RNA precursor and form a large complex, termed **spliceosome**. This, in turn, carries out dual steps of the RNA splicing, i.e. **breakage of the intron at the 5′-site,** and **joining of the exon sequences** together. **After removal of the introns, fully functional mature mRNA leaves the nucleus and passes into the cytosol.**

Mutations in the β-globin gene interfere with the removal of introns. This, in turn, leads to a condition called **β-thalassemia.**

- **Post-transcriptional modifications of the rRNA transcript in eukaryotes:** Ribosomal RNAs are synthesized from the long precursor molecules, called pre-rRNAs or 45S RNA, which contains sequences for 28S, 5.8S and 18S rRNAs. During post-transcriptional modifications, each pre-rRNA is cleaved to yield the required rRNA species (Fig. 15.15).

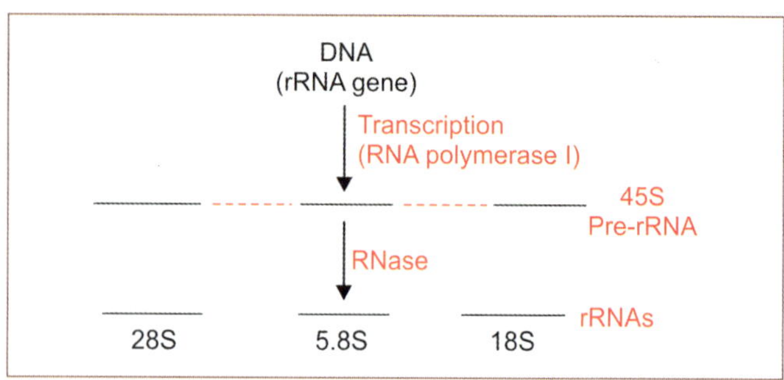

Fig. 15.15: Post-transcriptional processing of rRNA

Some of the proteins, which are destined to become components of ribosomes, also get associated with the pre-rRNAs, prior to and during post-transcriptional modifications in the nucleolus.

- **Post-transcriptional modifications of the tRNA transcript in eukaryotes: tRNA undergoes following modifications**
  - **Trimming:** The primary transcript of tRNA has large number of nucleotide sequences on both the ends which are removed, and the tRNA molecule is trimmed, nonspecifically.
    From the 5′-end, the primary tRNA transcript undergoes endonucleolytic cleavage by ribonuclease P (a ribozyme), while the 3′ extension is removed by the exonucleolytic cleavage.

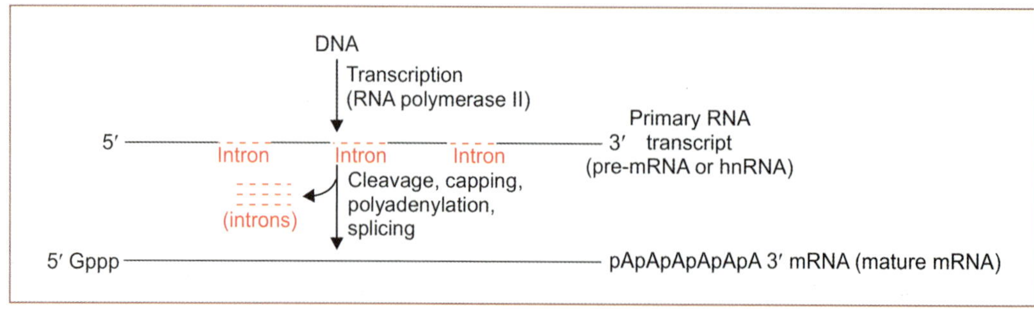

Fig. 15.14: Post-transcriptional processing of mRNA

15

Sometimes, the primary transcript may also contain introns, which are removed by the two-component enzyme system, whereas one of the enzymes removes introns, the other rejoins the remaining exon chains.

- **Addition of the terminal CCA sequence:** Each functional tRNA, both in the cytosol and the mitochondria, has a sequence of three nucleotides, CCA at the 3′ terminus. These nucleotides are added, sequentially, by the enzyme tRNA-nucleotidyltransferase.
- **Modifications of the bases:** As we know, the tRNA molecules have several modified nitrogenous bases.

  These modifications are done by various enzymes, which are either site specific or nucleotide sequence specific.

Inhibition of the Process of Transcription

Several antibiotics are known to inhibit the process of transcription. For example, rifampicin, used in the treatment of tuberculosis, inhibits RNA polymerase activity in several bacteria. Rifampicin inhibits the transcriptional machinery of bacteria by inhibiting the β-subunit of the bacterial RNA polymerase without much toxicity to the host.

RNA INTERFERENCE

Specific cellular mRNAs can be degraded by introducing mammalian cells to a **double-stranded RNA (dsRNA)**, derived from a virus or a transposon, or artificially prepared in the laboratory, in which one of the strands is complementary to the mRNA being targeted. Inside the cell, the dsRNA forms a **small interfering RNA (siRNA)** and the phenomenon is called **RNA interference (RNAi;** Chemistry to Clinics 15.4).

Chemistry to Clinics 15.4: RNA Interference

The siRNAs can be used as therapeutic agents. Several potential clinical applications of RNAi are currently being evaluated, e.g. the treatment of cancer, AIDS and other infections. Further, RNAi is currently the method of choice for eukaryotic gene inactivation. The consequences of loss of gene function reveal the role played by the gene product (RNA or protein) in the cell.

RNA interference is employed in **post-transcriptional gene silencing or gene knockdown,** as follows (Fig. 15.16).

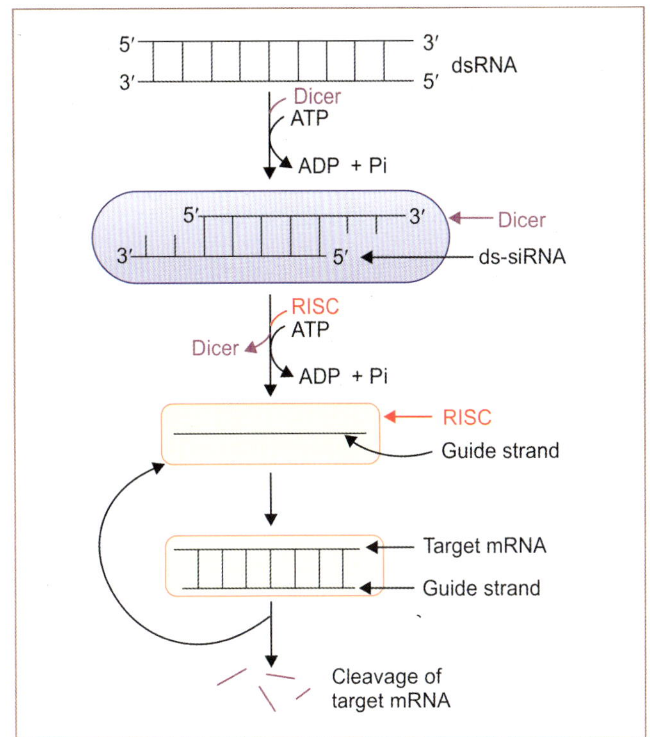

Fig. 15.16: RNA interference

- A dsRNA is introduced into a target cell. One strand of the dsRNA is designed to be an antisense RNA because its sequence is complementary to the RNA transcript of the gene selected for silencing.
- Inside the cell, an **ATP-dependent RNase III** called **dicer (riboendonuclease)**, catalyzes the cleavage of both strands to produce a **double-stranded small interfering RNA (ds-siRNA)**, 21–23 nucleotides long and having 2-nucleotides long 3′-overhangs on each strand.
- The ds-siRNA is passed onto another protein complex called **RNA-induced silencing complex (RISC)**.
- In an ATP-dependent manner, RISC unwinds the ds-siRNA and selects the antisense strand, now called the **guide strand**. The other strand called the **passenger strand** is discarded.
- RISC pairs the single guide strand with a complementary region on the target gene transcript (mRNA).
- The RNase H activity of RISC performs its **slicer** function by cleaving the RNA transcript so that it can no longer be translated by ribosomes.
- The guide strand remains associated with RISC, hence it can be used for **multiple cycles** of mRNA cleavage, i.e. post-transcriptional gene silencing.

15

TRANSLATION

The **process of protein biosynthesis** is called translation. It is the **biochemical translation of the genetic information, from the four-letter language of nucleotides to the twenty-letter language of amino acids,** as defined by the genetic code.

GENETIC CODE

Genetic code is **a dictionary** that gives a correspondence between the **sequences of four nucleotide bases** that are found in mRNA to the **corresponding sequence of 20 amino acids** present in peptides.

Each word of the genetic **code is composed of three letters (nucleotide bases),** referred to as **codon**.

This is due to the reason that if **one nucleotide** encodes **for an amino acid**, four nucleotides will code for $(4)^1$, i.e. **4 amino acids** only. If there are **2 nucleotides in a code**, it will translate $(4)^2$, i.e. **16 amino acids** only. Hence, a **3:1 correspondence of nucleotides to amino acids** forms $(4)^3$, i.e. 64 combinations, which are sufficient to code for **the 20 amino acids.**

These 64 combinations, of three bases each, define genetic code (Table 15.5).

Out of these 64 codons, 61 are known to code for 20 amino acids which are incorporated in proteins, while the remaining 3 codons are used as stop codons, i.e. they stop the process of translation.

Salient Features of the Genetic Code

Thus, codons, as mentioned above, are the permutations of four bases, which are taken in the sets of three. Salient features of the genetic code are shown in Table 15.6.

Table 15.6: Salient features of the genetic code

Degeneracy	Multiple codons code for the same amino acid
Unambiguous	A specific codon codes for only a single amino acid
Nonoverlapping	Reading of the genetic code occurs without overlapping
Punctuation	Message is read continuously without any break between the sequence of codons until a nonsense codon is reached
Universality	The same codon is used in all the living organisms with only few exceptions in the mitochondria

Wobble Hypothesis

The sequence of nucleotides (U, C, A and G) in **mRNA** is read from 5′-end to 3′-end in combination of three nucleotides at a time in the form of **codons.** On the other hand, as discussed in Chapter 14, **tRNA** has an anticodon arm that has a triplet nucleotide sequence

Table 15.5: Genetic code

	Middle-base								
5′-Base	**U**		**C**		**A**		**G**		**3′-Base**
U	UUU	Phe	UCU		UAU	Tyr	UGU	Cys	**U**
	UUC		UCC		UAC		UGC		
	UUA		UCA	Ser	UAA	Stop	UGA	Stop	
	UUG		UCG		UAG		UGG	Trp	
C	CUU		CCU		CAU	His	CGU		**C**
	CUC	Leu	CCC	Pro	CAC		CGC		
	CUA		CCA		CAA	Gln	CGA	Arg	
	CUG		CCG		CAG		CGG		
A	AUU		ACU		AAU	Asn	AGU	Ser	**A**
	AUC	Ile	ACC	Thr	AAC		AGC		
	AUA		ACA		AAA	Lys	AGA	Arg	
	AUG	Met	ACG		AAG		AGG		
G	GUU		GCU		GAU	Asp	GGU		**G**
	GUC		GCC	Ala	GAC		GGC		
	GUA	Val	GCA		GAA	Glu	GGA	Gly	
	GUG		GCG		GAG		GGG		

called **anticodon**, which is complementary to the codon present on mRNA. The anticodon is responsible for the specificity of a tRNA molecule and that each tRNA carries a specific amino acid only, which is defined by the sequence of three bases of the codon.

As discussed above, there are 61 codons which define 20 amino acids. At the same time, it is known that most of the cells have nearly 50 tRNA species. This, in turn, suggests that certain variations from the standard base pairing in codon–anticodon interactions occur and that all the codons may not be being used, equally, meaning thereby that some codons may be read more efficiently by an anticodon while some of the codons may be used less efficiently. This further suggests that many amino acids can be carried by more than one tRNA species while the degenerate codon can be read by more than one tRNA.

The possibility by which one anticodon recognizes more than one codon for the specific amino acid has been described by a hypothesis given by Crick. It is referred to as **Wobble hypothesis.**

The Wobble hypothesis explains that a **base at the 5′-end of the anticodon** (i.e. the first base of the anticodon or the third base of the codon) **is not as well defined with respect to its spatial configuration, as the other two bases.** Thus, the first two positions of the codon predominate in tRNA selection and that the third position, referred to as degenerate position, is less important in this regard.

PROCESS OF TRANSLATION IN EUKARYOTES

Protein synthesis (translation) requires mRNA, several tRNAs, ribosomes and various protein factors.

Besides the activation of amino acids, the process of protein synthesis occurs in three stages, i.e. **initiation, elongation and termination,** along with the release of a polypeptide.

Activation of Amino Acids

For their incorporation into the polypeptide chain, amino acids are first activated and attached to the appropriate tRNA carrier. **Linkage of the amino acid to its tRNA** requires ATP and is catalyzed by the enzyme referred to as **aminoacyl-tRNA synthetase.** Aminoacyl-tRNA synthetases consist of a group of enzymes, each one of which is specific for an amino acid and its appropriate tRNA.

During the process of amino acid activation, firstly a high-energy complex, referred to as **amino acid–AMP–enzyme complex** is formed as an intermediate. The enzyme, thereafter, recognizes the tRNA and transfers the amino acid, from the amino acid–AMP–enzyme complex to the corresponding tRNA (Fig. 15.17).

The enzyme (aminoacyl-**tRNA synthetase**) not only carries a correct amino acid but **also edits protein synthesis.** During this process, if there is a wrong acylated-tRNA it is recognized by the enzyme and removed.

Initiation of Protein Synthesis

Requirements: Initiation of protein synthesis involves assembly of various components of the translation system, i.e. 2 ribosomal subunits, mRNA to be translated, the aminoacyl-tRNA (specified by the first codon in the message), GTP and several initiation factors (IFs) that facilitate assembly of the initiation complex.

In **eukaryotes,** several initiation factors (**eIF**) participate in initiation. Further the **initiation codon** is **AUG**, which is recognized by the initiation tRNA that carries **methionine**, and requires eIF-2 (in humans).

The mRNA sequence is read in 5→3 direction and amino acids are incorporated from amino-terminal to carboxy-terminal in the peptide.

Assembly of the various components occurs as follows:

- First of all the **initiation codon** (AUG) is recognized by the initiation tRNA (that carries methionine). This is facilitated by **eIF-2a** (eukaryotic initiation factor-2a), which binds to **GTP** and **methioninyl-tRNA** (Met-tRNAi^{Met}), and **forms a ternary complex**.
- Subsequently, the ternary complex binds with **40S ribosomal subunit** (which is **associated with eIF-3**) and is placed over the initiation sequence in mRNA.
- The **pre-initiation complex** further binds to several other initiation factors, which include **eIF-4a, eIF-1b, cIF-4f** (also called cap-binding protein), **eIF-4d**

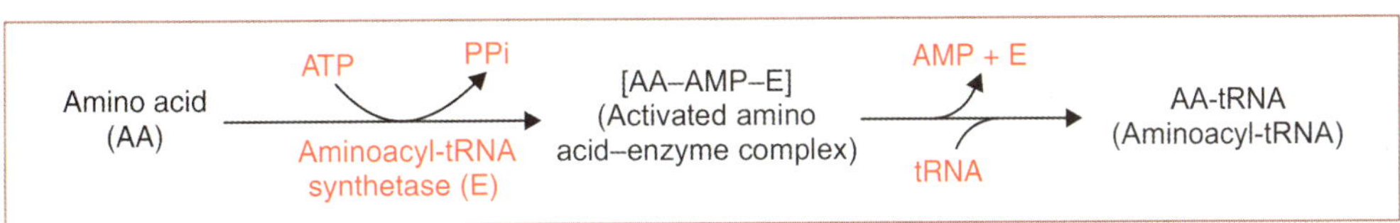

Fig. 15.17: Amino acid activation

and **eIF-5** and **60S ribosomal subunit**, to form 80S ribosome with mRNA and initiator tRNA (which is correctly positioned within the ribosome).

- **GTP is hydrolyzed**, and **eIF-2a–GDP**, **eIF-3** and **other factors are released.**
- The eIF-2a–GDP complex interacts with eIF-2b and GTP, to regenerate eIF-2a–GTP for another round (Fig. 15.18).

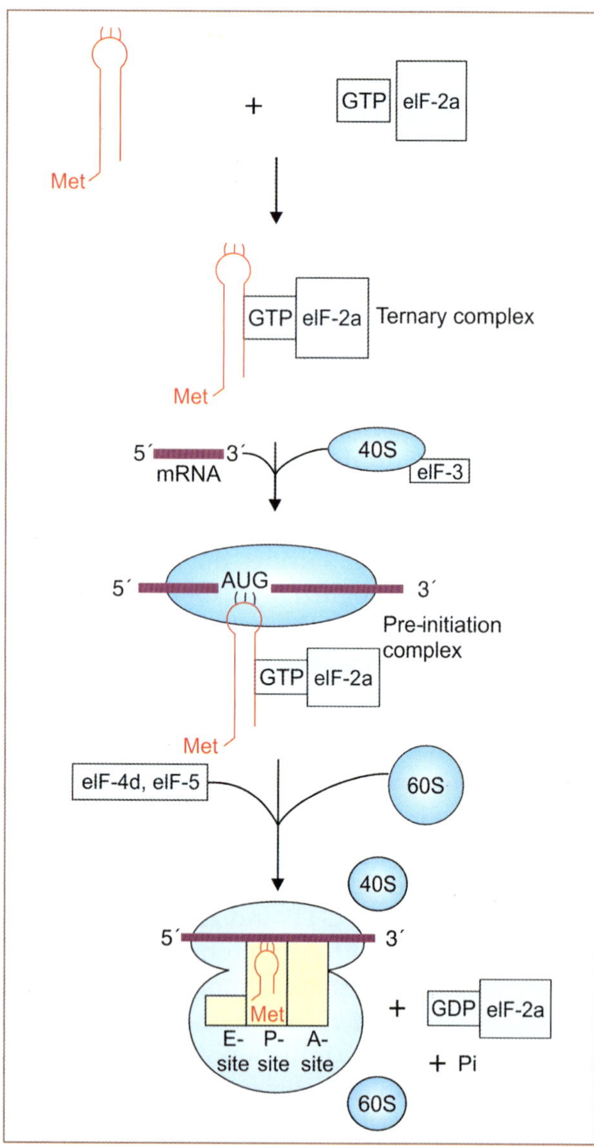

Fig. 15.18: Initiation of protein synthesis

In *E. coli*, binding and positioning of the mRNA on the 30S ribosomal subunit is facilitated by complementary base pairing between the pyrimidine-rich sequence of 8 nucleotides in the 16S RNA and a purine-rich sequence of 10 nucleotides (**Shine-Dalgarno sequence**), which is present on mRNA.

Chain Elongation

Chain elongation ensures selection of the proper aminoacyl-tRNAs and movement of the mRNA along with the associated tRNA, through the decoding region on the ribosome.

Cellular requirements for chain elongation: Chain elongation requires certain nonribosomal proteins called **elongation factors**, which utilize energy (liberated by GTP hydrolysis). This, in turn, ensures selection of the proper **aminoacyl-tRNA**, and movement of the mRNA and associated tRNAs through the decoding region of the ribosome. The tRNA molecules recognize and bind at the specific sites that are located on mRNA and span the ribosomal subunits.

Specific sites that span ribosomal subunits: During translation, up to three tRNA molecules may be bound at the specific sites that span the 2 ribosomal subunits.

- **P-site:** The initiating methionyl-tRNA is placed in such a position that it occupies a site referred to as **donor site**, also called **peptidyl site** or **P-site** of the ribosome, in the way that its methionyl residue may be donated (transferred) to the free α-amino group of the incoming aminoacyl-tRNA.
- **A-site:** The aminoacyl-tRNA, specified by the next codon of the mRNA, is bound at the other site referred to as **acceptor site**, also called **aminoacyl site** or **A-site** of the ribosome.

  The initiating methionyl-tRNA and the incoming aminoacyl-tRNA are now appropriately positioned in the manner that their anticodons are paired with the successive codons of the mRNA in the P- and the A-sites of the 40S subunit while their amino acids are besides one another at the peptidyl transferase site of the 60S subunit.
- **E-site:** After transfer of methionine to the amino group of the aminoacyl-tRNA, anticodon of the deacylated-tRNA remains in the P-site in the small subunit whereas the acceptor-end is shifted in the large subunit towards another site, wich may be referred to as the **exit site** or E-site (Fig. 15.19).

During the process of chain elongation:

- The initiating **methioninyl-tRNA** is placed at such a position that it occupies the **P-site** on the ribosome (so that its methioninyl residue can be transferred to the free α-amino group of the incoming aminoacyl-tRNA.
- Subsequently, **aminoacyl-tRNA** (specified by the next codon on the mRNA) is attached at the **A-site**. The selection of the correct aminoacyl-tRNA is done

15

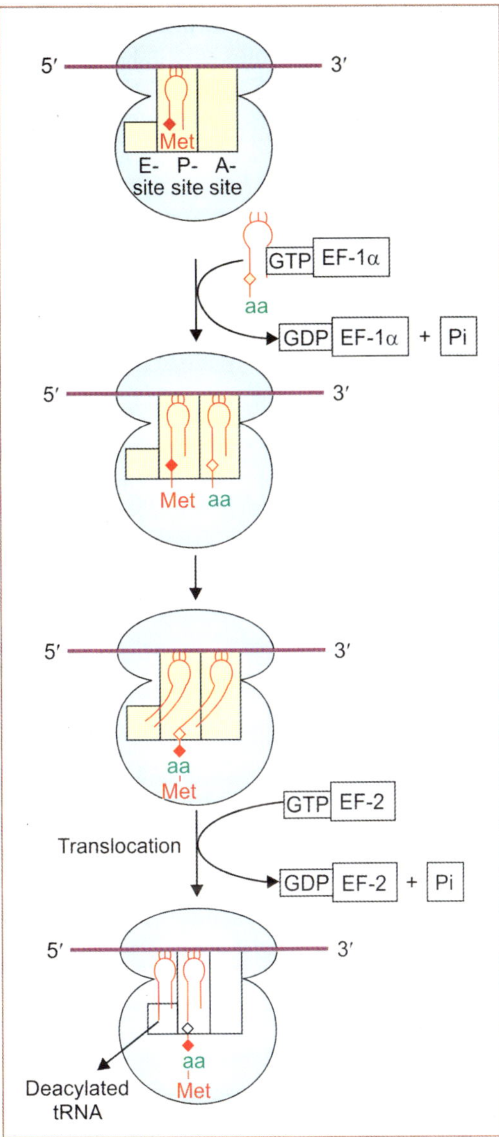

Fig. 15.19: Chain elongation

by a protein designated as **elongation factor 1** (**EF-1**), which has several components, including **EF-1α**. The **EF-1α** forms a **ternary complex** with the **aminoacyl-tRNA and GTP**. It is the **EF-1α-aminoacyl-tRNA–GTP ternary complex** that binds on the ribosome, and, if codon-anticodon interaction is correct, the **aminoacyl-tRNA** is placed at the **A-site.** During this process, **GTP is hydrolyzed** and **EF-1α–GDP complex is dissociated**.

- The initiating **methioninyl-tRNA** and the **incoming aminoacyl-tRNA** are now positioned on the ribosome on the **P-site** and **the A-site**, respectively. Their anticodons are paired with the successive codons on the mRNA (in the decoding region of the small subunits) while the amino acids are present on the peptidyltransferase site of the large subunit. For the formation of the peptide bond, **peptidyltransferase** catalyzes attachment of the α-amino group of the aminoacyl-tRNA to the carboxyl carbon of the methioninyl-tRNA. This, in turn, results in the transfer of methionine to the amino group of the aminoacyl-tRNA, which occupies a hybrid position on the ribosome. Whereas its anticodon remains in the 40S subunit on the A-site, the acceptor-end along with the attached polypeptide are present in the 60S subunit on the P-site. Further, **anticodon of the deacylated tRNA remains in the 40S on the P-site** while the **acceptor** is located **in the 60S,** towards the upper end in the **E-site**.
- The mRNA and the dipeptidyl-tRNA at the 40S subunit are now repositioned by another protein referred to as **elongation factor 2** (**EF-2**, also called **translocase**). **It also requires GTP, which is hydrolyzed**, and **mRNA and dipeptidyl-tRNA** move in the codon-anticodon register from A-site to P-site. As a result of it, the **A-site becomes vacant**. Simultaneously, the deacylated methionyl-tRNA also moves to the E-site (which, as discussed above, exists only in the 60S subunit).

Ribosomes now enter the new cycle. At each step, peptidyltransferase transfers the growing polypeptide from the carrier tRNA to the α-amino group of the amino acid residue of the aminoacyl-tRNA specified by the next codon, and with the hydrolysis of GTP, stepwise elongation of the chain results in completion of the polypeptide (Fig. 15.19).

Termination of Protein Synthesis

Presence of the chain-terminating codon (UAG, UAA, or UGA) on the A-site does not promote binding of the tRNA. Instead, a nonribosomal protein called **releasing factor (eRF)** binds at these sites on the ribosome as eRF–GTP complex**.**

With the hydrolysis of GTP, peptide-tRNA ester linkage is hydrolyzed by the enzyme **peptidyl-transferase**. **Polypeptide**, **tRNA** and the **ribosome** subunits are released to **re-enter the cycle** at the initiation stage (Fig. 15.20).

Differences in the Process of Protein Synthesis between Prokaryotes and Eukaryotes

Differences in the process of protein synthesis between prokaryotes and eukaryotes are shown in Table 15.7.

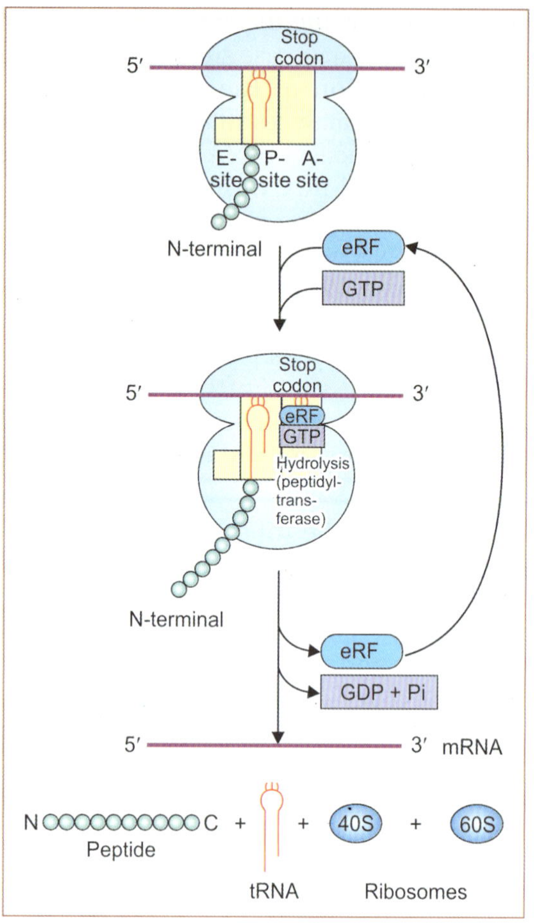

Fig. 15.20: Termination of protein synthesis

Table 15.7: Differences in the process of protein biosynthesis between prokaryotes and eukaryotes

Prokaryotes	Eukaryotes
The mRNA is usually polycistronic	The mRNA is monocistronic. It also contains a poly(A) tail
Ribosomes are present in the free form. They are 70S in size comprising 50S and 30S subunits	Ribosomes are present in the free form as well as bound to endoplasmic reticulum. They are 80S in size consisting of 60S and 40S subunits
Three initiation factors are required in the process	One initiation factor is known to participate in the process
N-Formylmethioninyl-tRNA binds to the start codon	Met-tRNA is not formylated
Three elongation factors are required. They are referred to as EF-Tu, EF-Ts, and EF-G	Two elongation factors are required. They are referred to as eEF-1 and eEF-2
Termination of the process requires three releasing factors, which are referred to as RF-1, RF-2 and RF-3	Termination of the process requires one releasing factor, which is designated as eRF

INHIBITORS OF PROTEIN BIOSYNTHESIS

Many antibiotics and toxins are known to inhibit the process of protein biosynthesis. They are useful in clinical practice as therapeutic agents (Table 15.8).

Antibiotics which Interfere with the Process of Initiation of Protein Synthesis

Streptomycin: It binds to the small subunit of the prokaryotic ribosome and interferes with initiation of protein synthesis. It also causes misreading of the mRNA.

Table 15.8: Inhibitors of the process of protein biosynthesis

Antibiotic/Inhibitor	Inhibitory effect in		Inhibits the process of
	Prokaryotes	Eukaryotes	
Streptomycin	30S subunit	—	Initiation and misreading of the mRNA
Tetracyclin	30S subunit	40S subunit	Binding of aminoacyl-tRNA
Puromycin/Chloramphenicol	70S ribosome	80S ribosome	Peptide transfer
Erythromycin	50S subunit	—	Translocation
Fusidic acid	EF-G	—	Translocation
Cycloheximide	—	80S ribosome	Elongation
Diphtheria toxin	—	60S subunit	Translocation
Ricin	—	60S subunit	Multiple processes in protein synthesis
α-Sarcin	—	60S subunit	Multiple processes in protein synthesis
Colicin E3	30S subunit	—	Initiation

Neomycin and Gentamycin: They interact with the small ribosomal subunit and cause mistranslation.

Tetracyclin: It binds directly to the ribosome and interferes in aminoacyl-tRNA binding.

Antibiotics that Interfere in Chain Elongation

Puromycin: It structurally resembles an aminoacyl-tRNA. It thus binds at the ribosomal A-site and acts as acceptor in peptidyltransferase reaction. Puromycin thus prematurely terminates translation, leading to release of peptidyl–puromycin complex.

Chloramphenicol: It directly inhibits peptidyl-transferase by binding the transferase.

Erythromycin: It interferes with the translocation process on prokaryotic ribosomes.

Fusidic acid: It interferes in the process of translocation by inhibiting EF-G (GTP-dependent translocase) in prokaryotes.

Cycloheximide: It inhibits elongation process in eukaryotes.

Diphtheria toxin: It is a protein, which is produced by *Corynebacterium diphtheriae* that inhibits the process of translocation in eukaryotes.

Toxins that Attack on RNAs and Inhibit Protein Synthesis

Ricin: It is obtained from the castor bean. It cleaves adenine from rRNA in the large subunit and thus inactivates the ribosome in eukaryotes.

α-Sarcin: It is a fungal toxin. It cleaves rRNA at the single site within the large subunit of the ribosome and inactivates the ribosome in eukaryotes.

Colicin E3: It is a toxin, which is obtained from *E. coli*. It has ribonuclease activity and cleaves 16S rRNA of the 30S ribosomal subunit near the mRNA-binding sequence and the decoding region. It thus inactivates small subunit of the ribosome and stops initiation of protein synthesis.

POST-TRANSLATIONAL MODIFICATIONS

After synthesis of the polypeptide chain, several proteins undergo various changes. Since these modifications occur after translation of the process, these changes are referred as **post-translational modifications.**

Post-translational modifications include partial proteolysis of the protein chain, or **covalent modification with the addition** of one or more groups on amino acids in the protein chain.

Partial Proteolysis of the Protein Chain

Some proteins, particularly, those destined for secretion from the cell, are synthesized as the large precursors that are not functionally active, e.g. insulin, several zymogens, etc. A small portion of the protein is removed by specialized endoproteases, which in turn results in the release of a biologically active protein.

Some of them are cleaved in endoplasmic reticulum or Golgi apparatus while others in developing secretory vesicles, or after secretion. For example:

Conversion of preproinsulin to insulin: Insulin is synthesized as preproinsulin, which enters endoplasmic reticulum where **signal peptidase cleaves the signal peptide** and converts it to proinsulin. **Proinsulin is then transported to the Golgi apparatus** where it is **packaged into the secretory granules.** The **C-peptide** (connecting-peptide) is **removed by proteolysis** and mature **insulin is secreted** (Fig. 15.21).

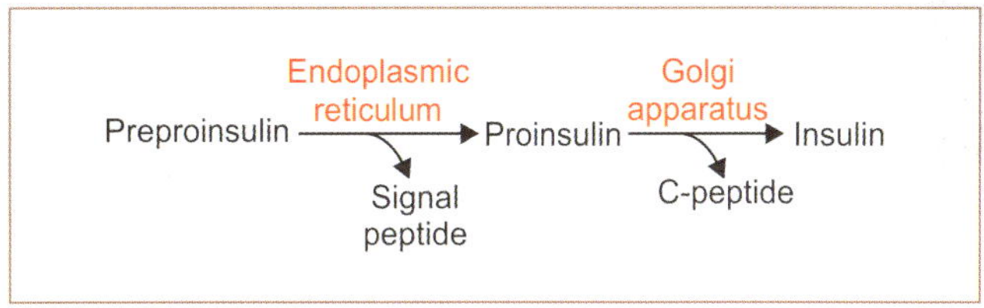

Fig. 15.21: Conversion of preproinsulin to insulin

Abnormally processed insulin (proinsulin) is **released into the circulation** in an autosomal dominant condition, referred to as **familial hyperproinsulinemia.**

Activation of the zymogen: Proteolysis also leads to **activation of the zymogen,** such as proteases. Inactive zymogen precursors are packaged in the storage granules and activated by proteolysis, e.g. trypsinogen is cleaved to trypsin, or chymotrypsinogen is converted to chymotrypsin.

Covalent Modifications

Though only 20 amino acids are encoded genetically, post-translational modifications, however, show the existence of many more amino acids in proteins. Modification of the amino acid may occur in several ways, such as:

Phosphorylation: Phosphorylation may occur on the hydroxyl group of serine or threonine, in a protein, e.g. reversible phosphorylation of glycogen phosphorylase and glycogen synthase by protein kinase and protein phosphatase, respectively.

Glycosylation: Plasma membrane proteins or some other proteins, which are to be secreted from the cell, have carbohydrate chains attached to the hydroxyl group of serine or threonine by O-linkage or to the NH_2 group of asparagine by N-linkage. Stepwise addition of sugar molecules (glucose, galactose, mannose, fucose, etc.) occurs in the endoplasmic reticulum and Golgi apparatus. Glycosylation of the protein thus forms a glycoprotein, such as membrane-bound glycoprotein.

Methylation: Methylation of the ε-amino group of lysine occurs in histones. This in turn modulates their interaction with the DNA.

Hydroxylation: Proline and lysine residues in collagen are extensively hydroxylated in the endoplasmic reticulum.

Table 15.9 lists some important conditions related to abnormal post-translational modifications of proteins.

Table 15.9: Conditions related to abnormal post-translational modifications
• **Familial hyper-proinsulinemia:** An autosomal dominant condition; abnormally processed insulin (proinsulin) enters the circulation.
• **Acute pancreatitis:** Premature activation of pancreatic zymogens.
• **Cancer:** Abnormal histone methylation alters their DNA binding and hence gene regulation.
• **Scurvy:** Vitamin C deficiency leading to abnormal processing of collagens.

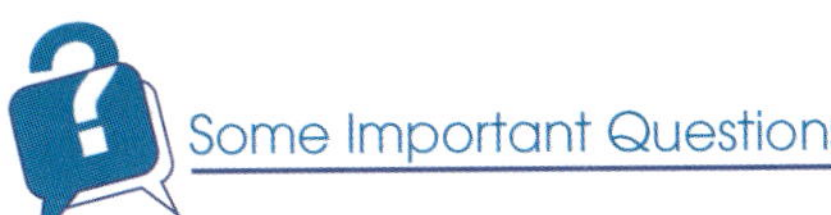

Some Important Questions

1. What is replication? Describe the process of DNA replication in prokaryotes. How does it differ in eukaryotes?

2. What are mutations? Describe different types of mutations.

3. Discuss the differences between DNA polymerases in prokaryotes and eukaryotes.

4. Describe the process of transcription in prokaryotes. How does it differ from eukaryotes?

5. Differentiate between RNA polymerases found in prokaryotes from those of eukaryotes.

6. Differentiate between the promoter regions in prokaryotes and eukaryotes.

7. Give a brief account of protein biosynthesis.

8. Explain the significance of post-translational modifications with examples.

9. Describe briefly:

i. Origin of replication
ii. Semiconservative replication of DNA
iii. Topoisomerase inhibitors
iv. Role of RNA primer in replication
v. Ter regions
vi. Replication of mitochondrial DNA
vii. Formation of nucleosomes

10. Write notes on:

i. DnaA protein
ii. Topoisomerases
iii. DNA polymerases
iv. Reverse transcriptase
v. Replication fork
vi. Okazaki fragments
vii. Primosome
viii. Telomeres
ix. Histones
x. DNA repair
xi. Xeroderma pigmentosum
xii. Single-stranded DNA-binding proteins
xiii. DNA helicases
xiv. Telomerases
xv. Promoter regions
xvi. RNA polymerases
xvii. Post-transcriptional modifications
xviii. DNA template
xix. Upstream nucleotide sequence
xx. Pribnow box
xxi. TATA box
xxii. Enhancers
xxiii. Rho-dependent termination of transcription
xxiv. Rho-independent termination of transcription
xxv. RNA interference
xxvi. Genetic code
xxvii. Wobble hypothesis
xxviii. Shine-Dalgarno sequence
xxix. Peptidyltransferase
xxx. Inhibitors of protein biosynthesis
xxxi. Diphtheria toxin

Multiple Choice Questions

1. The site of origin of DNA replication is rich in:

A. AT

B. GC

C. Any of the above

D. None of the above

2. The following is not involved in eukaryotic nuclear DNA synthesis:

A. DNA polymerase α

B. DNA polymerase β

C. DNA polymerase γ

D. DNA polymerase ε

3. DNA glycosylases participate in:

A. Base excision repair

B. Nucleotide excision repair

C. Mismatch repair

D. SOS repair

4. An AT$\rightarrow$GC mutation is an example of:

A. Point mutation, transition

B. Point mutation, transversion

C. Frame-shift mutation, insertion

D. Frame-shift mutation, deletion

5. In eukaryotes, the following enzyme is inhibited by high concentration of α-amanitin:

A. RNA polymerase I

B. RNA polymerase II

C. RNA polymerase III

D. mtRNA polymerase

6. Human mitochondrial RNase P is a:

A. Ribozyme B. Ribonucleoprotein

C. Protein D. RNA-DNA hybrid

7. RNA interference is not equivalent to:

A. Post-transcriptional gene silencing

B. Gene knockdown

C. Gene knockout

D. Aptamer-based gene silencing

8. The function of aminoacyl-tRNA synthetase is:

A. Activation of a specific amino acid

B. Transfer of amino acid to the corresponding tRNA

C. Deacylation of misacylated tRNA

D. All of the above

9. The peptidyltransferase activity resides in:

A. tRNA

B. mRNA

C. rRNA of large ribosomal subunit

D. rRNA of small ribosomal subunit

10. Chloramphenicol inhibits:

A. Aminoacyl-tRNA synthetase

B. Peptidyltransferase

C. Elongation factor 1

D. Elongation factor 2

CHAPTER 16

Gene Mutations and Regulation of Gene Expression

Competency Achievement: **The student should be able to:**

BI7.3 Describe gene mutations and basic mechanism of regulation of gene expression

GENE MUTATIONS

Mutations are **inheritable, irreparable** and **permanent alterations in DNA sequence** which may be phenotypically **silent (hidden)** or **expressed (visible)**. They can be detected only by gene sequence determination.

CAUSES OF GENE MUTATIONS

Mutations may arise by a number of means, such as due to an error in replication during proofreading by UV or ionizing radiation (X-rays and γ-rays) or by a chemical mutagen (an alkylating agent). Besides, DNA may also undergo certain spontaneous changes, such as deamination of cytosine (to form uracil), depurination, etc.

CLASSIFICATION OF GENE MUTATIONS

Mutations are classified into two categories, i.e. a point mutation and frameshift mutation.

Point Mutation

A point mutation involves a change in a **single base-pair** in the DNA, resulting in a single base change in the corresponding mRNA. This type of mutation may also be referred to as **base substitution mutation.** This may result in **transition** or **transversion** types of mutation (Fig. 16.1).

- **Transition mutation:** The substitution where a **purine-pyrimidine pair is replaced by another such pair** is called transition. It may occur spontaneously, induced chemically by a base analog (e.g. 5-bromouracil) or by a mutagen (such as nitrous acid). For example, if 5-bromouracil gets incorporated into DNA (in place of a thymine) it may induce AT→GC transition. On the other hand, treatment of DNA with nitrous acid may result in both AT→GC as well as GC→AT transitions.
- **Transversion mutation:** The substitution where a **purine-pyrimidine pair is replaced by a pyrimidine-**

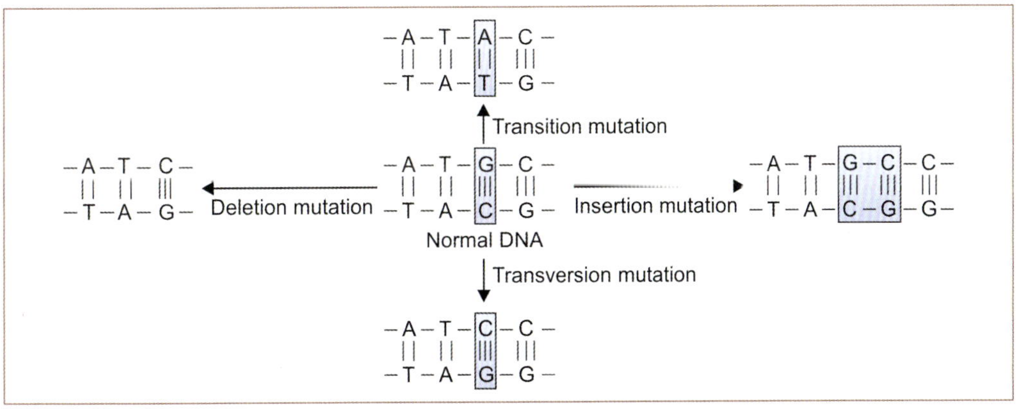

Fig. 16.1: Gene mutations

purine pair is called transversion. This may occur spontaneously and is common in human beings.

Frameshift Mutation

Frameshift mutations are the result of **insertion or deletion** of a base-pair.

- **Deletion:** Deletion of a base-pair from the DNA base sequence of the gene may **change its reading frame** and result in a nonfunctional gene product. For example, a frameshift mutation as a result of base deletion results in the production of abnormal hemoglobin such as **hemoglobin Wayne**. Deletion may be caused by deaminating agents.
- **Insertion:** Insertion of a base-pair into the gene sequence can lead to the synthesis of abnormal chain length of a protein. Some insertions can be caused by mutagens, such as acridines, ethidium bromide, etc.

EFFECTS OF GENE MUTATION

Mutations may be expressed phenotypically (visible) or remain silent.

Visible Mutation

A visible or expressed mutation may be a missense mutation or a nonsense mutation.

- **Missense mutation:** It is the result of a base change that causes the incorporation of a **different amino acid** in the encoded protein. An example of missense mutation is a change in second base of the codon GAA (or GAG) which codes for glutamate in the sixth position of the α-chain of hemoglobin. The change from A to U results in GUA (or GUG) which codes for valine. This, in turn, results in **sickle cell anemia**, one of the most common forms of hemoglobinopathies.
- **Nonsense mutation:** It may be a result of a change in the base of the codon, which may **destroy a termination codon,** or result in the formation of a **new termination codon**.
- **The formation of a new termination codon** may result in premature termination and thus reduce chain length of the protein. For example, the codon UAU or UAC normally encodes for tyrosine, as the 145th amino acid in the β-chain of hemoglobin. A single base mutation from UAU to UAA or UAC to UAG results in a termination codon, which in turn, reduces the chain length from 146 to 144 amino acids. This results in the synthesis of **hemoglobin McKees Rocks** which has a higher oxygen affinity and decreases oxygen delivery to the tissues.
- On the other hand, **mutation of a base in the termination codon to a codon which encodes an amino acid** results in a protein that has larger chain length than the normal. For example, a normal α-globin chain has 141 amino acid residues. When the stop codon UAA mutates, it results in the incorporation of an amino acid at 142nd position and increases the chain length to nearly 172 amino acids, i.e. until another stop codon is reached. Abnormally long α-globin chain has been shown to result in many instances of **α-thalassemias**.

Silent Mutation

This is a result of a base change that occurs in the **third position of a codon**, e.g. UUA to UUG. Since both the codons code for leucine and there is **no change in the specified amino acid**, such mutations are called silent mutations.

It is interesting to note that **certain mutations**, which may be otherwise silent, **require the presence of another mutation in a neighboring gene** to become clinically manifested, as observed in polycystic kidney disease. This is called the **two-hit hypothesis** (Chemistry to Clinics 16.1).

Chemistry to Clinics 16.1: Two-hit Hypothesis

Polycystic kidney disease (PKD) is a disorder in which numerous cysts (fluid-filled epithelial sacs) develop in both kidneys (Fig. 16.2).

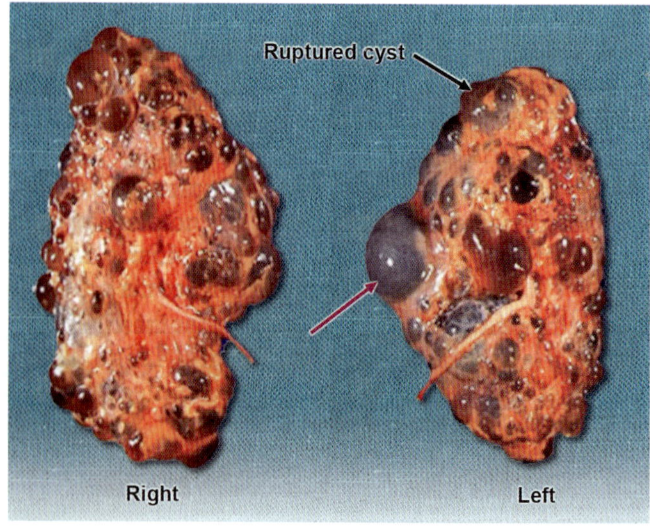

Fig. 16.2: Bilateral polycystic kidneys. Purple arrow indicates the largest cyst

The most common and severe form of the disease is **autosomal dominant PKD1** (ADPKD1), which is a **result of defective gene on chromosome 16**. The PKD1 gene encodes a large transmembrane protein called polycystin 1.

In ADPKD, the primary cilium is poorly developed, suggesting a link between abnormalities in this structure and the cystic phenotype. The phenotypic expression of ADPKD is variable. Some people show symptoms in childhood, whereas others may lead a long and healthy life with cystic kidneys detected only on autopsy. The usual pattern is for patients to develop symptoms (such as hypertension or pain in the back and sides) in their 30s and 40s. Extrarenal manifestations such as hepatic cysts are common. End-stage renal failure (requiring dialysis or a kidney transplantation) occurs in about 50% of patients by the age of 60.

Only 1% of nephrons produce cysts in ADPKD even though every renal cell has a mutant copy of a dominant gene. The **two-hit hypothesis** explains why the disease is so variable, and why only relatively a few nephrons produce cysts. According to this hypothesis, **production of a cyst requires a second (somatic) mutation**, so that the gene (allele) accompanying the inherited defective gene is also abnormal. Only when this happens, a cyst develops. It has been demonstrated that in many cysts in ADPKD, two abnormal genes are present.

REGULATION OF GENE EXPRESSION

A gene is a sequence of DNA that codes for a product which may be a protein as in the case of the majority of genes or RNA as in the case of genes that code for tRNA and rRNA. The crucial feature, however, is that the product diffuses away from its site of synthesis to act elsewhere. The process by which a gene gives rise to a product is called **gene expression**.

Gene expression is **controlled by several factors** that interact, specifically as well as nonspecifically, with DNA **such as various environmental factors**. For example, **supply of nutrients** can affect the rate of synthesis of some of the proteins in bacteria. Similarly, cells of the multicellular organism change substantially in shape, growth rate and other characteristics in **response to several hormones** and **growth factors**.

ORGANIZATION OF GENOME

Genome is a complete set of genetic instructions, i.e. the number, organization and functions of various genes in an organism. The apparent number of genes, like the overall quantity of DNA, roughly parallels complexity of the organism, e.g. *E. coli* has nearly 4300 genes, whereas the total number of genes is nearly 40,000 in humans. A large part of the genome consists of the potential **protein-coding sequences** with open-reading frames that are not interrupted by the stop codons. On the other hand, many genes have no known function and are referred to as **orphan genes**.

Gene Cluster

Genes are randomly distributed in a genome, i.e. no discrete proportion of the genome contains relatively more genes or genes related to a particular function than any other portion of the genome. However, **genes with related functions are found close together**, i.e. in clusters.

A set of genes descended by duplication and variation from some ancestral gene is called a **gene family**. Its members may be clustered together or dispersed on different chromosomes. Some gene families consist of identical members.

Clustering is a prerequisite for maintaining identity between genes, although clustered genes are not necessarily identical. Gene clusters range from extremes where duplication has generated an adjacent related gene to the cases where hundreds of identical genes lie in a tandem array. Extensive tandem repetition of a gene may occur when the product is needed in unusually large amounts, e.g. the genes for rRNA and histone proteins.

DNA in a gene **contains two types of sequences** called **control sites** and **coding regions.**

- The part of the DNA that is expressed via the production of mRNA to synthesize a protein is called the **coding region**.
- The **noncoding region** of the DNA contains several sequences that are called **nontranscribable sequences**. These sequences include the **regulatory sequences**, which separate individual genes and the sites that govern origin and termination of replication. The proportion of nontranscribed sequences varies greatly. For example, it may be about 10–20% in *E. coli* to as much as **98% in humans**. Much of the nontranscribed DNA in eukaryotes consists of **repetitive sequences**.

Repetitive sequences: Sequences that are **present in >1 copy in each genome** are called repetitive sequences. Repetitive DNA components consist of families of sequences that are not exactly the same but are related. DNA of most of the higher organisms contains several repetitive sequences. Repetitive DNA sequences may be of two types:

- **Highly repetitive sequences:** These are simple sequences that occur in tandem, ranging from 5 to 300 base-pairs (bp). They are repeated several times and occupy more than 50% of the total DNA. They are sometimes called **satellite DNA**. High concentration of repetitive DNA is located at the **centromeres** (the regions of the eukaryotic chromosomes that are attached to microtubular spindle during mitosis) and **telomeres** (ends of chromosomes). Highly repetitive DNA often forms discrete clusters.
- **Moderately repetitive sequences:** They are longer sequences and range from one-hundred to several thousands bp in length, and are quite variable. Some are clustered in one region of the genome while others are scattered throughout the DNA. Sometimes, a sequence is highly conserved from one repeat to another, while on the other hand different repeat units of the same sequence may have consider-able divergence. Moderately repetitive component includes a total length of 6×10^5 bp of DNA, repeated nearly 350 × per genome. Since they have no known function, these sequences form a part of the **selfish** or **junk DNA**. Neither of these classes represents a protein. These unexpressed sequences accumulate mutations at a greater rate than the expressed sequences.

THE OPERON

An operon is a **coordinated unit of gene expression**, i.e. a set of clustered genes in bacteria. An operon includes:

- The adjacent **structural genes** that **code for the related enzymes** or associated proteins.
- A **regulatory gene** that **encodes a repressor protein**, which binds to the operator site. The binding of the repressor to the operator prevents transcription of the structural genes.
- **Control elements** are the sites on DNA near the structural genes at which regulatory proteins act (Fig. 16.3).

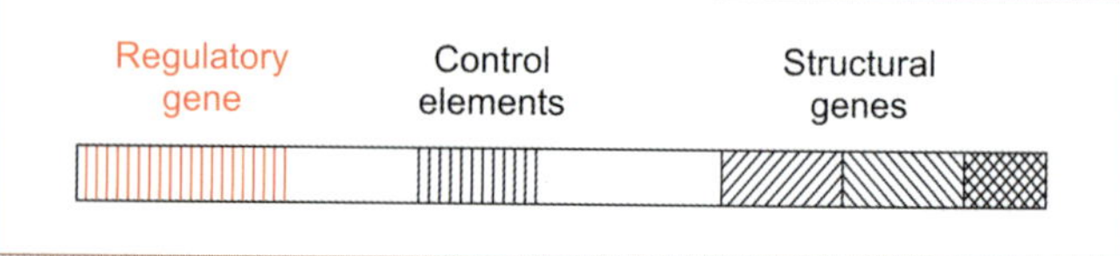

Fig. 16.3: The operon

TYPES OF REGULATION

There are two types of regulation of gene expression:

- **Induction:** It is the process of increase in expression of genes in response to the presence of a specific substrate called inducer.
- **Repression:** It is the process of turning-off transcription of a gene in response to the presence of a specific substrate called repressor.

REGULATION OF GENE EXPRESSION IN PROKARYOTES

In prokaryotes, the most common examples of regulation of gene expression include lac operon and trp operon.

LAC OPERON

The lac operon (lactose operon) contains several genes. These include:

- **Structural genes:** Lac operon contains three adjacent structural genes, designated as **lac Z**, **lac Y** and **lac A** (Fig. 16.4).
  - Lac Z codes for β-galactosidase
  - Lac Y for permease
  - Lac A for transacetylase.

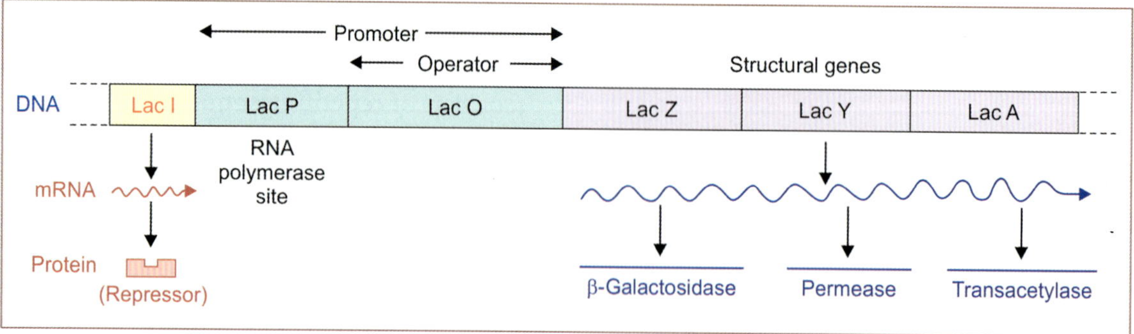

Fig. 16.4: Lac operon

16

All the three genes are transcribed to give a single mRNA molecule that encodes three proteins.

- **Regulatory gene:** Lac operon also contains a regulatory gene referred to as **lac I** that encodes a protein called **repressor**. It is located just in front of the controlling elements for the structural genes, i.e. the ZYA gene-cluster.
- **Control elements:** Lac operon also has two control elements, which are located in front of the three structural genes of the operon. These are referred to as an **operator site** (**lac O**) and a **promoter site** (**lac P**).
  Operator sequence is continuous with the promoter as well as structural genes while the **promoter is located immediately in front of the operator sequence.**
  The **promoter contains a recognition site for RNA polymerase**, and, in turn, directs the enzyme to occupy the correct transcription initiation site.

Utilization of Lactose by *E. coli*

Bacteria such as *E. coli*, usually, depend upon glucose as the source of carbon and energy. However, when glucose is lacking, *E. coli* can use lactose as the source of carbon. An **essential enzyme in the metabolism of lactose is β-galactosidase** that **converts lactose into its monosaccharides** (glucose and galactose). When *E. coli* is grown in a medium in the absence of lactose, it does not require β-galactosidase. On the other hand, when lactose is the sole source of carbon, several-fold increase in β-galactosidase occurs in the cell. Bacteria thus respond to the need to metabolize lactose by increasing the synthesis of β-galactosidase. Also, if lactose is removed from the medium, synthesis of the enzyme stops.

Besides β-galactosidase, two other proteins, namely **galactoside permease** and **thiogalactoside transacetylase** are also synthesized. **Permease is required for the transport of lactose across the bacterial cell membrane.** On the other hand, though **transacetylase** is not essential for lactose metabolism, it **plays an important role in acetylation and detoxification of the metabolite.**

This ability of bacteria to produce a series of proteins, only when needed for the utilization of a substrate, allows the bacteria to **adapt to the environment** without any need to continuously synthesize large quantities of the enzymes when these are not required.

Lac Repressor

The lac operon, as discussed above, contains a **regulatory gene lac I**. The **product of expression of this gene is a protein** called **repressor**, which **inhibits the synthesis of the three enzymes**. Repressor forms a tetramer, an active form of the protein.

- **In the absence of lactose, repressor recognizes the operator and binds to it. Binding of repressor to operator, prevents binding of RNA polymerase** and, thus, **blocks transcription of structural genes** (Fig. 16.5).
- **Addition of lactose** to the medium **leads to the formation of 1,6-allolactose (an analog of lactose,** where galactose and glucose are linked by α-1,6 linkage instead of β-1,4 linkage). It is a side product of the β-galactosidase reaction and **acts as an inducer**. The **inducer binds to the repressor** and forms **inducer–repressor complex**, which **cannot bind to the operator**. Accordingly, the **operator remains unoccupied** and **allows the transcription** and subsequent **translation of the enzymes** (Fig. 16.6).
  Lactose or its metabolite, since acts as an **inducer**; enhances synthesis of the three enzymes. **All the**

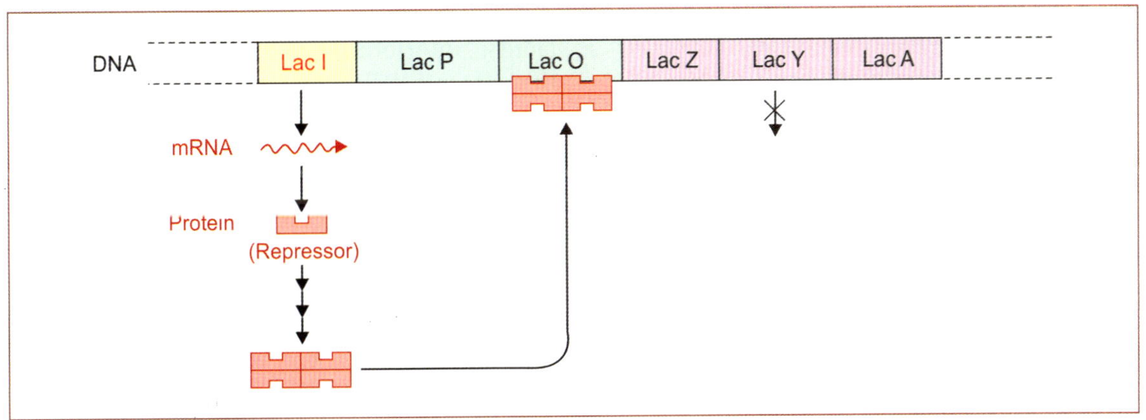

Fig. 16.5: Expression of lac operon in the absence of inducer (lactose)

16

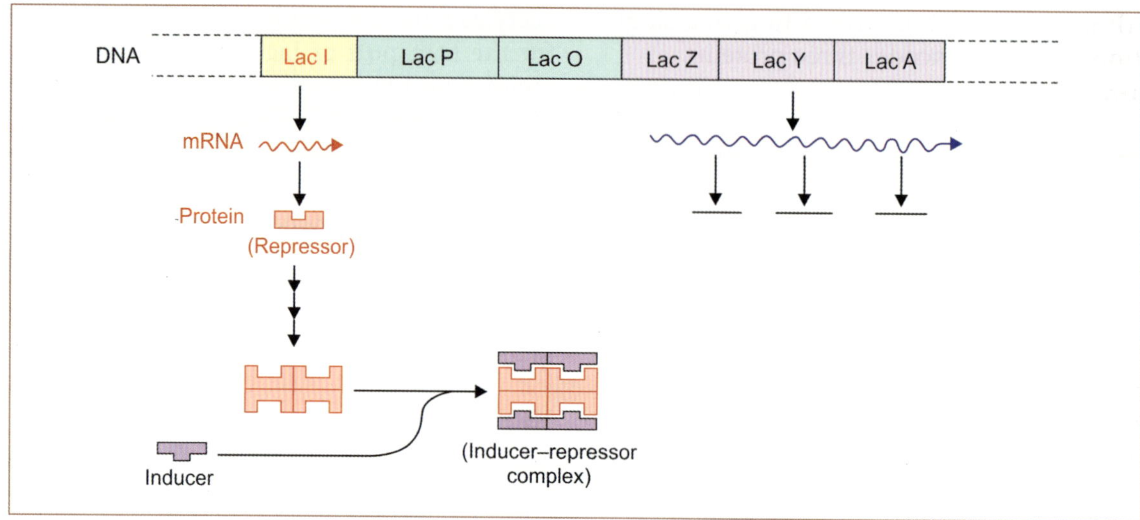

Fig. 16.6: Expression of lac operon in the presence of inducer (lactose)

three structural genes are coordinately expressed, i.e. either all the three are equally transcribed or none of these is transcribed. **The repressor, thus, inhibits (represses) the transcription, until the presence of lactose.**

Catabolite Repression

Besides, a binding site for RNA polymerase, **promoter also contains a recognition site for** another protein called **catabolite activator protein (CAP)**, a **DNA-binding protein**. CAP is **also called cAMP-response protein** (CRP), since CAP can bind to cAMP and form a complex with it. **It is, actually, the CAP–cAMP complex that binds to the promoter and not the CAP alone.**

As mentioned earlier, *E. coli* prefers glucose as a metabolic fuel instead of other sugars. For example, if both glucose and lactose are present in the medium in equal concentrations, bacteria will preferentially metabolize glucose. Only after all the glucose has been utilized, it will start utilizing lactose. This is because glucose lowers the intracellular concentration of cAMP. When glucose is absent from the medium, cAMP level increases. The CAP undergoes conformational changes and forms **CAP–cAMP complex** that **binds to the promoter and exerts a positive control on transcription.** The binding also facilitates the binding of RNA polymerase to the promoter and thereby results in transcription (Fig. 16.7).

On the other hand, when glucose is present, it inhibits the synthesis of cAMP whose level is reduced. The CAP–cAMP complex cannot be formed and a positive effect on RNA polymerase does not occur (Fig. 16.8).

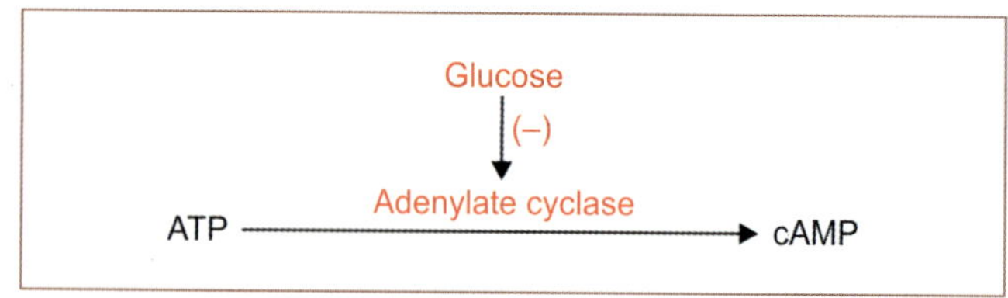

Fig. 16.8: Inhibition of cAMP synthesis by glucose

It is, therefore, clear that glucose, a catabolite of lactose, interferes with the induction of lac operon and this effect is called **catabolite repression.**

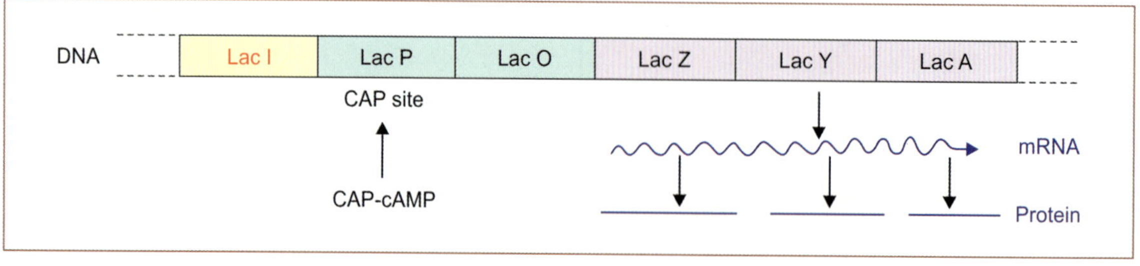

Fig. 16.7: Catabolite repression

16

The **CAP is a positive regulator** since it **turns the transcription on.** On the other hand, **lac repressor** is a **negative regulator** and **turns the transcription off**.

TRP OPERON

The trp operon (**tryptophan operon) is an anabolic operon**. Such operons exhibit an additional regulatory mechanism involving the formation of a secondary structure of the newly transcribed mRNA, which acts as an attenuator of transcription.

Tryptophan is synthesized in *E. coli* from chorismic acid in five steps by three different enzymes, since two of the enzymes, i.e. anthranilate synthetase and tryptophan synthetase, each have two different subunits.

Trp operon contains the following genes:

- **Trp operon** contains a **cluster of five structural genes** designated as **trp A, trp B, trp C, trp D and trp E**.
- **Upstream from this cluster of genes, is a promoter** (**trp P**), where transcription begins, and
- **An operator** (**trp O**) to which a repressor protein binds (Fig. 16.9).
- **Repressor:** Repressor is a **product of the R gene**, which is **not linked to trp operon**. It is a tetramer of four identical subunits.
  - The repressor **forms a complex with the corepressor** (a small molecule, such as **L-tryptophan**). **Repressor–corepressor complex binds to the operator and blocks binding of the RNA polymerase to the promoter**, resulting in decreased rate of transcription.
  - Besides, **repressor is also known to regulate transcription of its own gene**, i.e. the R gene.

Thus, when trp operon is actively transcribed, it is said to be de-repressed, as the repressor alone cannot prevent the binding of RNA polymerase with the promoter. On the other hand, when repressor forms a complex with the corepressor, trp operon gets repressed. Repression causes nearly 70-fold reduction in the rate of trp operon transcription.

- **Trp operon also contains additional regulatory elements** that impose further control on transcription.
  - **Secondary promoter:** One of these additional control sites is a **secondary promoter** which is located within the coding sequence of the trp D gene and is designated as trp P2. This secondary promoter is not regulated by the repressor but transcribes an mRNA that contains coding sequence for the last three genes of the operon (trp CBA).
  - **Attenuator:** Besides, there also exists an additional transcriptional control element, located upstream of the trp E gene, in the leader sequence (**trp L**). This control element is termed **attenuator**.

Regulatory elements of the tryptophan operon thus are the **primary promoter** (trp P), **operator** (trp O), **attenuator** (trp a), **secondary internal promoter** (trp P2) and **terminator** (trp t).

Attenuation

Attenuation is a prokaryotic mechanism for regulating transcription through modulation of the nascent RNA secondary structure. The **attenuator** is a short open-reading frame encoding a **14-amino acid leader peptide**, which contains two adjacent tryptophan residues in positions 10 and 11. RNA sequence of the attenuator region **contains four complementary segments**, referred to as segments 1, 2, 3 and 4,

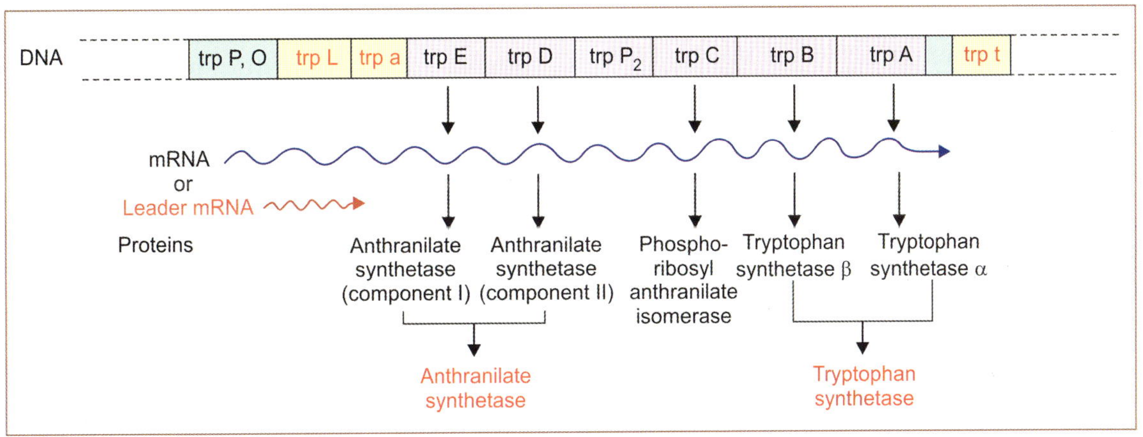

Fig. 16.9: Tryptophan operon of *E. coli*

16

respectively. These can adopt several possible secondary structures. Segments 3 and 4 together with the succeeding residues constitute a **transcription terminator** (a GC-rich hairpin, followed by several U residues). Transcription rarely proceeds beyond this site (termination site) unless tryptophan is in short supply.

During tryptophan deficiency, the entire polycistronic mRNA, inclusive of the trp L sequence, is synthesized. After tryptophan synthesis starts, rate of transcription decreases, since tryptophan binds to trp repressor. Tryptophan, in turn, results in premature termination of transcription. As a result of it, mRNA transcribes only the trp L segment.

Attenuation thus **regulates trp operon transcription according to the supply of tryptophan.**

REGULATION OF GENE EXPRESSION IN EUKARYOTES

Gene regulation in eukaryotes is more complex than in prokaryotes due to the reason that most of the DNA is packed in inaccessible structures called chromatin. Moreover, majority of DNA in multicellular organisms is not transcribed. In eukaryotes, gene expression is regulated at three distinct levels, i.e. at the transcriptional level, processing level and translational level.

Regulation at Transcriptional Level

Transcription of a particular gene is **controlled by transcription factors**, which are proteins that bind to specific sequences located beyond the gene's coding region. **The closest upstream regulatory sequence is the TATA box**, which is also the site of assembly of the pre-initiation complex. The activity of proteins at the TATA box depends on interactions with other proteins bound to other sites (e.g. various **response elements** or **enhancers**). Proteins bound to enhancers or promoters are brought into contact by loops in the DNA. Further, transcription factors contain at least **two domains**, one whose function is to recognize and bind to a specific DNA sequence, and another whose function is to regulate transcription (stimulate or inhibit) by interacting with other proteins. The transcription factor binds to DNA as homo- or heterodimers with the help of unique structural **DNA-binding motifs/domains**.

DNA-binding domains: DNA-binding domains are usually quite short and comprise only a small part of the protein structure. Several types of DNA-binding motifs are known to exist. These include:

- **Zinc finger motif:** It is a small group of conserved amino acids with a characteristic pattern of cysteine and histidine residues that **constitute the zinc binding site** (Fig. 16.10).

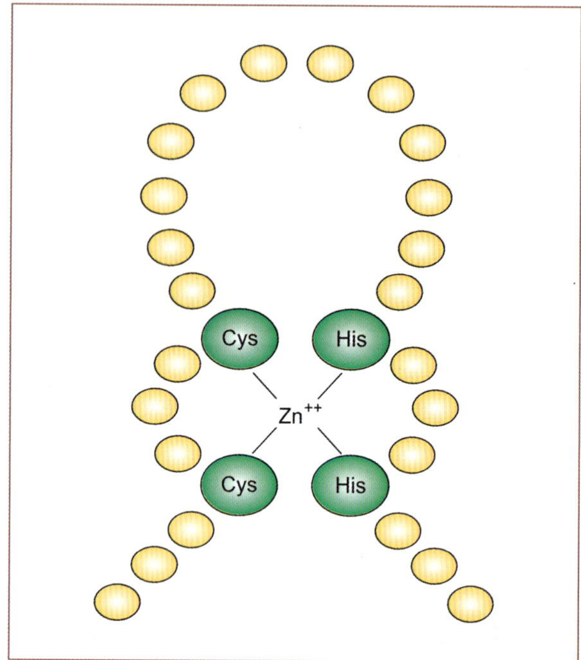

Fig. 16.10: A zinc finger. The motif takes its name from the loop of 12 amino acids (yellow) that protrudes from the zinc-binding site. Either 2 cysteine and 2 histidine residues (a cysteine-histidine zinc finger) or 4 cysteine residues (a cysteine-cysteine zinc finger) coordinate a zinc ion. The loop intercalates directly into the DNA helix. It was originally found in the factor TFIIIA, required for RNA Pol III to transcribe 5S rRNA genes

Zinc finger motifs are found in two types of DNA-binding proteins, such as the **zinc finger proteins** (e.g. TFIIIA) and some of the **steroid receptors** (e.g. estrogen receptors).

- **Homeodomains:** These domains bind related targets in DNA. The C-terminal region of the homeodomain, present in proteins of many eukaryotes, is homologous with the helix-turn-helix motif of prokaryotic repressors. Homeodomain proteins contain a sequence of 60 amino acids which can be either **transcriptional activators** or **repressors**. The homeodomain, particularly, **identifies genes concerned with the developmental regulation.**
- **Helix-loop-helix motif:** The amphipathic helix-loop-helix motif is found in some **developmental regulators** and in genes coding for the eukaryotic DNA-binding proteins. Each amphipathic helix presents a face of hydrophobic residues on one side and charged residues on the other side. The length

of the connecting loop varies from 12 to 28 amino acids. The motif **enables proteins to dimerize** and a basic region near this motif contacts DNA. These protein thus interact by combinatorial association.

- **Leucine zippers:** Leucine zippers consist of a stretch of amino acids with a leucine residue in every seventh position (Fig. 16.11).

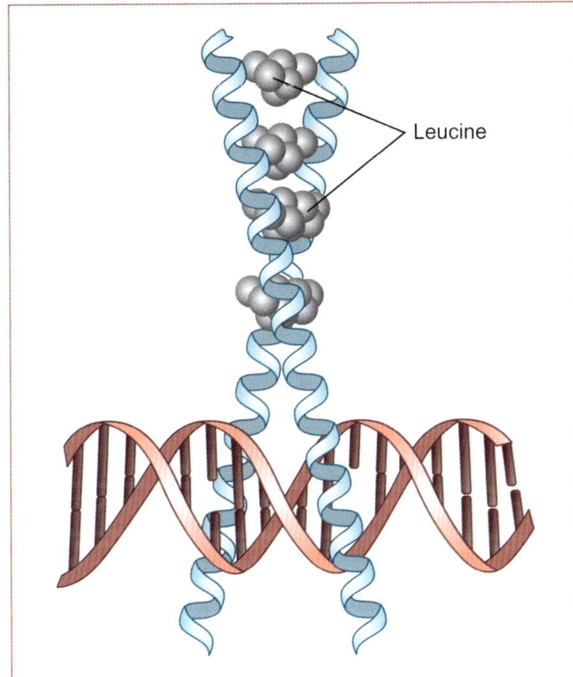

Fig. 16.11: The leucine zipper is a stretch of amino acids rich in leucine residues (grey) providing a dimerization motif. The zipper forms an amphipathic helix in which the leucines of the zipper on one protein (blue) protrude from the α-helix and interdigitate with the leucines of the zipper of another protein in parallel to form a coiled coil domain. The region adjacent to the leucine repeats is highly basic in each of the zipper proteins comprising of a DNA-binding site. The 2 leucine zippers form a Y-shaped structure, in which the zippers comprise the stem, and the 2 basic regions bifurcate symmetrically to form the arms that bind to DNA (red)

A **leucine zipper in one polypeptide interacts with a zipper in another polypeptide to form a dimer**. Adjacent to each zipper is a stretch of positively charged residues that is involved in its binding to DNA. Leucine zippers are found in the factors jun and fos, the products of the gene c-jun and c-fos, respectively.

Coactivators and Corepressors

Activation/repression of transcription is mediated by a number of large complexes that function as co-activators/corepressors. They serve as bridges between TF bound at upstream regulatory sites and the basal transcription machinery bound at the core promoter. Other specialized coactivators include **histone acetyl transferases (HATs),** which are responsible for the acetylation of core histones resulting in transcriptional activation, and chromatin remodeling complexes causing nucleosomes to slide along DNA.

- **Histone acetyl transferases (HATs):** As nucleosomes bind DNA tightly, it is not possible for RNA polymerase and its associated transcription factors to get access to promoter of the gene to initiate transcription. In order to alter the structure of chromatin and make it accessible for the transcription machinery, **histones are acetylated** in a controlled fashion. The ε-amino groups of Lys residues near the N-termini of histones H3 and H4 are acetylated by cytoplasmic HATs. There are two groups of HATs:

  Group A describes those **enzymes that are involved with transcription** while **group B** describes the **enzymes which are involved with nucleosome assembly**.

  Acetylation of histones thus occurs at both replication and transcription (Chemistry to Clinics 16.2).

Chemistry to Clinics 16.2: HATs as Drug Targets

A potential role of HATs in the pathology of cancer, asthma, chronic obstructive pulmonary disease (COPD) and viral infection has been described. Thus, specific HAT inhibitors may find therapeutic applications.

Histone acetylation decreases the affinity of histones for DNA, making additional genes accessible for transcription. On the other hand, a family of **histone deacetylases** removes the acetyl groups which were activated by histone acetylation. This silencing of genes facilitates the recruitment of RNA polymerase to other genes, so as to limit the amount of chromatin for scanning by the transcription factors. Deacetylation, in turn, contributes to transcriptional repression and conversely, repressors may be associated with deacetylases.

Methylation/Demethylation of DNA: In mammals, **transcriptionally silent DNA is highly methylated** than the DNA that is transcribed (Chemistry to Clinics 16.3).

Chemistry to Clinics 16.3: DNA Methylation in Health and Disease

DNA methylation is an epigenetic modification of the genome that is involved in embryonic development, transcription, X-chromosome inactivation, genomic imprinting, maintaining chromatin structure and chromosome stability. Altered DNA methylation is common in many conditions including cancer.

About 70% of the 5′-CpG-3′ sequences in mammalian genomes are methylated at the C5 position of cytosine. However, the distribution of these methylated cytosines varies depending upon the cell type. Methylation is catalyzed by **DNA methyltransferases** (Chemistry to Clinics 16.4).

Chemistry to Clinics 16.4: DNA Methyltransferase Inhibitor

Decitabine is a new anticancer drug which acts as false substrate to inhibit DNA methyltransferase. Reduced DNA methylation results in enhanced expression of antioncogenes thereby suppressing tumor growth.

The methyl group of 5-methylcytosine is projected into the major groove where it interferes with the binding of proteins that stimulate transcription. Relative absence of the 5-methylcytosine, near the start site, is referred to as **hypomethylation/under-methylation**. Only few sites are methylated in tissues in which the gene is expressed suggesting that an active gene may be undermethylated. The region of under-methylation coincides with the region of maximum sensitivity to DNase 1.

Demethylation at the promoter may be necessary to make it available for the initiation of transcription and is carried out by demethylases. The nucleosomes at the CpG-rich unmethylated islands in the 5′ regions also have a reduced content of histone H1.

Genomic imprinting: Another phenomenon associated with DNA methylation is genomic imprinting. Certain genes are active, or inactive, during early developmental stage, depending solely on whether they were brought into the zygote by the sperm or the egg/ovum, i.e. the **genes are imprinted according to their parental origin**. Genomic imprinting is an **epigenetic phenomenon** because the difference between alleles is based on parental inheritance and not on DNA sequence. It is the result of selective DNA methylation of one of the two alleles. Examples of imprinted genes include gene encoding a fetal growth factor called insulin-like growth factor 2 (**IGF 2**). It is active only on the chromosome transmitted from the father. On the other hand, gene encoding a specific K-channel (**KVLQT1**) is only active on the chromosome transmitted from the mother.

Disturbances in imprinting patterns are associated with specific diseases (Chemistry to Clinics 16.5).

16

Riboswitches: Riboswitches refers to conserved sequences of some mRNAs in the 5′ or 3′ untranslated region. These regions bind specific metabolites and regulate gene expression in response to changing concentrations of those metabolites.

Chemistry to Clinics 16.5: Syndromes Related to Genomic Imprinting

In Prader-Willi syndrome, several genes on chromosome 15 of paternal origin are nonexpressed or deleted. The maternal copy of the genes is imprinted and silenced. Children present with disturbances in physical and sexual development besides eating disorders.

The converse, i.e. nonexpressed genes on chromosome 15 of maternal origin and imprinted/silenced paternal copy of genes results in Angelman syndrome characterized by developmental delay, speech impairment and an apparently happy expression.

Regulation at Processing Level

Gene expression is regulated at the processing level by **alternative splicing** or **RNA editing**.

- **Alternative splicing:** It is a process whereby a **single gene can encode two or more related proteins**. Many primary transcripts can be processed by more than one pathway, producing mRNAs containing different combinations of exons. An example of alternative splicing occurs during the synthesis of a protein fibronectin, found in blood as well as the extracellular matrix (ECM). Fibronectin is produced by fibroblasts and retained in the ECM. It contains two extra peptides compared to the one produced by hepatocytes and secreted into the blood. The extra peptides are encoded by portions of the pre-mRNA that are retained during processing in the fibroblast but are removed during processing in the hepatocyte.
- **RNA editing:** It involves **changes in an RNA transcript by deaminating a base**. For example, an 'A'→'I' change (adenine to inosine; deamination at 6-position in a purine ring) can be catalyzed by adenosine deaminase. This changes the coding possibilities, since 'I' pairs with 'G' (instead of 'A' pairing with 'U', if editing had not occurred). Editing of RNA transcripts of **cerebral glutamate receptors** by this mechanism dramatically alters their ion-conductance properties.

Another example is a 'C'→'U' change (cytosine to uracil; deamination at 4-position in a pyrimidine ring) catalyzed by cytosine deaminase. This again changes the coding possibilities since 'U' pairs with 'A' (instead of 'C' pairing with 'G', if editing had not occurred). Editing of Apo B100 transcripts by this mechanism changes codon 2153 from CAA (encoding glutamine) to UAA (a stop codon), resulting in a shorter protein product Apo B48. This is the reason why **Apo B100** is formed in the **liver** and secreted in **VLDL** whereas **Apo B48** (consisting of only the N-terminal 48% of Apo B100) is formed in the **small intestine** and secreted in **chylomicrons**.

Regulation at Translational Level

Gene expression is regulated at the translational level by various processes including **mRNA localization, control of translation of existing mRNAs and mRNA longevity**. For example, in eukaryotes, genes encoding proteins that transport and store iron are regulated at the translational level. Iron response elements (IRE) present in certain mRNAs are bound by an IRE-binding protein when this protein is not bound with iron. Location of the IRE regulates expression of the gene, in response to changes in iron status of the cell.

Expression levels of ferritin (an iron storage protein found primarily in the liver and the kidney) and transferrin (a transport protein that carries iron in the serum) receptors, are reciprocally related in their responses to changes in iron level. When iron is deficient, the amount of transferrin receptors increases and little or no new ferritin is synthesized. An increase in the cellular iron level leads to the destruction of transferrin receptor mRNA and hence, a reduction in the production of transferrin receptor protein. The extent of mRNA synthesis for these proteins, however, does not change correspondingly. Instead, regulation takes place at the level of translation.

The **major regulatory points** of eukaryotic gene expression are highlighted in Fig. 16.12.

GENE EXPRESSION IN PROKARYOTES VERSUS EUKARYOTES

The overall control of gene expression is much more complex in eukaryotes and the major differences are presented in Table 16.1.

1. The genome being regulated is significantly **larger** in eukaryotes, e.g. the *E. coli* genome consists of a single circular chromosome containing 4.6×10^6 bases, compared to approximately 40,000 genes containing 3000×10^6 bases in human DNA.
2. Many eukaryotes have **different cell types**, e.g. the liver cells, the pancreatic cells, etc. These cells differ from others as their genes are differentially expressed.
3. Eukaryotic genes are **not organized into operons** but are spread widely across the genome.
4. In prokaryotes, transcription and translation are tightly coupled, i.e. protein synthesis starts on mRNA templates well before the mRNA has been completely synthesized. In eukaryotes, transcription and translation are distinct processes occurring in the nucleus and cytoplasm, respectively. Thus, **transcription and translation are uncoupled** in eukaryotes.
5. A large amount of **nontranscribable DNA** is present in eukaryotes.

Table 16.1: Differences in regulation of gene expression in prokaryotes and eukaryotes

Parameter	Prokaryotes	Eukaryotes
Genome size	Small; 4.6×10^6 bases in *E. coli*	Large; 3000×10^6 bases in humans
Cell types	Usually a single type	Different cell types (e.g. liver cells, pancreatic cells); each contains the same set of genes but in different cells they are expressed differently
Operons	Present	Absent
Transcription and translation	Coupled	Uncoupled
Untranscribed DNA	Very small amount	Large amount
Overall control of gene expression	Simple	Complex

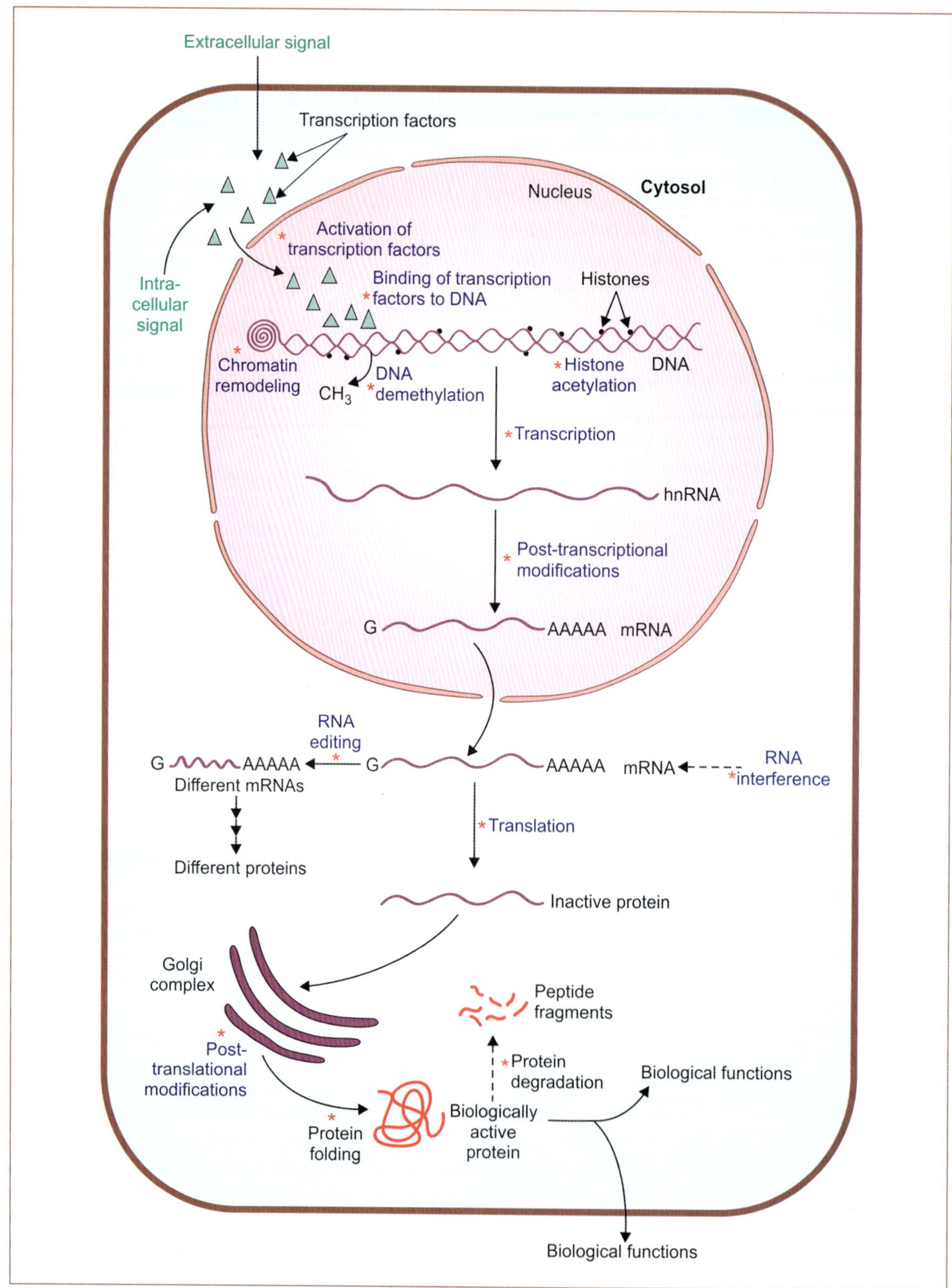

Fig. 16.12: Various steps (*) of regulation of eukaryotic gene expression: Chromatin remodeling, histone acetylation, DNA demethylation, activation of transcription factors, binding of transcription factors to DNA, transcription, post-transcriptional modifications, RNA editing, RNA interference, translation, post-translational modifications, protein folding and degradation

16

Some Important Questions

1. Describe regulation of gene expression in prokaryotes. How it differs from eukaryotes?

2. Discuss:

i. Types of regulation of gene expression
ii. Lac operon
iii. Catabolite repression
iv. Attenuation
v. Chromatin remodeling

3. Write notes on:

i. Gene cluster
ii. Nontranscribable DNA
iii. The operon
iv. Lac repressor
v. Tryptophan operon
vi. Replication of bacteriophage l
vii. DNA-binding domains
viii. Genomic imprinting
ix. Point mutation
x. Frameshift mutation
xi. Nonsense mutation
xii. Silent mutation
xiii. Two-hit hypothesis

Multiple Choice Questions

1. The nontranscribable DNA constitutes:

A. Regulatory sequences
B. Origin and termination of replication
C. Centromeres and telomeres
D. All of the above

2. The following is not a product of structural genes in lac operon:

A. β-Galactosidase
B. Permease
C. Lac repressor
D. Transacetylase

3. Following histone acetylation, the affinity of histones for DNA:

A. Remains unchanged
B. Decreases
C. Increases
D. Any of the above

4. The commonest methylated base in transcriptionally silent mammalian DNA is:

A. Adenine
B. Thymine
C. Guanine
D. Cytosine

5. The difference between apo B-48 and apo B-100 is due to:

A. Genomic imprinting
B. Alternative splicing
C. Frameshift mutation
D. RNA editing

16

CHAPTER 17

Applications of Molecular Technologies

Competency Achievement: **The student should be able to:**

BI7.4 Describe applications of molecular technologies like recombinant DNA technology, PCR in the diagnosis and treatment of diseases with genetic basis

RECOMBINANT DNA TECHNOLOGY

Recombinant DNA is a DNA molecule having different fragments from different sources. The science of various techniques used in the dissection of complex genomes into defined fragments, with complete analysis of the nucleotide sequences and functions is called **recombinant DNA technology** or **molecular cloning** or **genetic engineering**. The technology makes it possible to isolate, amplify and modify specific DNA sequences. This, in turn, allows the removal of a piece of DNA out of a larger molecule such as the genome of a virus or a human being and its amplification.

PALINDROME

In a palindromic DNA segment, the sequence of nucleotides is the same in each strand when the two strands of the palindrome are read in opposite directions, i.e. it has **two-fold symmetry**. These sequences are 4 to 6 nucleotides long and are the sites which are recognized and cleaved by restriction endonucleases. The recognized sequences are **completely symmetrical inverted repeats**, known as palindromes (Fig. 17.1).

Palindrome also serves as recognition sites for methylases that modify the host DNA by introducing methyl groups into two bases of a palindrome. Once these bases are methylated, the palindrome cannot be recognized by the corresponding restriction endonuclease and thus the DNA gets protected from cleavage.

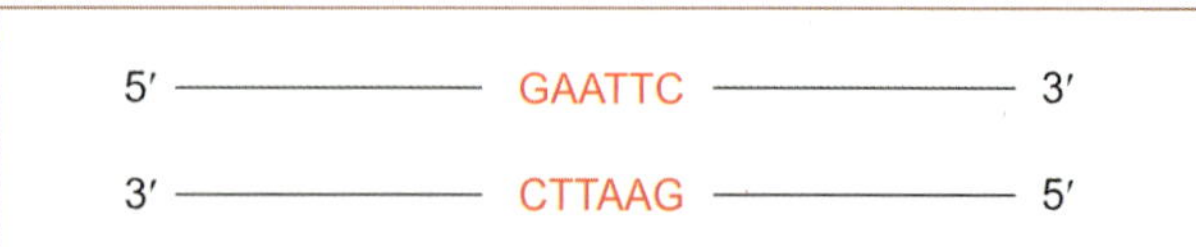

Fig. 17.1: A palindrome

RESTRICTION ENDONUCLEASES

Restriction endonucleases (**restriction enzymes**) are the enzymes that recognize and cleave specific DNA sequences which are symmetrical inverted repeats, known as palindromes. Salient features of restriction endonucleases are shown in Table 17.1.

Table 17.1: Salient features of restriction endonucleases
• Isolated from bacteria
• Recognize and cleave specific DNA sequences (palindromes)
• Generate sticky ends or blunt ends
• Some are isoschizomers
• Used to prepare restriction digest
• Used to prepare restriction map

Salient Characteristics of Restriction Endonucleases

- Highly **specific** enzymes which make **two cuts**, one in each strand of the double-stranded DNA and generate a 3′-OH terminus and a 5′-p-terminus. They are named according to the bacterial source from which they are isolated: The first letter of the genus and first two letters of the species of the bacterium that produces it, followed by its serotype or strain, if any. There may also be a Roman numeral if the bacterium contains more than one type of the restriction enzymes.

- Classified into **three categories**, i.e. as types I, II and III. Types I and III make cuts in the vicinity of the recognition sites in an unpredictable manner. Type II specifically cuts DNA within the recognition sequences. Type II enzymes are very useful in the laboratory for the reconstruction of a genetic map. A large number of restriction enzymes with various recognition sequences have been characterized, such as EcoRI, the enzyme isolated from *E. coli* RY13.
- Most of the restriction endonucleases cleave two strands of a DNA in a staggered manner and produce fragments with single-stranded regions at their 5′- and 3′-ends, called the **sticky ends or cohesive ends**. DNA fragments generated from different molecules with the same restriction endonuclease have complementary single-stranded ends which can be annealed and covalently linked together with a DNA ligase, producing a recombinant DNA molecule.

  Some of the restriction endonucleases cut both the strands symmetrically and produce restriction fragments with base-paired ends, called the **flush ends or blunt ends**. Enzymatically, a poly(dA) tail is added to one of the species of the blunt-ended DNA while a poly(dT) tail is added to the blunt-ended DNA of the other species. These two DNA fragments with complementary tails can then be annealed and ligated (Fig. 17.2).
- Confer **protection** to the host bacteria against invading bacteriophages (viruses that are specific for bacteria). Bacterial DNA sequences normally recognized by a restriction endonuclease may be protected from cleavage by methylation of certain nucleotide-specific sequences of its own DNA (enzyme recognized palindromes) by methylases. On the other hand, viral DNA that has not been methylated on at least one of its two strands is recognized as foreign and is hydrolyzed by the restriction endonuclease.
- Sometimes, different restriction enzymes recognize and cleave within identical target sequences. They are referred to as **isoschizomers**, meaning that they cut at the same site. For example, EcoRII and AtuI are isoschizomers cutting at ↓CCAGG.
- Treatment of the DNA molecule with a restriction endonuclease results in the production of a series of precisely **defined fragments** that can be separated according to their size by gel electrophoresis and visualized by an appropriate technique, such as staining, fluorescence or radioactive labelling. A particular enzyme thus generates a unique family of fragments for any given DNA molecule. The product of fragmentation is called **'restriction digest'**.
- Restriction endonucleases are used to construct a new type of genetic map, referred to as a **restriction map**.

RESTRICTION MAP

Restriction map is a **diagrammatic representation** of a DNA molecule, showing the sites recognized by restriction endonuclease. It is constructed by the analysis of the fragments which are generated by the digestion of the DNA with a restriction endonuclease. In a restriction map, sites of the enzymatic cleavage within the DNA are also defined (Fig. 17.3).

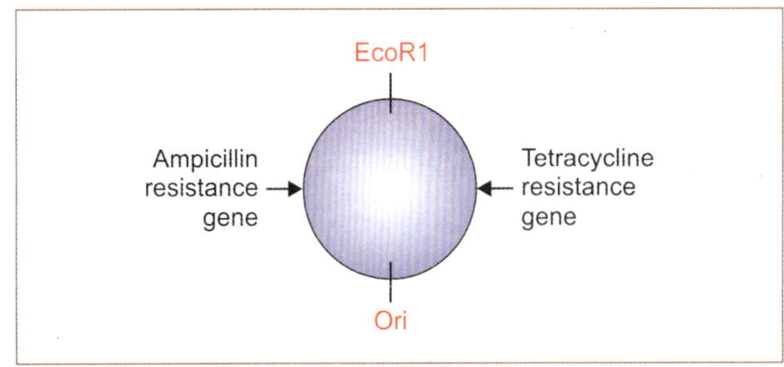

Fig. 17.3: A restriction map

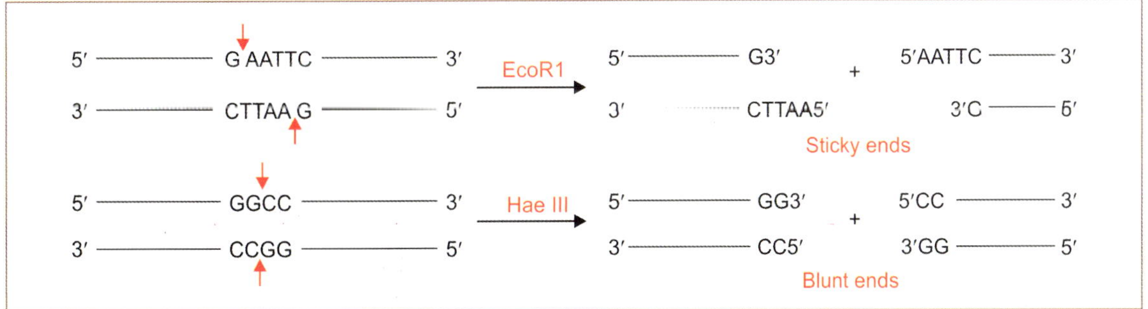

Fig. 17.2: Action of type II restriction endonucleases

17

Technique of Mapping

For the restriction endonuclease mapping of DNA, the purified DNA is subjected to a restriction endonuclease digestion for varying times which generates partially-to-fully cleaved DNA fragments. These fragments are separated by agarose gel electrophoresis and stained with ethidium bromide. Sizes of the DNA fragments are determined by their relative migration through the gel. DNA bands are visualized with a UV light source and photographed. The relative size of each fragment within the DNA molecule is deduced from the size of the incompletely hydrolyzed fragments.

Uses of Restriction Maps

Restriction maps are the convenient frameworks locating particular base sequences on a chromosome, and for comparing different chromosomes. Restriction maps can be used to:

- Demonstrate **sequence diversity** of the organelles DNA, such as mitochondrial DNA within the species.
- Detect **deletion mutations**.
- For **cloning and sequencing** of the genes and their flanking DNA regions.

CLONING

A clone is the collection of identical cells arising from a common ancestor. Cloning is a technique for the production of **multiple identical copies** of a DNA segment or a cell of an organism that contains the desired DNA. Various small autonomously replicating DNA molecules are used as cloning vectors.

Vector

A vector (a cloning vector) is a molecule of **carrier DNA** to which the fragment of foreign DNA, to be cloned, can be attached. A vector must:

- Be capable of autonomous replication.
- Contain at least one specific nucleotide sequence recognizable by a restriction endonuclease.
- Carry at least one gene that confers its ability as a vector.

Commonly used vectors include a plasmid, a bacteriophage, a cosmid, or yeast artificial chromosome.

- **Plasmid:** Plasmids are small circular DNA molecules of only a few thousand base-pairs, found in **prokaryotes**. Plasmids replicate independently of replication of the main bacterial chromosome. They replicate easily, carry genes that confer resistance to one or more antibiotics and have several restriction sites where foreign DNA can be easily inserted. Bacterial plasmids are most suited as recombinant DNA vectors. These are, however, useful to clone DNA segments of up to 10 kb-pairs only.
- **Bacteriophage λ:** Bacteriophage λ (phage 1) is a type of **virus** (phage particle) that infects and replicates in bacteria. It is a cloning vector that can accommodate DNA inserts of up to 16 kb-pairs. The λ phage selectively infects bacteria and can replicate by either a lytic or a lysogenic (nonlytic) pathway. It contains a self-complementary 12 bases long single-stranded tail, called the cohesive termini (cos sites) at both the ends of its double-stranded DNA molecule.

  During infection by the phage, DNA contained in the head of the phage particle enters the bacteria where it is replicated nearly hundred-times and packaged to form progeny phage particles. The part of the phage particle which is not required for infection can be replaced by foreign DNA. Such a recombinant DNA, also called chimeric DNA, is packaged into phage particles and can be introduced into the host cell.
- **Cosmid:** Cosmid vectors are a **cross between plasmid and bacteriophage**. Cosmids contain an antibiotic resistance gene for the selection of a recombinant DNA molecule, an origin of replication for propagation in bacteria and a cos site for packaging of the recombinant molecules in the bacteriophages. A cosmid vector can accommodate foreign DNA insert of up to nearly 45 kb-pairs.
- **Yeast artificial chromosomes:** Yeast artificial chromosomes are linear DNA molecules that contain all the chromosomal structures required for normal replication and segregation during **yeast cell division**. Much large DNA segments (up to several hundred kb-pairs) can be cloned in these vectors.

GENOMIC LIBRARY

Genomic library is a **set of cloned DNA fragments representing the entire genome of the organism**. When a complex mixture of thousands of genes, arranged on different chromosomes (such as in the human genome), is subjected to hydrolysis with a single restriction endonuclease, it results in the generation of a large number of DNA fragments. These DNA fragments are annealed with a vector which has also been cleaved with the same restriction enzyme. Usually, only one of the DNA fragment out of the large number, is inserted into each vector. Bacteria are transformed with the recombinant molecules in such a way that only one plasmid is taken up by a single bacterium. Each recombinant molecule gets replicated within the bacterium. Since each bacterium progeny carries multiple copies of the recombinant DNA, the total population of bacteria now contains fragments of DNA that may represent the entire human genome.

Complementary DNA and cDNA Library

Transcription of a functional eukaryotic mRNA with the use of RNA-dependent DNA polymerase (**reverse transcriptase**) in the presence of the four dNTPs, results in the formation of a complementary strand of DNA, called complementary DNA (cDNA). The collection of cloned cDNAs synthesized from the total mRNA, in a given tissue or cell type is called a cDNA library, such as liver cDNA library, reticulocyte cDNA library, etc. A cDNA library thus **represents the population of mRNAs** in a tissue.

The cDNA libraries are prepared by first isolating all the mRNAs in a tissue and then copying these molecules into double-stranded DNA using the enzymes reverse transcriptase and DNA polymerase. For the construction of a recombinant DNA, the cloning vector and the foreign DNA are cut by the same restriction endonuclease. The complementary ends of the two DNAs, i.e. the vector and the foreign DNA fragments form base-pairs (anneal) and are covalently joined (ligated) by the action of DNA ligase. This, in turn, results in the formation of a chimeric DNA containing a portion of the foreign DNA inserted into the vector (Fig. 17.4).

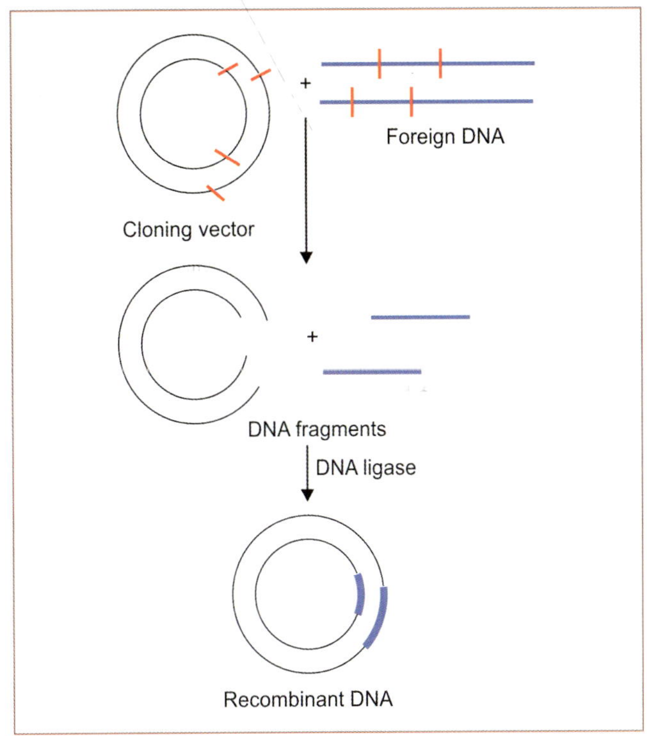

Fig. 17.4: Construction of a recombinant (chimeric) DNA

Directional Cloning Versus Shotgun Cloning

DNA molecules whose ends have different overhangs can be used to form chimeric constructs in which the foreign DNA can enter the plasmid in only one orientation, not randomly. For this, the **foreign DNA** is digested with **two different restriction enzymes**. The **same two enzymes** are used to digest the **plasmid** followed by ligation. This is **directional cloning**.

A particular gene constitutes a very small part of the genome so that it is cumbersome to attempt to recover such sequences from the isolated DNA. Instead, a genomic library is prepared by isolating total DNA, digesting it into fragments of suitable sizes and cloning them into an appropriate vector. This approach is called **shotgun cloning,** because it does not target a particular gene but instead **clones all the genes at one time**. The idea is that at least one clone will contain at least some part of the gene of interest. For this, the DNA is only partly digested so that not every restriction site is cleaved in every DNA molecule. Therefore, even if the gene of interest contains a susceptible restriction site, some intact genes are still present in the digest.

Functional Cloning versus Positional Cloning

In a disease, if an **abnormal protein is already identified**, functionally characterized and sequenced, it is possible to develop probes which can identify and locate the corresponding gene on the chromosome. This is **functional cloning** through which the **gene for hemophilia A** was identified.

On the other hand, the **abnormal protein may be unknown** but genetic mapping in affected families identifies the chromosomal position of the gene and ultimately the gene itself. Thus, the amino acid sequence may be deduced followed by its functional characterization and link with the disease. This is **positional cloning** through which the gene and **mutated protein for cystic fibrosis** were identified (Fig. 17.5).

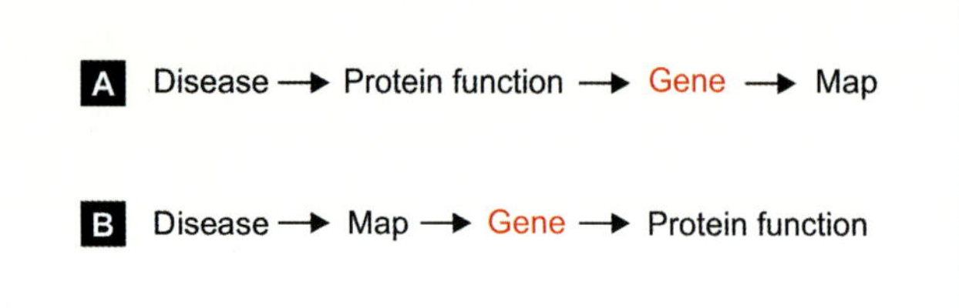

Fig. 17.5: Functional cloning (A) and positional cloning (B)

STEPS IN RECOMBINANT DNA TECHNOLOGY

Recombinant DNA technology involves several steps:

1. A fragment of DNA of the appropriate size is generated by using restriction endonuclease.
2. The fragment is isolated and incorporated into another DNA molecule known as a vector which contains sequences necessary to direct DNA replication.
3. The vector, with the DNA of interest, is introduced into the cells where it is replicated.
4. Finally, cells containing the desired DNA are identified.

Restriction Fragment Length Polymorphism (RFLP)

The human genome is extremely heterogeneous. A variation which affects **<1%** of a population is called a **genetic variant**, whereas that affecting **≥1%** of the population is termed as **genetic polymorphism**. A high degree of genetic polymorphism describes individuality in human and other species. There are inherited differences in DNA sequences among the members of the same species. These differences, in turn, lead to variations in the sites of cleavage of DNA by particular restriction endonucleases producing DNA fragments of different lengths.

The length of the restriction fragment is altered if the genetic variant alters the DNA, so as to create or abolish a site of restriction endonuclease cleavage. RFLPs can be used to detect human genetic defects, e.g. in prospective parents or in fetal tissue. As homologous human chromosomes differ in sequences, these genetic differences result in different restriction sites. For example, whole human genomic DNA isolated from two individuals and digested with a restriction endonuclease when transferred (blotted) to a nitrocellulose filter and hybridized with a probe showed different pattern of bands. Individual A presented a normal pattern while individual B had a high molecular weight band (Fig. 17.6).

The action of a restriction enzyme on two homologous chromosomes (DNA) thus results in the formation of **fragments with different lengths due to the altered DNA**, i.e. the two DNA molecules show restriction fragment length polymorphism (RFLP: Chemistry to Clinics 17.1).

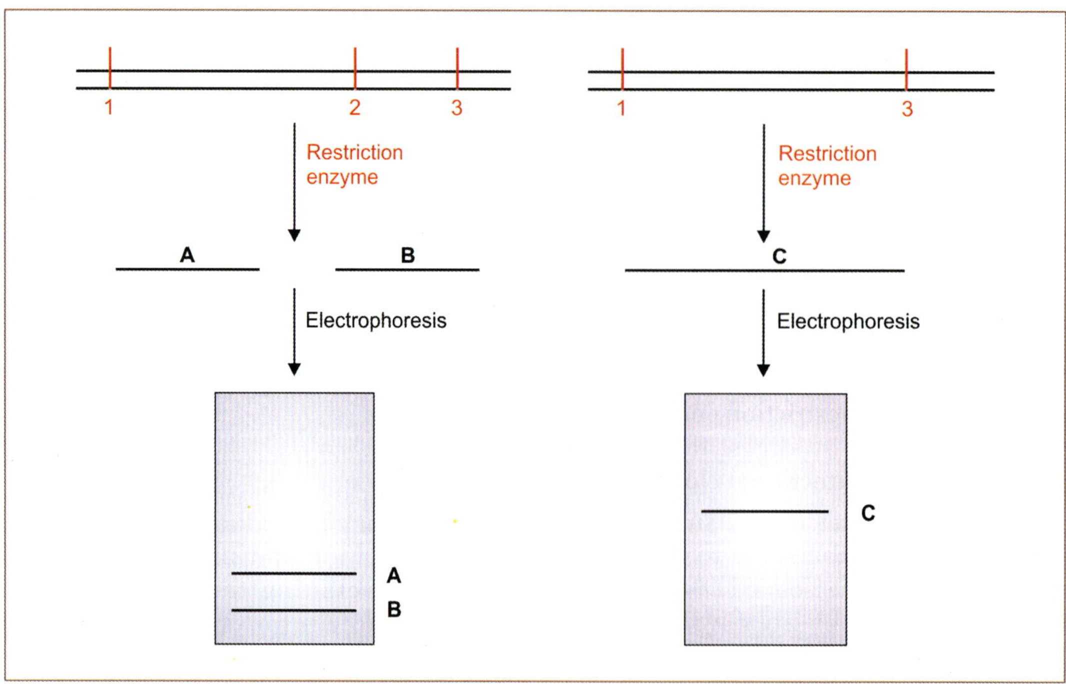

Fig. 17.6: RFLP analysis of two homologous chromosomes

17

Chemistry to Clinics 17.1: Restriction Fragment Length Polymorphism (RFLP)

RFLP is useful in the diagnosis of those inherited disorders for which a molecular defect is not known, such as to define the clonal origin of tumors. If a particular RFLP is closely linked to a defective gene, the detection of such an RFLP in an individual indicates high probability of inheritance of such a defective gene.

Chromosome Walking

The technique is used either to analyze long stretches of DNA or when the sequence is known but the **location of a particular gene is unknown**. It involves the following steps:

- A clone is selected from a genomic library and a small fragment from one end is subcloned.
- The subclone is hybridized with other clones and a second clone is identified that hybridizes with the previous subclone.
- The end of the second clone is then subcloned and used similarly for hybridization.
- The process is repeated and restriction map of each selected clone is constructed at each step and compared to know the region of overlap, equivalent to **'walking along the chromosome'**. The **cystic fibrosis gene** was identified by this technique (Fig. 17.7).

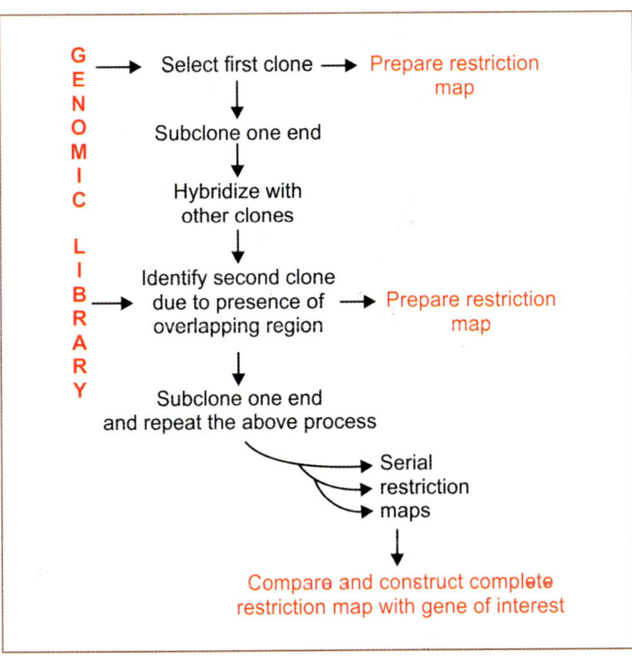

Fig. 17.7: Chromosome walking

DNA Sequencing

The process of determining the **sequence of nucleotides** in DNA is designated as DNA sequencing. The sequence, in turn, also highlights the sequences of their encoded proteins. DNA sequencing also reveals information about the regulation of genes. Once known, a nucleic acid sequence can be duplicated, modified and expressed. This facilitates the study of proteins that could not otherwise by obtained in large quantities.

For determining the sequence of a small polynucleotide, it is partially digested with snake venom phosphodiesterase which breaks phosphodiester bonds between the nucleotide residues starting at the 3′-end of the nucleotide. This, in turn, results in a mixture of fragments of all lengths which can be separated. By comparing the base composition of a pair of fragments that differ in length by one nucleotide, the identity of the 3′-terminal nucleotide in the larger fragment can be established. Analysis of each pair of fragments thus reveals the sequence of the original polynucleotide (Fig. 17.8).

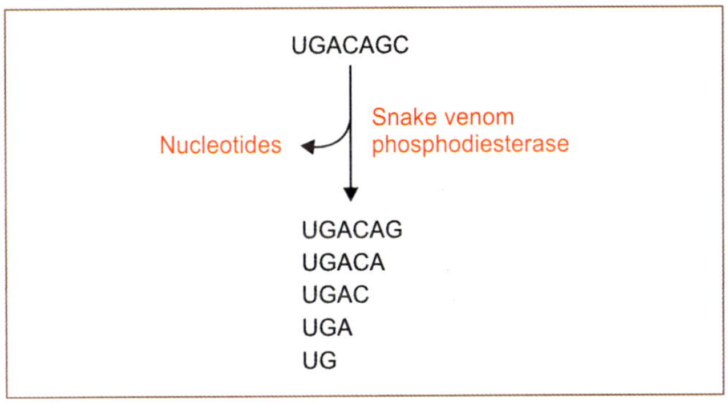

Fig. 17.8: DNA sequencing

POLYMERASE CHAIN REACTION

Polymerase chain reaction (**PCR**) is a procedure for **amplifying a segment of DNA by repeated rounds of replication** centered between primers that hybridize with the two ends of DNA segment of interest.

The PCR requires two nucleotide oligomers that can hybridize to the complementary DNA sequences in a region of interest. These oligomers serve as primers for DNA polymerase, the enzyme that extends each strand:

- In order to initiate the process, DNA sample is heated to 90°C to dissociate the two strands of DNA and cooled in the presence of excess amounts of two different complementary oligomers that hybridize to the known vector DNA, flanking the foreign DNA insert.
- A new cycle of DNA replication is initiated in the presence of DNA polymerase and all the four dNTPs.
- In the presence of sufficient quantities of dNTPs, DNA polymerase directs the synthesis of the

complementary strands. DNA polymerase used for DNA amplification by PCR is a heat-stable DNA polymerase such as Taq DNA polymerase which is isolated from *Thermus aquatics*. Being heat stable, this enzyme eliminates the need for fresh enzyme after each cycle.

- The product of PCR is a double-stranded DNA molecule and the reaction is completed in each cycle, when all the template molecules have been copied (Fig. 17.9).

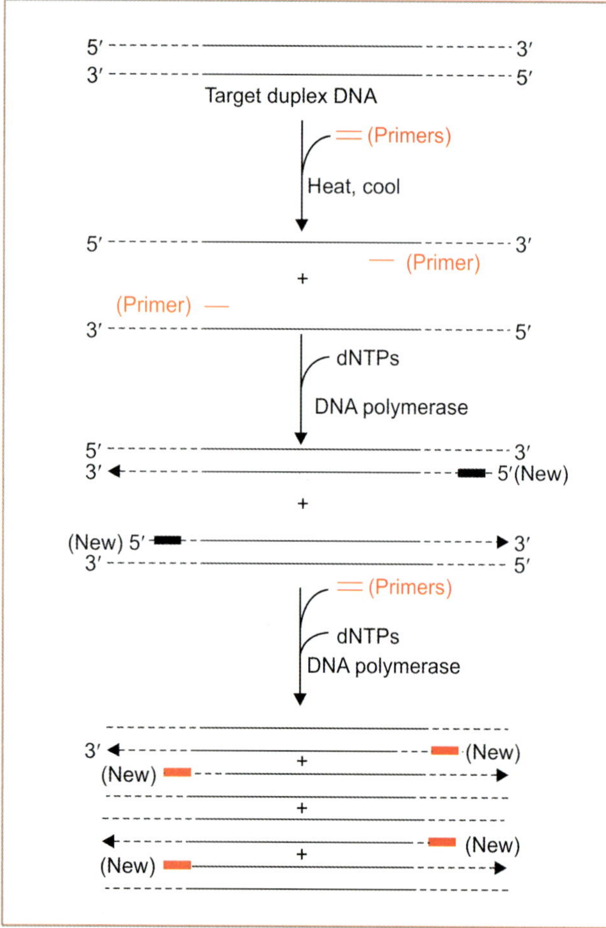

Fig. 17.9: Polymerase chain reaction (PCR)

- Multiple cycles of this process, each doubling the amount of the target DNA, geometrically amplify DNA to the extent that twenty cycles of PCR increase the amount of the target sequence by nearly one million-fold.

Advantages of PCR

17

1. PCR amplification has become an indispensable tool in biotechnology with several applications (Chemistry to Clinics 17.2).

Chemistry to Clinics 17.2: Applications of Polymerase Chain Reaction (PCR)

1. PCR amplification of potential DNA sequences from various infectious pathogens, such as *Mycobacterium tuberculosis*, human immunodeficiency virus, hepatitis B virus, etc. helps in identification of the infectious agent.
2. To detect rare pathological changes, such as mutations leading to cancer.
3. In forensic investigations where only a very small quantity of the DNA is available, such as a drop of dried blood, semen or a single hair. The DNA from such a material is amplified by PCR and its RFLPs can be used to identify the source/donor with the preserved biological material.

2. PCR amplification of a specific DNA sequence can be accomplished with a purified DNA sample or a small region within a complex mixture of DNA.
3. The major advantages of PCR over cloning, as a mechanism of amplifying a specific DNA sequence, are its sensitivity and speed.

Reverse Transcriptase Polymerase Chain Reaction (RT-PCR)

Reverse transcriptase polymerase chain reaction (**RT-PCR**) is a variation of the PCR (basic PCR) technique and is useful when the nucleic acid to be amplified is **RNA instead of DNA**. The enzyme **reverse transcriptase** is employed to synthesize a cDNA strand complementary to the RNA and this cDNA serves as the template for further cycles of conventional PCR. However, it has several **drawbacks** as:

- It is time consuming.
- It has low sensitivity.
- It is semiquantitative.

Real-time PCR (qRT-PCR or Q-PCR)

The Q-PCR enables detection with simultaneous quantification besides numerous other **advantages** (Table 17.2).

Table 17.2: Advantages of real-time PCR (Q-PCR)
• Completely automated process and minimizes user intervention
• Time-saving
• Sensitive
• Inbuilt controls avoid false-positive diagnosis
• Provides a quantitative estimate of amplification in every cycle
• Applicable to detect and quantify DNA as well as RNA (qRT-PCR)

PROBE

The probe is a **labeled single-stranded DNA or RNA** segment whose sequence is **complementary** to a portion of the DNA of interest (**target DNA**). A probe is used to pick up a specific gene/DNA sequence of interest, out of the large number of DNA fragments which are obtained after cleavage of the large DNA molecule by restriction endonucleases. A probe may be a synthetic oligonucleotide of 20 to 30 nucleotides, usually labeled with a radioisotope, an antibody or a nonradioactive biotin-coupled oligonucleotide.

The probe, in turn, hybridizes with the target DNA or RNA of interest in a screening procedure. After washing away the unbound probe, presence of the probe on the nitrocellulose is detected by a technique such as autoradiography. Only those colonies or plaques containing the desired gene bind the probe and are detected. Using this technique, a human genomic library of nearly one million clones can be readily screened for the presence of one particular DNA segment.

Probes are used in laboratory diagnosis of many genetic diseases such as sickle cell anemia phenylketonuria, or certain types of cancers.

DNA CHIP TECHNOLOGY (DNA MICROARRAY TECHNOLOGY)

It is a small device in which thousands of nucleotide sequences are attached to a chip in a **grid pattern**. The chip has a solid surface of glass or silicon (gene chip) and contains a chemical matrix of polyacrylamide or lysine to which the sequences are covalently linked by a technique called **surface engineering**. These sequences act as probes to detect whether a test sample contains a particular DNA or RNA sequence. For example:

- The mRNAs are isolated from normal and suspected cancerous tissue and processed as shown in Fig. 17.10.
- By reverse transcription, cDNAs are prepared and labeled with separate colored fluorescent labels. The labeled cDNAs are mixed and added to the chip containing an array of 60,000 or more different DNA sequences, each single-stranded and nearly 20 nucleotides long. Thus, each strand represents a tiny but unique region of a gene in the genome.
- The cDNAs that are complementary to the probes on the chip hybridize and adhere to that location. Unbound cDNAs are washed away.

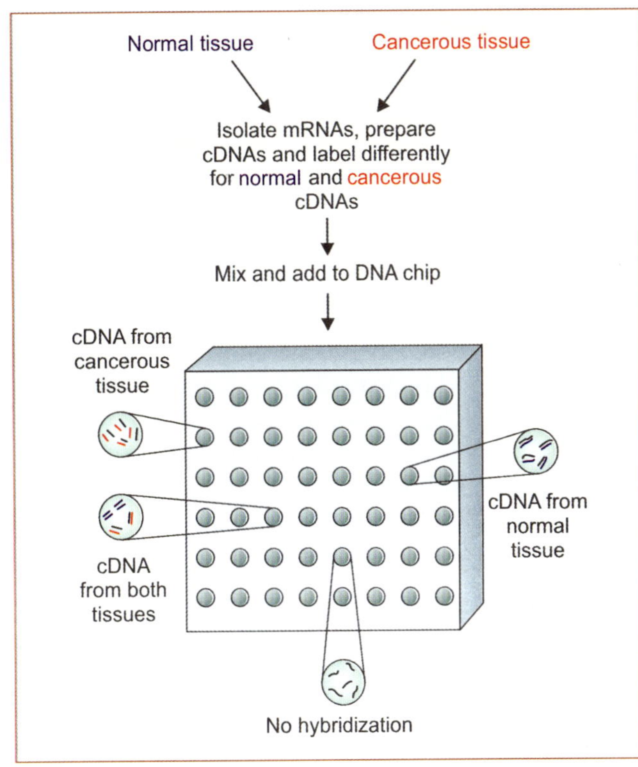

Fig. 17.10: DNA chip technology

- A scanner detects the **patterns of hybridization** by sensing the **color signals which differ** depending on the presence or absence of specific cDNAs (Fig. 17.10; Chemistry to Clinics 17.3).

Chemistry to Clinics 17.3: Applications of DNA Microarray

- Each area of the chip represents a known DNA sequence corresponding to a known gene, hence the identities of the hybridizing cDNAs reveal which genes are expressed in cancerous versus normal tissue.
- Based on the genes expressed, specific treatment strategies can be planned.
- Many genetic tests can be performed rapidly and in parallel.

PEPTIDE NUCLEIC ACIDS (PNAs)

These are **analogs of DNA or RNA** where the sugar-phosphate backbone is replaced artificially by a **peptide backbone** made up of repeating units of N-(2-aminoethyl)-glycine residues linked by peptide bonds. The PNAs are resistant to nucleases as well as proteases and are therefore **highly stable**. They are used as **probes** that bind to specific DNA/RNA sequences. They are also used for **antisense drug therapy**.

17

SOUTHERN BLOTTING

Southern blotting is a procedure for **identifying a DNA sequence** after electrophoresis, through its ability to **hybridize** with a complementary single-stranded segment of the labeled DNA or RNA. This technique is used to detect mutations in DNA and involves the use of restriction enzyme in combination with the DNA probes. The technique is named after its inventor Edward Southern.

- DNA is extracted from the cells, e.g. a patient's leucocytes, and is cleaved into several fragments by using a restriction endonuclease.
- These fragments are separated on the basis of their size by **electrophoresis** as the large fragments move slower than the smaller fragments.
- The fragments of interest are identified by a probe.
- The DNA is denatured and transferred onto the nitrocellulose membrane. Radioactive probe hybridizes with the restriction fragments and produces dark bands on the exposed X-ray film (Fig. 17.11).

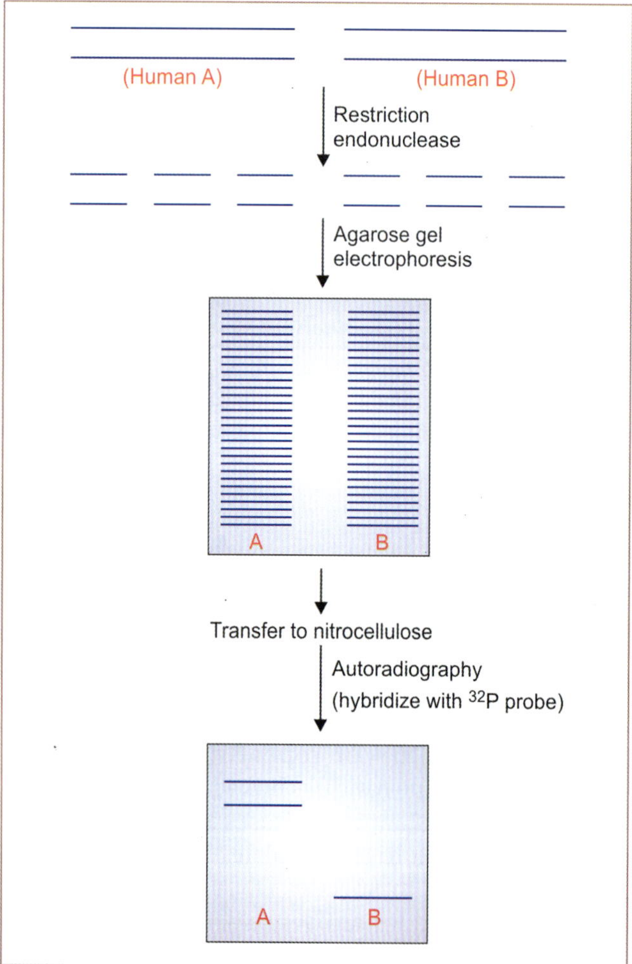

Fig. 17.11: Southern blotting

- The patterns observed on Southern blot analysis depend upon the specific restriction endonuclease as well as the probe used to visualize the restriction fragments. The presence of a mutation affecting a restriction site causes the pattern of bands to differ from those seen with a normal gene.

NORTHERN BLOTTING

Specific **RNA sequences** are detected through a variation of the Southern blot, by the technique referred to as Northern blotting. It is a procedure for identifying RNA containing a particular base sequence through its ability to hybridize with a complementary single-stranded segment of the DNA or the RNA.

WESTERN BLOTTING

A specific **protein** is analogously detected by the technique called Western blotting. Immunoblotting is a technique in which a molecule immobilized on a membrane filter can be detected through its ability to bind to an antibody directed against it. A Western blot is an **immunoblot** to detect an immobilized protein after electrophoresis.

Northern blot or Western blot, however, do not relate to the name of an individual like the Southern blot but are referred only traditionally.

TRANSGENIC ANIMALS

Animals that develop from a fertilized egg when foreign genes are inserted into the genome of a fertilized egg, carry that gene in every cell. Such multicellular organisms expressing a foreign gene (gene from another organism) are said to be transgenic and the foreign gene which is transplanted is called **transgene**. For the change to be permanent, a **transgene gets integrated into the germ cell** of the organism. Transgenic mice and other animals as well as transgenic plants have been developed successfully. Transgenic animals are useful for:

- Analysis of tissue-specific gene expression.
- Studying results of gene overexpression/silencing.
- Discovering genes involved in development.
- Correction of genetic deficiencies.

DNA FINGERPRINTING

The use of **DNA restriction analysis to identify individuals** is called DNA fingerprinting. It is a variation of RFLP analysis in which the probe hybridizes to sequences between restriction enzyme sites that are highly polymorphic. These highly polymorphic sites are called **hypervariable regions** and are made up of tandem repeats of short sequences of 10–60 bp. The number of repeats may vary considerably between individuals and often are called **variable number of tandem repeats (VNTRs)**. The sequence of each repeat may be unique and detected by a single locus probe or have core regions common to many other hypervariable regions that may be detected by a multilocus probe.

The hybridization pattern detected by a **Southern blot** analysis with different probes is generally specific to an individual, just like a fingerprint. The hypervariable regions show a high degree of variability between individuals. This, in turn, can serve as a **DNA fingerprint** that is **unique to the individual** (Fig. 17.11).

DNA fingerprinting can be used for forensic identification, identifying parentage or for the evaluation of the success of bone marrow transplants.

DNA FOOTPRINTING

It is a technique to **identify the nucleotide sequence in DNA where a specific protein binds**, e.g. the promoter sequence bound by RNA polymerase holoenzyme. The DNA is suitably labeled at one end and the labeled DNA–protein complex is incubated with DNase 1. Subsequently, the DNA is denatured and the sets of labeled fragments are subjected to **gel electrophoresis**. Labeled naked DNA (without bound protein) is treated similarly for comparison. The protein binding site is revealed by the **absence of some fragments on the gel** (Fig. 17.12).

REPORTER GENE

Functional aspects of promoters can be studied by using reporter genes. Regulatory sequences such as promoters can be investigated by placing them into plasmids upstream of a gene, called a reporter gene, whose expression is easy to measure. Such chimeric plasmids are introduced into cells of choice to assess the function of the promoter sequence because the expression of the reporter gene serves as a **report** on the effectiveness of the promoter.

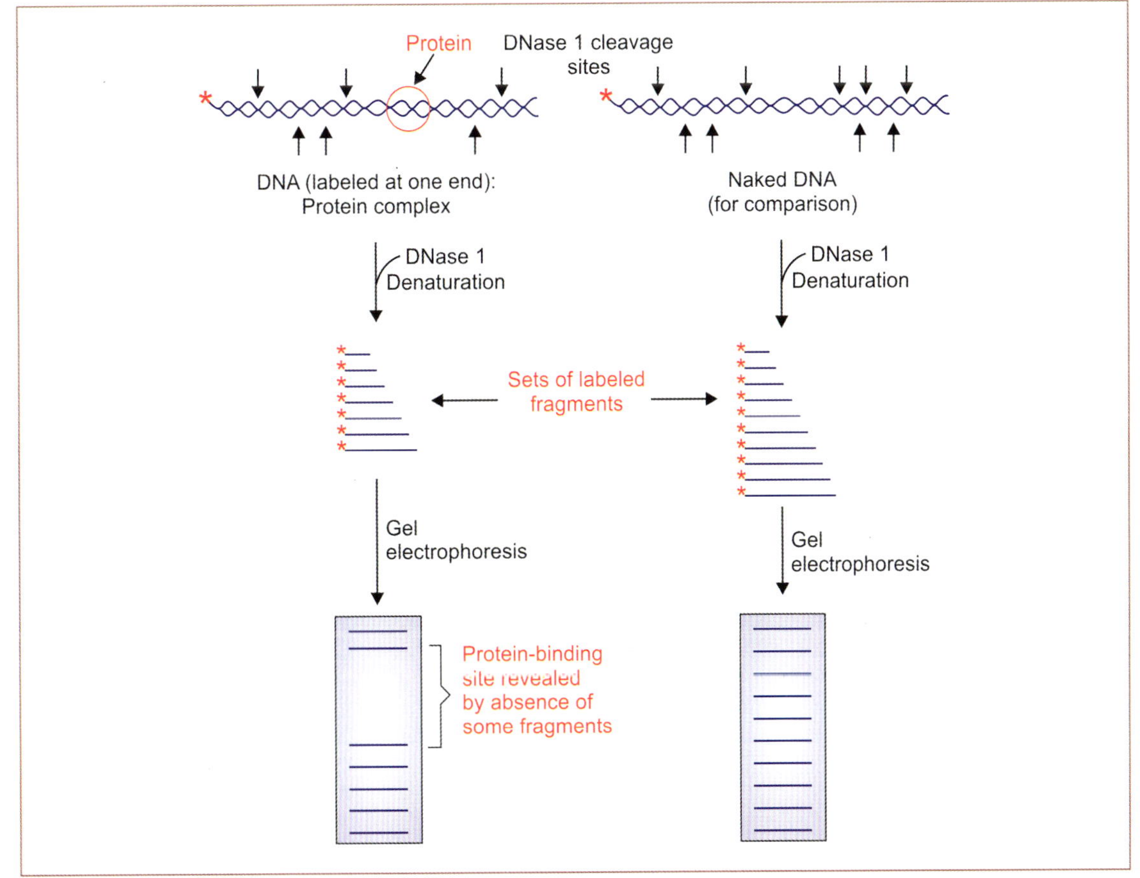

Fig. 17.12: DNA footprinting

17

APPLICATIONS OF RECOMBINANT DNA TECHNOLOGY

Recombinant DNA methodologies are useful for numerous biological disciplines, such as in the study of evolution, forensic biology, clinical medicine and agriculture. Some of its major applications are discussed below.

1. **Understanding gene structure and function:** Treatment of a particular DNA segment with a specific restriction endonuclease produces a set of fragments. Analysis of fragments produced by different enzymes gives a **restriction map** of the gene. It is in this way, the structure of the globin gene was determined (Fig. 17.13).
2. **Molecular analysis including pedigree analysis:** It has become possible to determine the cause of many diseases at the grass-root level, i.e. the fundamental molecular defects leading to disease processes and often being inheritable (Fig. 17.14).
3. **Recombinant DNA techniques such as RFLP, DNA fingerprinting and chromosome walking are used to:**
   - Establish the **perfect genetic identity** of an individual in medicolegal cases to identify criminals and settle issues of disputed paternity.
   - Study various races and ethnic populations, i.e. **population genetics**.
   - Perform **linkage studies** in cases where the exact genetic defect in a disease is unknown. For example, linkage analysis in patients from many families affected with cystic fibrosis revealed two RFLPs flanking a particular gene comprising 1.5 million base pairs on chromosome 7. By chromosome walking, the exact mutation site was identified, i.e. DF508 leading to a malfunctioning of cystic fibrosis transmembrane receptor (CFTR) protein. A similar approach proved that Duchenne muscular dystrophy was due to a mutation in dystrophin gene on the X-chromosome. Other examples include α-thalassemia (chromosome 16), β-thalassemia (chromosome 11), adenosine deaminase deficiency (chromosome 20) and phenylketonuria (chromosome 12).

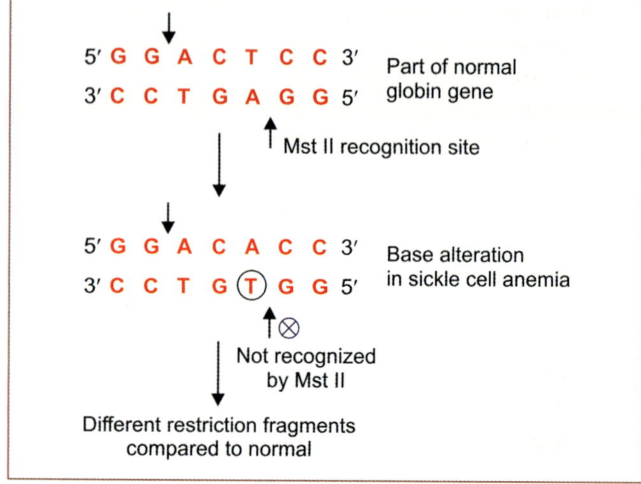

Fig. 17.13: Molecular diagnosis of sickle cell anemia

4. **Disease prevention:** This has been achieved through:
   - **Preclinical diagnosis** and carrier detection in case of hepatitis B, AIDS and tuberculosis.
   - **Prenatal diagnosis** where the disease is detected in the unborn (fetus), providing an option to the parents to terminate the pregnancy if deemed necessary. Genetic markers are available for several diseases (Table 17.3).

Table 17.3: Diseases where prenatal diagnosis is possible

Autosomal dominant	Autosomal recessive	X-linked
Myotonic dystrophy Huntington's chorea	Cystic fibrosis Phenylketonuria	Hemophilia Duchenne muscular dystrophy Becker's dystrophy Fragile X mental retardation syndrome

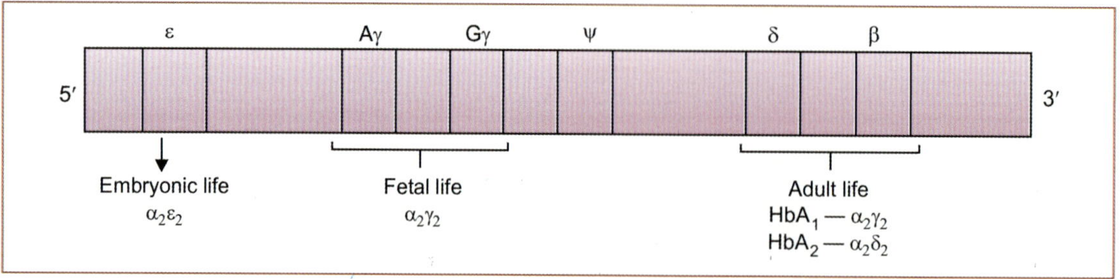

Fig. 17.14: Structure of globin gene

5. **Production of recombinant DNA products:** A cloned gene is inserted into an expression vector (plasmid) that contains properly positioned transcriptional and translational control sequences. A genetically engineered organism thus can produce large quantities of the desired protein. Such organisms are called **overproducers**. A wide range of proteins are commercially being produced to ease the life of patients suffering from many diseases (Table 17.4).

Table 17.4: Diseases being treated by recombinant DNA protein products

Recombinant protein	Target disease
Human insulin	Diabetes mellitus
Human growth hormone	Dwarfism
Somatostatin	Acromegaly
Tissue plasminogen activator	Myocardial infarction
Coagulation factors VIII and IX	Hemophilia A and B
Erythropoietin	Anemia of chronic renal failure
Colony-stimulating factor	Severe immunodeficiency
Growth factors	Extensive nonhealing wounds
Interferons, interleukins	Cancer, advanced viral infections
Monoclonal antibodies	Cancer
Superoxide dismutase	Reperfusion injury in cardiac surgery
Vaccines	Hepatitis B

6. **Gene therapy:** It is the transfer of genetic material to the cells of an individual in order to produce a therapeutic effect. Gene therapy retains considerable promise for treating >4000 known genetic diseases, particularly those with no alternative treatment.

   Guidelines for gene therapy
   - Only somatic cells should be employed to avoid alterations in germ cell lines.
   - Lethal genetic diseases should be selected.
   - The normal gene must be identified and cloned.
   - Single-gene disorders should be chosen.
   - Feasibility and benefits should be documented in properly conducted animal experiments prior to undertaking human trials.

Types of gene therapy

i. **Gene replacement:** To replace the defective gene with the normal gene.

ii. **Gene augmentation:** It is the most popular technique involving the introduction of a foreign gene into the cell to mask the results of the defective gene. Methods of augmentation therapy include:
- Calcium–DNA precipitates
- Electroporation
- Microinjection
- Retroviral vectors
- Adenoviral vectors
- Plasmid–DNA complexes
- Naked DNA (DNA vaccines)
- Site-directed recombination

iii. **Genome editing:** It refers to correction of mutation by selectively removing and replacing defective lengths of DNA. Zinc finger nucleases (artificial restriction enzymes prepared by fusing a zinc finger DNA-binding domain to a DNA-cleavage domain) are employed to target the desired DNA sequence. By taking advantage of the usual DNA repair mechanisms, the sequence is successfully altered. Compared with simple gene replacement therapy, genome editing carries lower risk of random insertion into the genome.

Disease candidates for gene therapy
- **Globin chain disorders:** Hemoglobinopathies.
- **Immunodeficiency disorders:** AIDS, adenosine deaminase (ADA) deficiency, nucleoside phosphorylase deficiency, leucocyte adhesion deficiency. Gene for ADA has been successfully introduced into children with ADA deficiency.
- **Metabolic disorders:** Urea cycle enzyme deficiency, Lesch-Nyhan syndrome, phenyl-ketonuria, lysosomal storage diseases, familial hypercholesterolemia, atherosclerosis.
- **Organ system disorders:** Duchenne muscular dystrophy, cystic fibrosis, α_1-antitrypsin deficiency, Huntington's disease, cancers.
- **Coagulation disorders:** Hemophilia A and B.

Some Important Questions

1. What is recombinant DNA technology? Discuss its applications.

2. Describe briefly:

i. Restriction endonucleases
ii. Cloning
iii. Complementary DNA and cDNA library
iv. RFLPs
v. DNA sequencing
vi. Polymerase chain reaction

3. Write notes on:

i. Palindrome
ii. Restriction map
iii. Vector
iv. Plasmid
v. Cosmid
vi. Genomic library
vii. Southern blotting
viii. Probe
ix. Northern blotting
x. Western blotting
xi. Immunoblot
xii. Transgenic animals
xiii. Gene therapy
xiv. DNA fingerprinting
xv. DNA footprinting

Multiple Choice Questions

1. The small size of cloned DNA fragments is a major limitation with:

A. Yeast artificial chromosomes
B. Bacteriophages
C. Plasmids
D. Cosmids

2. When the DNA sequence is known but the location of the gene is unknown, the following is the most suitable approach to find the same:

A. Shotgun cloning
B. RFLP analysis
C. SNP analysis
D. Chromosome walking

3. An RNA sequence may be determined by:

A. Southern blot B. Northern blot
C. Western blot D. Any of the above

4. Prenatal diagnosis is possible for:

A. Myotonic dystrophy
B. Huntington's chorea
C. Cystic fibrosis
D. All of the above

5. The principles of gene therapy include the following *except*:

A. Normal gene must be identified and cloned
B. Lethal genetic disease should be selected
C. Germline cells must be employed
D. Single gene disorders should be chosen

17

CHAPTER

18

Xenobiotics

Competency Achievement: The student should be able to:

BI7.5 Describe the role of xenobiotics in disease

Xenobiotic means **foreign to life**. It includes any foreign substance or exogenous chemicals, excluding antigen, which the body does not recognize, such as drugs, pollutants, as well as some food additives and cosmetics. It enters the body by various routes such as by inhalation of the polluted air, e.g. industrial chemicals and automobile exhaust; ingestion of contaminated food, such as those contaminated with pesticides, insecticides or herbicides; food additives including colors and sweeteners like butter yellow, azo dye or saccharin; cosmetics such as hair dyes, sprays or lipstick and drugs such as aspirin, tranquilizers or oral contraceptives.

Besides, xenobiotics also include some of the toxic metabolites which are formed by the action of bacteria on food in the gastrointestinal tract, such as amines produced by the decarboxylation of the unabsorbed amino acids (Table 18.1).

On December 3, 1984, thousands of people died (and even more lie affected till today) in Bhopal (Madhya Pradesh, India) following exposure to the gas methyl isocyanate. The gas, normally used to prepare a pesticide called carbaryl, leaked from a chemical factory in the city. The Bhopal tragedy is known as the **Hiroshima of the Chemical Industry**.

There are also certain endogenous substances which are produced in the body, i.e. bilirubin produced during normal metabolism of the red blood cells or phenols produced in the large intestine by the action of bacteria on tryptophan. Most of these compounds are highly lipophilic. These may accumulate within the cells and interfere with cellular functions over a period of time.

Table 18.1: Sources of xenobiotics

Sources	Examples
Industrial chemicals	Solvents (benzene, carbon tetrachloride) Detergents Bleaching agents
Air pollutants Food additives and contaminants	Tobacco smoke Colors (butter yellow, azo dye) Sweeteners (saccharin) Insecticides
Bacterial metabolites Cosmetics Drugs	Bacterial toxins Lipstick, hair dyes, body sprays Aspirin, tranquilizers, oral contraceptives

Biotransformation (B)

The ability of the body to convert a xenobiotic into its excretory metabolite is called **biotransformation** (Fig. 18.1).

Biotransformation (B) includes all those biochemical changes which convert a xenobiotic (not ordinarily utilized) to the excretory product. Though not always true, majority of these metabolites are **more acidic, less toxic and more water soluble** than the xenobiotics themselves. Because the **toxicity** of the original xenobiotic is **abolished or reduced**, the process of biotransformation is sometimes also referred to as **detoxification (D)**.

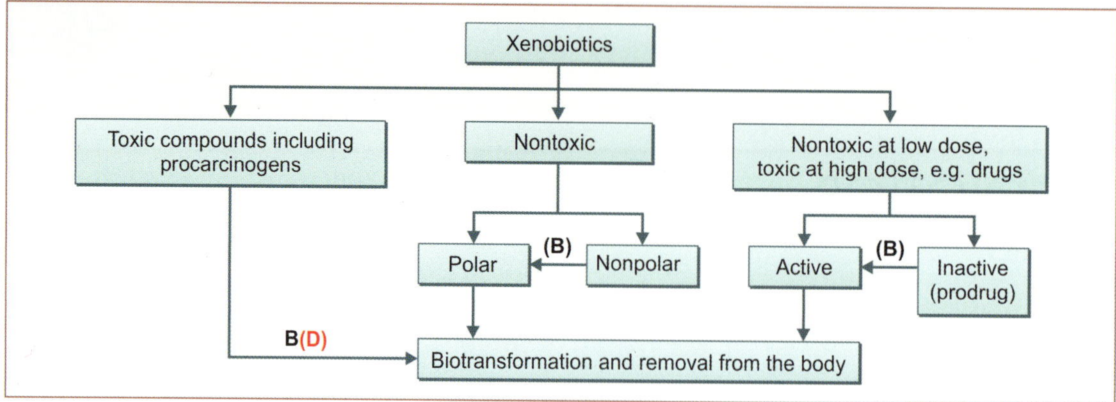

Fig. 18.1: Biotransformation (B)/detoxification (D) of xenobiotics

METABOLISM OF XENOBIOTICS

Site of Metabolism of Xenobiotics

The tissues at the portal of entry into or exit from the body are important in the detoxification of xenobiotics, with **liver being the major organ** (Fig. 18.2).

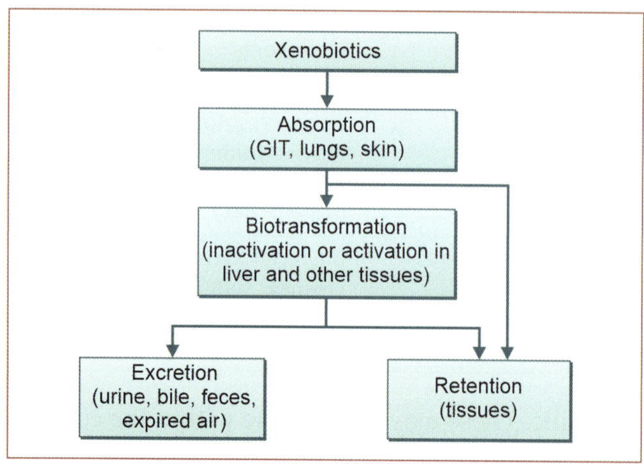

Fig. 18.2: Sites of metabolism of xenobiotics

Generally, metabolites produced by the liver are relatively more water soluble and pass via blood to the kidney for excretion. Some of the metabolites may also be excreted via feces, bile or the expired air. A small portion of the metabolite may also return to the intestine, by enterohepatic circulation. A xenobiotic or its metabolite may also bind to a cellular macromolecule such as DNA, RNA or protein and may be retained in the tissues. The binding of a xenobiotic or its metabolite, however, can cause serious consequences, such as mutations.

Mechanisms of Metabolism of Xenobiotics

Xenobiotic metabolizing enzymes can be divided into phase I and phase II.

Phase I: Lipophilic xenobiotics are often first metabolized by **phase I** enzymes, which function to make xenobiotics more polar and provide sites for conjugation reactions.

Phase II: Phase II enzymes are conjugating enzymes and can directly interact with xenobiotics but more commonly interact with metabolites produced by phase I enzymes.

Through both passive and active transport, these more polar metabolites are eliminated. Most xenobiotics are cleared through multiple enzymes and pathways (Fig. 18.3).

Phase I reactions: A xenobiotic may undergo oxidation (hydroxylation), reduction or hydrolysis during phase I of reaction and the metabolite so produced may either be excreted as such or undergoes phase II of metabolism.

- **Oxidation:** Compounds detoxified by the oxidative processes include alcohols, aldehydes, amines and their derivatives, aromatic hydrocarbons, and certain drugs.
  - **Alcohols:** Aliphatic as well as aromatic alcohols are oxidized to their corresponding acids.

    Methanol → Formic acid

    Ethanol → Acetic acid

    Benzyl alcohol → Benzoic acid (Fig. 18.4)
  - **Aldehydes:** These are also oxidized to their corresponding acids.

    Benzaldehyde → Benzoic acid

    Trichloroaldehyde → Trichloroacetic acid
  - **Amines:** ***Primary aliphatic amines*** are oxidized to their acids and liberate ammonia.

    $RCH_2\text{-}NH_2 \rightarrow R\text{-}COOH + \text{Ammonia}$
  - On the other hand, ***aromatic amines*** are oxidized to phenols (Fig. 18.5)

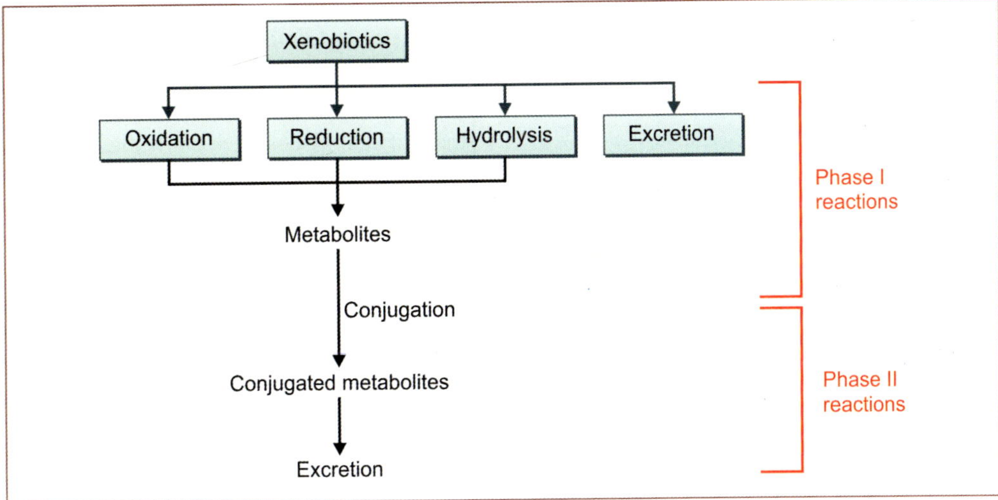

Fig. 18.3: Mechanisms of biotransformation of xenobiotics

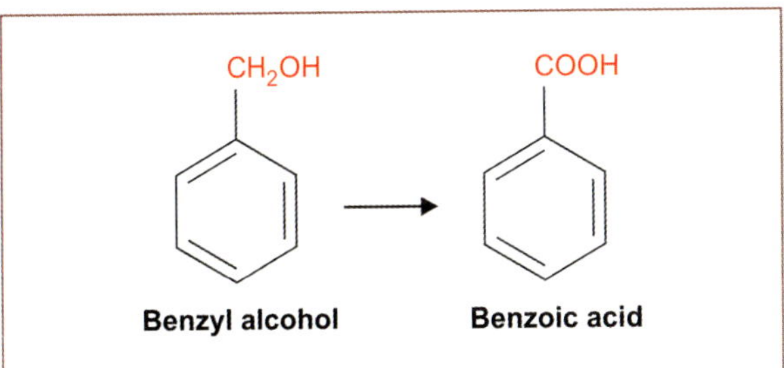

Fig. 18.4: Oxidation of an aromatic alcohol to acid

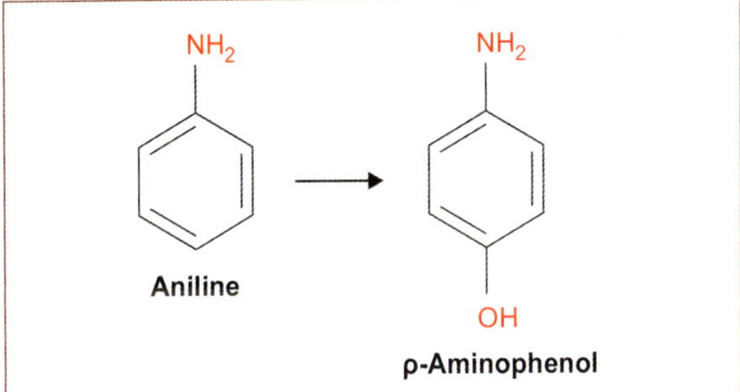

Fig. 18.5: Oxidation of an aromatic amine to alcohol

- **Anilides:** These are oxidized to the corresponding phenols, e.g. acetanilide to *p*-acetylaminophenol.
- **Aromatic hydrocarbons:** These are oxidized to phenols, e.g. oxidation of benzene produces several aromatic alcohols, such as phenols, quinols and catechols. The process thus involves the introduction of an –OH group (hydroxylation) onto the aromatic ring. This, in turn, provides a site for the attachment of a conjugating group in the phase II reaction.

  Some **epoxides** formed during the oxidation of xenobiotics are strong electrophiles and hence are very reactive. These may be converted to relatively inactive hydroxyl compounds by the enzyme epoxide hydrolase, which in turn, provides an –OH group for the conjugating molecule (Fig. 18.6).
- **Drugs:** Some drugs may be oxidized to their hydroxy derivatives, e.g.

  Meprobamate → Hydroxymeprobamate

Cytochrome P450 and its Role in Oxidative Metabolism of Xenobiotics

Oxidation of xenobiotics is mainly dependent upon a special class of cytochromes collectively referred to as cytochrome P450 whose salient features include:

Fig. 18.6: Oxidation of aromatic hydrocarbon

1. These are **hemoproteins**.
2. The number **450 refers to the absorption peak**, as the enzyme when exposed to carbon monoxide, exhibits a distinct peak at 450 nm.
3. Cytochrome P450 **oxidizes a variety of xenobiotics**, particularly lipophilic compounds such as drugs, carcinogens, pesticides, petroleum products and pollutants.
4. Due to subtle differences in their protein moiety, **multiple forms** of cytochrome P450 are known to exist.
5. All forms of cytochrome P450 are **monooxygenases** requiring atmospheric oxygen and NADPH, i.e. the enzyme utilizes one atom of oxygen to form water while the other atom of oxygen is used to form an oxidized derivative of the xenobiotic. Due to their dual function, as well as dual fate of oxygen, these monooxygenases are also designated as **mixed function oxidases**. The addition of a hydroxyl group to the substrate makes the compound more polar.
6. Cytochrome P450 is located in the **smooth endoplasmic reticulum** in most of the tissues but **liver** contains it in highest amount.
7. These monooxygenases often exhibit **broad substrate specificity** and many of these are **inducible** enzymes, i.e. these are synthesized by cells in response to the nature of a chemical inducing their formation (Chemistry to Clinics 18.1).

Chemistry to Clinics 18.1: Drug Interactions due to Enzyme Induction

Hydroxylation is the main metabolic pathway for ethinyl estradiol, one of the constituents of oral contraceptive pills (OCPs). Rifampicin, an antitubercular drug, induces cytochrome P450 enzymes in the liver, which results in increased hepatic hydroxylation of estrogens. This reduces plasma estradiol levels and thus its efficacy. It may result in contraceptive failure in female patients suffering from tuberculosis, taking rifampicin and OCPs concomitantly.

8. In addition to hydroxylation, cytochrome P450 is also involved in deamination, desulfuration, epoxidation and peroxygenation of certain xenobiotics.

Cytochrome P448: Metabolism of polycyclic aromatic hydrocarbons and related molecules require another isoform of cytochrome P450 called cytochrome P448. These enzymes are also designated as aromatic hydrocarbon hydroxylases (Chemistry to Clinics 18.2).

18

- **Reduction:** Some of the xenobiotics during the course of their detoxification undergo reduction, e.g.

Chemistry to Clinics 18.2: Tobacco Smoking and Cytochrome P448

Smokers have higher levels of cytochrome P448 enzymes in some of their tissues particularly the lungs because it is involved in the conversion of an inactive polycyclic aromatic hydrocarbon (procarcinogen) inhaled with smoke, to active carcinogen by the hydroxylation reaction in the lungs.

Picric acid → Picramic acid

Trichloroacetaldehyde → Trichloroethanol

Sometimes, a reduced metabolite may be more toxic than the original xenobiotic, e.g. prontosil (an azo red dye) is reduced to the more toxic sulfanilamide.

- **Hydrolysis:** Some of the xenobiotics, particularly certain therapeutic compounds, undergo hydrolysis during the course of their detoxification, e.g. aspirin, procaine, etc.

Aspirin (acetylsalicylic acid) → Acetate + Salicylic acid

Procaine → ρ-Aminobenzoic acid + Diethyl-aminoethanol

Aspirin (acetylsalicylic acid) undergoes hydrolysis and produces acetate and salicylic acid. Acetate so formed may be either oxidized or used for the synthesis of various physiological compounds. On the other hand, salicylic acid is excreted by the kidneys after conjugation with glucuronic acid.

Though some xenobiotics may undergo conjugation directly and the conjugate, so produced, is excreted as such without undergoing a preliminary reaction in phase I but conjugation, more often, occurs as a phase II reaction (Fig. 18.3).

Phase II reactions: A metabolite of the phase-I reaction is subsequently conjugated with some other compound (such as glycine) or group (like a methyl group). Conjugation makes the molecule **more polar and highly water soluble** which can be easily excreted from the body. Most of the conjugation reactions are synthetic processes and thus require energy.

The conjugation of a xenobiotic (X) with the conjugating molecule (Y) can occur via two different pathways, i.e. either the X or the Y gets activated and subsequently conjugates with the other molecule:

$$X \rightarrow X\sim \rightarrow X\sim Y$$
$$Y \rightarrow \sim Y \rightarrow X\sim Y$$

Compounds Used for Conjugation in Phase II

Compounds used for conjugation in phase II include readily available reactants, such as glutathione, amino acids like glycine or glutamine, glucuronate (as UDP glucuronic acid), a sulfate group, an acetyl group or a methyl group:

- **Glucuronic acid:** Glucuronic acid is an oxidation product of glucose. It participates in detoxification reactions as UDP glucuronic acid which gets conjugated with a xenobiotic (X-OH) and forms a highly soluble excretory glucuronide (X-O-glucuronide). The reaction is catalyzed by **UDP-glucuronyl transferase** present both in the endoplasmic reticulum as well as cytosol of many tissues but mainly in the liver (Fig. 18.7).

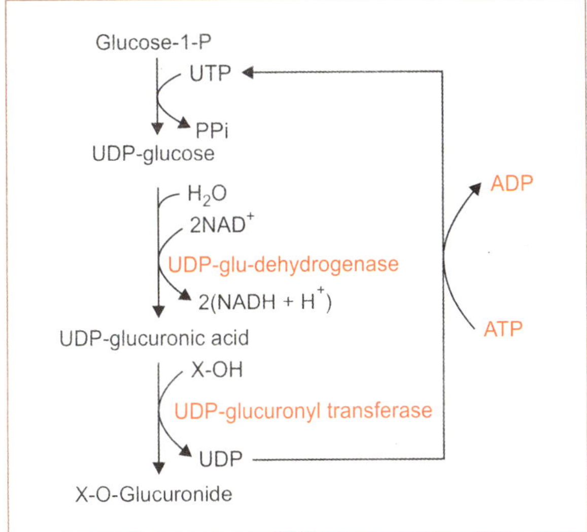

Fig. 18.7: Conjugation of xenobiotic (X-OH) with glucuronic acid

Various compounds, such as benzoic acid, morphine, methanol and camphor are excreted in conjugation with glucuronic acid. Endogenously produced bilirubin is also conjugated in the liver with glucuronic acid.

Benzoic acid + UDP-glucuronic acid → Benzoyl glucuronide + UDP

Bilirubin + UDP-glucuronic acid → Bilirubin monoglucuronide

Bilirubin monoglucuronide + UDP-glucuronic acid → Bilirubin diglucuronide + UDP

- **Glutathione:** A wide range of organic compounds which are toxic electrophiles such as aromatic halogenated compounds, aliphatic halides, sulfates, nitrocompounds and carcinogenic epoxides (formed from polycyclic hydrocarbons) are excreted after conjugation with the cysteinyl moiety of glutathione (a tripeptide of glutamate, cysteine and glycine). A xenobiotic (H-X) after conjugation with glutathione, forms mercapturic acid. The reaction is catalyzed by a group of enzymes referred to as glutathione-S-transferases. These are present in various tissues with high amounts in the liver cytosol.
  - In the initial reaction, reduced glutathione (GSH) reacts with an electrophilic center on the xenobiotic.
  - The glutamyl and glycinyl groups are sequentially removed.
  - Subsequently, an acetyl group is added (from acetyl-CoA) to the amino group of the remaining cysteinyl residue which is bound to the xenobiotic (X-cysteine).
  - The resulting compound, a mercapturic acid, i.e. a conjugate of acetylcysteine, is excreted in the urine (Fig. 18.8).

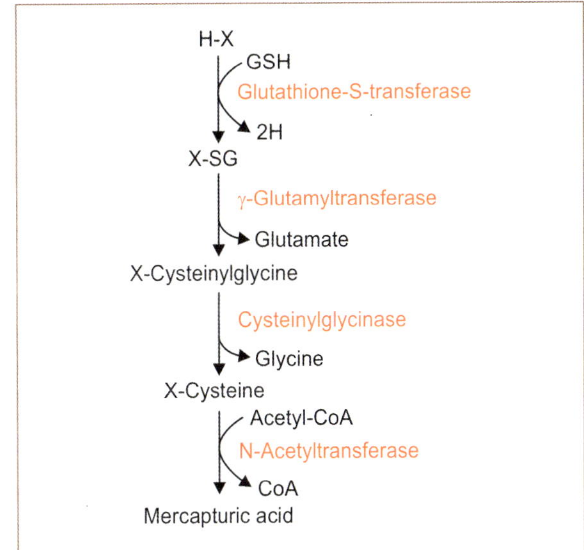

Fig. 18.8: Conjugation of xenobiotic (H-X) with glutathione (GSH)

Due to conjugation with glutathione, large doses of some of the drugs such as paracetamol, leads to depletion of glutathione in the liver (Chemistry to Clinics 18.3).

Chemistry to Clinics 18.3: Paracetamol Poisoning

Paracetamol is the most popular antipyretic (a drug used to treat pyrexia, i.e. fever). It is metabolized mainly in the liver. An overdose of paracetamol generates excess of free radicals in the hepatocytes. Reduced glutathione (GSH), the most important intracellular antioxidant, is depleted in its effort to detoxify the free radicals because it gets oxidized in the process (forming oxidized glutathione, GSSG). The free radicals thus cause widespread cell injury which may be fatal if not timely treated. Prompt administration of N-acetylcysteine, a sulfhydryl (–SH) donor, replenishes the intracellular pool of GSH, thereby restoring the antioxidant capacity of hepatocytes. This helps to recover from paracetamol poisoning.

- **Glycine:** Glycine conjugates with many aromatic carboxylic acids, e.g. benzoic acid, cholic acid, etc. Glycine conjugates are harmless compounds and are excreted in the urine.

  Benzoic acid + Glycine → Benzoyl glycine (hippuric acid)

  Cholic acid + Glycine → Glycocholic acid
- **Glutamine:** Phenylacetic acid is detoxified by conjugation with glutamine.

  Phenylacetic acid + Glutamine → Phenylacetyl-glutamine
- **Sulfate:** Biosynthesis of a sulfate ester requires a high energy sulfate donor, i.e. 3′-phosphoadenosine-5′-phosphosulfate (**PAPS** or **active sulfate)**. Transfer of sulfate group from active sulfate to various acceptors such as phenol and indole, is catalyzed by specific sulftransferases.
- **Acetate:** As for other acetylation reactions, active acetate (acetyl-CoA) is used as an acetyl donor. Acetylation of a xenobiotic is catalyzed by acetyl-transferases present in the cytosol of various tissues, mainly in the liver. Many drugs such as sulfanilamide and isoniazid are metabolized by acetylation (Chemistry to Clinics 18.4).

Chemistry to Clinics 18.4: Acetylation and Drug Toxicity

1. Some of the acetylated products of the drugs such as acetyl sulfanilamide are less soluble than the xenobiotic (sulfanilamide) itself. It gets deposited in the kidney and may cause renal failure.
2. Isoniazid (isonicotinic acid hydrazide, INH), an antitubercular drug, is inactivated in the liver via acetylation. The rate of acetylation is genetically determined. Fast acetylation leads to higher plasma levels of the toxic metabolite acetyl isoniazid and thus to an increase in toxic reactions, e.g. hepatitis which is more common than in slow acetylators. On the other hand, patients with the slow acetylator genotype have higher plasma INH levels and tend to develop neuropathy.

- **Methyl group:** The methyl group of S-adenosylmethionine (**SAM or active methionine**) is used by methyltransferases to methylate a xenobiotic, mainly various pyridine derivatives. Many of the methylated products though are less toxic than the parent xenobiotic, some of these however, are more toxic, e.g. excess dose of nicotinamide after methylation is converted to a more toxic product (methyl-nicotinamide).

LIMITATIONS OF BIOTRANSFORMATION: GLOBAL WARMING

The above discussion does not imply an indefinite capacity of tissues such as the liver, to handle and biotransform xenobiotics such as industrial pollutants, which continue to increase day by day. Global warming refers to the adverse climate change caused by the trapping of **greenhouse gases**, affecting the entire ecosystem and posing serious health hazards. Naturally occurring greenhouse gases, such as carbon dioxide, water vapor, methane, nitrous oxide and ozone should be present at optimum levels in the atmosphere to keep the earth warm enough to sustain life. This is called the **normal greenhouse effect**. However, certain human activities lead to an **enhanced greenhouse effect** and contribute to **global warming**. These include the burning of fossil fuels (coal, oil and natural gas), solid waste and wood; deforestation; and industrial production of perfluorocarbons and sulfur hexafluoride.

Major health hazards of global warming include:

1. An increase in the incidence of infectious diseases especially those which are vector-borne.
2. Since the cardiovascular system has to work harder to keep the body cool under hot climatic conditions, cardiovascular diseases, heat stroke and renal stones are likely to increase.
3. High air temperature increases the ozone concentration at ground level and ozone is a known respiratory pollutant.
4. Adverse effects on agriculture and rise in sea level may encourage malnutrition and the extinction of those species who fail to adapt to the changing climatic conditions. In fact, the long-term serious consequences to human health may threaten our very existence on this planet.

Countermeasures to facilitate living in hotter temperature actually consume more electricity from power plants that consume fossil fuels. This adds on to the global warming and initiates a vicious cycle. The only **practical remedies** are:

1. To economize the use of fossil fuels.
2. Use energy-efficient products such as compact fluorescent bulbs and solar heaters.
3. Planting more trees.
4. Recycling papers and plastics.
5. Avoid wastage of food and water.

The first global agreement, known as the **Copenhagen Accord**, to comprehensively influence the flow and share of natural resources, was agreed upon by more than 25 countries in December 2009 at Copenhagen, Denmark.

ROLE OF XENOBIOTICS IN DISEASE

As discussed above, xenobiotics include compounds that act as foreign chemicals to human and animal cells. Due to their recalcitrant nature they can produce many diseases in humans and other living systems. Furthermore, particularly, for metal pollutants, the hypothesis about the role exerted by impaired mitochondrial function is gaining a leading causative role. Mitochondrial dysfunction plays an important role in the pathophysiology of age-related chronic diseases such as metabolic syndrome, diabetes, coronary artery disease, acute coronary syndrome, stroke, Alzheimer's disease, Parkinson's disease, depression and cancer.

Fatty Liver Disease

Fatty liver disease is a major public health burden affecting a large population throughout the world. It is the result of accumulation of fat (steatosis) in hepatocytes. The diagnosis of steatosis is made when fat in the liver exceeds 5–10% by weight. Fatty liver disease has been classified into two categories, as **alcoholic steatohepatitis** (ASH) or **nonalcoholic steatohepatitis** (NASH).

- In **alcoholic steatohepatitis** chronic alcohol consumption results in fatty liver due to production of toxic metabolites of alcohol including aldehydes.
- In **nonalcoholic steatohepatitis** multiple (nonalcohol) factors including nutritional, drugs and hepatic-toxicants and metabolic disorders have been identified in the initiation and progression of the disease.

  Recent studies have suggested a **link between xenobiotic exposure** (including pharmaceuticals and nonpharmaceutical chemicals) **and initiation and progression of the clinical course of nonalcoholic fatty liver disease** (NAFL). Since, liver is the major organ for the metabolism of drugs and environmental agents, it has been demonstrated that exposure to some of these agents may lead to lipid accumulation in hepatocytes through increased fatty acid biosynthesis, mitochondrial dysfunction, modulation of nuclear receptor activation (NR modulation), insulin resistance and impaired lipid excretion (Fig. 18.9).

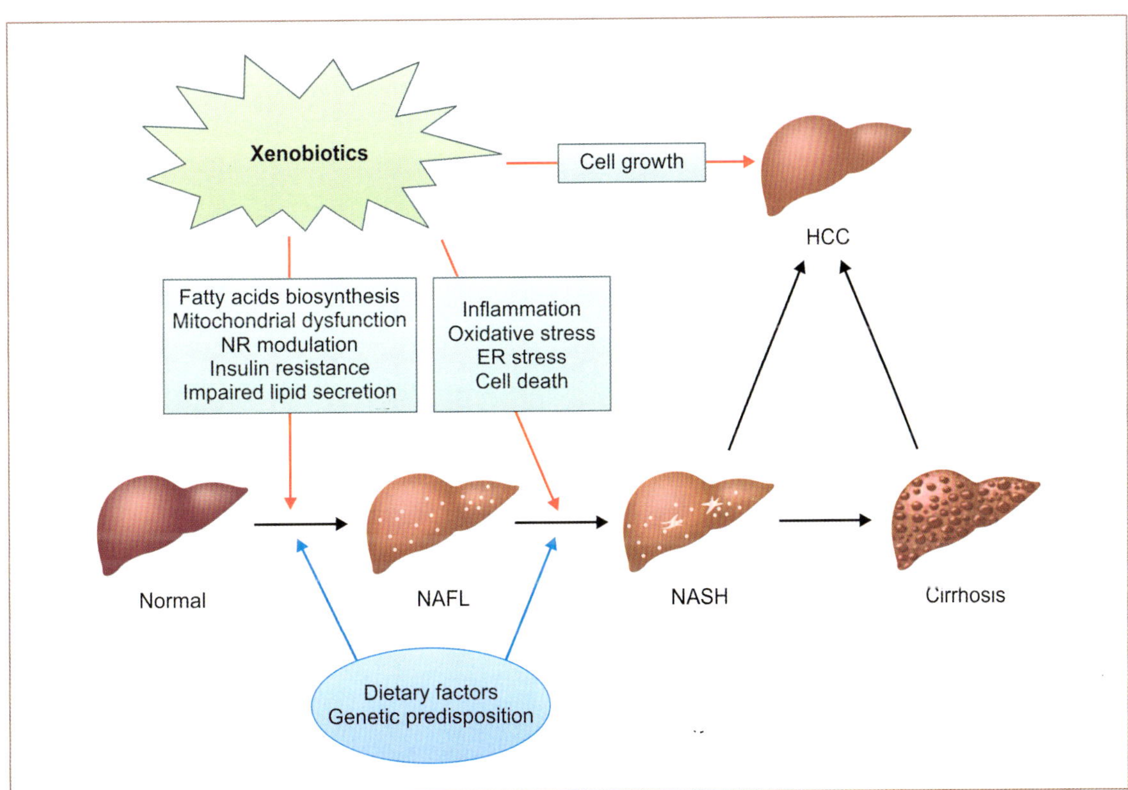

Fig. 18.9: Potential roles of xenobiotics in nonalcoholic fatty liver diseases

Moreover, progression from simple steatosis to steatohepatitis may be induced by xenobiotics *via* oxidative stress, inflammation, endoplasmic reticulum stress (ER stress) and cell death. Finally, exposure to chemicals may stimulate cell growth in the liver, which further increases the chance of developing hepatocellular carcinoma (HCC) in patients with NASH.

Cancer

- The National Cancer Institute and the American Cancer Society have reported an association between **diesel exhaust exposure** and **increased risk of lung and other cancers** including **cancers of bladder, larynx (voice box), esophagus, stomach and pancreas**.

  Diesel exhaust has been classified as **Group 1A carcinogen**. Transition metals such as Fe, Zn, Cr, Pb, V and Ni, and polycyclic aromatic hydrocarbons (PAHs) amounts are high in diesel exposure. These chemicals trigger lung disease and cancer.
- Epidemiologic studies have suggested an association with the **increased risk of several cancers** and **high consumption of red meat**. It is suggested that chemicals such as heterocyclic amines are formed when meat is cooked at high temperature. These amines have strong carcinogenic potential in animals. Accordingly, **red meat** has been classified as **Group 2A, probably carcinogenic to human**.
- Another important xenobiotic is **acrylamide**. It is reported that when refined grain is exposed to high temperature during bread production, acrylamide is formed in bread. **Acrylamide** has been shown to be carcinogenic in animals, and is classified as **likely to be carcinogenic to humans**. It is suggested that whole grain bread should be consumed to reduce the risk.
- World Health Organization has emphasized that the consumption of **unsafe food**, particularly vegetables and fruits, that contain harmful bacteria, viruses, parasites and chemical substances such as **pesticide residues**, cause more than 200 diseases ranging from diarrhea to cancers.
- Food-contact materials cause food to be exposed to chemicals such as polycarbonate-plastics derivatives, e.g. **bisphenol A**. United States Environmental Protection Agency advised to protect sensitive populations, particularly, infants and young children against bisphenol A exposure.

Infertility

It is known that several xenobiotics and toxic metals cause DNA damage. Infertile patients with high levels of oxidative stress may be more susceptible. The occupational and environmental exposure to certain pollutants can act as hormone disruptors and could be a cause of unexplained infertility.

Some Important Questions

1. What are xenobiotics? Discuss various mechanisms of xenobiotics metabolism.

2. Write notes on:

i. Biotransformation of xenobiotics
ii. Mechanisms of xenobiotics detoxification
iii. Role of cytochrome P450 in oxidative metabolism of xenobiotics
iv. Cytochrome P448
v. Phase II reactions of xenobiotics detoxification
vi. Role of glucuronic acid in xenobiotics metabolism
vii. Role of glutathione in xenobiotics metabolism
viii. Acetylation and drug toxicity

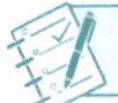

Multiple Choice Questions

1. Bhopal gas tragedy is attributed to the inhalation of:

A. Hydrogen sulphide
B. Dichloromethane
C. Methyl isocyanate
D. Carbon monoxide

2. During phase I xenobiotics metabolism, aromatic hydrocarbons are converted to:

A. Ketones B. Aldehydes
C. Acids D. Phenols

3. Cytochrome P450 participates in:

A. Hydroxylation
B. Deamination
C. Desulphuration
D. All of the above

4. The following moiety of GSH is involved in conjugation reactions to form mercapturic acid:

A. Cysteine
B. Glutamate
C. Glycine
D. Any of the above

5. The following is a hazard of global warming:

A. Vector-borne infectious diseases
B. Renal stones
C. Heat stroke
D. All of the above

18

CHAPTER 19

Antioxidant Defense System and Oxidative Stress

Competency Achievement: The student should be able to:

BI7.6 Describe the antioxidant defense systems in the body

BI7.7 Describe the role of oxidative stress in the pathogenesis of conditions such as cancer, complications of diabetes mellitus and atherosclerosis

Antioxidants are the compounds that inhibit oxidation, a chemical reaction that can produce free radicals.

FREE RADICALS

Oxygen is one of the important components of aerobic life. However, in some circumstances, this oxygen may be a killer of cells when it generates reactive species that causes necrosis and ultimately the cell death. About 90% of the elemental oxygen (O_2) is used via oxidative phosphorylation while 5–8% in enzymatic hydroxylation and oxygenation reactions. A small fraction of the oxygen (<5%) has the ability to become part of potentially harmful and damaging molecules called free radicals.

Free radicals are reactive chemical entities that are short lived species containing one or more unpaired electrons, thereby, leading to chain reactions that may damage the cells of organisms. They induce damage to cells by passing the unpaired electron resulting in oxidation of cell components and molecules. They are, generally, very unstable and very much reactive and are a source of chronic damage to biomolecules within the tissues.

Both exogenous and endogenous substances produce free radicals in cells and its surroundings. They can be produced from nonenzymatic reactions of organic compounds with oxygen as well as those initiated by ionizing radiations. This process may also occur in mitochondria by oxidative phosphorylation. Free radicals include reactive oxygen species (ROS) and reactive nitrogen species (RNS).

- **Reactive oxygen species:** In biological redox reactions, oxygen is activated by redox active metal ions, such as iron and copper, which are present in metalloenzymes and other proteins, e.g. hemoglobin, myoglobin, etc. These metal ions provide one electron at a time to oxygen and activate it to strong oxidizing forms. A number of ROS, including free radicals and nonradicals, are formed from partial reduction of molecular oxygen (Fig. 19.1).
  - The first product is the **superoxide anion** free radical (**$O_2^{\bullet -}$**).
  - Reduction of superoxide yields **hydrogen peroxide (H_2O_2, a nonradical ROS)**.
  - Reduction of H_2O_2 causes a cleavage reaction that releases **hydroxyl free radical ($OH^{\bullet -}$)**.

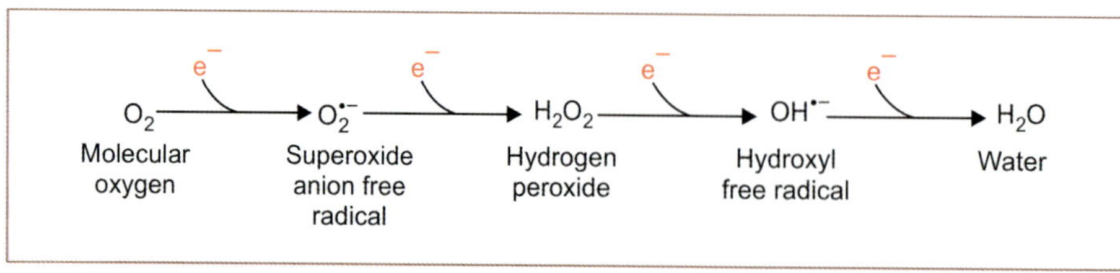

Fig. 19.1: Formation of reactive oxygen species from molecular oxygen (e^- = electron)

- The end product of complete reduction of oxygen is **water**.

- **Reactive nitrogen species:** Similar to ROS, nitrogen-based reactive species, called reactive nitrogen species (RNS) are also produced in the body. Peroxynitrite ($ONOO^-$) and nitric oxide (NO) are important examples, which in turn, are responsible for **nitrosative stress**.

  Increased production of free oxygen radicals and free nitrogen radicals damage lipids, proteins and DNA structures in the cells, and cause apoptosis, inflammation and cancer.

Sources of ROS and RNS

ROS and RNS are continuously produced within the cells, particularly, as:

i. A result of the electron transfer processes in the mitochondria, and
ii. The activity of several inflammation-linked enzymes, such as NADPH oxidase, nitric oxide synthase (NOS), xanthine oxidase, myeloperoxidase (MPO), lipoxygenase (LOX) and cyclooxygenase (COX).

Nature of Oxygen Radical Damage

One of the most sensitive sites of free radical damage is the cell membrane, which is rich in readily oxidizable polyunsaturated fatty acids.

- The $^{\bullet}OH$ extracts a hydrogen atom from a polyunsaturated fatty acid, setting-off a chain of lipid peroxidation reactions.
- Lipid peroxides formed in this reaction degrade to form characteristic products such as **malondialdehyde (MDA)**.
- These compounds react with proteins to form adducts and cross links, known as **advanced lipoxidation end products** (**ALE**).
- Further, ROS also react with carbohydrates to form dicarbonyl compounds that, in turn, react with proteins to form cross links and adducts, known as glycoxidation products or **advanced glycation end products** (**AGE**).
- ROS also damage the genome, in the form of mutations in DNA (Fig. 19.2).

  As a result of oxidative stress, MDA adducts (ALE and AGE) increase in several chronic conditions such as atherosclerosis, Alzheimer's disease and diabetes mellitus.

ANTIOXIDANT DEFENSE SYSTEM

In order to scavenge the deleterious effects of free radicals, the body has different mechanisms to produce **antioxidants**, which neutralize the elevated amount of free radicals and keep the cells protected against their toxic effects, contributing towards the prevention of

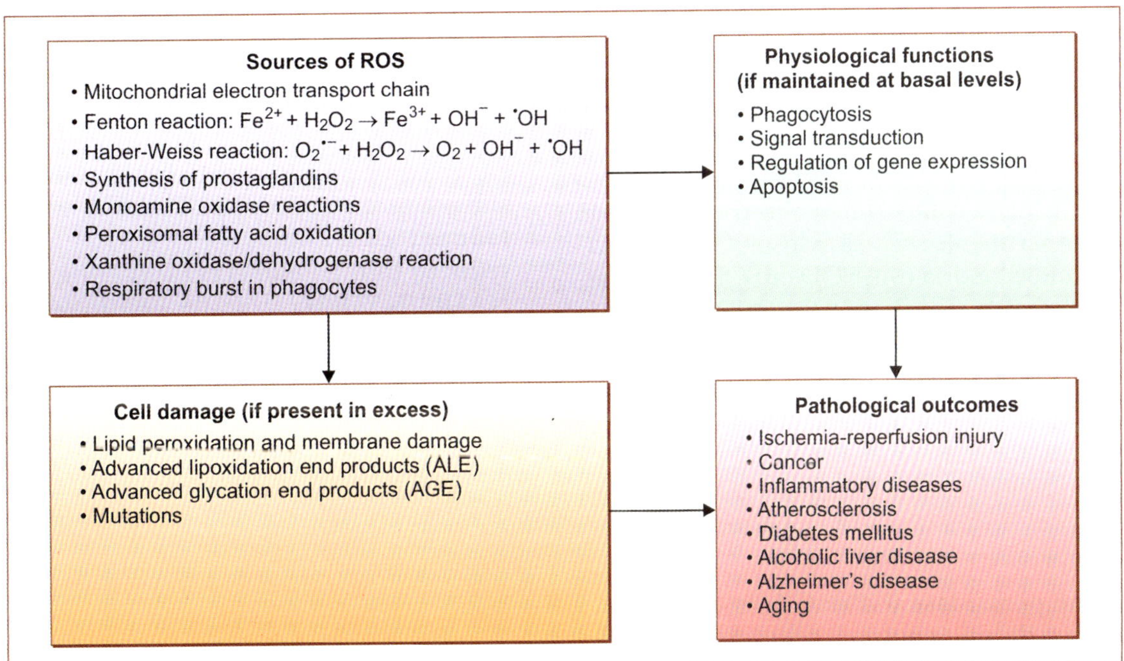

Fig. 19.2: Reactive oxygen species (ROS): Sources, functions and pathological outcomes

19

diseases. Cells contain both **enzymatic** and **non-enzymatic antioxidants** that work together to regulate ROS and RNS concentrations.

Antioxidant Enzymes

There is a group of enzymes that act to detoxify ROS. The primary **antioxidant enzymes** in tissues that are able to detoxify directly oxidizing species include superoxide dismutase (SOD), glutathione peroxidase (Gpx) and catalase (CAT). Other fundamental antioxidant enzymes, such as glutathione reductase (GR) and thioredoxin reductase (TrxR), also contribute to cellular protection by reducing oxidized critical thiols in key enzymes/proteins and maintaining the suitable intracellular redox state.

- **Catalase:** It is present in peroxisomes and detoxifies H_2O_2 (Fig. 19.3).

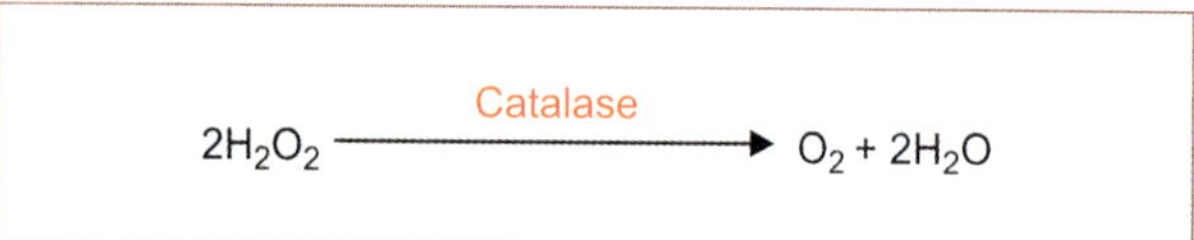

Fig. 19.3: Detoxification of H_2O_2 by catalase

- **Superoxide dismutase (SOD):** SOD detoxifies $O_2^{\bullet-}$ (Fig. 19.4).

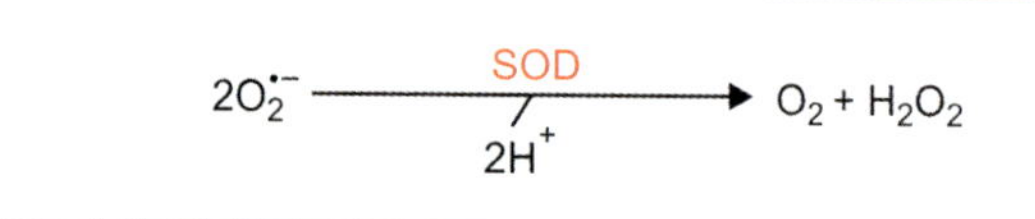

Fig. 19.4: Detoxification of $O_2^{\bullet-}$ by superoxide dismutase (SOD)

Superoxide dismutases are a group of metalloenzymes which are compartmentalized in different cellular compartments such as cytosol (Cu-Zn-SOD or SOD_1), mitochondria (Mn-SOD or SOD_2) and the extracellular matrix (Cu-Zn-SOD or SOD_3).

All the three SODs contribute to control ROS intracellular concentration and, in conjunction with CAT and GPx, to maintain the flux of H_2O_2 suitable for redox regulation of intracellular signaling. Mutation in SOD_1 results in failure to adequately protect against ROS such as in amyotrophic lateral sclerosis (Chemistry to Clinics 19.1).

- **Glutathione peroxidase (GPx):** GPx is an enzyme dependent on the micronutrient selenium and plays a crucial role in the reduction of lipid oxidation and peroxide detoxification. Moreover, together with glutathione reductase (GR), it plays a critical role in GSH metabolism, reducing glutathione disulfide (GSSG) to GSH, by the NADPH-dependent mechanism (Fig. 19.5).

> **Chemistry to Clinics 19.1: Amyotrophic Lateral Sclerosis**
>
> It is the commonest form of motor neuron disease characterized by weakness, atrophy, fasciculation and stiffness of muscles. Besides difficulty in movement, there is compromise in speech, swallowing and breathing. Mutation in SOD_1 results in failure to adequately protect against ROS. Aggregation of the abnormal SOD chains also interferes with normal cellular functions.

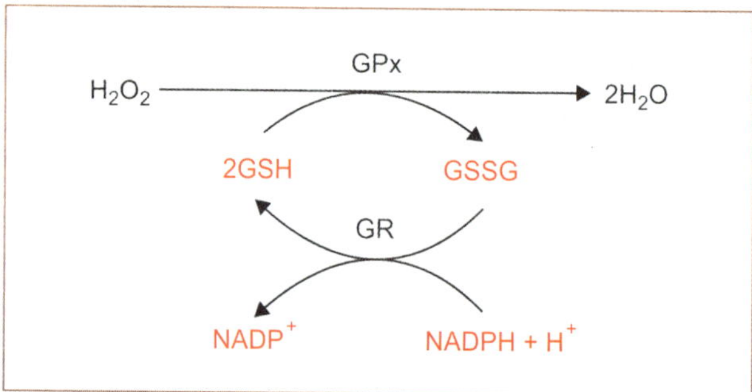

Fig. 19.5: Detoxification of H_2O_2 by glutathione peroxidase (GPx) catalyzed reaction with reduced glutathione (GSH). Oxidized glutathione (GSSG) is reduced by glutathione reductase (GR) to regenerate GSH

- **Thioredoxin reductase:** Thioredoxin reductase (**TrxR**) has catalytic redox-active cysteines and catalyzes the reduction of protein mixed disulfides. Thioredoxin, in particular, has function in DNA and protein repair by reducing ribonucleotide reductase as well as methionine sulfoxide reductases.

  Some of these antioxidants, proteins, and redox enzymes belong to a network connected through substrates and products. Together with **oxidized/reduced glutathione** (GSH/GSSG) and **oxidized/reduced thioredoxin** (Trx/TrxR), the **redox couple NADP⁺/NADPH** is crucial for the intracellular redox homeostasis.

Nonenzymatic System

The **nonenzymatic system** includes low molecular weight endogenous compounds such as reduced glutathione (GSH), uric acid, bilirubin and ceruloplasmin, as well as dietary low molecular weight compounds, such as vitamins (vitamins A, C, and E), β-carotene, flavonoids, polyphenols, and zinc and selenium. They are fundamental antioxidant molecules because they can directly detoxify ROS and RNS, and repair oxidized biological targets.

- **Glutathione (GSH** or reduced glutathione) is a tripeptide-thiol (γ-glutamylcysteinylglycine) containing glutamate, cysteine and glycine. It is the major cellular redox buffer, universally used as an indicator of the cellular redox environment. Reduced glutathione reacts with several oxidizing species, including •OH, HClO, and $ONOO^-$, and is the substrate of glutathione peroxidase (GPx) in its peroxide detoxification activity. During this process, GSH is oxidized to GSSG (oxidized glutathione), which is not protective. The cell regenerates GSH from GSSG by an NADPH-dependent enzyme called **glutathione reductase**. **NADPH** is produced by the pentose phosphate pathway. The erythrocytes are, particularly, equipped with the GSH:NADPH-based antioxidant defense system, which prevents membrane lipid peroxidation and hemolysis.
  The main source of intracellular NADPH is the oxidative branch of the pentose phosphate pathway, with the cofactor being produced by the rate-limiting glucose-6-phosphate dehydrogenase and 6-phosphogluconate dehydrogenase.
- **Reduced thioredoxin** (TrxR) provides reducing equivalents for thioredoxin reductase, which is also involved in H_2O_2 removal, in maintaining the suitable thiol/disulfide intracellular equilibrium linked to redox signaling.
- **Antioxidant vitamins:** Three vitamins, i.e. **vitamins A, C and E**, provide the other line of defense against oxidative damage and are called **antioxidant vitamins** or the **big three antioxidants**.
  - **Vitamin A** is a lipophilic antioxidant. It is a potent singlet oxygen scavenger and protects against damage from sunlight in the retina and skin.
  - **Vitamin C** or ascorbic acid is a biologically ubiquitous and water-soluble antioxidant, which donates an electron to potentially damaging oxidizing radicals, such as •OH, alkoxyl radical (RO•), peroxyl radical (ROO•) and tocopheroxyl radicals (TO•). It has been shown that physiological concentrations of ascorbic acid inhibit oxidation of LDL, lipids and proteins. An important feature of ascorbic acid is acting synergistically with vitamin E and protecting this vitamin from the oxidative modifications.
  - **Vitamin E** is lipid soluble, primary antioxidant in LDL and lipid membrane. There are eight naturally occurring vitamin E isoforms, amongst which its one-electron oxidation product, the α-tocoperoxyl radical, can be reduced by ascorbic acid. Vitamin E acts as a radical-scavenging antioxidant against lipid peroxidation by scavenging lipid-centered ROO• before it attacks lipid in other molecules to yield lipid hydroperoxide (LOOH), and a lipid radical (L•), which propagates the chain oxidation.
- **β-Carotene** is a powerful singlet oxygen quencher and exhibits additional, strong antioxidant properties. It is very reactive to peroxyl radicals and DNA damage, but less so to •OH and $\mathbf{O_2^{\bullet-}}$.
- **Uric acid** is synthesized, mainly, in the liver, intestine and the vascular endothelium, as the end product of an exogenous pool of purines, is a strong ROS and RNS scavenger (such as •OH, $ONOO^-$, and HClO), and has metal-chelating properties in blood plasma and saliva.
- **Bilirubin** has been proved to be a powerful antioxidant in human blood plasma, both in its unconjugated form and complexed with serum albumin. In addition to its ability to inhibit membrane lipid peroxidation acting in synergy with the membrane-bound α-tocopherol, bilirubin can scavenge both ROS and RNS and protect proteins from ROS- and RNS-mediated oxidative damage.
- **Other antioxidants:** Besides, lycopene, flavonoids, serum albumin (containing –SH groups), bilirubin, uric acid, etc. are also a part of the antioxidant defense system.

OXIDATIVE STRESS

Oxidative stress can be defined as any **disturbance in the balance of antioxidants and pro-oxidants**, in favor of the later, due to different factors such as aging, drug actions and toxicity, inflammation and/or addiction. Excess formation or/and insufficient removal of free radicals lead to the irreversible oxidation of proteins, lipids and nucleic acids in the cells, resulting in free radicals-induced cell injury.

ROLE OF OXIDATIVE STRESS IN PATHOGENESIS OF CERTAIN CLINICAL CONDITIONS

Oxidative stress has been implicated in a number of pathological processes including metabolic, degenerative and inflammatory diseases such as cancer, complications of diabetes mellitus, atherosclerosis and ischemia-reperfusion injury.

ROLE OF OXIDATIVE STRESS IN THE PATHOGENESIS OF CANCER

Many studies have demonstrated **direct relationship between chronic inflammation and carcinogenesis**.

- **Inflammation:** The **main chemical effectors** of these effects of the inflammatory response **are free radical species** derived from oxidative stress induced by inflammation. RONS may directly or indirectly damage other chemical or structural components in target cells or recruit other inflammatory cells leading to additional production of RONS that amplifies the damage. In particular, **RONS and inflammatory cytokines** such as TNF-α, **activate transcription factor** NFκB which **induces the expression of genes involved in cell proliferation, apoptosis and carcinogenesis**.
- **Angiogenesis:** Chronic inflammation is also associated with **angiogenesis** (another characteristic of cancer), because RONS can also increase expression of transcriptional factors (i.e. c-fos and c-jun), which are involved in neoplastic transformation and enhancement of cancer angiogenesis. Moreover, macrophages, platelets, fibroblasts and cancer cells are a major source of angiogenic factors (i.e. fibroblast growth factor, vascular endothelial growth factor, and prostaglandins E1 and E2) which increase the production of RONS and, subsequently, increase the risk of cancer.
- **DNA damage:** The mutagenic/carcinogenic potential of RONS is due to **their capability of reacting with DNA** and chemically modifying it. In particular, **ROS-induced DNA damage can result in transcriptional arrest**, induction/replication errors or genomic instability, all of which are **associated with carcinogenesis**.
- **Age-dependent escalation in cancer risk and increased oxidative stress:** Oxidative stress and the damages caused by it, over a lifetime, may be responsible for this phenomenon. In fact, there is an accumulation of RONS-induced DNA damages with age, which is confirmed by the **progressive and significant increase in the levels of certain metabolites**, such as 7,8-dihydro-8-oxo-22-deoxyguanosine (8oxodG), which are observed with aging. Among oxidized-DNA products, 8-oxodG and 8-nitroguanine are considered as biomarkers for inflammation-induced carcinogenesis. Thus, chronic inflammation and oxidative stress are high risk factors for cancer, especially in elderly people.

ROLE OF OXIDATIVE STRESS IN THE PATHOGENESIS OF COMPLICATIONS OF DIABETES MELLITUS

19

Diabetes mellitus is a metabolic disease **associated with increased formation of free radicals** and decreased antioxidant potential, **leading to macro- and microvascular complications.** Oxidant stress in type 2 diabetes promotes prothrombotic reactions leading to cardiovascular complications. Thus, diabetes damages can be considered as tissue oxidative damaging effects of **chronic hyperglycemia**.

Increased intracellular concentration of glucose leads to increased production of RONS which exceeds antioxidant capability of the cell to neutralize them. In this way, **RONS induce activation of four important molecular pathways involved in hyperglycemia-induced oxidative tissue**, i.e.:

- **Activation of protein kinase C** (PKC)
- **Increased hexosamine pathway flux**
- **Increased AGEs**
- **Increased polyol pathway flux**.

In particular, the activation of the AGEs pathway can damage cells, modifying the regulation of gene transcription, the signaling between the matrix and other cells, and blood proteins (e.g. albumin), causing them to bind to AGE-receptors (R-AGEs) on macrophages/mesangial cells and increase the production of growth factors and proinflammatory cytokines. AGEs and R-AGEs interaction elicits oxidative stress generation in various types of cells and subsequently, evokes proliferative, inflammatory and thrombogenic reactions, playing an important role in the development and progression of diabetes-associated disorders.

- Free radical and oxidative stress-induced complications from diabetes mellitus include **coronary artery disease, nephropathy, retinopathy** and **stroke.**
- Increase in the levels of glucose and insulin along **with dyslipidemia** in patients suffering from diabetes develops **macroangiopathies** that cause oxidative stress **leading to atherosclerosis**.

Biomarkers of protein glycation in type 2 diabetes is glycated-hemoglobin (HbA1c), which is more negatively charged than hemoglobin and has a higher oxygen affinity, therefore reducing gaseous exchange to tissues.

ROLE OF OXIDATIVE STRESS IN THE PATHOGENESIS OF ATHEROSCLEROSIS

Cardiovascular diseases are a leading cause of morbidity and mortality in the elderly, and atherosclerosis plays a crucial role as main causal event. Several studies have proven that heart tolerance to oxidative stress decreases **with age** because of a

reduction in the concentrations of the antioxidant enzymes (i.e. GSH-Px and SOD), contributing to the development of cardiovascular alterations.

The evidence, currently available, links atherosclerosis with **oxidized LDL-cholesterol** (oxLDL) as the compound, mainly, responsible for it. The increase of oxLDL may amplify LDL atherogenicity because of the pro-oxidant and proinflammatory environments that characterize elderly subjects. Moreover, the development of oxidative stress contributes to vascular endothelial dysfunction with aging. Endothelial dysfunction and vascular remodeling are recognized as early determinants in the development of hypertension and atherosclerosis.

ROLE OF OXIDATIVE STRESS IN THE PATHOGENESIS OF ISCHEMIA-REPERFUSION INJURY

Ischemia is defined as a condition of reduced oxygen availability to a tissue as a result of reduced blood flow, although it can arise from any condition in which the oxygen demand of the tissue is greater than its oxygen supply. In the heart, this most often occurs acutely by the development of an obstruction in one of the major coronary arteries, usually from a blood clot in the area of an advanced or ruptured atherosclerotic plaque. Ischemia cannot be tolerated for long in myocardial tissue. Immediately at the onset of ischemia, the affected myocardial tissue becomes acontractile (unable to contract). Within one hour, the oxygen-dependent cellular ionic and water balance mechanisms fail and the tissues swell, with a further loss of membrane integrity. Calcium extrusion mechanisms fail, and the resultant increase in intracellular Ca^{2+} activates enzymes that destroy myocardial tissue. If acute ischemia involves enough myocardial tissue, the initial loss of contractile ability may be sufficient to cause acute failure of the heart and circulatory collapse (cardiogenic shock). However, even with small ischemic episodes, the resulting tissue damage within hours after the initial insult may be enough to cause death from cardiac failure.

Reperfusion

The best course of action to reduce ischemic damage in the heart is to restore myocardial blood flow as quickly as possible and/or to change hemodynamic variables in such a way as to reduce myocardial oxygen demand. If the ischemia results from a blood clot in a major coronary artery, clot-lysing drugs, such as streptokinase or tissue-type plasminogen activator, are injected through a catheter into the major coronary artery, affected by the clot. These drugs dissolve the clot and restore flow. However, in reality, restoration of blood flow is often associated with induction of additional damage to the myocardium instead of restoration of cell viability. This phenomenon is called **ischemia-reperfusion injury**. It happens because during the ischemic period, the arterioles downstream from the coronary arterial obstruction dilate through myogenic and metabolic mechanisms, lowering vascular resistance. On removal of the obstruction, this lowered resistance allows for a substantial reactive hyperemia, which floods the previously ischemic area with blood-derived inflammatory cells and oxygen. This hyperemia is associated with cell death from necrosis and apoptosis.

Tissue damage from ischemia-reperfusion injury results from **increased generation of oxygen free radicals in the myocardium and endothelium**, as well as from infiltrating neutrophils. Myocardial sources may result from ischemic conversion of xanthine dehydrogenase to xanthine oxidase, which produces superoxide anion radical from xanthine. Damaged mitochondria also act as a source of oxygen free radicals. Further, the radicals impair mitochondrial recovery and ATP generation, which leads to cell death. The accompanying neutrophil infiltration sets up a local inflammatory response which produces damaging cytokines, production of additional reactive oxygen species in the tissues and complement activation.

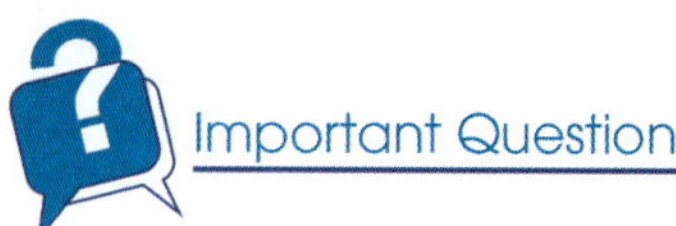

1. **Write notes on:**
   i. Reactive oxygen species
   ii. Oxidative stress
   iii. Free radicals
   iv. Antioxidant defenses
   v. Antioxidant vitamins
   vi. Ischemia-reperfusion injury

Multiple Choice Questions

1. The reactive oxygen species are implicated in the pathogenesis of:

A. Ischemia-reperfusion injury
B. Alzheimer's disease
C. Diabetes mellitus
D. All of the above

2. The following physiological process involves reactive oxygen species:

A. Phagocytosis
B. Regulation of gene expression
C. Apoptosis
D. All of the above

3. The following is not a physiological source of reactive oxygen species:

A. Xanthine oxidase reaction
B. Pyruvate kinase reaction
C. Oxidative phosphorylation
D. Peroxisomal fatty acid oxidation

4. The following detoxifies both H_2O_2 and lipid hydroperoxides:

A. Superoxide dismutase
B. Catalase
C. Glutathione peroxidase
D. Vitamin C

5. The following helps to maintain the levels of vitamin E:

A. Vitamin C
B. Reduced glutathione
C. β-Carotene
D. All of the above

CHAPTER 20

Nutrition

Competency Achievement: The student should be able to:

BI8.1	Discuss the importance of various dietary components and explain importance of dietary fiber
BI8.2	Describe the types and causes of protein energy malnutrition and its effects
BI8.3	Provide dietary advice for optimal health in childhood and adult, in disease conditions like diabetes mellitus, coronary artery disease and in pregnancy
BI8.4	Describe the causes (including dietary habits), effects and health risks associated with being overweight/obesity
BI8.5	Summarize the nutritional importance of commonly used items of food including fruits and vegetables. (Macromolecules and its importance)
IM23.1	Discuss and describe the methods of nutritional assessment in an adult and calculation of caloric requirements during illnesses
IM23.2	Discuss and describe the causes and consequences of protein caloric malnutrition in the hospital
IM23.4	Enumerate the indications for enteral and parenteral nutrition in critically ill patients
IM24.22	Describe and discuss the etiopathogenesis, clinical presentation, complications, assessment and management of nutritional disorders in the elderly
PA12.2	Describe the pathogenesis of disorders caused by protein calorie malnutrition and starvation
PE9.1	Describe the age-related nutritional needs of infants, children and adolescents including micronutrients and vitamins
PE9.3	Explain the calorific value of common Indian foods
PE11.1	Describe the common etiology, clinical features and management of obesity in children
PE11.2	Discuss the risk approach for obesity and discuss the prevention strategies

Nutrition is the study of nutrients and their relationship with food and living beings, i.e. it is a science of food and its relationship to health.

Nutrition interprets the interaction of nutrients and other substances in food, in relation to maintenance, growth, reproduction, health and disease of an organism. It includes food intake, and absorption, assimilation and catabolism of nutrients, and excretion of waste products.

DIETARY COMPONENTS OF NUTRITION

Dietary components refer to all the organic and inorganic substances that are obtained from the food, which we eat. These are also referred to as **accessory food factors** or **nutrients**. Dietary components of nutrition are, generally, divided into two groups, as **macronutrients** and **micronutrients**.

- **Macronutrients:** Macronutrients include **carbohydrates, fats** and **proteins**. They are needed in relatively large amounts and are also referred to as proximate principles of food. These are oxidized in the body to provide energy. Lipids are also essential for the formation of cell membrane. They also act as signaling molecules. Proteins also provide structural material. Together with **water**, carbohydrates, fats and proteins form bulk of an Indian diet (Table 20.1).
- **Micronutrients:** Micronutrients mainly include **vitamins** and **minerals**. They are required in smaller quantities, from milligrams to few grams, and may also be referred to as protective foods. Besides, vitamins and minerals, antioxidants and phytochemicals, too, may be said as micronutrients, since these are also known to influence (or protect) some body systems. However, their necessity is not as well established, as that of the vitamins and minerals.

Table 20.1: Dietary components of nutrition (macro- and micronutrients) with their importance

Dietary component	Importance
Carbohydrates	Major source of energy
Lipids	Provide large amount of energy, insulation, fat soluble vitamins and essential fatty acids
Proteins	Building and maintenance of tissues, antibodies, enzymes, hormones and other compounds
Vitamins	Facilitate use of other nutrients, used in regulation of growth and several metabolites
Minerals	Help in building bones and teeth, maintenance of acid–base balance, muscle functions and nervous system activity
Water	Dissolves and carries nutrients, removes waste products, regulates body temperature

CARBOHYDRATES

Carbohydrates are the most significant sources of energy in Indian diets. Being a cheap source of energy, carbohydrates form the bulk of an Indian diet. Dietary carbohydrates are classified into two groups:

1. **Available or digestible carbohydrates:** These are digestible by the enzymes present in the GIT and thus, serve as a source of energy. Carbohydrates are at the forefront and most efficient sources of energy. According to ICMR-NIN (2020) 55–60% of the dietary energy should be available from carbohydrates. Any carbohydrate in excess of that needed for energy is converted to glycogen and triacylglycerols for storage in the body. Principal sources of carbohydrates in the diet include starch (cereals, pulses and potatoes), lactose (milk), and sucrose (table sugar). Glucose though is specifically required by many tissues but may not form an essential part of the diet since starch and other dietary carbohydrates are readily converted to glucose in the body. A significant source of starch is potato. Compared to potato, the starch content of wheat is about 70% while that of pulses is 60%.
2. **Dietary fiber:** Dietary fiber (also called nonstarch polysaccharides) refers to the unavailable or indigestible carbohydrates that are **not digestible** by enzymes in the GIT and thus do not serve as source ICMR-NIN (2020) Expert Group has suggested that on an average dietary fiber intake should be 15 g/1000 kcal/day.
3. **Resistant starch:** Small fractions of starch that escape digestion and absorption are called resistant starch. It is found in whole legumes, raw potatoes and unripe bananas. Like fibers, they promote bowel movement in the colon but do not reduce blood cholesterol since they cannot bind to bile salts.

20

FATS

Dietary fats include triglycerides, cholesterol, phospholipids and other complex lipids. Over 90% of the dietary fat includes **triacylglycerols** (triglycerides). Fat is a **concentrated source of energy**. It provides, nearly, more than twice the energy supplied by carbohydrates or proteins per unit weight (9 kcal/g from lipids compared to 4 kcal/g from carbohydrates or proteins). Thus, lipids reduce bulk of the food. Dietary lipids are also important for palatability of food, ability to impart a sense of satiety, for forming membrane structures and absorption of lipid-soluble vitamins, etc. ICMR-NIN (2020) Expert Group has recommended that not more than 20–30% of dietary energy should be made available from fat.

Plant Fats Versus Animal Fats

Fat included in the diet should preferably be derived from **vegetable sources**, since it is rich in polyunsaturated fatty acids (PUFA) and serves as a source of **essential fatty acids** for the body. This is not only lower in cost but also superior in quality as compared to the animal fat. Sunflower oil, cottonseed oil, wheat-germ oil, soybean oil and corn oil are some of the vegetable oils in common use. These oils have more than 50% of the fat as PUFAs. Hydrogenation of the vegetable oil reduces the quantity of PUFAs, originally present in the oil.

Predominant fatty acids in **animal fats**, such as in meat, are saturated. Animal fat also contains phospholipids and cholesterol. **Phospholipids** are essential for the functioning of the nervous tissue. **Cholesterol** is an important precursor of vitamin D, steroid hormones and bile acids. **Excess consumption of saturated fat**, such as from animal sources and of cholesterol, such as from eggs is associated with **hypercholesterolemia** and **atherosclerosis.** Eggs have highest concentration of cholesterol. Cholesterol content of the skimmed-milk is lower than the whole milk. Pulses do not contain cholesterol.

As discussed above, fat should not provide more than 20–30% of the daily energy requirement. Out of this, about 10% of the calorie intake should be available from **invisible fat**, such as from milk, cereals, pulses and legumes (pulses and legumes can provide nearly 5% fat). As per ICMR-NIN (2020) not more than 10% of dietary energy should be consumed in the form of visible fat, such as from ghee, butter or oil, etc. ***Trans* fat should be avoided**.

Compared to the cost of carbohydrates which are the cheapest sources of energy, dietary fats are costlier. Thus, it is appropriately said that people who require more fat cannot afford it but those who can afford it should not consume it.

Essential Fatty Acids

Two of the polyunsaturated fatty acids have been recognized as essential in the diet of men. These are **linolenic acid and arachidonic acid**, and are called essential fatty acids. Essential fatty acids are needed for lowering serum cholesterol, for maintaining the function and integrity of membrane structure, and for the synthesis of eicosanoids. The most common symptom of essential fatty acids deficiency is scaly dermatitis.

PROTEINS

Proteins have more physiological roles than other any nutrient. They are essential **structural components of the cell**. Proteins are also important for maintaining output of essential secretions, such as digestive **enzymes** and peptide or **protein hormones**. Amino acids, the hydrolyzed product of protein, are required for the synthesis of **plasma proteins**, which are essential for the maintenance of osmotic balance, transport of substances through blood and for maintaining immunity. Excess of the protein may also be used as a **source of energy**, with the glucogenic amino acids being converted to glucose while the ketogenic amino acids being converted to fatty acids and ketone bodies.

Normally, the contribution of protein to energy value in a balanced diet should be 10 to 15% of the total calorie intake. Daily protein requirement for an adult man has been suggested as 0.64 g/kg/day. Among the various dietary sources, meat, eggs, soybean and milk are good choices.

Protein Quality

Quality of the dietary protein can be assessed by several criteria, such as biological value, digestibility, net-protein utilization, amino acid score or chemical score. Biological value, digestibility or net-protein utilization can be assessed by knowing the amount of protein-nitrogen that is ingested, absorbed and retained by the body.

Biological value (BV) of a protein refers to the proportion of the absorbed protein nitrogen retained by the body.

Amino acid score refers to the total amino acid content in the protein relative to that present in the same quantity of a reference protein, expressed as percentage.

Chemical score refers to the content of each essential amino acid in the protein relative to that present in the same quantity of a reference protein, expressed as percentage.

Nitrogen balance: Nitrogen balance is a comparison between intake of nitrogen as protein and its excretion through various routes, chiefly as undigested protein in feces, and urea and ammonia in urine (Fig. 20.1).

Protein status of the body can be assessed by calculating the nitrogen balance of an individual. A

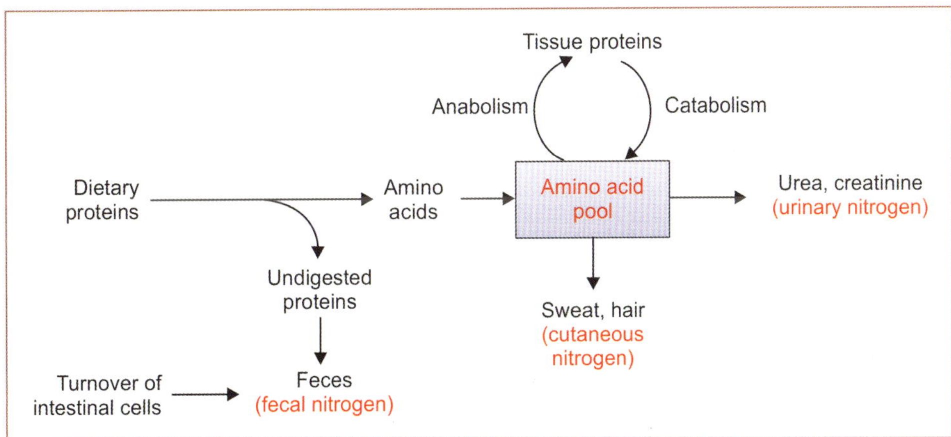

Fig. 20.1: Nitrogen balance

20

subject is said to be in nitrogen equilibrium, i.e. **zero nitrogen balance**, when daily nitrogen intake equals excretion, i.e. the output through the urine, feces and skin. A growing child should be in a **positive nitrogen balance**. Other conditions like pregnancy, lactation and convalescence (recovery from metabolic stress or acute illness) should also be associated with positive nitrogen balance. On the other hand, injury, chronic diseases (such as tuberculosis, rheumatoid arthritis, cancer), increased muscular activity, inadequate protein intake, lack of essential amino acids and increased metabolic stress lead to a **negative nitrogen balance** (Table 20.2).

Table 20.2: Type of nitrogen balance and examples of the prevailing conditions

Nitrogen balance	Protein intake (I)/output (O)	Condition
Equilibrium	I = O	Normal/healthy individuals
Positive	I > O	Growth, pregnancy, convalescence
Negative	I < O	↓ Protein intake, trauma, chronic illness (e.g. tuberculosis)

Essential Amino Acids

Dietary protein is an important source of amino acids required for the growth in children and for the maintenance of nitrogen balance in adults. As growth slows down, the need for protein declines. The requirement of protein is not only with respect to the quantity of protein in the diet but also the quality. An adult human body can maintain its nitrogen equilibrium on a mixture of 8 amino acids as the sole source of nitrogen. These are called essential amino acids.

Essential amino acids include **isoleucine, leucine, lysine, methionine, phenylalanine, threonine, tryptophan** and **valine**. In addition, **histidine** and **arginine** are also needed in extra amounts by infants during growth and by females during pregnancy and lactation. Accordingly, these two amino acids are called **semiessential amino acids**. The remaining amino acids are dietary nonessential.

Complete and Incomplete Proteins

Most of the **animal proteins**, such as egg albumin, milk casein, etc. generally, contain all the **essential amino acids.** These are called **complete proteins**. On the other hand, **vegetable proteins**, e.g. proteins from cereals and pulses, often lack one or more essential amino acids. They are called **incomplete proteins**.

Supplementary Action of Proteins

For vegetarians, though pulses are an important source of protein but, as mentioned above, most of the **vegetative proteins** are of **poor biological value,** because they are **limiting** in **some of the essential amino acids**. For example, wheat is limiting in lysine, pulses lack methionine, maize (corn) is deficient in lysine, methionine as well as tryptophan.

In general, it is known that cereals are deficient in lysine and threonine, but they contain sufficiently high amounts of methionine. On the other hand, legumes and pulses are good sources of lysine and threonine but are poor in methionine. When the proteins from the two sources are taken together in the diet, the amino acids present in excess in pulses can effectively supplement the limiting amino acids of the cereals, and vice versa. This is known as **supplementary action of proteins**.

It provides a strong biochemical basis for the **traditional Indian dietary habit** of taking rice or wheat-bread with pulses.

Biological Value of Proteins

As mentioned above, since different types of dietary proteins contain different amounts and combinations of amino acids, dietary proteins are divided into two categories:

- **High quality proteins:** These are mainly obtained from animal sources, e.g. meat, fish, eggs, dairy products, etc. They contain full range of all the essential amino acids, which are needed by human body. These are also referred to as the proteins of high biological value.
- **Low quality proteins:** These are obtained mainly, from plant sources. They have low biological value, since they lack one or more essential amino acids.

VITAMINS

Vitamins are a group of organic compounds, which perform a variety of functions in the body. Every vitamin is chemically different from each other. Though they do not yield energy but enable the body to use other nutrients. Since body is, generally, unable to synthesize most of the vitamins, hence, they must be provided by food. As discussed in Chapter 8, vitamins are divided into two groups, as:

i. **Fat-soluble vitamins**, which include vitamins A, D, E and K.

ii. **Water-soluble vitamins**, which include B vitamins and vitamin C.

Though recommended daily allowance for each vitamin differs, but it is important to consume all the vitamins, each day, to keep our body healthy.

- Vitamins are required by the body in small amounts, for a variety of essential processes.
- Most vitamins cannot be made by the body, so need to be provided in the diet.
- Vitamin D can be made by the body in the skin when it is exposed to sunlight.
- Requirements for vitamins change across life stages.

MINERALS

Minerals are the inorganic substances required by the body in small amounts, for a variety of functions, such as:

- Formation of bones and teeth
- To form essential constituents of body fluids and tissues
- Coenzyme, required with several enzymes, and
- For normal nerve functions.

As discussed in Chapter 11, our body requires different amounts of each mineral. Accordingly, minerals are divided into two groups (Table 20.3).

- **Major minerals** such as sodium, potassium, calcium, phosphorus, magnesium, sulfur and chloride, which are required in large amounts (grams or milligrams).
- **Trace minerals** (trace elements) like copper, fluoride, zinc, iron, chromium, selenium, iodine, molybdenum and manganese, which are needed in small amounts (micrograms to milligrams).

All the minerals and trace elements are present in healthy tissues, where their concentration remains relatively constant. Elements, like nickel, vanadium, tin, boron, etc. have not been shown to have any function in the human body and are not considered to be dietary essential.

Table 20.3: Essential minerals and trace elements required by human body

Minerals	Trace elements
Calcium	Copper
Phosphorus	Chromium
Magnesium	Manganese
Sodium	Molybdenum
Potassium	Selenium
Iron	Iodine
Zinc	Fluoride

WATER

Water is essential for life. Although human can survive for a number of weeks without food, one cannot live without fluid for more than 2 or 3 days. On an average, water makes up nearly 60% of body weight and is essential for normal functioning of all the cells in the body. **Though, amount of fluid needed varies according to age, time of the year, climate conditions, diet and level of physical activity,** ICMR-NIN (2020) has suggested daily water intake, based on the energy requirement and the WHO Guidelines, as 1.5 mL per Kcal.

It is a major nutritional element that helps to

- Regulate body temperature
- Lubricate joints
- Protect major organs and tissues
- Transport important substances.

We can obtain our fluid requirements from a number of sources, such as water and other drinks, as well as the food we eat (*see* Chapter 10).

DIETARY FIBER

Dietary fiber comprises:

i. **Insoluble fiber**, also called crude fiber or roughage), include cellulose and hemicellulose. Their functions include:
   - Retention of water during intestinal transit thereby preventing constipation.
   - Binding various dietary toxins thereby reducing the incidence of colon cancer.
   - Imparting a sense of early satiety (fullness of stomach) thereby helping to reduce calorie intake and thus to control obesity and diabetes mellitus.

   Insoluble fibers are abundant in vegetable grains. It is worth mentioning that insoluble fibers also include some nonpolysaccharides, e.g. lignins (carrots, strawberry seeds), cutins and tannins.

ii. **Soluble fiber**, e.g. gums and pectins found in legumes, fruits and oats. Their functions include:
   - Binding cholesterol and bile salts thereby reducing their enterohepatic circulation and enhancing the conversion of cholesterol into bile salts, lowering plasma cholesterol levels.
   - Reducing gastric emptying thereby delaying the postprandial rise in blood glucose of diabetic patients.

Importance of Dietary Fiber

High intake of **dietary fiber has many health benefits.** For example, diets rich in fiber decreases risk of obesity, type 2 diabetes, colon cancer, cardiovascular disease and gastrointestinal disorders:

- Diets rich in fiber are, usually, low in fat and provide lesser calories. Since such a diet forms bulk of the food, which takes longer to eat, and gives a feeling of fullness. Dietary fiber not only regulates body weight but also **lowers the risk of obesity**.
- Higher intake of soluble fiber also delays stomach emptying and, thus, regulates blood glucose level. This, in turn, also **reduces the risk of type 2 diabetes.**
- Diet rich in fiber also lowers the risk of certain types of cancer. It is due to the reason that food with large amounts of fruits and vegetables, provides antioxidants, which protect our body against cell damage and **cancer**.
- Soluble fiber also lowers serum cholesterol, thus, **reduces the risk of a cardiovascular disease**.
- Diet rich in insoluble fiber also adds bulk to feces and softens stool for its easy passage. Thus, dietary fiber **helps in prevention of constipation and hemorrhoids**, particularly, when fluid intake is high.

PROTEIN ENERGY MALNUTRITION

Protein energy malnutrition **(PEM)**, also referred to as **protein calorie malnutrition** (PCM), refers to the form of malnutrition due to inadequate intake of calories and/or protein. PEM, though, can occur at any stage of life, it is most common during childhood, when extra protein is needed for rapid growth. PEM occurs in all parts of the world, but is most commonty in Southeast Asia, Africa, South and Central America, and Middle East countries. It is seen, most often, in population living in poverty, elderly people and hospitalized patients having some associated condition, such as anorexia nervosa, AIDS, cancer or malabsorption syndrome. Two common forms of PEM include kwashiorkor and marasmus. This classification of PEM is based on deficit in body weight for age and presence or absence of edema (Fig. 20.2).

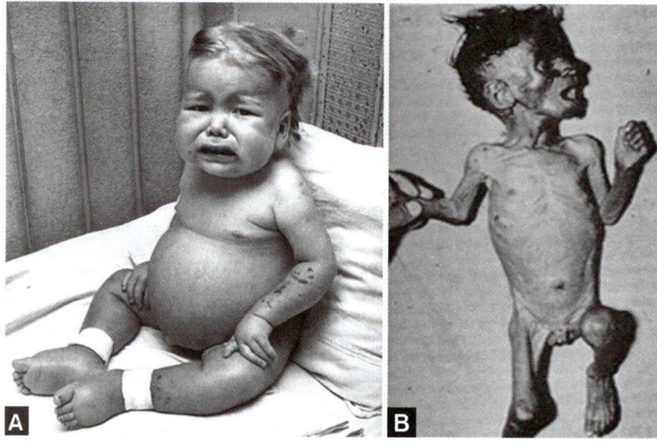

Fig. 20.2: The two extremes of the spectrum of protein energy malnutrition. (A) Kwashiorkor; (B) Marasmus

KWASHIORKOR

The term kwashiorkor comes from a word used in Ghana, which means a disease of a baby deposed from the breast when the next one is born. It is said that kwashiorkor, usually, develops when a baby is weaned from the protein-rich breast milk and switched to a protein-poor food. Today, it is the most serious and prevalent form of malnutrition in the world, especially, in industrially underdeveloped countries. Kwashiorkor, typically, occurs at about 1 year of age, after infants are weaned from breast milk to a protein-deficient diet, but can develop at any time during the formative years (Fig. 20.3).

Signs and Symptoms

Signs and symptoms of kwashiorkor include:

- Edema with swollen legs
- Pot belly (enlarged liver)
- Mild-to-moderate growth retardation
- Some weight loss and low subcutaneous fat
- Muscle atrophy
- Round face (moon face)
- Dry, flaky peeling skin
- Thin, dry and easily plucked hair

MARASMUS

Marasmus occurs due to the deficient intake of both protein and calories, i.e. total food, generally, due to early weaning. It differs from kwashiorkor with respect to the subcutaneous fat which disappears in marasmus but not in kwashiorkor. A marasmic infant thus generally has a thin, wasted appearance and is small-for-age. Marasmus occurs most often in infants and children between 6 and 18 months of age, particularly in those who are given diluted milk (Fig. 20.4).

Signs and Symptoms

- Severe weight loss
- No edema
- Severe growth failure

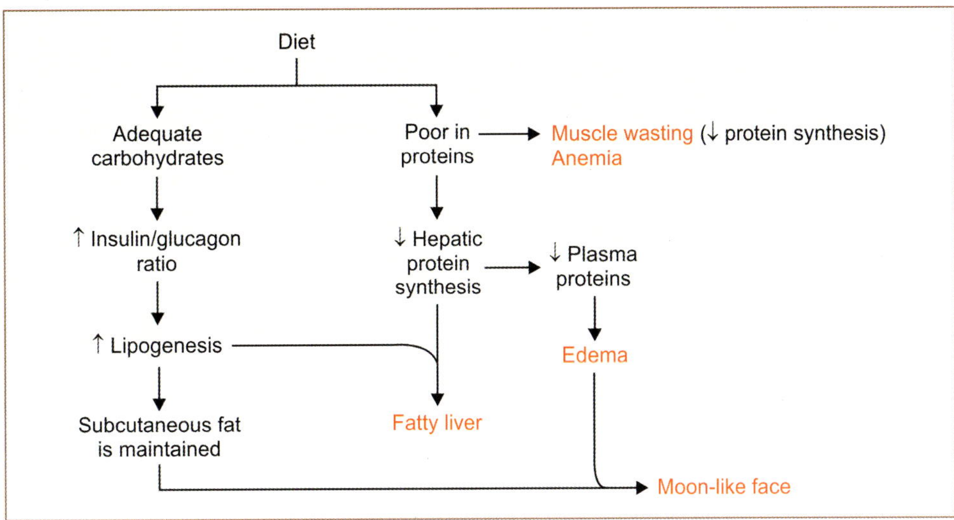

Fig. 20.3: Biochemical–clinical correlations in kwashiorkor

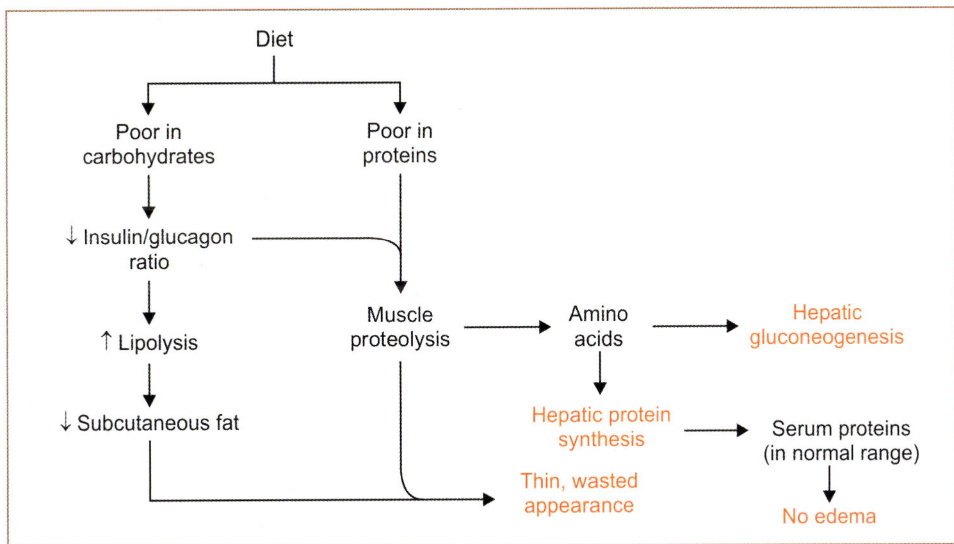

Fig. 20.4: Biochemical–clinical correlations in marasmus

- Severe loss of subcutaneous fat
- Weight loss up to 40%
- Severe muscle atrophy
- Wrinkled face (old man's face)
- Rare skin changes
- Common hair changes

Differences between Kwashiorkor and Marasmus

Marasmus can be distinguished from **kwashiorkor** in the way that, kwashiorkor is protein deficiency with adequate energy intake, whereas **marasmus** is inadequate energy intake in all forms, including protein.

Besides, there are other differences between the two conditions, as shown in Table 20.4.

Table 20.4: Differences between kwashiorkor and marasmus

Kwashiorkor	Marasmus
• Scaly skin	• Severe muscle wasting (particularly, loss of fat from buttocks and thighs)
• Distended abdomen (pot belly)	• Old person's face
• Swollen ankles (edema)	• Hair loss

20

DIETARY ADVICE FOR OPTIMAL HEALTH

In nutrition, **diet** is the sum of food consumed by a person, or other organism. The word diet often implies the use of specific intake of nutrients for optimal health and weight management.

The **Nutrients Advisory Committee** of the **Indian Council of Medical Research** (ICMR) is the body for giving dietary advice for Indians. Based on the recommendations of the ICMR-NIN (2020) Expert Group, recommended dietary allowances for Indians, for different age groups are shown in Tables 20.5 to 20.7.

Balanced Diet

A balanced diet is defined as a diet which provides, quantitatively as well as qualitatively, adequate amounts of all the dietary components for maintaining an optimum health. As a general rule, the following criteria should be met in a balanced diet:

1. **Calorie distribution:** Nearly 55–60% of the calories should be derived from carbohydrates, 20–30% from lipids and 10–15% from proteins.
2. **Carbohydrates:** It should include both digestible as well as indigestible (fibers) carbohydrates.
3. **Lipids:** It should mainly be from the vegetable sources. Diet should be rich in polyunsaturated fatty acids (PUFAs) but low in cholesterol.
4. **Proteins:** It should be of high biological value and easily digestible.
5. **Vitamins and minerals:** Green-leafy vegetables, fruits and milk should be included to provide the required amounts of vitamins and minerals.
6. **Water:** Adequate water intake is a must for all the aspects of metabolism, besides elimination of toxic wastes.

Table 20.5: Recommended daily allowlances of macronutrients for Indians (ICMR-NIN, 2020)

Population/ Group	Category of worker/ Period	Carbohydrates (g)	Dietary Fiber* (g)	Visible fat (g)	Protein (g)
Adult men (18+)	Sedentary	100	30	25	
	Moderate	100	40	30	54
	Heavy	100	50	40	
Adult women (18+)	Sedentary	100	25	20	
	Moderate	100	30	25	46
	Heavy	100	40	30	
Pregnant women	2nd Trimester	135		30	(+) 9.5
	3rd Trimester	135		30	(+) 22
Lactating women	0–6 Months	155		30	(+) 16.9
	7–12 Months	155		30	(+) 13.2
Infants	0–6 Months**	55*			8
	7–12 Months	95*		25	10.5
Children	1–3 Years	100	15	25	12.5
	4–6 Years	100	20	25	16
	7–9 Years	100	26	30	23
Adolescents	Boys 10–12 Yrs	100	33	35	32
	Boys 13–15 Yrs	100	43	45	45
	Boys 16–18 Yrs	100	50	50	55
	Girls 10–12 Yrs	100	30	35	33
	Girls 13–15 Yrs	100	36	40	43
	Girls 16–18 Yrs	100	38	35	46

*Estimated Average Requirement (EAR)

**Adequate Intake (AI)

Table 20.6: Recommended daily allowances of vitamins for Indians (ICMR-NIN, 2020)

Population/ Group	Category of worker/Period (mg)	Thiamine (mg)	Riboflavin (mg)	Niacin (mg)	Pantothenic acid* (mg)	Pyridoxine (mg)	Biotin* (µg)	Folate* (µg)	B12 (µg)	Vitamin C (mg)	Vitamin A (µg)	Vitamin D (IU)
Adult men (18+)	Sedentary	1.4	2	14	5	1.9	25	300	2.2	80	1000	600
	Moderate	1.8	2.5	18	5	2.4	25	300	2.2	80	1000	600
	Heavy	2.3	3.2	23	5	3.1	25	300	2.2	80	1000	600
Adult women (18+)	Sedentary	1.4	1.9	11	5	1.9	25	220	2.2	65	840	600
	Moderate	1.7	2.4	14	5	1.9	25	220	2.2	65	840	600
	Heavy	2.2	3.1	18	5	2.4	25	220	2.2	65	840	600
Pregnant women	2nd Trimester	2	2.7	(+) 2	5	2.3	25	570	(+) 0.25	(+)15	900	600
	3rd Trimester	2	2.7	(+) 2	5	2.3	25	570	(+) 0.25	(+) 15	900	600
Lactating women	0–6 Months	2.1	3	(+) 5	(+) 2	(+) 0.26	(+) 5	330	(+) 1	(+) 50	950	600
	7–12 Months	2.1	2.9	(+) 5	(+) 2	(+) 0.17	(+) 5	330	(+) 1	(+) 50	950	600
Infants	0–6 Months*	0.2*	0.4*	2*	2	0.1*	4	25*	1.2	20*	350*	400*
	7–12 Months	0.4*	0.6*	5*	2	0.6*	5	85	1.2	30*	350	400*
Children	1–3 Years	0.7	1.1	7	2	0.9	7	120	1.2	30	390	600
	4–6 Years	0.9	1.3	9	3	1.2	9	135	2.2	35	510	600
	7–9 Years	1.1	1.6	11	4	1.5	12	170	2.2	45	630	600
Adolescents	Boys 10–12 Yrs	1.5	2.1	15	5	2	15	220	2.2	55	770	600
	Girls 10–12 Yrs	1.4	1.9	14	5	1.9	16	225	2.2	50	790	600
	Boys 13–15 Yrs	1.9	2.7	19	5	2.6	20	285	2.2	70	930	600
	Girls 13–15 Yrs	1.6	2.2	16	5	2.2	20	245	2.2	65	890	600
	Boys 16–18 Yrs	2.2	3.1	22	5	3	25	340	2.2	85	1000	600
	Girls 16–18 Yrs	1.7	2.3	17	5	2.3	25	270	2.2	70	860	600

*Adequate Intake

Table 20.7: Recommended daily allowances of minerals and not vitamins for Indians (ICMR-NIN, 2020

Population/ Group	Category of worker/(mg) Period	Calcium phorus (mg)	Phos- esium (mg)	Magn- (mg)	Sodium* (mg)	Potassium* (mg)	Iron (mg)	Zinc (mg)	Copper mium (mg)	Chro- genese (mg)	Man- (mg)	Selenium (µg)	Iodine (µg)
Adult men (+18)	Sedentary	1000	1000	440	2000	3500	19	17	1.7	50	4	40	140
	Moderate	1000	1000	440	2000	3500	19	17	1.7	50	4	40	140
	Heavy	1000	1000	440	2000	3500	19	17	1.7	50	4	40	140
Addult women (18+)	Sedentary	1000	1000	370	2000	3500	29	13	1.5	50	4	40	140
	Moderate	1000	1000	370	2000	3500	29	13	1.5	50	4	40	140
	Heavy	1000	1000	370	2000	3500	29	13	1.5	50	4	40	140
Pregnant	2nd Trimester	1000	1000	440	2000	3500	27	14.5					220
women	3rd Trimester	1000	1000	440	2000	3500	27	14.5					
Lactating	0–6 Months	1200	1200	400	2000	3500	23	14.1					280
women	7–12 Months	1200	1200	400	2000	3500	23	14.1					
Infants	0–6 Months	300**	450**	30**	500	900							100**
	7–12 Months	300**	450**	75**	650	1100	3	2.5					130**
Children	1–3 Years	500	500	90	1000	1750	8	3.3	0.6	22	1.8	16–18	90
	4–6 Years	550	550	125	1300	2250	11	4.5	0.9	28	2.9	29–32	90
	7–9 Years	650	650	175	1600	2825	15	5.9	1	31	3.6	36–42	90
Adolescents	Boys 10–12 Yrs	850	850	240	2000	3500	16	8.5	1.28	36	4.7	51	100
	Girls 10–12 Yrs	850	850	250	2000	3500	28	8.5	1.15	34	4.1	45	100
	Boys 13–15 Yrs	1000	1000	345	2000	3500	22	14.3	1.43	41	5.1	58	140
	Girls 13–15 Yrs	1000	1000	340	2000	3500	30	12.8	1.3	37	4.6	52	140
	Boys 16–18 Yrs	1050	1050	440	2000	3500	26	17.6	1.8	44	6.1	71	140
	Girls 16–18 Yrs	1050	1050	380	2000	3500	32	14.2	1.54	38	4.7	55	140

*Safe intake

** Adequate intake

7. **Economy:** The diet should have a variety of items from different sources, best possible within one's own budget.

DIETARY ADVICE FOR OPTIMAL HEALTH FOR INFANTS

During First 6 Months of Age

- **Energy:** For infants with the average body weight of 5.8 kg, **adequate intake** of energy has been suggested as **530 kcal/d.**
- **Fat:** Minimum level of total fat has been suggested as **40–60% of the total energy intake.**
- **Protein:** **RDA** for protein has been suggested as **8.0 g/d.**
- **Vitamins:**
  - **Thiamine—RDA** for thiamine has been suggested as 0.2 mg/d.
  - **Riboflavin—RDA** for riboflavin has been suggested as **0.4 mg/d.**
  - **Niacin—RDA** for niacin has been suggested as **2.0 mg/d.**
  - **Vitamin B_6—RDA** for vitamin B_6 has been suggested as **0.1 mg/d.**
  - **Folate—RDA** for folate has been suggested as **25 µg/d.**
  - **Vitamin B_{12}—RDA** for vitamin B_{12} has been suggested as **1.2 µg/d.**
  - **Vitamin C—RDA** for vitamin C has been suggested as **20 mg/d.**
  - **Vitamin A—RDA** for vitamin A has been suggested as **350 µg/d.**
  - **Vitamin D—RDA** for vitamin D has been suggested as **400 IU/d.**
- **Minerals**
  - **Calcium-RDA** for calcium has been suggested as **300 mg/d.**
  - **Magnesium-RDA** for magnesium has been suggested as **30 mg/d.**
  - **Iodine-RDA** for iodine has been suggested as **100 µg/d.**
- **Water:** Total water requirement has been suggested as 600 mL/d, which is available from breast milk.

  Further, it has also been suggested that, since **breast milk contains all these nutrients** which are essentially **required for infants, and that the requirements of these nutrients, for infants between 0–6 months of age, can be met from breast milk,** thus, breast-feeding should, essentially, be promoted at least for six months.
- Breast milk also **provides several special components** such as **growth factors, enzymes, hormones and anti-infective factors.**
- It also has a **high content of DHA** (docosahexaenoic acid) which plays an important role in brain development.
- Breast milk also provides **IgA** (immunoglobulin A), **lactoferrin, lacto-peroxidase and complements** which provide immunity and protects the infant from several types of infections.
- Besides breast milk, **colostrum** (the milk secreted during the first 3–4 days after child birth) **is also rich in proteins, minerals, vitamins** (especially vitamin A) and **antibodies.**

During 6–12 months of age

- **Energy:** For infants above 6 months of age, with the average body weight of 8.5 kg, **adequate intake** of energy has been suggested as **680 kcal/d.**
- **Fat:** Minimum level of total fat has been suggested as **35% of energy.**

  It is further suggested that **visible fat intake should be 25 g/d.**
- **Protein:** **RDA** for protein has been suggested as **10.5 g/d.**
- **Vitamins:**
  - **Thiamine—RDA** for thiamine has been suggested as **0.4 mg/d.**
  - **Riboflavin—RDA** for riboflavin has been suggested as **0.6 mg/d.**
  - **Niacin—RDA** for niacin has been suggested as **5.0 mg/d.**
  - **Vitamin B_6—RDA** for vitamin B_6 has been suggested as **0.6 mg/d.**
  - **Folate—RDA** for folate has been suggested as **85 µg/d.**
  - **Vitamin B_{12}—RDA** for vitamin B_{12} has been suggested as **1.2 µg/d.**
  - **Vitamin C—RDA** for vitamin C has been suggested as **30 mg/d.**
  - **Vitamin A—RDA** for vitamin A has been suggested as **350 µg/d.**
  - **Vitamin D—RDA** for vitamin D has been suggested as **400 IU/d.**
- **Minerals:**
  - **Calcium—RDA** for calcium has been suggested as **300 mg/d.**

- **Magnesium—RDA** for magnesium has been suggested as **75 mg/d**.
- **Iron—RDA** for iron has been suggested as **3 mg/d**.
- **Zinc—RDA** for magnesium has been suggested as **2.5 mg/d**.
- **Iodine—RDA** for iodine has been suggested as **130 µg/d**.

- **Water:** Total water requirement has been suggested as 1000 mL/d. It can be met from breast milk, water and other fluids.

  Further it has been suggested that these requirements should, partially, be met from breast milk. Accordingly, along with the breast milk, these infants, after six months of age, should be given home-based semi-solid foods. For this purpose:
  - In addition to breast milk, **they should be provided the supplementary or complementary foods such as** liquids (like **milk**), semisolids (like **khichdi and kheer**) and solid preparations like **rice**, etc.
  - **These can be low-cost food supplements which can be prepared, at home, from commonly used ingredients**, such as cereals (wheat, rice, ragi. jowar, bajra, etc.), pulses (grams and dals), nuts and oilseeds (groundnut, sesame, etc.), vegetable oils (groundnut oil, sesame oil, etc.), and sugar and jaggery. These foods, in turn, will provide **good quality protein, adequate calories and several protective nutrients**.
  - In addition, these infants should also be **given fruits and green leafy vegetables** which are rich sources of vitamins and minerals. However, these should be well cleaned before cooking.

During Childhood and Adolescence

Childhood and adolescence are the **periods of continuous growth and development**.

- **During the second-year**, a **child increases in height by 7–8 cm** and **gains body weight**, approximately, **to 4 times of its birth weight**.
- **During the pre-adolescent period**, a **child grows, on an average. by 6–7 cm in height** and **1.5–3.0 kg in body weight, every year** and simultaneously, development and maturation of the various tissues and organs takes place.
- **Adolescent period** (teenage) **is spread almost over a decade** and is **characterized by rapid increase in height and weight** along with the hormonal changes, sexual maturation and wide swing in emotions.
  - Adolescent **growth spurt starts at about 10–12 years in girls** and **two years later in boys**.
  - **Annual peak rates for increase in height and weight are 9–10 cm and 8–10 kg**, respectively.
  - During this period, development of the critical bone mass is essential as this forms the ground for maintaining mineral integrity of bone in later life.
  - Pattern and proportion of various body components, like body water, muscle mass, bone and fat, increase during the entire childhood and adolescence to reach adult values by about 18 years.
  - **Adolescent girls** are at greater physiological stress than boys because of menstruation. Their **nutritional needs are of particular importance** as they have to prepare for motherhood. All these rapid anabolic changes require more nutrients per unit body weight.

Accordingly, it is advised that:

- **Growing children and adolescents require more calcium**. It is recommended that they **should consume calcium rich foods** like **milk and milk products, ragi** (fox tail millet) and **til** (sesame seed), etc.
- **Young children**, below 5 years of age, **should be given** less bulky **foods** but are **rich in energy and protein**, such as **legumes, pulses, nuts, edible oil/ghee, sugar, milk and eggs**.
- **Vegetables**, including **green leafy vegetables, and** locally available **seasonal fruits** should be a part of their daily menu.
- Older children and adolescents **should also consume plenty of milk** to fulfil high calcium requirements.
- They should consume, nearly, **25–50 g of cooking oils/ghee**.
- **Excessive salt intake should be avoided,** particularly, by children having a family history of hypertension.

DIETARY ADVICE FOR OPTIMAL HEALTH FOR ADULTS

Based on the recommendations of the ICMR-NIN (2020), RDA for various nutrients, for adult moderate workers are described below:

- **Energy: RDA for calories for adult moderate workers** has been suggested as **2710 kcal/day for males** and **2130 kcal/d for females**.
- It is further suggested that since 70–80% of the total dietary calories in India are derived from carbohydrates that are present in plant foods such as cereals, millets and pulses, the **recommendation** for **cereals and millets is 400 g** and for **pulses 80 g/day**.
- **Carbohydrates:** It is recommended that a **minimum of 100–130 g of carbohydrates should be consumed per day**.

- **Dietary fiber: Safe intake of dietary fiber** has been suggested as **15 g per 1000 kcal/d.**
- **Fats:** The **upper limit for visible fat intake for healthy adult moderate workers has been suggested as 30 g for males** and **25 g/d** for **females.**
- **Protein: Safe intake of protein** has been suggested as **0.83 g/kg/d.**
- **Vitamins:**
  - **Thiamin—RDA for thiamine for** adult moderate workers has been suggested as **1.8 mg/d for males** and **1.7 mg/d for females.**
  - **Riboflavin—RDA for riboflavin** for adult moderate workers has been suggested as **2.5 mg/d for males** and 2.4 **mg/d for females.**
  - **Niacin—RDA for niacin (NE)** for adult moderate workers has been suggested as **18 mg/d for males** and **14 mg/d for females.**
  - **Pyridoxine—RDA for pyridoxine** for adult moderate workers has been suggested as **2.5 mg/d for males** and **1.9 mg/d for females.**
  - **Folate—RDA for folate** for adult moderate worker has been suggested as **300 µg/d for males** and **220 µg/d for females.**
  - **Vitamin B_{12}—RDA for** vitamin B_{12} for adult moderate male and female workers has been suggested as **2.2 µg/d.**
  - **Vitamin C—RDA for vitamin C** for adult moderate workers has been suggested as **80 mg/d for males** and **65 mg/d for females.**
  - **Vitamin A–RDA for vitamin A** (RE) for adult moderate workers has been suggested as **1000 µg/d for males and 840 µg/d for females.**
- **Minerals:**
  - **Calcium** and **phosphorus—**RDA for calcium for adult moderate workers has been suggested as **1000 mg/day** for males and females.
    Additional 200 mg per day has been suggested **for women during post-menopause.**
    Similar values have been recommended for phosphorus.
  - **Magnesium—estimated average requirement** for magnesium for adult moderate workers has been recommended as **440 mg/d for males** and **370 mg/d for females.**
  - **Sodium** and **potassium—safe intake of sodium** has been suggested as **2000 mg/day.** Accordingly, the **salt intake** has been recommended as **5 g/day.**
  - **Potassium** intake has been suggested as **3500 mg/day.**
  - **Iron—RDA for iron** for adult moderate workers has been suggested as **19 mg/d for males and 29 mg/d for females.**
- **Water : Total water requirement** for adult moderate workers has been suggested as **4050 mL/d for males** and **3200 mL/d for females.**

For elderly persons

As one grows old, his/her **body composition changes.** In general:

- Elderly person **loses lean body mass** and **gains fat mass.**
- **Loss of lean tissue compromises strength, reduces resting energy expenditure** and increases the **risk of osteoporosis.**
- **Perception of taste** also **declines with age,** which also contributes to **loss of appetite** and **poor food intake.**
- **Reduction in acid and enzymes secretions** further affect nutrient absorption.
- **Immune functions also decline** with age.
- **Absorption, transport, storage and metabolism of fat-soluble vitamins are also affected** by aging.
  Thus, aging causes **multiple physiological changes,** which, accordingly, **affect our nutrients need as well as nutritional status.**

Accordingly, **ICMR-NIN (2020)** has recommended that, **to maintain regular physical activity, elders should consume nutrient-dense foods,** such as **nuts, oilseeds, fruits, vegetables, legumes and flesh-foods,** to meet their daily requirements of vitamins and minerals.

Recommendations of the Group for various nutrients for the elderly persons (more than 60 years of age) are shown in Table 20.8.

- **Energy:** Due to a reduction in BMR and the sedentary lifestyle, the Group has **suggested** RDA for energy in terms of **estimated average requirement** (EAR).
  EAR for energy has been suggested as **1700 Kcal/day for elderly males** (with average body weight of 65 Kg) and **1500 Kal for elderly females** (with average body weight of 55 Kg).
- **Dietary fiber:** RDA for dietary fiber has been suggested as **30 g/d for elderly males** and **25 g/d for elderly females.**
- **Protein:** RDA for protein has been suggested as **54 g/d for elderly males** and **46 g/d for elderly females.**
- **Vitamins:**
  - **Thiamine—**RDA for thiamine has been suggested as **1.4 mg/d for elderly males as well as females.**
  - **Riboflavin—**RDA for riboflavin has been suggested as **2.0 mg/d for elderly males** and **1.9 mg/d for elderly females.**

Table 20.8: Recommended dietary allowances of macro- and micronutrients for the elderly (ICMR-NIN, 2020)

Dietary nutrient	Male (60+)	Female (60+)
Energy (Kcal)	1700	1500
Dietary Fiber (g)	32	25
Proteins (g)	54	46
Thiamine (mg)	1.4	1.4
Riboflavin (mg)	2	1.9
Niacin (mg)	12	9
Vitamin B_6 (mg)	1.9	1.9
Folate (µg)	300	200
Vitamin B_{12} (µg)	2.2	2.2
Vitamin C (mg)	80	65
Vitamin A (µg)	1000	840
Vitamin D (IU)*	800	800
Calcium (mg)	1200	1200
Magnesium (mg)	440	370
Iron (mg)	19	19
Zinc (mg)	17	13
Iodine (µg)	150	150

* Adequate intake

- **Niacin**—RDA for niacin (NE) has been suggested as **14 mg/d for** elderly **males** and **11 mg/d for elderly females**.
- **Vitamin B_6**—RDA for vitamin B_6 has been suggested as **1.9 mg/d for elderly males as well as females**.
- **Folate**—RDA for dietary folate has been suggested as **300 µg/d for elderly males** and **200 µg/d for elderly females**.
- **Vitamin B_{12}**—RDA for vitamin B_{12} has been suggested as **2.2 µg/day for elderly males as well as females**.
- **Vitamin C**—RDA for vitamin C has been suggested as **80 mg/d for elderly males** and **65 mg/d for elderly females**.
- **Vitamin A**—RDA for vitamin A (RE) has been suggested as **1000 µg/d for elderly males** and **840 µg/d for elderly females**.
- **Vitamin D**—RDA for vitamin D has been suggested as **800 IU/d for** elderly **males as well as females**.

20

- **Minerals:**
  - **Calcium**—RDA for calcium has been suggested as **1200 mg/d for elderly males as well as females**.
  - **Magnesium**—RDA for magnesium has been suggested as **440 mg/d for elderly males** and **370 mg/d for elderly females**.
  - **Iron**—RDA for iron has been suggested as **19 µg/d for elderly males as well as females**.
  - **Zinc**—RDA for zinc has been suggested as **17 mg/d for elderly males** and **13 mg/d for elderly females**.
  - **Iodine**—RDA for iodine has been suggested as **140 µg/d for elderly males as well as females**.
- **Water:** Water is essential for various body functions. In elderly persons, decreased thirst response and reduced concentrating capacity of the kidney may lead to dehydration. Moreover, use of diuretics, alcohol and caffeine increase fluid excretion and further contribute to dehydration. With the increasing dietary fiber intake, it is also essential to consume adequate fluid, ideally water, to avoid dehydration and constipation.

  Accordingly, total water requirement has been suggested as 2800 mL/d for elderly males and 2550 mL/d for elderly females.

DIETARY ADVICE FOR OPTIMAL HEALTH IN DIABETES MELLITUS

Diabetes mellitus is a group of diseases characterized by high blood glucose concentration, resulting from defects in insulin secretion and/or its action. People with diabetes have nearly double the risk of being overweight (obese) and heart disease. They are also at a greater risk of developing mental health disorders such as depression. The dietary advice for diabetic patients, therefore, depends on the:

- Presence or absence of obesity
- Response to a weight-reduction diet
- Stage of progression of β-cell dysfunction.

Thus, the dietary advices for the individuals with diabetes are flexible and patient centered. The **American Diabetes Association** (ADA), **American Association of Clinical Endocrinologists** (AACE) and **Indian Council of Medical Research** (ICMR) have recommended that to promote and support healthful eating patterns, one should consume a variety of nutrient dense foods in appropriate portion sizes in order to improve overall health and:

- Achieve and maintain body weight goals

- Attain individualized glycemic, blood pressure and lipid goals
- Delay or prevent complications of diabetes.

- **Calories:** To lose weight, one need to eat fewer calories and replace less healthy foods with foods low in calories, fat and sugar. Calories obtained from fructose (found in sugary beverages such as soda, energy and sports drinks, coffee and processed foods like doughnuts, muffins, cereal, candy and granola bars, etc.) are more likely to add weight around the abdomen.
- **Carbohydrates:** As carbohydrates have a big impact on blood sugar levels, more so than fats and proteins, so one need to be smart about what types of carbohydrates to eat. Limit refined carbohydrates like white bread, pasta and rice as well as soda, candy, packaged meals and snack foods. One should focus on high fiber complex carbohydrates, also known as slow-release carbohydrates, since they are digested more slowly and prevent body from producing too much insulin.

  The total amount of carbohydrate consumed also has strongest influence on glycemic response. The majority of persons with DM should eat moderate amounts of carbohydrate (~45% of total energy intake).

  People with diabetes and those at risk are advised to avoid sugar-sweetened beverages (including fruit juices) in order to control glycemia and weight, and reduce their risk for cardiovascular disease and fatty liver, and should minimize the consumption of foods with added sugar that have the capacity to displace healthier, more nutrient-dense food choices. They should also limit or avoid intake of high-fructose corn syrup and sucrose, to reduce risk for weight gain and worsening of cardiometabolic risk profile.
- **Dietary fiber:** Patients with DM should consume 20 to 35 g of fiber from raw vegetables and unprocessed grains. High fiber containing carbohydrate sources include legumes, whole grain breads and cereals, whole fruits and vegetables, which should be included as part of the daily carbohydrate intake. These **unrefined carbohydrate sources have low glycemic index and** are important for people prone to diabetes because they help keep blood sugar levels in check. One should consume small amounts of potatoes. Instead, they should try brown rice or less well-known grains like wheat berries, millet, hulled barley or quinoa. Strive to include a variety of fresh fruits and vegetables in meals every day.

GLYCEMIC INDEX AND GLYCEMIC LOAD

Glycemic index (GI) refers to the scale that ranks carbohydrate rich foods by how much they raise blood glucose levels. It has been demonstrated that high fiber, low GI foods can help delay the absorption of glucose into the bloodstream, consequently helping to control blood glucose levels. As a rule, refined grain products and potatoes have a higher GI, legumes and whole grains have a moderate GI, and nonstarchy fruits and vegetables have a low GI. Substituting low-glycemic load foods for high-glycemic load foods may modestly improve glycemic control.

- **Proteins:** Persons with diabetes, but normal renal functions, can have usual protein intake. The proteins consumed, however, should primarily, come from plant sources such as tofu, legumes or meat alternative products. One however, should be aware of possible higher sodium content.
- **Fats:** Limit intake of saturated fats by cutting back on processed and fast foods, red meat, and full-fat dairy foods. Try replacing red meat with beans, nuts, skinless poultry and fish, whenever possible, and switching from whole milk and other full-fat dairy foods to lower fat versions. In place of butter or margarine, use liquid vegetable oils rich in polyunsaturated and monounsaturated fats in cooking and at the table. Eat one or more good sources of omega-3 fats every day, such as fatty fish, walnuts, soybean oil, ground flax seeds or flaxseed oil. Intake of fried foods, and foods high in saturated and trans-fat should be limited.
- **Vitamins and minerals:** They should consume whole grains, and fruits and vegetables to meet the required amounts of vitamins and minerals. Since type 2 diabetes is a state of increased oxidative stress, one should consume **large doses of antioxidant vitamins**. Diabetics should **limit sodium consumption** to 2,300 mg/day. There is some evidence that **higher dietary intake of magnesium** may help prevent type 2 diabetes. Several studies have also demonstrated a potential role for **chromium supplementation** in the management of insulin resistance and type 2 diabetes.

DIETARY ADVICE FOR OPTIMAL HEALTH IN CORONARY HEART DISEASE

Coronary heart disease (CHD) occurs when fatty deposits, known as plaque, build up in the arteries. This causes them to narrow, restricting blood supply to the heart and brain. In some cases, these deposits may eventually block the artery entirely, resulting in a heart attack or stroke.

Risk Factors for CAD

A number of factors are associated with the build up of fatty deposits in the coronary arteries, including **cigarette smoking, lack of physical activity** and **a family history of the disease**. Some of the common risk factors are:

- **Obesity:** Many overweight and obese people have diets high in fat, particularly, saturated fat. A person who carries the bulk of their body fat around their stomach (**apple shaped body**) is at greater risk of heart disease than someone whose body fat tends to settle around their bottom, hips and thighs (pear shaped body).
- **Hypertension:** Blood pressure is the amount of pressure within the arteries (blood vessels that carry blood around the body). High blood pressure, or hypertension, means that the pressure in the arteries is higher than normal. This may be because the arteries are less elastic, there is more blood volume or more blood is being pumped out of the heart.
- **Uncontrolled diabetes and impaired glucose tolerance:** In healthy people, insulin keeps the blood sugar level relatively constant. However, for those vulnerable to type 2 diabetes, the body gradually loses its sensitivity to insulin. This leads to chronically elevated blood sugar levels, also known as impaired glucose tolerance. Uncontrolled diabetes can damage the artery walls and contribute to coronary heart disease.

Dietary Advice for CAD

There is no single food to decrease the risk of developing heart disease but one need to eat a healthy diet and have plenty of exercise. Dietary advice for optimal health in CAD include:

- **Fat:** Limiting saturated and trans fat is an important step to reduce blood cholesterol and lower the risk of coronary artery disease. A high blood cholesterol level can lead to a build up of plaques in arteries, called atherosclerosis, which can increase the risk of heart attack and stroke. Because plaque is mostly made of harmful low density lipoproteins (LDL), the first tenet of a successful diet for coronary artery disease is **avoiding foods that raise LDL cholesterol**, namely those that are **rich in saturated and trans fats**. Common sources of saturated fats include animal products (butter, meat fat, beef, lamb, chicken skin and full cream dairy foods) and processed foods like pastries and biscuits. Trans fats are formed when monounsaturated or polyunsaturated vegetable oils are hydrogenated and hardened to form margarines.

  Choose **unsaturated fats**, such as olive oil or canola oil. They are naturally low in saturated and trans fats, but rich in heart-friendly unsaturated fats. **Polyunsaturated fats** found in certain fish, avocados, nuts and seeds, also are good choices for a heart-healthy diet. **Oily fish**, such as tuna, salmon and herring, contain **omega-3 fatty acids**, which decrease triglycerides, increase HDL-cholesterol, improve blood vessel elasticity and thin the blood, making it less likely to clot and block blood flow.

  Vegetable oils, such as corn oil, soybeans oil and safflower oil are rich in **omega-6 fatty acid**, while canola oil and olive oil are rich in omega-3 fatty acid.
- **Fiber: Wholegrain cereals**, and **fruit and vegetables** are rich in fiber and other nutrients that play a role in regulating blood pressure and heart health. One can increase the amount of whole grains in the diet by making substitutions for the refined grain products. Eating more fruits and vegetables also help cut back on higher calorie foods, such as meat, cheese and snacks.

  Oats are rich in β-glucan, a fiber that blocks the absorption of cholesterol from the digestive tract. **Beans** reduce the amount of cholesterol absorption from food. **Nuts, like** almonds, pistachios, walnuts, etc. are rich in arginine that keeps blood vessels relaxed and help in free blood flow throughout the body.
- **Protein: Choose low-fat protein sources**. As we know, lean meat, poultry and fish, and low-fat dairy products and eggs are some of the best sources of protein. But one should be careful to choose lower fat options, such as skim milk rather than whole milk, and skinless chicken breasts rather than fried chicken patties. Besides, legumes (beans, peas and lentils) are also good sources of protein. They contain less fat and no cholesterol, making them good substitutes for meat. Substituting plant protein for animal protein, e.g. a soy or bean burger for a hamburger will reduce fat and cholesterol intake and increase fiber intake.
- **Vitamins and minerals:** Fruits and vegetables are good sources of vitamins and minerals. For example, **folate** helps lower the blood levels of the amino acid homocysteine that is linked to increased risk of heart disease. **Vitamin E** also acts as an antioxidant and help to protect against bad cholesterol. **Foods containing vitamin E** include avocados, dark green vegetables, vegetable oils and wholegrain products. Fruits and vegetables also contain antioxidants, which further offer protection against a heart disease.

Reduce the sodium in food. Eating a lot of sodium can contribute to high blood pressure, a risk factor for cardiovascular disease. One should not have more than 2,300 mg of sodium a day.

- **Other advices:** In addition to dietary advice, **lifestyle** also plays an important role in managing coronary artery disease, so we should also **maintain a healthy body weight** and **exercise regularly**. Besides, antioxidants in **tea** also help and prevent the build-up of fatty deposits in the arteries. Antioxidants also act as an antiblood clotting agent and improve blood vessel dilation to allow increased blood flow. High intake of **alcohol** increases blood pressure and tends to increase triglycerides in the blood, increasing the risk of heart disease. Allicin, present in fresh **garlic**, has also been shown to lower blood cholesterol. A daily intake of 2–3 g of phytosterols/stanols lowers LDL cholesterol. Phytosterol-enriched foods include margarine spreads, reduced-fat yoghurts, milk and breakfast cereals. **Live tobacco free,** do not smoke or use tobacco or nicotine products, and avoid smoke vapor.

DIETARY ADVICE FOR OPTIMAL HEALTH DURING PREGNANCY AND LACTATION

Pregnancy is the time of **tremendous physiological changes** that **demands healthful dietary** and **lifestyle choices**. This is also a **process of growth and development that affects both, the mother as well as the foetus.**

Guided by the changing levels of hormones, **body of the mother undergoes various changes** during pregnancy. Various maternal tissues, including the **breast, uterus and adipose stores increase in size,** and **blood volume is expanded.** At the same time, **gastrointestinal motility is slow,** as a result of which food moves more slowly through the intestinal tract. Further, **due to vomiting and loss of appetite during the early months of pregnancy food intake is** also, generally, **reduced.**

Thus, **additional food is required for gestational weight gain of** nearly 10–14 kg **and the full-term birth weight** of the **fetus of about 3.3 kg.** Besides some micronutrients (**vitamins and minerals) are also required in extra amounts** during these physiological stages.

Accordingly, the **daily diet of a pregnant woman should contain additional amounts of:**

- **Energy:** Due to change in body weight during pregnancy, the Group has suggested a proportionate increase in energy requirement.

  In case of lactation, an increase in energy requirement has been suggested because of utilization of energy in milk production. Accordingly,
  - **Additional 350 kcal/d** have been suggested **during pregnancy.**
  - **Additional** energy requirement of a women who exclusively breast feed, has been recommended as **600 kcal/d during the first 6 months of lactation** and **520 Kcal/d during 7–12 months of lactation.**
- **Carbohydrates:** Carbohydrate intake has been suggested as **135 g/d during pregnancy** and **155 g/d during lactation.**
- **Fat: Total visible fat intake** has been suggested as **30 g/d during pregnancy** as well as **lactation.**
- **Protein: Additional requirement** of protein has been recommended as **9.5 g/d during the second trimester** and **22 g/d during the third trimester of pregnancy.**

Additional protein **requirement for lactating women** has been recommended as **16.9 g/d during the first 6 months** and **13.2 g/d during 7–12 months of lactation.**

- **Vitamins**
  - **Thiamine:** RDA for thiamine has been suggested as **2.0 mg/d during pregnancy, and 2.1 mg/d during lactation.**
  - **Riboflavin:** RDA for riboflavin has been suggested as **2.7 mg/d during pregnancy.**

    RDA during lactation has been suggested as 3.0 mg/d during the first 6 months and **2.9 mg/d during 7–12 months.**
  - **Niacin—additional 2 mg/d** of niacin has been suggested **during pregnancy.**

    Additional 5 mg/d of niacin has been suggested during lactation.
  - **Pantothenic acid—**RDA for pantothenic acid is suggested as **5.0 mg/d during pregnancy.**

    Additional 2.0 mg/d has been recommended **during lactation.**
  - **Vitamin B_6—**RDA for vitamin B_6 has been suggested as **2.3 mg/d during pregnancy.**

    Additional recommendations of **0.26 mg/d during 0–6 months of lactation** and **0.17 mg/d during 7–12 months of lactation** have been made.

    Biotin RDA for biotin has been suggested as **25 µg/d during pregnancy.**

    Additional 5.0 µg/d has been suggested **during lactation.**
  - **Folate—additional** intake of dietary folate has been suggested as **270 µg/d during pregnancy.** Further, it is recommended that to reduce the risk of congenital malformations and increase in birth

weight of the fetus, folate should be taken throughout the pregnancy

Additional intake of dietary folate has been suggested as **110 µg/d during lactation**.

- **Vitamin B_{12}—additional** intake of vitamin B_{12} has been suggested **0.25 µg/d during pregnancy** and **1.0 µg/d during lactation**.
- **Vitamin C – Additional** intake of vitamin C has been suggested as **15 mg/d during pregnancy** and **50 mg during lactation**.
- **Vitamin A - RDA** of vitamin A has been suggested as **900 µg/d during pregnancy** and **950 µg/d during lactation.**

  It is further suggested that during pregnancy and lactation a **minimum 50% of the vitamin A** (retinol equivalent, RE) requirement **should be met from animal sources**.
- **Vitamin D – RDA** of vitamin D has been suggested as **600 IU/d during pregnancy and lactation**.

• **Minerals:**
  - **Calcium**—It is well known that calcium is essential, both during pregnancy as well as lactation for proper formation of bones and teeth of the offspring, besides its secretion in breast milk as well as to prevent osteoporosis in mothers.

    RDA for calcium has been suggested as **1000 mg/d during pregnancy.**

    An **additional 200 mg/d** has been suggested **during lactation**.
  - **Phosphorus**—recommendations for phosphorus is **similar to that for calcium**.
  - **Magnesium—RDA for magnesium has been suggested as 440 mg/d during pregnancy** and **400 mg/d during lactation**.
  - **Iron**—Extra iron is required by the mother as well as the growing fetus to meet the increased demand for erythropoiesis (formation of RBC).

    Accordingly, RDA for iron has been suggested as **27 mg/d during pregnancy** and **23 mg/d during lactation**.
  - **Zinc—RDA** for zinc has been suggested as **14–15 mg/d during pregnancy as well as lactation**.
  - **Iodine—RDA** for iodine has been suggested as **220 µg/d during pregnancy** and **280 µg/d during lactation**.

• **Water :** Total water requirement has been suggested as 3700 mL/d during pregnancy and 4100 mL/d during lactation.

20

The group has further suggested that, **to meet the above requirements, pregnant and lactating women should eat a wide variety of foods** to make sure that her own nutritional needs as well as those of the growing fetus are met. Though, there is no particular need to modify the usual dietary pattern, the quantity and frequency of usage of different foods should be increased. Furthermore, it is suggested that:

• Maximum amount of **energy can be derived from rice, wheat and millets**.

• A **proper combination of cereals, pulses and nuts can be used to provide adequate protein**.

• **Mineral and vitamin requirements can be met by consuming** a variety of seasonal vegetables, particularly, **green leafy vegetables, milk and fresh fruits**.

• In addition, they are also advised to take daily **supplement of iron, folic acid, vitamin B** and **calcium**.

• These women should also choose **foods rich in dietary fiber**, like whole grain cereals, pulses and vegetables, to avoid constipation.

• Besides, they should take **plenty of fluids**, including 8–12 glasses of water per day.

• **Salt intake should also be restricted** to prevent pregnancy-induced hypertension and pre-eclampsia.

OVERWEIGHT AND OBESITY

Obesity is the commonest form of malnutrition worldwide, characterized by a **body mass index (BMI, i.e. weight in kg/height in m^2) >30 kg/m^2**. A BMI of 20–25 is considered normal whereas 25–30 is considered overweight.

Types of Obesity

• *Based on the time of onset and histological features:* It is of two types, i.e. **hyperplastic or juvenile-onset obesity** characterized by increase in adipocyte number, and **hypertrophic or adult-onset obesity** characterized by increase in adipocyte size mainly. Adipocyte number, once attained and largely fixed at puberty, cannot be reduced by weight-reduction programs, hence currently the attention is heavily directed towards early detection of hyperplastic obesity.

• *Based on the distribution of body fat:* It is again of two types, i.e. central obesity and pear-like obesity. **Central obesity** refers to excess intra-abdominal fat deposition around the organs. It is also called **apple-like obesity** and **android ('man-like') obesity**. It generally affects men and postmenopausal women. The central body fat cells are larger and more insulin-resistant than the lower body fat cells. Hence, it is associated with diabetes mellitus and cardiovascular diseases, besides some cancers. On the other hand, lower body fat around the hips and thighs is called **pear-like obesity** and **gynoid ('woman-like') obesity**. It is common in women in their reproductive years and poses less of health problems.

Causes of Obesity

It is multifactorial, involving a complex interplay between:

Genetic factors: **Leptin**, a protein product of *ob* gene, is secreted from adipose tissue and gastric mucosa (Chemistry to Clinics 20.1).

High blood leptin levels are indicative of adequate stores of triacylglycerol (well-fed state) thereby abolishing the neural signals to eat more, and vice versa. It is thus a **lipostat** that acts through cerebral receptors and other local hormones in the CNS such as neuropeptide Y (NPY), to regulate the **feeding behavior** (Fig. 20.5).

Mutations in *ob* gene result in suboptimal leptin levels with a persistent signal to eat more.

Chemistry to Clinics 20.1: Leptin and Peptic Ulcer Disease

Many cases of peptic ulcer disease have an infectious etiology attributed to the bacteria *Helicobacter pylori* (*H. pylori*). Infection-induced gastritis is associated with high gastric leptin expression resulting in reduced food intake and partly serves to explain the weight loss in these patients. Cure of infection restores the normal body weight.

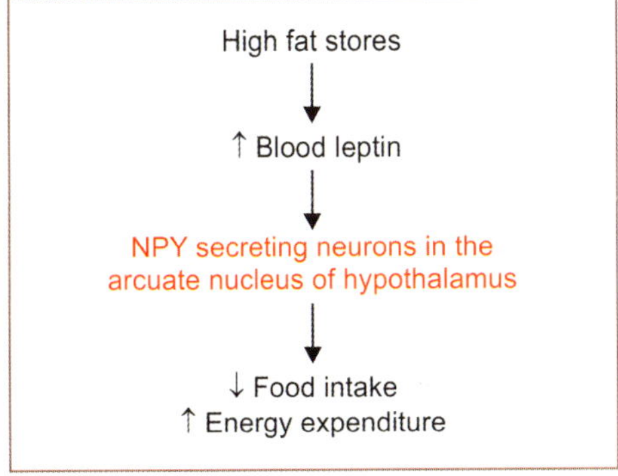

Fig. 20.5: Regulation of feeding behavior by leptin

Environmental Factors

i. ***External environment:*** High calorie intake versus reduced physical exercise.
   - **Social influences:** Social factors have important influence on the development of obesity. Abundance of calories, highly palatable food and social enjoyment of eating, create pressure to overeat and lead to obesity.
   - **Age and lifestyle:** People gain most of the body weight between 25 and 35 years of age. Exercise patterns also influence development of obesity, which is associated with reduced physical activity.
   - **Sex:** Obesity is more prevalent in women than men. Women often develop obesity after pregnancy and menopause.
   - Beside, race, ethnicity, socioeconomic status and psychological factors also contribute to obesity.

ii. ***Internal environment:*** Low content of brown adipose tissue with or without specific endocrine disorders, e.g. diabetes mellitus, Cushing's syndrome, hypothyroidism, etc.

Food Habits and Obesity

Foods that contain energy/calories (from carbohydrate and/or fat) but lack protein, vitamins and minerals are known as '**empty calorie foods**'. A popular synonym is '**junk food**'. Examples are potato chips, candies, colas, alcohol, etc. A preference for such foods during childhood and adolescence along with lack of adequate physical activity is a major factor contributing to premature obesity and other health problems. Therefore, the **ABC of good health** should be remembered and followed—**a**im for fitness, **b**uild a healthy base, **c**hoose sensibly (food guide pyramid, Fig. 20.6).

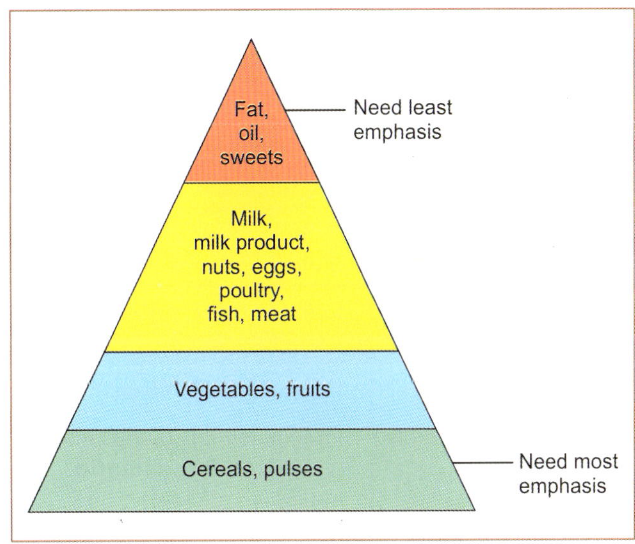

Fig. 20.6: Food guide pyramid

Health Hazards of Obesity

Besides considered to be a social stigma, the adverse clinical outcomes of obesity include:

- Type 2 diabetes mellitus (Chemistry to Clinics 20.2)

Chemistry to Clinics 20.2: Metabolic Syndrome

Obesity is very often associated with an insulin-resistant state owing to downregulation of insulin receptors (decrease in the number of insulin receptors or their affinity for insulin or both) resulting in various metabolic aberrations (Fig. 20.7). Further, obesity and insulin resistance may coexist with dyslipidemia and hypertension. Such combination is called '**metabolic syndrome**' or '**syndrome X**' and is associated with increased risk of cardiovascular disease.

- Hypertension and related cardiovascular disorders
- Osteoarthritis
- Gall stones
- Endometrial carcinoma
- Hypoventilation (Pickwickian syndrome).

NUTRITIONAL IMPORTANCE OF COMMONLY USED FOOD ITEMS

Nutritional importance of commonly used food items is shown in Table 20.9.

Table 20.9: Nutritional importance of commonly used food items

Food items	Nutritional importance
Cereals and millets	Carbohydrates, protein, water-soluble vitamins and minerals
Pulses and legumes	Protein, water-soluble vitamins and minerals
Vegetables	Protein, water-soluble vitamins and minerals
Roots and tubers	Carbohydrates, small amounts of protein and vitamin C
Fruits	Carbohydrates and water-soluble vitamins
Fats and oils	Fat and fat-soluble vitamins
Milk and milk products	Protein, fat, fat-soluble vitamins, water-soluble vitamins and minerals
Meat, fish and eggs	Protein, fat, fat-soluble vitamins, water-soluble vitamins and minerals

Whole Grain Cereals and Millets

- **Cereals**, such as **rice and wheat**, and **millets**, like jowar, bajra, ragi, etc. are the most widely eaten staple foods in India.
  - These are the cheapest **sources of calories** and constitute as much as 70–80% of the calories in the diet of majority of population in our country.
  - Most cereal grains also contain 6–12% **proteins**. In general, cereal proteins are deficient in the essential amino acid lysine. Rice protein, however, is rich in lysine, compared to other cereals.
  - Whole grain cereals are also important sources of **B vitamins**, especially, **thiamine** and **nicotinic acid**, which are present in the outer bran layer of the grain. Excessive milling and polishing of rice removes the outer covering and, hence, decreases its thiamine content.
  - Cereal grains do not contain vitamin A, except yellow maize, which contains some amount of **β-carotene**.
  - Total fat content in cereals varies from 2–5%.
  - On an average, 400 g of cereals are consumed per person, per day, in India.
  - Commonly used legumes include **grams, peas** and **beans**.
  - Dried **pulses and legumes** are rich in **protein** (about 19–24%). They are good sources of **lysine** and **threonine**, which are deficient in most of the cereals. Pulses are, however, poor source of sulfur-containing amino acids.
  - Pulses are also good sources of several B vitamins and minerals, such as **thiamin, riboflavin** and **phosphorus**.
  - Legumes, however, contain some **natural toxins** that can be removed by soaking and normal cooking procedures. The cooking procedures, however, result in loss of some B vitamins.
  - Legumes are **good for young children** provided these are cooked, finely mashed and mixed with other food items.
  - Germination or **sprouting increases vitamin C**, riboflavin and niacin contents of legumes.

Nuts and Oilseeds

- Nuts and oilseeds, such as peanut (groundnut), soybean and oilseeds, are rich sources of **protein**. They contain about 18–40% protein. They are also rich sources of **fat**, several **B vitamins** and **vitamin E**.
  - **Groundnut** contains about 20–30% protein and 40–50% oil. Though limiting in lysine, threonine

and methionine, groundnut is a good source of **thiamin, niacin, pantothenic acid** and **phosphorus**. When harvested under moist conditions, groundnut gets contaminated with *Aspergillus flavus*, which produces **aflatoxin**. Roasting destroys trypsin inhibitors and improves its nutritive value.

- **Soybeans** contain nearly 35–45% protein and 15–20% fat. Soybean proteins are good sources of all **essential amino acids** except methionine. It is also a good source of **thiamin** and **niacin**. Soybean, however, contains hemagglutinins and trypsin, and certain growth inhibitors, which can be inactivated by pressure cooking. Soybean is mainly used in soy-flour, milk substitutes and infant foods.

Vegetables

- Vegetables are broadly classified into 3 groups, as green-leafy vegetables, roots and tubers, and other vegetables.
  - **Green-leafy vegetables:** Many types of green leaves, such as spinach (palak), amaranth, fenugreek leaves (methi), drumstick leaves, mint, coriander, mustard leaves, colocasia leaves, radish and turnip leaves, and bathua, are rich sources of iron, β-carotene, vitamin C, riboflavin, folic acid and calcium. They also provide dietary fiber and antioxidants, and proteins (about 2–7%). Green-leafy vegetables, however, contain oxalic acid, which, in turn, interferes with the absorption of calcium.
  - **Roots and tubers:** Roots and tubers, such as potatoes, sweet potatoes, carrots, etc. are good sources of starch. They also contain small amount of protein, some B vitamins and vitamin C. Yellow sweet potatoes and carrots are also rich sources of carotene.
  - **Other vegetables:** These include green peas and beans, pumpkin, gourds, ladies finger, brinjal, etc. Green peas and beans are good sources of protein and some B vitamins. They are also fair sources of vitamin C and certain minerals.
- **Fruits:** Fruits are good sources of different carbohydrates, vitamins and minerals.
  - Fresh fruits are, generally, good sources of vitamins. **Amla** (gooseberry), is, especially, rich in **vitamin C**.
  - **Yellow fruits**, like mango and papaya, contain β-carotene.
  - **Dried fruits**, like dates and raisins, are rich sources of **iron**.
  - Banana is rich in carbohydrates. Some fruits contain glucose, while others contain fructose or pentose.
  - Most of the fruits are also good sources of potassium.
  - Fruits also contain pectins, which provide bulk to the diet and helps in bowel movement.
  - Drying of fruits results in loss of carotene. Other procedures cause loss of thiamin. Canning of fruit juice results in loss of vitamin C.

  Since, fruit and vegetables provide vitamins, minerals and fiber, they should be included in meals and snacks each day. Choose a variety of fruits and vegetables (including different colors, textures and flavors) to provide a wide range of vitamins and minerals.

Milk and Milk Products

Milk is either used as such or in the preparation of several products, such as curd, cheese, ice cream, butter, ghee and a variety of sweets. Milk is an ideal food for infants and children. It is also a good supplementary food for adults. Milk contains good quality proteins (3.2–4.3%). It is also rich in calcium and several other nutrients in proper proportions, and thus milk is considered to be a complete food. Milk is, however, deficient in vitamin C and iron. Composition of milk varies widely, from its source. For example, human milk contains more lactose, while buffalo milk contains more fat.

Milk, yoghurt and cheese are the most common dairy foods, and main dietary sources of calcium. Having enough calcium is important for healthy bones and teeth. Full-cream plain milk is recommended for children aged 1 to 2 years, while reduced-fat plain milk is suitable for adults.

Pasteurization results in loss of vitamin C, while prolonged boiling results in loss of thiamin, vitamin B_6 and vitamin B_{12}.

Eggs and Poultry

- **Eggs** contain about 13% proteins and 13% fat. Egg proteins are good sources of all essential amino acids and have high nutritive value. Egg is also a rich source of vitamin A and some B vitamins. Egg, however, does not contain vitamin C and is a poor source of calcium. Egg consists of egg white and egg yolk.
  - **Egg white** contains about 11% protein, mainly **albumin**. Besides, egg white is also a good source

20

of **riboflavin** but devoid of fat and vitamin A. Raw egg white also contains a heat labile factor, called **avidin**, which binds with biotin and makes it unavailable.
- **Egg yolk** contains about 15% proteins and 30% fat. It is a rich source of riboflavin, vitamin A, iron and phosphorus. Egg yolk is also rich in cholesterol. It is used as a supplement to the diet of infants.
- **Poultry meat** is a good source of proteins, containing all essential amino acids.

Meat and Fish

- This group includes red meat (such as beef and lamb), white meat (such as pork and chicken) and fish. They are rich in protein, iron and zinc.
  - Protein content of **flesh foods** is around 20%. Meat is also a good source of several B vitamins, particularly, vitamin B_{12}, iron and phosphorus. Flesh foods, generally, are not good sources of vitamin A with the exception of liver, which is very rich in vitamin A.
  - **Fish** contains polyunsaturated fatty acids, which protect against cardiovascular diseases. Fish is also rich in protein, but a fair source of B vitamins. Fatty fish also contains vitamins A and D. Small fishes are good source of calcium, since these are eaten with bones. Large fishes are rich in phosphorus.

  Canning of meat and poultry results in loss of various B vitamins, particularly thiamin.

Fat and Oils

- Fats and oils are the main sources of energy as well as essential fatty acids and fat-soluble vitamins.
  - **Fats of animal origin** contain cholesterol, but poor source of vitamin E and essential fatty acids.
  - On the other hand, **fats of vegetable origin**, such as sunflower oil, soybeans oil, cottonseed oil, etc., are good sources of essential fatty acids and vitamin E.
  - Frying destroys vitamin A, vitamin E and essential fatty acids.
  - Rancidity results in the formation of peroxides, which, in turn, affect intestinal flora and have irritating effects on the intestine.

Condiments and Spices

- Condiments and spices are used as seasoning or flavoring agents in food to increase its acceptability. Since condiments and spices are used in small quantities, they do not add, substantially, to the nutritive value of the food, but improve taste and flavor of the cooked food. They also act on the mucous membranes of mouth, stomach and intestine, and stimulate secretion of digestive juices.
  - Some of the condiments, like chilies and coriander, are good sources of carotene.
  - Green chilies supply vitamin C.
  - Turmeric and tamarind are fair sources of antioxidants and iron.
  - Some of the spices, such as garlic, also have their effect on intestinal flora and prevent flatulence.
  - Others, such as chilies, black pepper, etc. are very pungent. Their excessive use can cause irritation of the mucous membrane, resulting in peptic and duodenal ulcers.

Beverages

- Various beverages have different effects.
  - **Coffee and tea** contain caffeine, which stimulates gastric secretion and may aid in the digestion. Excess of caffeine produces insomnia, causes irritability and rapid heart action, and increases excitability of the nervous system. Tea, however, is also a rich source of oxalic acid. Hence, excessive consumption of tea may lead to the development of renal calculi.
  - **Fruit juices** contain sugar, vitamin C, small amounts of other vitamins and some of the minerals.
  - Beverages, such as **sugarcane juice**, contain nearly 9% sugar, while sweetened carbonated beverages contain about 10–15% sugar.
  - **Alcoholic beverages** contain varying amounts of alcohol (from 4 to 40%). Alcohol in moderate doses stimulates gastric secretion and serves as a source of energy. Excessive consumption of alcohol causes severe depression and incoordination of movements, and loss of consciousness, due to its depressant action on the nervous system.

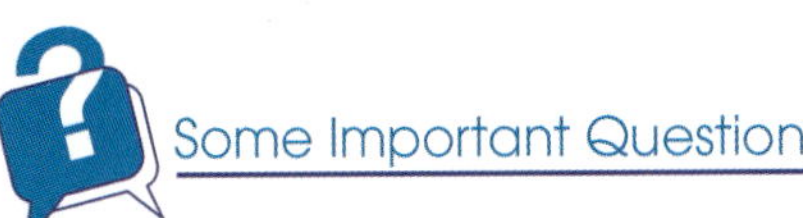

Some Important Questions

1. Discuss:

i. Importance of dietary fiber
ii. Importance of carbohydrates in human nutrition
iii. Supplementary action of proteins
iv. Protein energy malnutrition

2. Write notes on:

i. Biological value of proteins
ii. Balanced diet
iii. Essential fatty acids
iv. Essential amino acids
v. Nitrogen balance

Multiple Choice Questions

1. Juvenile-onset obesity is mainly:

A. Hypoplastic
B. Hyperplastic
C. Atrophic
D. Hypertrophic

2. Metabolic syndrome includes:

A. Obesity and dyslipidemia
B. Insulin resistance
C. Hypertension
D. All of the above

3. Edema, enlarged fatty liver and hair 'flag sign' are characteristic of:

A. Marasmus
B. Obesity
C. Nephrotic syndrome
D. Kwashiorkor

4. The following is required more during pregnancy than during lactation:

A. Iron
B. Calcium
C. Vitamin D
D. Vitamin A

5. Children with marasmus have:

A. Pot belly
B. Edema
C. Moon-like face
D. Severe weight loss

CHAPTER

21

Extracellular Matrix

Competency Achievement: **The student should be able to:**

BI9.1 List the functions and components of the extracellular matrix (ECM)

BI9.2 Discuss the involvement of ECM components in health and disease

BI9.3 Describe protein targeting and sorting along with its associated disorders

Extracellular matrix (ECM) is a three-dimensional network of extracellular macromolecules, such as collagen and glycoproteins, that provide structural and biochemical support to the surrounding cells. ECM **determines the structure and function of tissue through a complex network of macromolecules.**

The extracellular matrix can be divided into two groups, each with a specific structure. The first are called **interstitial matrices** and surround cells while the second are termed **pericellular matrices** and are cell-associated.

Interstitial matrix is present between various animal cells, i.e. in the intercellular spaces. Gels of polysaccharides and fibrous proteins fill the interstitial space and act as a compression buffer against the stress placed on the ECM.

Basement membranes are sheet-like depositions of ECM on which various epithelial cells rest. The basement membrane is an important example of a pericellular matrix found between the functional and connective tissue. The structure provides an anchoring layer that keeps functional tissue cells together. The cells embedded within the extracellular matrix interact through surface receptors and integrate signals from the matrix that are associated with their function.

FUNCTIONS OF THE EXTRACELLULAR MATRIX

Due to its diverse nature and composition, ECM serves many functions, such as **providing support, segregating tissues from one another** and **regulating intercellular communication**. In addition, ECM sequesters a wide range of cellular growth factors and acts as a local store for them. The stiffness and elasticity of the ECM have important implications in cell migration, gene expression and differentiation. Cells actively sense ECM rigidity and migrate, preferentially, towards stiffer surfaces, in a phenomenon called durotaxis. They also detect elasticity and adjust their gene expression, accordingly. This has its impact on differentiation and cancer progression.

CELL ADHESION

Cell adhesion can occur in two ways, i.e. by **focal adhesions** (connecting the ECM to actin filaments of the cell) and **hemidesmosomes** (connecting the ECM to intermediate filaments such as keratin).

Focal adhesions occur at the attachment site of the cell cytoskeleton and the fibronectin glycoprotein. This type of attachment anchors the cell and facilitates signaling across the plasma membrane.

Hemidesmosomes connect intermediate filaments to the basal laminae of epithelial cells, thereby supplying a rigid structure to epithelial tissue.

Cell Adhesion Proteins

Cell-to-ECM adhesion is regulated by specific **cell-surface cellular adhesion molecules** (CAM), known as **integrins.** Integrins are cell-surface proteins that bind cells to ECM structures (such as **fibronectin** and **laminin)** and also to **integrin proteins** on the surface of the other cells. Integrins have weak ligand interactions, suggesting that multiple adhesions to ECM-protein binding sites are required. This weak interaction is particularly advantageous for migrating cells.

Fibronectin: Fibronectins are glycoproteins that connect cells with collagen fibres in the ECM, allowing cells to move through the ECM. They are secreted by the cells in unfolded, inactive forms. Fibronectins bind to ECM macromolecules and facilitate their binding to transmembrane integrins. Binding to integrins unfolds fibronectin molecules, allowing them to form dimers, so that they can function properly. The attachment of fibronectin to the extracellular domain initiates intracellular signaling pathways as well as its association with the cellular cytoskeleton, via a set of adaptor molecules such as **actin**. Fibronectins also help at the site of tissue injury by binding to platelets during blood clotting and facilitating cell movement to the affected area, during wound healing.

Laminin: Laminins are proteins found in the basal laminae of, virtually, all animals. Rather than forming collagen-like fibers, laminins form networks of web-like structures that resist tensile forces in the basal lamina. Laminins also assist in cell adhesion and bind other ECM components, such as collagens and nidogens.

TISSUE REPAIR AND GROWTH

The mechanism for repairing damaged tissue is also dependent on the ECM. The regulation of cell types, within the ECM, allows for mobilization in areas requiring rebuilt tissue. The ECM proteins, fibrin, fibronectin and collagen, provide structural integrity during the repair, with the fibrin-fibronectin interaction acting as a foundation for cell adhesion and migration. The freshly deposited ECM can be remodeled to form normal tissue through the cross-linking of collagen fibrils.

The interaction between the cell and the ECM also affects the level of acute inflammation, re-epithelialization and contraction, when tissue is damaged. These factors promote rapid wound closure meaning that these biological responses, for minimizing the risk of infection, are dependent on the ECM.

The ability to control cell–ECM interaction, locally, is also an attractive therapeutic target. The proteins (matricellular proteins) found within the ECM provide signals that trigger specific cell activities within the wound. These proteins are expressed in high frequencies during development but are absent in normal adult tissues.

ECM proteins are also commonly used in **cell culture systems** to maintain stem and precursor cells in an undifferentiated state during cell culture and function to induce differentiation of epithelial, endothelial and smooth muscle cells *in vitro*. They can also be used to support 3D cell culture for modeling tumor development. It is suggested that ECM promotes constructive remodeling of tissue and that matrix-bound nanovesicles (MBVs) are a key player in the healing process.

Matrix-bound nanovesicles: Matrix-bound nanovesicles (MBVs) are an integral and functional key component of ECM bioscaffolds. MBVs shape and size are consistent with exosomes. MBVs cargo includes different protein molecules, lipids, DNA, fragments and miRNAs. Similar to ECM bioscaffolds, MBVs can modify the activation state of macrophages and alter different cellular properties such as proliferation, migration and cell cycle.

COMPONENTS OF THE EXTRACELLULAR MATRIX

Components of the extracellular matrix (ECM) are produced, intracellularly by resident cells and secreted into the ECM via exocytosis. Once secreted, they aggregate with the existing matrix. Major components of the extracellular matrix include collagens, elastin, proteoglycans and a variety of other proteins.

COLLAGENS

Collagen (COL) is the most abundant protein in the human body and accounts for 90% of bone matrix protein content. Collagens are present in the ECM as fibrillar proteins and give structural support to resident cells. Collagen is exocytosed in precursor form (**procollagen**), which is then cleaved by procollagen proteases to allow extracellular assembly.

A collagen molecule has a long rigid structure in which three polypeptides, called α-chains, are wound around one another in a **rope-like triple helix**. It is a superfamily of proteins, which includes, at least, **27 distinct types**. Although there are many differences among the members of the collagen family, all share at least two important structural features:

1. All collagen molecules are trimers, consisting of three polypeptide chains called α-chains.
2. All three polypeptide chains are wound around each other to form a unique, rod-like triple helix, e.g. collagen type I is αI2α2 (i.e. it has two αI and one α2-chains), type II collagen is αI3 (containing 3 αI-chains), etc.

Types of Collagens

Based on their locations and functions in the body, collagens are organized into three groups:

1. **Fibril-forming collagens:** Fibril-forming collagens (fibrillar) are linear polymers with characteristic bonding patterns. They have rope-like triple-stranded helix, e.g. type I, type II and type III. **Type I collagen fibers** are found in supporting elements of high tensile strength, such as in the skin, bone, tendon, blood vessels and cornea. **Type II fibers** are found in cartilaginous structures, such as cartilage, intervertebral disc and vitreous body. **Type III collagens** occur in more distensible tissues, such as blood vessels and fetal skin.
2. **Network-forming collagens:** Network-forming collagens form a three-dimensional mesh, e.g. type IV and type VII collagens. **Type IV collagens** are thin, sheet or mesh-like structures that function as semipermeable basement membrane, such as found in the kidneys and the lungs. **Type VII collagens** are found beneath stratified squamous epithelia.
3. **Fibril-associated collagens:** Fibril-associated collagens link collagen fibrils to one another as well as to other components in the ECM, e.g. type IX and type XII collagens. **Type IX collagens** are found in cartilage, whereas **type XII collagens** occur in tendons and ligaments.

Structure and Composition of Collagens

A collagen molecule is a fibrous protein, which has an elongated triple-helical structure (Fig. 21.1).

Collagens are rich in proline and glycine, both of which are important in the formation of the triple-stranded helix. **Proline** facilitates formation of the helical conformation of each α-chain because of its ring structure that causes kinks in the peptide chain. **Glycine** is found in every third position of the polypeptide chain, forming a part of the repeating sequence **Gly-X-Y**. It is due to the reason that glycine is the smallest amino acid and fits into the restricted space where three chains of the helix come together. X is frequently proline while Y may be proline or lysine, which gets hydroxylated, and occur as hydroxyproline and hydroxylysine.

Biosynthesis of Collagens

1. Polypeptide precursors of the collagens are formed in fibroblasts (or osteoblasts of bone and chondroblasts of cartilage) and secreted into the ECM. The newly synthesized polypeptide precursors of α-chains (preprocollagens) contain a special amino acid sequence at the N-terminal end. This signal sequence facilitates the binding of ribosomes to the rough endoplasmic reticulum (RER) and directs the passage of the polypeptide chain into the cisternae of the RER. The signal sequence is rapidly cleaved in the endoplasmic reticulum to yield a precursor called pro-α-chain.
2. The pro-α-chain is processed by a number of enzymes within the lumen of the RER while the polypeptides are still being synthesized. Proline and lysine residues, found in the Y-position, are hydroxylated by prolylhydroxylase and lysylhydroxylase, respectively. This is a **post-translational modification** and the hydroxylation reactions require molecular oxygen and **vitamin C**. **Hydroxyproline is important in stabilizing the triple-helical structure** of collagens, because it maximizes interchain hydrogen bond formation.
3. Some hydroxylysine residues are enzymatically glycosylated.
4. After hydroxylation and glycosylation, pro-α-chains form procollagen, which are translocated to the Golgi

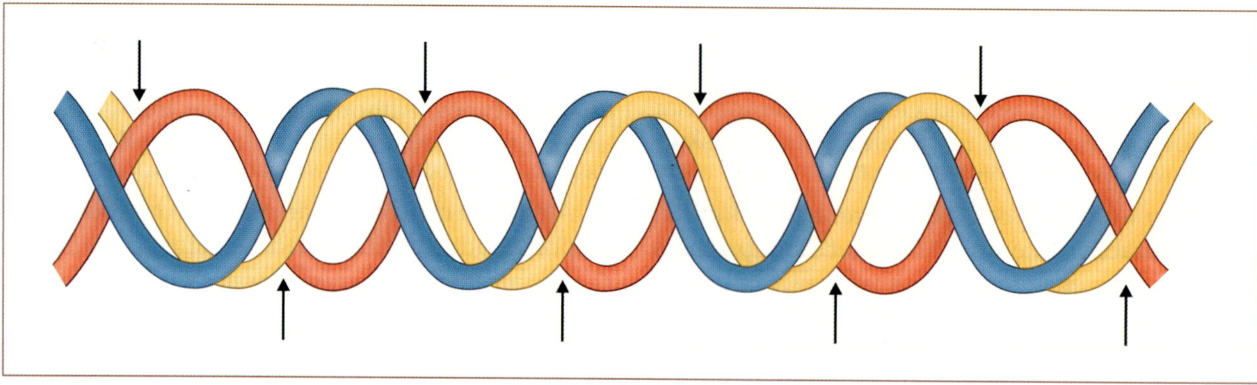

Fig. 21.1: Triple-helical structure of collagen, arrows indicate the sites where the three chains are very close to each other. Glycine is invariably present at these sites

apparatus, where they are packed in the secretory vesicles. These vesicles fuse with the cell membrane, causing the release of procollagen into the extra-cellular space.

5. After their release, the procollagen molecules are cleaved by the N- and C-procollagen peptidases, which remove the terminal propeptides, releasing triple-helical molecules.
6. Individual collagen molecules spontaneously associate to form fibrils.
7. Lysyloxidase, oxidatively deaminates some of the lysyl- and hydroxylysyl residues resulting in the formation of allysine and hydroxyallysine. These reactive aldehydes condense with lysyl- and hydroxylysyl residues, in the neighboring collagen molecules, to form covalent cross-links of mature collagen, called tropocollagen (Fig. 21.2).

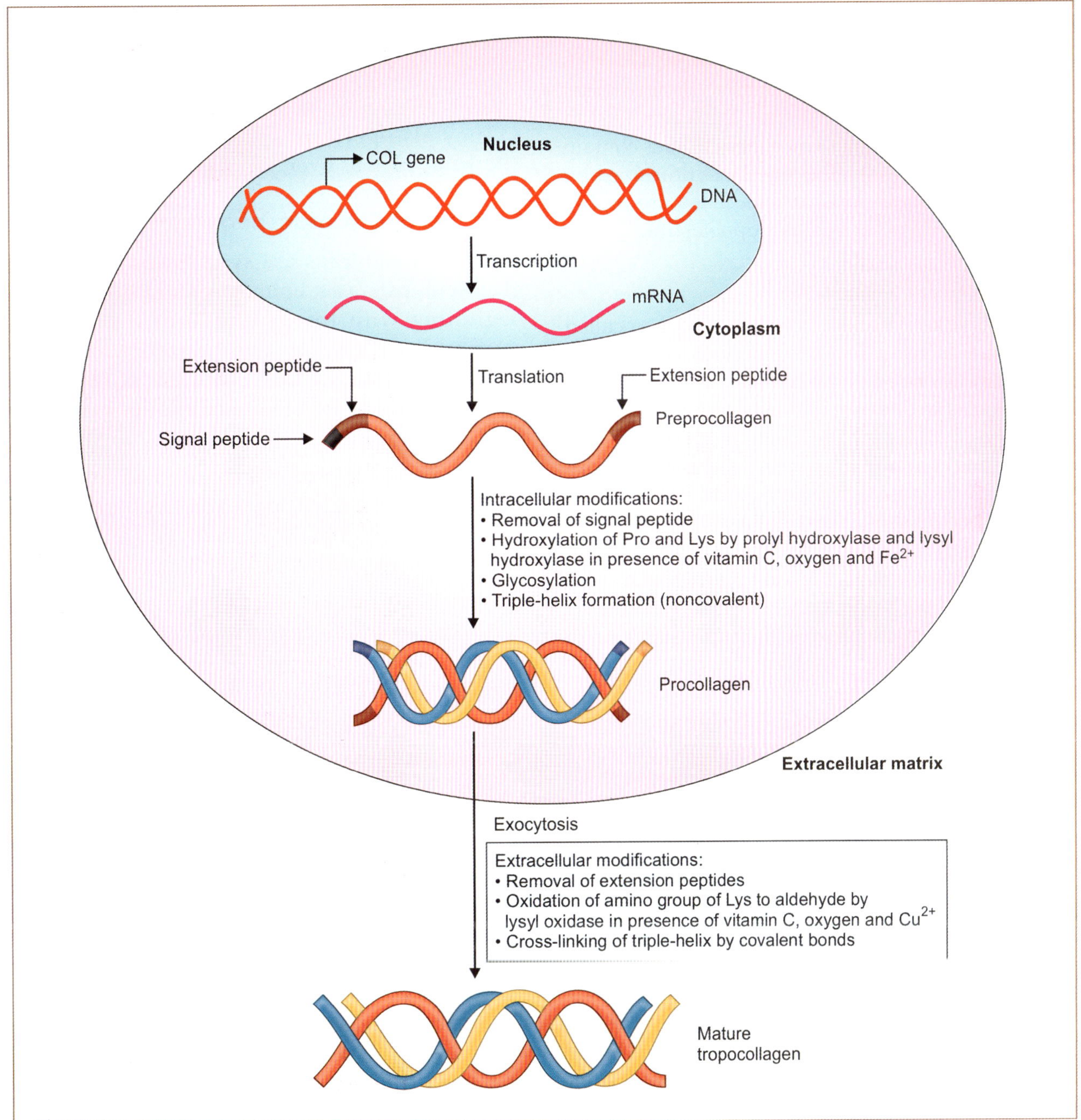

Fig. 21.2: Biosynthesis of collagen by a fibroblast, showing the extensive post-translational modifications

21

Degradation of Collagen

Normal collagens are highly stable molecules. However, connective tissue is constantly being remodeled, often in response to growth or injury of the tissue. Collagen fibrils are broken down with the help of specific matrix metalloproteinases, called **collagenases**. These enzymes cleave the molecules into the smaller fragments, which are further degraded to the constituent amino acids by other matrix proteinases.

ELASTIN

Elastins give elasticity to tissues, allowing them to stretch, when needed and then return to their original state. This is useful in blood vessels, the lungs, in skin and the ligamentum nuchae, since these tissues contain high amounts of elastins. Elastins are synthesized by fibroblasts and smooth muscle cells. They are highly insoluble and are synthesized as tropoelastins.

Structure and Synthesis of Elastin

Elastin is a polymer synthesized from a precursor called **tropoelastin**, which is a linear polypeptide synthesized on the RER and secreted by the cell into the extracellular space. Tropoelastin does not undergo post-translational modifications, but during the assembly process, some of the lysyl-side chains of the tropoelastin polypeptides are oxidatively deaminated by lysyl oxidase, generating **allysine** in specific sequences. The reactive aldehyde of allysine condenses with other allysine, or with unmodified lysine, from the same or on different tropoelastin polypeptide chains, to form **desmosine** cross-linked heterocyclic structures. As a result, elastin can stretch in any direction giving elasticity to the connective tissues.

Elastin is rich in **glycine, proline, lysine** and **valine**. One in every seven of its amino acids is valine. Its primary structure consists of alternating hydrophilic and hydrophobic lysine and valine-rich domains. Lysines are involved in intermolecular cross-linking, while the weak interactions between valine residues in the hydrophobic domains impart elasticity to the molecule.

GLYCOSAMINOGLYCANS

21

Glycosaminoglycans (**GAGs**; originally designated as **mucopolysaccharides**) are large complexes of negatively charged heteropolysaccharides associated with a small amount of protein, forming **proteoglycans**, which are the gel forming components of the extracellular matrices. The GAGs are unbranched polysaccharides and consist of alternating **uronic acid** and **hexosamine** residues. Solutions of GAGs have slimy, mucus like consistency, due to their high viscosity and elasticity.

Classification and structures of various glycosaminoglycans are described in Chapter 3.

Functions of Glycosaminoglacans

1. GAGs provide structural support to tissues, especially, cartilage and connective tissue.
2. They also enable the tissues to withstand torsion and shock.
3. GAGs also provide a balance between integrity and flexibility.
4. They also perform specific functions in certain organs, such as liver, kidney, cornea, etc.

Synthesis of Glycosaminoglycans

Glycosaminoglycans are synthesized by a series of glycosyltransferases, epimerases and sulftransferases, beginning with the synthesis of the core oligosaccharides. These are synthesized while the core protein is still in the RER. Synthesis of the repeating oligosaccharides and other modifications take place in the Golgi apparatus.

- Polysaccharide chains are elongated by sequential addition of alternating acidic and amino sugars, donated by their UDP-derivatives (UDP-glucuronic acid is produced by the oxidation of UDP-glucose).
- After D-glucuronic acid has been incorporated into the carbohydrate chain, some of the D-glucuronic acid units are converted to L-iduronic acid. Epimerization of the D-sugar alcohol to the L-sugar alcohol is caused by the enzyme uronosyl-5-epimerase.
- Sulfation of the carbohydrate chain occurs after the monosaccharide (to be sulfated) has been incorporated into the growing oligosaccharide chain. 3′-Phosphoadenosyl-5′-phosphosulfate (**PAPS** or **active sulfate**) is the source of the sulfate moiety, which is transferred at specific sites to cause sulfation of the carbohydrate by the sulftransferases.

Degradation of Glycosaminoglycans

Glycosaminoglycans are degraded by the sequential action of several lysosomal acid hydrolases, including exoglycosidases and sulfatases, beginning from the external end of the glycan chain. This may involve removal of the sulfate by a sulfatase, then removal of the terminal sugar by a specific glycosidase, and so on.

The ECM is directly connected to the cells, it surrounds. Some of the key connectors are the proteins called **integrins**, which are embedded in the plasma membrane. Other proteins in the ECM, like the **fibronectin** molecules, act as bridges between the integrins and other ECM proteins, such as collagen. On the inner side of the membrane, integrins are linked to the cytoskeleton.

INVOLVEMENT OF ECM COMPONENTS IN HEALTH AND DISEASE

Extracellular components are involved in several diseases.

SCURVY

As we know that scurvy results from the deficiency of vitamin C. It is characterized by inflammed gums and tooth loss, poor wound healing, brittle bones and weakening of the lining of blood vessels, causing internal bleeding.

As a result of vitamin C deficiency, collagen fibers cannot be cross-linked, greatly, decreasing the tensile strength of the assembled fiber.

INHERITED DISORDERS OF COLLAGEN SYNTHESIS

Osteogenesis Imperfecta (Brittle Bone Syndrome)

Mutations in the gene for either the pro-I- or pro-2-α chains of type I collagen can result in structurally abnormal pro-α-chains that can prevent folding of the protein into a triple-helical conformation. Extremely fragile bones that easily bend and fracture, thin skin and ***weak tendons characterize it. Type I osteogenesis imperfecta, called osteogenesis*** imperfecta tarda, presents in early infancy with fractures secondary to minor trauma. ***Type II*** osteogenesis imperfecta, called ***osteogenesis imperfecta congenita,*** is more severe and patients die *in utero* or in the neonatal period due to pulmonary hypoplasia.

Ehlers-Danlos Syndrome

It is characterized by a deficiency of any collagen processing enzyme, e.g. lysyl hydroxylase or pro-collagen peptidase. The defect involves the fibrillar collagen types I and III. The patients have hypermobile joints and hyperextensible skin (Fig. 21.3).

Alport's Syndrome

A renal disease in which the glomerular basement membrane is disrupted due to mutation in type IV collagen gene.

DISORDERS OF ELASTIN METABOLISM

Marfan Syndrome

It is due to mutations in the fibrillin gene. Patients have a typically tall stature, long arms and legs, and long spidery fingers (arachnodactyly, Fig. 21.4).

The disease in a mild form causes loose joints, deformed spine, floppy mitral valves and lens dislocation. In severely affected individuals, the aortic wall is prone to rupture.

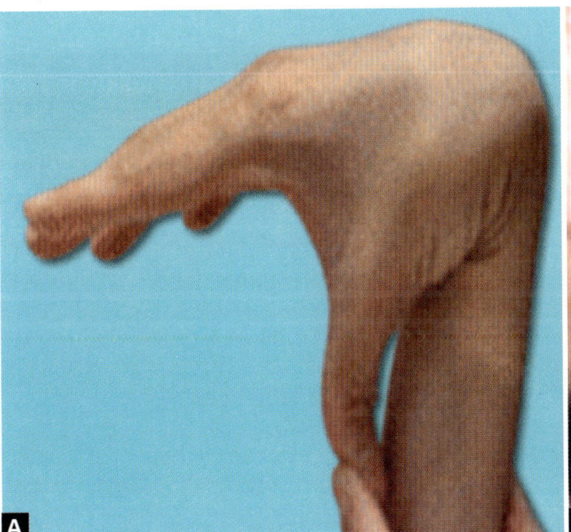

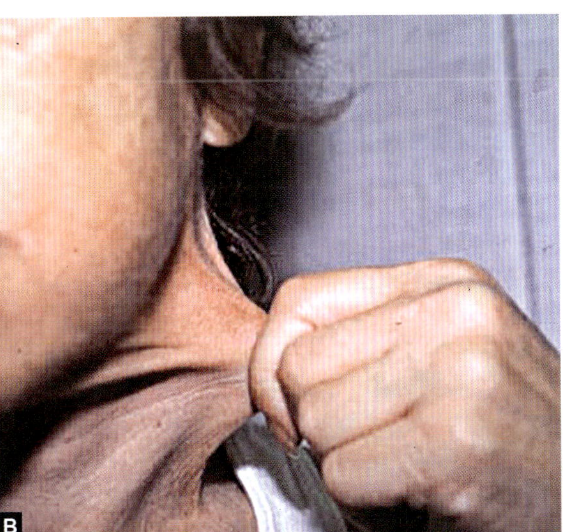

Fig. 21.3: Ehlers-Danlos syndrome. (A) Hypermobile joints; (B) Hyperextensible skin

21

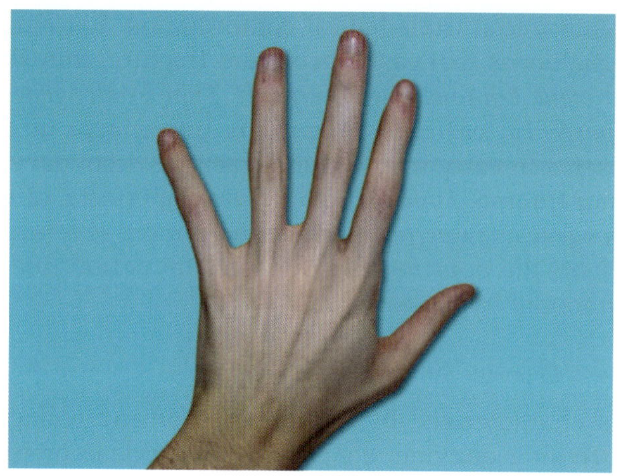

Fig. 21.4: Marfan syndrome: Arachnodactyly (long, slender, **spider-like** fingers)

Emphysema

Elastin is degraded by the enzyme elastase. Elastase is a powerful protease that is released from neutrophils (especially, during inflammation) into the extracellular space and can degrade elastin of alveolar walls and other structural proteins in a variety of tissues. However, α_1-antitrypsin (α_1-AT), produced primarily, by liver and other cells, such as monocytes and alveolar macrophages, inhibits a number of proteolytic enzymes, including elastase. This, in turn, prevents elastin degradation in the alveolar walls and maintains elastase/antielastase balance.

A **deficiency of α_1-AT causes emphysema**, results from the destruction of the connective tissue of alveolar walls, due to **elastase/antielastase imbalance**. World-wide, it is an important form of chronic obstructive pulmonary disease (COPD). The deficiency may be genetic (mutation in α_1-AT gene) or acquired as a result of damage to α_1-AT by reactive oxygen species present in tobacco smoke.

DEFECTS OF GLYCOSAMINOGLYCAN DEGRADATION

If one of the enzymes involved in the stepwise degradation pathway is missing, the entire degradation process is halted at that point. As a result of it, the undegraded GAG molecule accumulates in the lysosomes, causing **lysosomal storage diseases (lysosomal storage disorders)**. The defects of glycosaminoglycans degradation are also referred to as **mucopolysaccharidoses** (Table 21.1).

Lysosomal Storage Disorders

Lysosomes are responsible for the intracellular digestion of the extracellular and the intracellular substances. They contain a number of hydrolyzing enzymes (hydrolases) for the hydrolysis of proteins, lipids, carbohydrates and nucleic acids. These hydrolases are most active at acidic pH and split complex molecules into simple low molecular weight compounds that can be reutilized.

In a number of genetic disorders, classified as lysosomal storage diseases, individual lysosomal enzymes are missing, leading to accumulation of the substrate of the missing enzyme. The lysosomes become enlarged with undigested material, thereby

Table 21.1: The mucopolysaccharidoses

Syndrome	Deficient enzyme	Product (accumulate in lysosomes and excrete in urine)
Hunter syndrome	Iduronate sulfatase	Heparan sulfate and dermatan sulfate
Hurler syndrome	α-L-Iduronidase	–do–
Morquio syndromes		
A	Galactose-6-sulfatase	Keratan sulfate
B	β-Galactosidase	–do–
Sanfilippo syndrome		
A	Heparan sulfamidase	Heparan sulfate
B	N-Acetylglycosaminidase	–do–
C	Acetyl-CoA: Glucosaminide-N-acetyl-transferase	–do–
D	N-Acetylglucosamine-6-sulfate-sulfatase	–do–
Sly syndrome	β-Glucuronidase	Dermatan sulfate and heparan sulfate

interfering with the normal cell processes. Several lysosomal storage diseases are known to exist, e.g. sphingolipidoses, mucopolysaccharidoses, etc.

- All the deficiencies are autosomal and recessively inherited except Hunter syndrome, which is X-linked.
- They are characterized by the accumulation of GAGs in various tissues, causing varied symptoms such as skeletal and extracellular matrix deformities and mental retardation. Children who are homozygous for one of these diseases are apparently normal at birth and then gradually deteriorate. In most severe cases, death occurs in childhood.
- These diseases can be diagnosed by the identification of the specific glycosaminoglycan chains in the urine, followed by the assay of the specific hydrolases in leukocytes or fibroblasts.

DEFECTS OF SPHINGOLIPID DEGRADATION

This is a group of lipid storage diseases caused by the deficiency of the specific lysosomal hydrolytic enzyme that causes defects in the degradation of sphingolipids, also referred to as **sphingolipidoses**.

Due to a genetic error when activity of any of the hydrolytic enzymes is markedly reduced, substrate for the defective enzyme accumulates and gets deposited within the lysosomes of the tissue responsible for the catabolism of that sphingolipid. Usually, only a single sphingolipid, which is the substrate for the deficient enzyme, accumulates in the involved organs in each disease, such as Niemann-Pick disease, Gaucher's disease and Tay-Sachs disease. These are the autosomal recessive diseases that can be diagnosed by measuring enzyme activity in cultured fibroblasts or peripheral leukocytes.

Niemann-Pick Disease

It results from a deficiency of the enzyme sphingomyelinase which leads to accumulation of sphingomyelin in lysosomes. It is characterized by hepatosplenomegaly.

Gaucher's Disease

It is a lysosomal storage disease where the enzyme glucocerebrosidase is missing. It is characterized by hepatomegaly, long bone osteoporosis and neuro degeneration.

Tay-Sachs Disease

It is due to lack of the enzyme hexosaminidase. It is the most common form of GM_2 gangliosidosis. Ganglion cells of the cerebral cortex are swollen due to the deposition of GM_2 gangliosides. The disease is characterized by neurodegeneration, blindness, cherry-red macula, muscular weakness and seizures.

Matrix Biomarkers

Various matrix components are not only emerging as biomarkers for chronic inflammatory, metabolic and cardiovascular diseases, but also act as a prognostic marker.

Osteonectin acts as a very promising prognostic marker in HER-2 negative breast cancer. Increased level of **osteopontin**, in plasma, helps in detecting pancreatic duct adenocarcinoma. Increased level of **tenacin-C** is associated with poor recovery in patients of heart failure. **Thrombospondin-1** is associated with solid tumors of bladder and breast.

PROTEIN TARGETING AND PROTEIN SORTING

PROTEIN TARGETING

A typical mammalian cell contains numerous kinds of proteins. Besides, several proteins are also present in the endoplasmic reticulum (ER), mitochondria, Golgi apparatus, peroxisomes, nucleus, cytosol and the membranes of all the cellular organelles. As mentioned in Chapter 1, **free ribosomes synthesize proteins that remain within the cell** and perform their functions either within the cytoplasm or in the organelles, such as nucleus or mitochondria. On the other hand, **ribosomes that are bound to the endoplasmic reticulum** (rough endoplasmic reticulum)**, usually, synthesize proteins** which are either **incorporated into the cell membrane** or **destined to leave the cell,** except a few of them that are synthesized within the mitochondria. Accordingly, proteins are selectively transported into the appropriate organelles inside the cell as well as across the plasma membrane for secretion outside the cell. Some of them are carried into the membrane-bound vesicles, which bud-off from an organelle and are transported in definite pathways. Different destinations of different **proteins require sophisticated system for labeling and sorting of the newly synthesized proteins**, ensuring that they reach proper places. Transportation of proteins to their final destinations is called **protein targeting**.

Protein targeting is carried out, based on the information contained within the protein itself. This information is present in the form of amino acids sequence, in the polypeptide chain, called **signal peptides** (**targeting peptides** or **signal sequences**). The targeting signal is the information, which enables the cellular transport machinery to correctly position a protein, inside or outside the cell. There are two types of targeting peptides, called **presequences** and the **internal targeting peptides**. The presequences of the targeting peptides are, often, found as the N-terminal extensions. In addition, protein modifications, like glycosylations, can induce targeting.

Peptide targeting signals interact with the specific receptors, which are present either on the target organelle or the carrier protein. In the absence of the targeting signal, the newly synthesized protein remains within the cytoplasm. If the synthesized protein belongs to some other organelle, it is transported there in either of two ways, i.e. as **cotranslational translocation** (translocation during the process of translation) or **post-translational translocation** (translocation after the process of translation is complete).

Cotranslational Translocation

Most proteins that are secretory, membrane-bound or reside in the ER, Golgi apparatus or endosomes, use the cotranslational translocation pathway. This process begins with the N-terminal signal peptide of the protein being recognized by a **signal recognition particle** (SRP), while the protein is still being synthesized on the ribosomes.

- **In secretory proteins and type I transmembrane proteins**, the signal sequence is immediately cleaved from the nascent polypeptide, once it has been translocated into the membrane of the ER, by the signal peptidase.
- The signal sequences of **type II membrane proteins** are not cleaved off. These sequences are referred to as **signal anchor sequences**.

  Within the ER, the designated protein is first **covered by a chaperone protein** to protect it from the high concentrations of other proteins in the ER, giving it time to fold correctly. Once folded, the protein is modified, as may be needed (e.g. by glycosylation), transported to the Golgi for further processing and goes to the target organelles, or is retained in the ER.

Post-translational Translocation

Some of the secretory proteins are translated in the cytosol. They are later transported to the ER by a post-translational system. For example, proteins targeted to
21 the mitochondria or the peroxisomes. Proteins targeted to the nucleus are also translocated by this process. These proteins pass through the nuclear envelope via nuclear pores.

PROTEIN SORTING

The process by which proteins are identified as belonging to a particular compartment and then correctly delivered to that destination is known as **protein sorting**. As a protein is synthesized, it passes step by step, through a shipping decision tree. At each stage, the protein is checked for molecular tags, to see if it needs to be rerouted to a different pathway or destination.

The first major branch point comes shortly after translation starts. At this point, the protein will either remain in the cytosol for the rest of translation or fed into the endoplasmic reticulum (ER). For example, proteins destined for any part of the endomembrane system, or outside of the cell, are brought to the ER during translation and fed in, as they are made, if they have an address label.

Address Labels

Address labels, also referred to as **sorting signals**, **signal sequences** or **leader sequences,** indicates the destination or cellular compartment the proteins are destined for. Most of the sorting signals are the **short stretches of amino acid sequences**, which comprises 13–35 amino acids that form a part of the amino acid sequence of the protein. The sorting sequence is the first to be synthesized during translation, and is mostly, present at the amino-terminal (N-terminal) of the protein chain. They are, literally, the address labels that indicate where the protein should be sent. Different cellular compartments have different address labels.

The address label on the ribosome is recognized by a protein complex called **signal-recognition particle (SRP)**, which takes the ribosome to the ER. The SRP binds to the signal sequence of the nascent protein as soon as it emerges out of the ribosome and directs it towards the ER membrane. The binding of the SRP with the signal sequence stops further synthesis of the SRP protein chain, when it is about 70 amino acids long to prevent it from folding. As the growing polypeptide chain emerges into the ER lumen, the signal sequence is cleaved by a peptide called **signal peptidase**. Once inside the lumen of the ER, the **destined protein undergoes folding** and several other modifications (such as glycation, etc.), for which the ER lumen contains a number of enzymes and chaperone proteins. **Glycosylation** refers to the addition of the carbohydrate(s) to the protein chain. After glycosylation, many proteins are further folded and stabilized by the formation of disulfide bonds (–S–S–), catalyzed by protein disulphide isomerase (PDI).

Mechanisms of Protein Targeting and Sorting

The mechanisms by which proteins cross membranes to get into different organelles vary. Some proteins are further sorted to a subcompartment within the target organelle. For this purpose, a **second signal sequence** is present, **behind the first signal sequence**, which is later cleaved. These proteins that carry proteins inside the membrane bound vesicles are called **cargo proteins**.

- **Proteins going into the ER** enters the lumen through **protein translocators** in the ER membrane. In this case, the protein enters in an **unfolded form**, since the dimensions of the translocator does not allow a folded protein to pass through.
- **Proteins going into the nucleus** are transported through pores in the nuclear membranes with the help of **nuclear transporter proteins in their folded state**.
- A third mechanism encloses **proteins inside a membrane vesicle**, which travels to the target organelle, and **fuses with the membrane of the target**. The vesicle buds-off from the ER and fuses with the *cis*-compartment (cisternae), or the receiving compartment of Golgi. In this process, cargo proteins are delivered into the lumen of Golgi and the membrane proteins become part of the membrane of the target vesicles. The proteins are later glycosylated, folded, modified and sorted in the ER, and the process continues in the successive Golgi cisternae. Starting from the *cis*-compartment to medial compartment and lastly, to *trans*-Golgi network (TGN), proteins are exported to the end target. In the TGN, proteins are further sorted, to be delivered to the lysosomes, for secretion outside the cell and to plasma membrane, according to the signals present in the nascent proteins.

Targeting of Proteins to Lysosomes

The lysosomal enzymes and lysosomal membrane proteins are synthesized in the rough ER (RER) and transported to the Golgi cisternae and, ultimately, to the lysosomes. The sorting signal that directs the lysosomal enzymes from the TGN to the lysosomes, is mannose-6-phosphate (M6P), since wall of the TGN contains M6P receptors. The M6P receptors bind only to the lysosomal proteins. Attachment of M6P to the lysosomal proteins (enzymes) prevents their further modifications. Separation of M6P-bearing lysosomal enzymes from other proteins takes place in the TGN. The vesicles containing the receptor-bearing proteins bud-off from the TGN. Low pH of the lysosomes triggers dissociation of the proteins (enzymes) from the receptors, which are recycled back to the TNG.

Lysosomes contain hydrolyzing proteolytic enzyme, which digests proteins meant for degradation. A protein, called ubiquitin, present in all the eukaryotic cells, marks the proteins which are meant for destruction.

The proteins meant for secretion travel from the TNG to the plasma membrane. Transportation of vesicles from the RER to the *cis*-face of Golgi, to successive levels of Golgi, and onto their final destinations, requires high level of specificity in targeting. Transport of the vesicles, to the wrong destination may lead to cellular chaos.

Targeting of Proteins to Mitochondria

Although, **mitochondria** possess their own DNA, ribosomes and mRNA, and **synthesize a few proteins, most of the proteins required in mitochondria are synthesized in the cytosol**, by the nuclear DNA, and then transported into the mitochondria. These proteins have more than one successive N-terminal targeting signal sequence. The first signal sequence imports the protein into matrix and the second signal redirects the protein into the membranes, or the intermembrane space.

Targeting and translocation of the mitochondrial proteins involve a series of **receptors**, **import pores** and **molecular machinery** located in four intra-mitochondrial locations, i.e. **the outer and inner mitochondrial membranes, the intermembrane space** (IMS) and **the matrix**.

Most of the mitochondrial proteins are synthesized as cytosolic precursors, containing uptake peptide signals called **preproteins**. Cytosolic **chaperones**, such as heat shock proteins (e.g. Hsp70), deliver the preproteins to the channel-linked receptors in the mitochondrial membrane, where they bind to the **receptors** and the **general import pores** (GIP). The receptors and the GIP are collectively referred to as **translocase of the outer membrane** (TOM). The preprotein is translocated through TOM as hairpin loops. From there, they are sorted to their final destination by the combined action of the translocation machinery and the targeting information encoded within the protein. Within the matrix, the targeting sequence is cleaved off by mtHsp70.

Targeting of Proteins into the Nucleus

The proteins that are to be imported into the nucleus are in fully folded state and do not require any chaprones. They have targeting signal sequences on them, called **nuclear localization signals** (**NLS**). Each NLS is a stretch of positively charged 4–8 amino acids like lysine and arginine. NLS is an internal (not terminal) sequence that is not cleaved from the protein. This serves as the label that marks the protein for delivery to the nucleus. The nuclear proteins must cross the nuclear envelope to get inside the nucleus.

- The **nuclear envelope** is made up of two membranes (each with a regular phospholipid bilayer structure) called outer and inner membranes, which are separated by the intermembranous space that is connected to the lumen of the endoplasmic reticulum.
- The **inner membrane** of the nuclear envelope has an underlying meshwork of protein filaments called the **nuclear lamina** which provide structural support to the nuclear envelope.
- The **outer membrane** is continuous with the ER and has ribosomes on it. Proteins for the nucleus are synthesized on free ribosomes in the cytosol and imported into the nucleus through nuclear pores, which are the special gates.
- The **nuclear pore** is a channel through which large molecules, like RNA and protein, get across the nuclear envelope. Each nuclear pore is made up of a large number of proteins, and controls the traffic of molecules into and out of the nucleus. There are thousands of such pores through the nuclear envelope.

There are two steps in the process by which proteins with a nuclear localization signal get into the nucleus:

1. The nuclear localization signal is recognized by another protein called **nuclear transport receptor** or **importin**. The importin binds to the nuclear localization signal and brings the protein (to be transported) to the nuclear pore. The **receptor–cargo complex** (consisting of the transport receptor and its cargo) then moves through the nuclear pore into the nucleus.
2. In the nucleus, a **transport protein** called **Ran** (bound to **GTP**) binds to the receptor–cargo complex. This makes the transporter release the cargo protein into the nucleus. The transporter (Ran-GTP) returns to the cytosol, where Ran is released and the GTP is hydrolyzed.

Targeting of Proteins into the Membranes

The proteins embedded in different membranes may have single transmembrane domain, which is a segment of 20–25 amino acids. Other proteins may have many transmembrane domains connected by loops on both sides of the membrane. These proteins are called multipass orientation proteins.

DISORDERS ASSOCIATED WITH PROTEIN TARGETING AND SORTING

As discussed above, although most of the proteins are synthesized by the same set of cytosolic ribosomes, each protein has a specific subcellular location in which it resides and functions properly. In addition to specific targeting and compartmentalization within the cell, proteins also undergo post-translational modifications, such as processing, folding and oligomerization. Errors in any of the steps that proteins must go through, before they become fully active in their proper location, can result in a disease.

PYRUVATE DEHYDROGENASE DEFICIENCY

Pyruvate dehydrogenase complex (PDH) is an enzyme which catalyzes oxidative decarboxylation of pyruvate to acetyl-CoA. Its deficiency is one of the most common causes of primary lactic acidosis in infants and children. PDH deficiency can be due to a **variation in the mitochondrial targeting signals, a defect in the X-linked PDH-E1α subunit**. This, in turn, leads to structural abnormalities of the central nervous system, including microcephaly and cerebral atrophy.

PRIMARY HYPEROXALURIA TYPE 1

Primary hyperoxaluria type I (PH1) is due to the deficiency of the enzyme alanine/glyoxylate aminotransferase 1 (AGT). AGT catalyzes the conversion of glyoxylate to glycine in the peroxisomes of hepatocytes. AGT deficiency can be caused by its **mistargeting to mitochondria rather than peroxisomes**, an autosomal recessive disease caused by **mutations in the *AGXT*-gene coding for the liver-specific peroxisomal enzyme**. The mistargeting of AGT disrupts peroxisomal function, leading to glyoxylate being oxidized to oxalate and the deposition of calcium oxalate in the kidney and urinary tract. This, in turn, may lead to kidney failure, and the deposition of calcium oxalate in almost every organ and tissue in the body.

SEVERE ALCOHOLIC LIVER DISEASE

Superoxide anions, generated as a result of oxidative phosphorylation, are converted to hydrogen peroxide by manganese superoxide dismutase (MnSOD) and then reduced to water by glutathione peroxidase (GPX). Alcohol consumption is known to increase reactive oxygen species in the mitochondria, which are detoxified by MnSOD and GPX.

MnSOD is synthesized in the cytosol by the nuclear DNA and then targeted into the mitochondrial matrix cleavable amino-terminal targeting signal. The **increased import of Ala-allele at the MnSOD-locus** (Ala-MnSOD), leads to an **imbalance between MnSOD and GPX** and results in a **build up of hydrogen peroxide**. An **increase in oxidative stress** has been shown to damage mitochondria, promote both apoptotic and necrotic cell death, and contribute to alcohol-induced liver diseases. This, in turn, suggests that even if proteins are correctly targeted to the mitochondria, it is important that they must also be properly imported and sorted to one of the four intra-mitochondrial locations.

HUMAN DEAFNESS DYSTONIA SYNDROME

Human deafness dystonia syndrome (**DDS**, also known as **Mohr-Tranebjaerg syndrome**) is characterized by postlingual progressive sensorineural deafness, dystonia, spasticity, dysphagia, mental deterioration, paranoia and cortical blindness.

It is an X-linked neurodegenerative disorder, due to **defects in the mitochondrial import and processing machinery**. DDS is caused by **mutations in the intermembrane space (IMS) protein deafness dystonia peptide 1 (DDP1/Tim8)**, which is homologous to the fungal protein Tim8. The complete absence of the DDP1/Tim8 protein has been described in a DDS patient with a missense mutation (G→C transversion in nucleotide position 38) of the first exon.

ZELLWEGER SYNDROME

Zellweger syndrome is due to the **accumulation of very long chain fatty acids** (VLCFA) and **branched-chain fatty acids** (BCFA) **in different tissues and cells**. Accumulation of these fatty acids impairs the normal functions of the multiple organ systems. In addition, these individuals also show deficient levels of plasmalogens (ether phospholipids) that are, especially, important for brain and lung function.

Zellweger syndrome is a result of impaired peroxisome functions. It is an **autosomal recessive disorder caused by mutations in the genes that encode peroxins**, the **proteins required for the normal assembly of peroxisomes**. In almost all cases, patients have mutations that inactivate or greatly reduce the **activity of both the maternal and paternal copies of the *PEX* genes**.

ADRENOLEUKODYSTROPHY

Adrenoleukodystrophy (ALD) is a **disorder of peroxisomal fatty acid beta oxidation**. This, in turn, results in the **accumulation of unbranched, saturated, very long chain fatty acids**, particularly, cerotic acid (26:0), in tissues throughout the body. The most severely affected tissues are the myelin in the central nervous system, the adrenal cortex and the Leydig cells in the testes. Accumulation of these fatty acids causes damage to the myelin sheath of the nerves, resulting in seizures and hyperactivity, besides problems with speaking, listening and understanding verbal instructions. ALD is caused by **mutations in ABCD1 gene** (located on the X chromosome) **that codes for ALD**, a **peroxisomal membrane transporter protein**, which is responsible for transporting very long chain fatty acid substrate into the peroxisomes for degradation.

REFSUM DISEASE

Refsum disease (RD) is a neurocutaneous syndrome that is characterized by the **accumulation of phytanic acid** in plasma and tissues. Patients with Refsum disease are unable to degrade phytanic acid because of a **deficient activity of phytanoyl-CoA hydroxylase** (PhyH), a **peroxisomal enzyme** catalyzing the first step of phytanic acid α-oxidation. The accumulation of phytanic acid is toxic to cells.

Refsum disease can be classified as a peroxisome biogenesis disorder, which is inherited as an **autosomal recessive trait due to mutations in either the PHYH or *PEX7* gene**. It is characterized by altered peroxisome assembly, resulting in multiple peroxisome enzyme deficiencies, complex developmental sequelae and progressive disabilities. The disease, usually, begins in adulthood with increasing night blindness due to degeneration of the retina (retinitis pigmentosa). If the disease progresses, other symptoms may include deafness, loss of the sense of smell (anosmia), problems with balance and coordination (ataxia), dry and scaly skin (ichthyosis), and heartbeat abnormalities (cardiac arrhythmias). Some individuals also have shortened bones in their fingers or toes, or a visibly shortened fourth toe.

PARKINSON DISEASE

Parkinson disease (PD) is a devastating incurable disease in which degeneration of dopamine neurons in the brainstem leads to **tremors** and **problems with movement and coordination**. An increasing proportion of the patients have been shown to be genetically predisposed, where the disease has been shown to be associated with the **accumulation of the presynaptic protein α-synuclein, a block in ER-Golgi transport**. It has been suggested that the **VPS35 mutation** is the genetic determinant of the late-onset PD and that perturbation of retromer-mediated protein sorting is linked with neurodegeneration.

Recent studies have further suggested that **retromer sorting defects are also associated with Alzheimer disease.**

NEPHROGENIC DIABETES INSIPIDUS

Nephrogenic diabetes insipidus (NDI) is a water balance disease characterized by the **incapacity to concentrate urine**, resulting in severe polyuria and polydipsia. This may lead to dehydration, electrolyte imbalance (hypernatremia), and growth and mental retardation. Persistent polyuria can also result in urologic complications, from slight dilation of the urinary tract to severe hydronephrosis. The X-linked form of congenital NDI is caused by **loss-of-function mutations in the *AVPR2* gene**, which is essential for the control of water balance, mediated by the **peptide hormone arginine-vasopressin** (AVP), resulting in insensitivity of principal cells of the collecting duct to AVP. These mutations cause **misfolding of the protein, its retention in the ER and degradation**.

Future Prospectives

The fact that the mislocalized proteins result in loss of its respective function laid a ground for the researchers to find ways to cause therapeutic manipulation of localization of various proteins and, thereby, inhibit their functions. Therapeutic mislocalization of oncoproteins as a treatment strategy for carcinomas is under research.

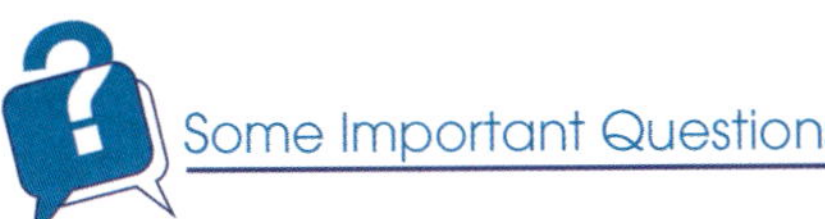

Some Important Questions

1. **What are collagens? How they are synthesized? Describe some abnormalities of biosynthesis of collagens.**
2. **What are glycosaminoglycans? Describe functions of glycosaminoglycans.**
3. **Write notes on:**
   i. Extracellular matrix
   ii. Collagens
   iii. Osteogenesis imperfecta
   iv. Ehlers-Danlos syndrome
   v. Elastin
   vi. Marfan syndrome
   vii. Glycosaminoglycans
   viii. Lysosomal storage disorders
   ix. Tay-Sachs disease
   x. Emphysema

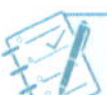

Multiple Choice Questions

1. **The following is not true for collagens:**
   A. Fibrous proteins
   B. Extracellular
   C. Glycoproteins
   D. Lack quaternary structure
2. **The commonest amino acid in collagens is:**
   A. Glycine B. Proline
   C. Hydroxyproline D. Lysine
3. **The formation of interchain H-bonds in collagens depends on the presence of:**
   A. Glycine
   B. Proline
   C. Hydroxyproline
   D. Lysine
4. **The formation of interchain covalent bonds in collagens depends on the presence of:**
   A. Glycine
   B. Proline
   C. Hydroxyproline
   D. Hydroxylysine
5. **Lysyl hydroxylase requires:**
   A. Oxygen B. Ferrous ions
   C. Ascorbic acid D. All of the above
6. **The following is true for extension peptides in procollagen:**
   A. Completely retained in mature collagens
   B. Removed intracellularly
   C. Removed extracellularly
   D. Partly retained in mature collagens
7. **Osteogenesis imperfecta involves collagen type:**
   A. I B. II
   C. III D. IV
8. **Desmosine cross-links are found in:**
   A. Collagens B. Elastin
   C. Fibrillin D. Fibronectin
9. **The following is true for Marfan syndrome:**
   A. Floppy mitral valves
   B. Arachnodactyly
   C. Fibrillin gene mutation
   D. All of the above
10. **The enzyme deficient in Hunter syndrome is:**
    A. Iduronate sulfatase
    B. α-L-Iduronidase
    C. Galactose-6-sulfatase
    D. β-Galactosidase

CHAPTER 22

Oncogenesis

Competency Achievement: **The student should be able to:**

BI10.1 Describe the cancer initiation, promotion oncogenes and oncogene activation. Also focus on p53 and apoptosis

BI10.2 Describe various biochemical tumor markers and the biochemical basis of cancer therapy

Cancer is a genetic disease and, mainly, arises due to a number of reasons including **activation of oncogenes**, **malfunction of tumor suppressor genes**, or **mutagenesis due to** external factors, such as **chemicals** and **radiation**, etc. It is a most serious disease affecting human beings of all ages, universally, and is the **second most common cause of death** (first being the cardiac diseases).

NEOPLASM

In common medical usage, a neoplasm (**new growth**) is defined as a tumor (an abnormal tissue growth), which may be benign or malignant.

Benign Tumor

A tumor is said to be benign when its microscopic and gross characteristics are relatively **constant**. Further, it remains **localized** within a limited area and, normally, does not spread to other sites. Benign tumors are, generally, designated by the suffix **'-oma'**, to the cell type from which a tumor arises, e.g. a benign tumor of the **fibrous tissue** is referred to as a **fibroma**.

Malignant Tumor

Malignant tumor means a lesion that can **invade**, **destroy adjacent structures**, **spread to different sites** and **cause death**. Malignant tumors are collectively referred to as **cancers**, a descriptive term to cover the conditions in which cells proliferate, for whatever the reason, in a more or less **uncontrolled manner**, meaning that cancer cells have **lost usual growth control**. These cells invade adjacent tissues and set up **satellite growth** in other organs. The process, if left undisturbed, may lead to **death** of the host.

Malignant neoplasms of epithelial origin are referred to as **carcinomas**, while those arising in **mesenchymal tissues** are termed **sarcomas**. Sarcomas (solid tumors) could be transferred from one animal to another using Rous sarcoma virus. Tumors could be caused either by the addition or by expression of genetic material to normal cells.

Comparison of a Benign and a Malignant Tumor

A tumor cell is distinguished from a normal cell by its **immortality**, **morphological transformation** and ability to undergo **metastasis**. Comparison of a benign tumor and a malignant tumor is given in Table 22.1.

Table 22.1: Comparison of a benign and a malignant tumor

Benign tumor	Malignant tumor
Usually small in size	Comparatively large in size
Well demarcated	Poorly demarcated
Slow growing	Erratic, slow/rapidly growing with numerous and abnormal mitotic figures
Noninvasive	Locally invasive
No metastasis	Frequent metastasis
Well differentiated	Poorly differentiated
Easily managed by chemotherapy/surgery, mortality low or nil	Treatment is difficult in many cases. May require a combination of chemotherapy/surgery/radiotherapy; mortality moderate to high

METASTASIS

Some tumors adopt the ability to **escape the site of their origin** and **intrude other parts of the body**, where it **grows as a secondary tumor** by progressive infiltration, invasion, destruction and penetration, is referred to as metastasis. It, thus, marks the development of secondary implants (called **secondaries**), discontinuous with the primary tumor, in remote tissues. It is a complex phenomenon, due to a failure in cell–cell interaction and is a major problem presented by the disease.

EPIDEMIOLOGY OF CANCER

Epidemiological studies have correlated several environmental, racial and cultural influences to the occurrence of specific neoplasms. For example:

1. **Smoking:** Though all smokers may not get cancer, a close link between smoking and **lung cancer** has been well established. Moreover, the risk increases with the increasing number of cigarettes/bidis smoked per day as well as the duration of smoking.
2. **Diet:** A **high-fat low-fiber diet** has been shown to be a causative factor in **colon cancer**.
3. **Age:** The frequency of occurrence of many types of cancer increases with age due to accumulation of somatic mutations, a decline in immune competence and age-related hormonal changes (e.g. **prostate cancer**).
4. **Inherited susceptibility:** It plays a role in the genesis of several types of cancer, such as **retinoblastoma**.
5. **Preneoplastic disorders:** These are conditions which predispose to the development of malignant neoplasia, e.g. **leukoplakia of the oral cavity** has been shown to increase the risk of **squamous cell carcinoma**.

CARCINOGENESIS

Carcinogenesis, also called **oncogenesis** or **tumorigenesis,** is the formation of a cancer, whereby normal cells are transformed into cancer cells. The process is characterized by changes at the cellular, genetic and epigenetic levels and abnormal cell division.

An agent that causes cancer is termed as **carcinogen,** which may act **directly or indirectly** to change the genotype of the cell. Carcinogenesis is a multistep process, where three types of changes occur:

1. ***Immortalization*:** It is the property of indefinite growth without other changes in the phenotype.
2. ***Transformation*:** It means failure to observe normal constraints of growth, e.g. transformed cells become independent of growth factors, which are, usually, needed for cell growth.
3. ***Metastasis*:** It is the stage at which cancer cells gain the ability to invade normal tissues, so that they can move away from the tissue of origin and establish a new colony/colonies elsewhere in the body.

INITIATION AND PROMOTION OF CANCER

Sometimes, carcinogens are divided into those that initiate and those that promote tumor formation, implying the existence of difference stages in cancer development.

INITIATION OF CANCER

It involves mutation, a small but significant change in DNA of the cell. Initiation is an **irreversible** process. Such cells may remain dormant for years within the body without undergoing proliferation. This period is a gap between the exposure to a carcinogen (**initiator**) and the appearance of a full-blown tumor and is referred to as the **latent period**, which may vary from 5 to 6 years for the induction of leukemia by radiation to as long as 35–40 years for the asbestos-induced lung cancer. Reasons for this long lag period are not known.

PROMOTION OF CANCER

Carcinogenicity of an initiator may be **augmented** by the subsequent administration of some other agent(s) called **promoter**, e.g. croton oil (which contains phorbol ester, a promoter of carcinogenesis), if applied after benzopyrene (mutagen) application, results in tumor.

A promoter has a **little or no carcinogenic activity** of its own. To be effective, application of a mutagen (an initiator) must follow repeated exposures of the promoter. For example:

- If skin of a mice is painted with an **initiator**, such as benzo(a)pyrene, and **no subsequent treatment** is given, **tumor does not develop**.
- But, if this application of the **initiator** is followed by **several applications of the promoter (like croton oil)**, a **tumor** subsequently **develops**.
- Application of the **promoter alone** also **does not cause tumor formation:**

  An application of initiator (I) → No tumor

  An application of promoter (P) → No tumor

  An application of I followed by several applications of P → Tumor

An application of P followed by several applications of I → No tumor.

It is due to the reason that **application of the initiator**, as mentioned above, causes mutational activation of some cells and converts them to **potential tumor cells. Subsequent applications of the promoter** lead to **clonal expansion** of the initiated (mutated) cells to **produce a tumor** (Fig. 22.1).

The mutated cells, subsequently, acquire many characteristics, which make them **autonomous** (free from regulatory controls). For example, these cells acquire the ability to invade and destroy surrounding tissues, and to spread to other parts of the body. Their requirement for growth factors is reduced and that they become less responsive to growth inhibitory signals. They expand their energy solely for the uncontrolled growth and, eventually, develop into a malignant tumor.

As mentioned above, cancer arises due to a number of reasons, including **mutagenesis due to** factors such as **chemicals** and **radiation**, besides genetic factors which include **activation of oncogenes** or **malfunction of the tumor suppressor genes**, etc.

CHEMICAL CARCINOGENS

Nearly 80% of human cancers are caused by environmental factors, mainly chemicals. Exposure to such chemicals can be due to a person's occupation, diet, lifestyle or use of therapeutic drugs. While some of the carcinogens are direct reacting substances, majority of them are indirect reacting substances (Table 22.2).

- **Direct reacting substances:** These are referred to as direct carcinogens, since they do not undergo any metabolic transformation to become a carcinogen. As these substances enter the body in the mutagenic form, they are also referred to as **mutagens**, e.g. cyclophosphamide, nitrosourea, etc. The carcinogenic potential of a mutagen can be tested by the Ames test.

Table 22.2: Some chemical carcinogens

Directly reacting substances
• Cyclophosphamide, nitrosourea
• Alkylating agents
• Acylating agents
Indirectly reacting procarcinogens
• Polycyclic/heterocyclic aromatic hydrocarbons
– Benzo(a)pyrene
• Aromatic amines, amides, azo dyes
– 2-Naphthylamine
– 2-Acetylaminofluorene
– Dimethylaminoazobenzene
• Plant and microbial products
– Aflatoxin B_1
– Griseofulvin
– Betel nuts
• Others
– Nitrosoamines and amides
– Vinyl chloride, nickel, chromium
– Insecticides, fungicides
– Polychlorinated biphenyls
– Arsenic
– Asbestos

Ames Test

Ames test is the test to know mutagenicity of a compound. For this purpose, a specially constituted strain of *Salmonella typhimurium* (**His$^-$**), which has a mutation in the gene, encoding one of the enzymes for histidine biosynthesis, is used. Since His$^-$ bacteria cannot synthesize histidine, the amino acid (histidine) has to be added in the medium, for optimum growth of the bacteria. Reversion of the mutation (back conversion), caused by the carcinogen, at the same site of the genome (i.e. at the His$^-$ site), restores its reading sequence and, thus, **reverts the bacteria to His$^+$**. The progeny of bacteria containing such a **reverse mutation** can now synthesize histidine and grow in the medium lacking histidine. This **conversion** (from His$^-$ to His$^+$) **proves mutagenicity** of the tested chemical.

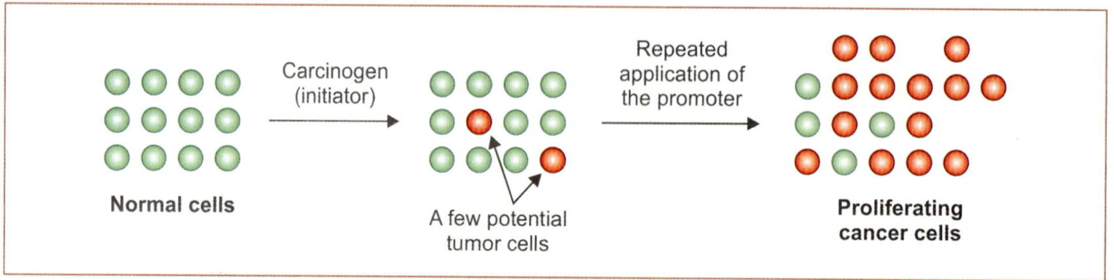

Fig. 22.1: Role of initiator and promoter in tumor development

- **Indirect reacting substances:** Indirect reacting substances are also called **indirect carcinogens** or **procarcinogens**. These are not mutagenic in the form in which they enter the body, but are converted in the liver to a more reactive form by a family of enzymes referred to as **mixed function oxidases**, through an intermediate called **proximate carcinogen**. The final product of the conversion of procarcinogen, via proximate carcinogen, is called **ultimate carcinogen** (Fig. 22.2).

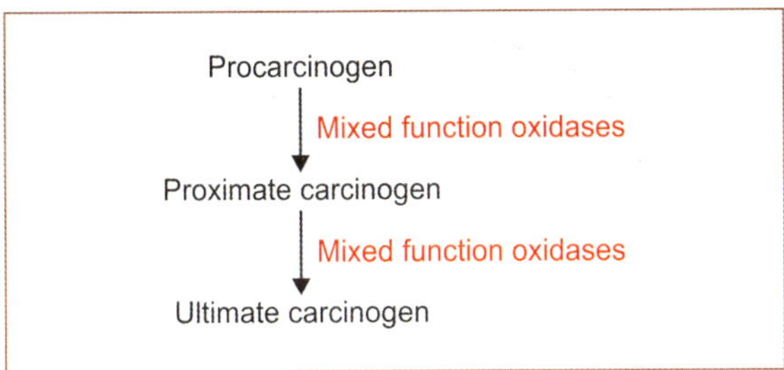

Fig. 22.2: Activation of a procarcinogen

The ultimate carcinogen adducts with DNA and, subsequently, mutates it. Several procarcinogens are present in the environment, at the work place, or in the food (Chemistry to Clinics 22.1).

The indirect carcinogens can also be tested by the Ames test, if the medium is supplemented with the liver extract, which serves as a source of mixed function oxidases.

Chemistry to Clinics 22.1: Procarcinogens

Several compounds may act as procarcinogens, e.g.:

- **Polycyclic hydrocarbons:** Polycyclic hydrocarbons such as benzo(a)pyrene are produced during high temperature combustion of tobacco. These substances have been implicated in the causation of **lung cancer** in the smokers as well as in the nonsmokers who are exposed to environmental tobacco smoke (passive smokers). Such compounds can also be produced from animal fats (e.g. in smoked cheese, meat or fish) and may be the risk factors for **colon cancer**.
- **Aromatic amines, amides and azo dyes:** Aromatic amines, amides and azo dyes are present in the dyes and detergents. They increase the incidence of **urinary bladder cancer** in workers in the aniline, dye and rubber industries (an occupational hazard).
- **Food additives** and **toxins:** Food additives and toxins such as colors (butter yellow), sweeteners (saccharin), or certain plant and microbial toxins (such as aflatoxin B1) may produce **hepatocellular carcinoma**.
- **Nitrosamines** and **amides:** Nitrosamines and amides are endogenously formed in the acidic environment of the stomach and may lead to **gastric carcinoma**.

Indirect carcinogens can also be tested by the Ames test, provided the medium is supplemented with the liver extract, which serves as a source of mixed function oxidases.

RADIATION

Radiation, from whatever the source it may be (UV rays of sunlight, X-rays, nuclear fission or radionuclides), is strongly carcinogenic. It causes various **mutagenic effects**, e.g. chromosomal break, translocation or point mutation, etc. Radiation may lead to **leukemia, cancer of the skin, lungs, thyroid gland, breast** or **colon**.

Besides, UV rays can also exhibit other biological effects such as that it can cause DNA damage by forming pyrimidine dimers. Apart from its direct effect on DNA, radiation also leads to the formation of **free radicals**, which, in turn, can interact with DNA and other macromolecules, thereby leading to their damage that further contributes to the process of carcinogenesis.

ONCOGENIC VIRUSES

Viruses which cause cancer are called oncogenic viruses or **tumor viruses**. These may be DNA or RNA viruses (Table 22.3).

These viruses infect the host either by inserting oncogenes in host chromosome, interfering proto-oncogene transcription factors/regulators or by inserting homologous sequences corresponding to normal proto-oncogene of host.

Table 22.3: Oncogenic viruses

Type of virus	Associated tumors
DNA virus	
Epstein-Barr virus (EBV)	Nasopharyngeal carcinoma, Burkitt's lymphoma, B cell lymphomas
Hepatitis B virus	Hepatocellular carcinoma
Human papillomavirus	Anogenital cancer
RNA virus	
Human T cell leukemia-lymphoma virus type 1 (HTLL-1)	Adult T cell leukemia

ONCOGENES

Oncogenes are the tumor-causing genes and have important role in development of many cancers. These genes are called oncogenes due to their ability to convert the normal cells to the oncogenic (tumorigenic) state. Oncogenes are carried by viruses that cause transformation of their target (host) cells. The viral oncogenes have their cellular counterparts (in the host cells), which are involved in normal cell functions and are called **proto-oncogenes** (Table 22.4).

Table 22.4: Examples of proto-oncogenes or oncogenes associated with tumors

Proto-oncogene	Tumor
ras	Carcinoma of colon, lung, pancreas, genitourinary tract, acute lymphoblastic leukemia
erb	Squamous cell carcinoma
myc	Carcinoma of lung, breast
bcl-2	B cell lymphoma

Nomenclature of the Oncogenes

Genomes of the acute transforming retroviruses (which cause rapid induction of tumor in animals) contain unique transforming sequences (genes) referred to as **viral oncogenes (v-onc)**. The v-onc sequences are not found in the genome of the nontransforming retroviruses. Each v-onc is designated by the three letters that relates the v-onc to the virus from which it was isolated, e.g. v-onc contained in the **si**mian **s**arcoma virus is referred to as **v-sis**, whereas the v-onc in **fe**line **s**arcoma virus is designated as **v-fes**.

The cellular counterparts of these genes (proto-oncogenes isolated from the host cells) are named by using the prefix '**c**', instead of the prefix 'v'. For example, the oncogene carried by Rous sarcoma virus is called v-src, whereas the proto-oncogene related to it, in the cellular genome is referred to as **c-src**.

ONCOGENESIS

Oncogenesis refers to the expression of oncogenes. Oncogenes are activated through two mechanisms, i.e. either by the infection of the cells by the tumor viruses or by mutation of the cellular proto-oncogenes (which are usually normal). During infection, the **transducing virus** carries with it the **cellular gene**(s) that have been obtained by the recombination event. Thus, they mimic the behavior of **'gain-of-function' in proto-oncogenes**. On the other hand, when they **specify proteins that inactivate tumor suppressor genes**, their action, in part, mimics **'loss-of-function' of the tumor suppressor genes**.

ACTIVATION OF PROTO-ONCOGENES TO ONCOGENES

Oncogenes are the deregulated form of the normal proto-oncogenes, which are required for cell division, differentiation and regulation. As a result of some mutation in the otherwise normal proto-oncogenes, their deregulation occurs and uncontrolled proliferation of cells starts, and leads to cancer. For example, as a result of gene duplication, addition, insertion, deletion or chromosomal translocation, the chromosomal rearrangement of certain proto-oncogenes can alter their function and convert them into oncogenes. These mutations overexpress the protein to an uncontrolled level, which may lead to tumor. Any of the following processes can result in the activation of a proto-oncogene to oncogene:

- **Point mutation: Substitution in the coding sequence** can **convert** a cellular **proto-oncogene** into an **oncogene**. Any mutation at either position 12 or 61 has been shown to convert a **c-ras proto-oncogene** into an **active oncogene**. For example, DNA sequences of c-ras proto-oncogenes (from normal human cells) and that from the human urinary bladder cancer cells have been shown to differ solely in one base. Besides, a large number of other human tumors are also known to carry ras mutations, e.g. carcinoma of the pancreas, colon, lungs and thyroid.
- **Chromosomal translocation:** When **a piece of one chromosome is split-off** and **joins the other chromosome**, it is called chromosomal translocation. It is a **reciprocal** event that **exchanges parts of the two chromosomes**. Chromosomal translocation results in **overexpression of the proto-oncogene**, such as in certain cases of Burkitt's lymphoma. Translocation has been shown to **activate** the human **c-myc proto-oncogene**.

  Translocation in B cell tumors, usually, involves chromosome 8, which carries c-myc and chromosome 14, which carries immunoglobulin heavy chain locus. When there occurs a break of a segment from an end of the q arm of the chromosome 8 (containing myc gene) and is translocated to chromosome 14 (containing gene for the heavy chain of IgG). This, in turn, results in the transcription of the heavy chain of IgG. Synthesis of the increased amount of DNA-binding protein coded by the myc gene forces the cell towards malignancy (Fig. 22.3).
- **Gene amplification: Amplification of the DNA sequence** may also result in the **activation of a proto-oncogene**. The **c-myc gene in neuroblastoma** and **c-erb B_2 gene in breast cancer** are the examples of the activation of their proto-oncogenes, as a result of amplification of their DNA sequences.
- **Insertion of promoter/enhancer:** Certain retroviruses, e.g. avian leukemia virus when infect a cell, the DNA copy of their RNA genome (called cDNA) is synthesized by reverse transcriptase and gets integrated into the genome of the host. The inte-

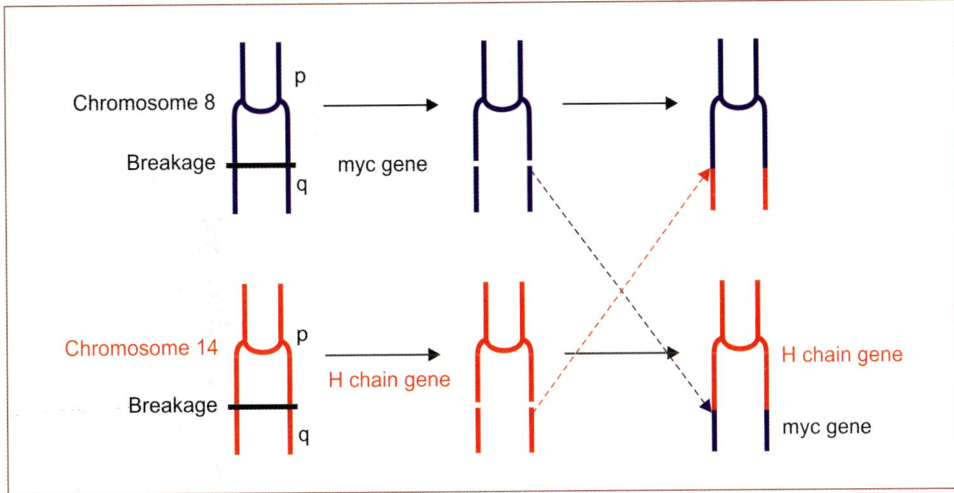

Fig. 22.3: Chromosomal translocation

grated double-stranded DNA is called provirus. These cDNA copies of the retroviruses are flanked at both the ends by the sequences termed as **long terminal repeats** (LTR), which **are important in the integration of a provirus**. Following infection of chicken B lymphocytes by the avian leukemia virus, the **provirus becomes integrated near the myc gene** and **acts as a promoter**. This, in turn, **promotes transcription of the corresponding myc RNA** and subsequent **translation of the gene product** in such cells (Fig. 22.4).

The transforming potential of the avian leukemia virus (a retrovirus) is due to the ability of the LTR of the integrated form to cause expression of cellular gene(s). In some cases, the provirus may be inserted downstream as an enhancer, instead of the upstream (Fig. 22.4).

Types and Classification of Oncogenes

Protein products of the oncogenes are called **oncoproteins**. Their common feature is that they trigger general changes in the cell phenotype either by initiating or responding to changes associated with the cell growth or by changing gene expression, directly.

Based on the protein products formed by mutation or deregulation of proto-oncogenes, oncogenes can be classified into different classes. Oncoproteins include growth factors, growth factor receptors (GFRs), serine/threonine kinases, GTPase molecules and transcription factors (Table 22.5).

- **Growth factors:** Mutations in the growth factors can lead to several types of cancers such as fibrosarcoma, glioblastoma (brain cancer), osteosarcoma (bone cancer), etc.

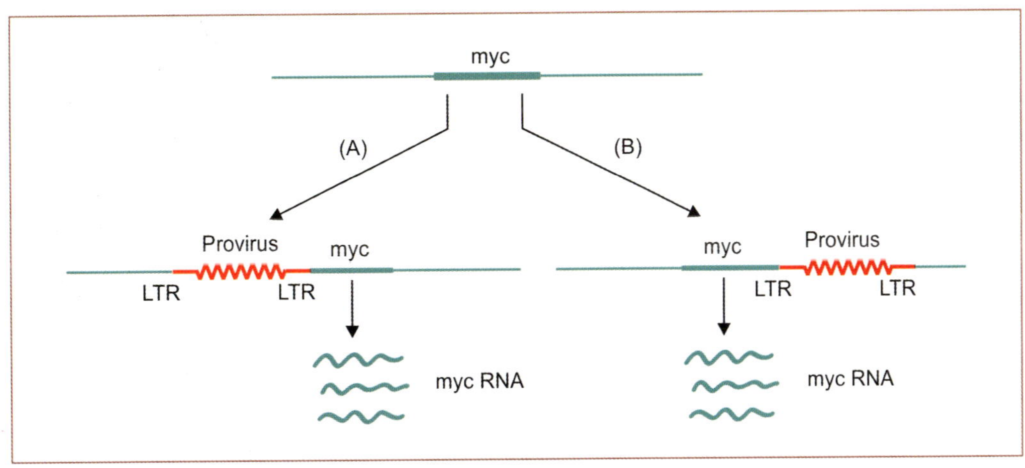

Fig. 22.4: Insertion of a promoter (A) or an enhancer (B)

22

Table 22.5: Oncoproteins (protein products of oncogenes)

Protein function	Example	Result of activation
Growth factor	PDGF-β	Astrocytoma
Growth factor receptor	EGF receptor	Squamous cell lung carcinoma
Regulation of signal transduction	Tyrosine kinase	Leukemia
Regulation of nuclear transcription and cell cycle	Cyclins	Breast cancer

PDGF-β: Platelet derived growth factor-β; EGF: Epidermal growth factor.

- **Growth factor receptors:** Ligand-binding domain deletions of epidermal growth factor receptors (GFRs) cause successive activation of the receptors, even in absence of ligand by transmembrane protein carrying tyrosine kinase activity. This activation further causes interaction with cytoplasmic proteins, like SRC domain, and leads to the deregulation of numerous signaling pathways. GFR mutations are seen in the gastrointestinal, breast and lung cancers.
- **Kinases:** Overexpression of Raf-1 kinase or cyclin-dependent kinases, due to uncontrolled phosphorylation, may cause many cancers, such as thyroid and ovarian cancers.
- **GTPases:** Deregulated activation of GTPases, such as Ras, causes activation of MAPK pathway. Uncontrolled signaling and division of the cells cause several cancers, such as myeloid leukemia.
- **Transcription factors:** Mutation, translocation or rearrangement of the transcription factors proteins causes overexpression of the gene. Unwanted consecutive transcription of the target gene may lead to many types of cancers, such as pancreatic and lung cancer.

TUMOR SUPPRESSOR GENES

Other than expression of oncogenes, cancer may also arise due to the **loss or damage of tumor suppressor genes**, which check and control the cell growth.

Tumor suppressor genes, also called **cancer suppressor genes**, **antioncogenes** or **recessive oncogenes**, play their role by inhibiting cellular proliferation and tumor development. **Inactivation of the tumor suppressor genes** eliminates negative regulation of these genes and leads to abnormal cell proliferation, causing cancer. Tumor suppressor genes have **loss of function** mutations because they develop cancer by inactivating their inhibitory effect on cell proliferation. For a tumor suppressor gene to promote tumor development, both copies of the gene must be inactivated because one copy is sufficient for controlling cell proliferation. These mutations act recessively. Tumor suppressor genes can be studied at the levels of DNA, mRNA and proteins in the normal and cancerous cells using various methods.

Several tumor suppressor genes regulate cell cycle progression through a specific stage, e.g. protein products of Rb and p53 genes.

Retinoblastoma Gene

Mutation in **retinoblastoma** (**RB**) gene is involved in the genesis of retinoblastoma, the tumor of the eye. It results in inactivation of its protein product, designated as **pRB**. Loss of the negative regulatory effect of pRB on cell division leads to increased cell multiplication, as seen in tumor originating from retina, bone and connective tissue.

Two mutagenic events are required for retinoblastoma development in sporadic cases, whereas only one mutagenic event is needed in individuals with inherited form of the disease, in which it displays autosomal dominant inheritance. In normal cells, CDK2 and cyclin D complexes regulate the entry through the constraint point, thereby phosphorylating and inactivating pRB. The pRB also impedes entry through constraint point in the G_1 phase of the cell cycle by repressing the transcription of many genes involved in cell cycle advancement.

p53 Tumor Suppressor Gene

The ***TP53* gene** is located on the short arm of chromosome 17. The name **p53** tumor suppressor **gene** was given to it due to the reason that it encodes a **53 kDa protein**, also known as p53, **cellular tumor antigen p53**, **tumor suppressor p53**, **antigen NY-CO-13**, or **transformation-related protein 53** (TRP53). The p53 is a **proline-rich phosphoprotein** and has been described as the **guardian of the genome**, because of its role in conserving stability by preventing genome mutation.

It has now been shown that the human *TP53* gene encodes at least 15 protein isoforms, called the p53 isoforms. This homolog, originally thought to be, and often spoken of as a single protein, is crucial in multicellular organisms, where it prevents cancer formation, and, thus, functions as a tumor suppressor.

The p53 can arrest the cell cycle upon DNA damage. It allows the DNA to repair or cause apoptosis (programmed cell death). Mutation in p53 in tumorigenic cells results in uncontrolled cell proliferation and inefficient DNA repair. The p53 plays a role in regulation or progression through the cell cycle, apoptosis and genomic stability by means of several mechanisms:

- Transcriptional regulation of certain genes involved in cell division.
- Activation of DNA repairs proteins, when DNA has sustained damage.
- Participation in the initiation of apoptosis (programmed cell death), if DNA damage proves to be irreparable.
- Interaction with other antioncogenes. The p53 has a tissue-level anticancer effect that works by inhibiting angiogenesis.

Levels of p53 play an important role in the maintenance of stem cells throughout development and the rest of the human life. If the *TP53* gene is damaged, tumor suppression is severely compromised, since mutations in p53 gene may result in many tumors, e.g. tumors of the lungs, skin, pancreas, etc.

Protein Products of the Cancer Suppressor Genes

Tumor suppressor genes encode proteins, which form various components of the growth inhibitory pathway. These include growth inhibitory factors, molecules that regulate cell adhesion, signal transduction, nuclear transcription and cell cycle (Table 22.6).

DNA REPAIR GENES

There are several inherited disorders in which genes that encode proteins needed in DNA repair are defective. Individuals born with such inherited mutations are at increased risk of developing cancer (Chemistry to Clinics 22.2).

Chemistry to Clinics 22.2: Defective DNA Repair and Cancer

Due to a defect in DNA repair, patients with xeroderma pigmentosum are at increased risk for the development of cancer of the skin due to exposure to ultraviolet light contained in sunrays. Hereditary nonpolyposis colon carcinoma (HNPCC) is another disorder resulting from defects in genes involved in DNA repair.

APOPTOSIS

The term **programmed cell death** was introduced in 1964, proposing that cell death during development is not of accidental nature but follows a sequence of controlled steps leading to locally and temporally defined self-destruction. Eventually, the term **apoptosis** was coined to describe the morphological processes leading to **controlled cellular self-destruction** and was first introduced in a publication by Kerr, Wyllie and Currie in 1972. **Apoptosis** is of **Greek origin**, meaning **falling off** or **dropping off**, in analogy to leaves falling off trees or petals dropping off flowers. It emphasizes that the death of living matter is an integral and necessary part of the life cycle of organisms. **Apoptosis differs from necrosis** in several aspects related to the cell size, membrane changes and inflammatory response.

Biochemical Mechanism of Apoptosis

Apoptosis can be triggered by various stimuli known as **death signals** that may be initiated **outside the cell** (such as the binding of specific 'death' ligands to membrane 'death' receptors, exposure to radiation or cytotoxic drugs) or **within the cell** (such as faulty DNA repair, improper control of the cell cycle check points) (Fig. 22.5).

Table 22.6: Protein products of cancer suppressor genes

Protein function	Example	Result of mutation
Growth inhibition	BRCA-1	Breast cancer
Regulation of cell-cell and cell-matrix adhesion	DCC	Colon cancer
Regulation of signal transduction	NF-1	Neurofibroma
Regulation of nuclear transcription and cell cycle	Rb p53	Retinoblastoma Lung cancer

BRCA-1: Breast cancer 1; DCC: Deleted in colon carcinoma; NF-1: Neurofibromin 1.

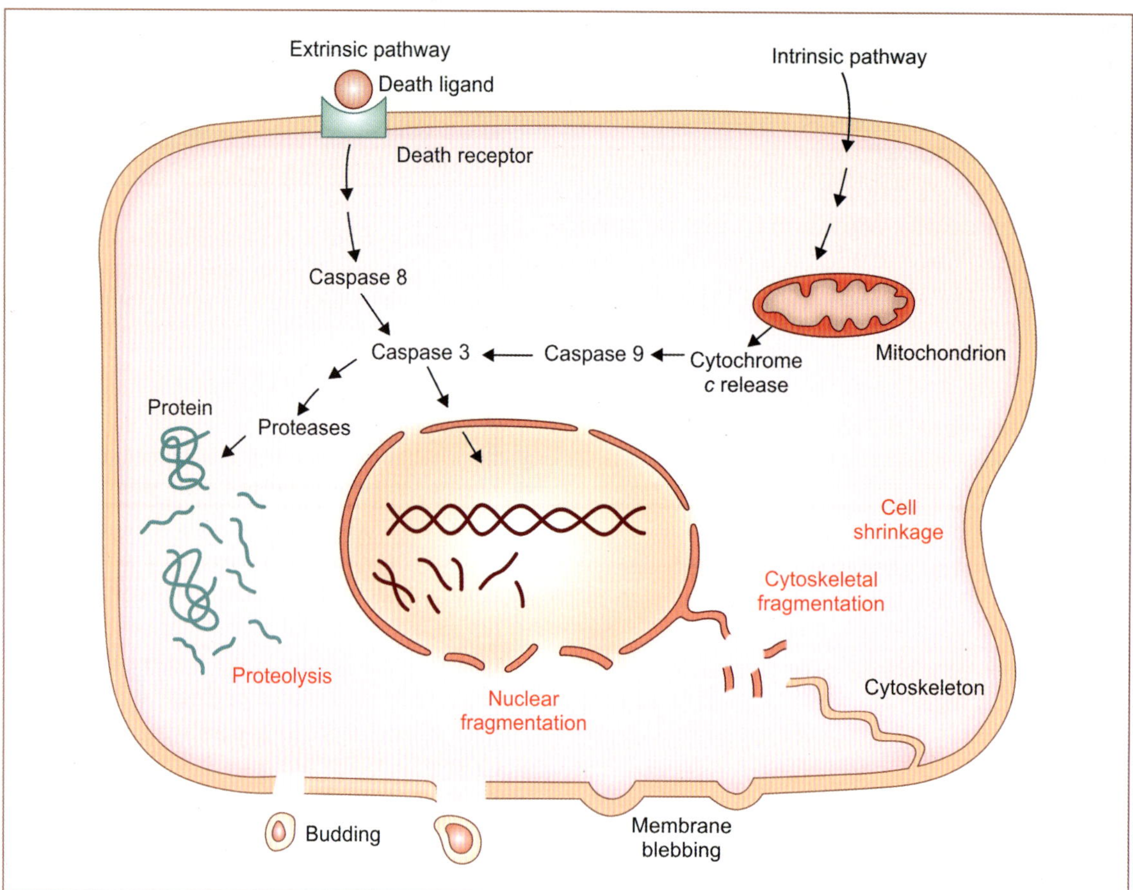

Fig. 22.5: Apoptosis

The death ligand-receptor-mediated biochemical mechanisms are said to follow the extrinsic apoptotic pathway; others follow the intrinsic apoptotic pathway. However, death signals of diverse origin eventually activate a common cell death machinery followed by apoptosis.

- ***Extrinsic apoptotic pathway*:** A hallmark of this pathway is the execution of cells mediated by the enzymes called **caspases**. The term is derived from 'cysteine-dependent **a**spartate-**sp**ecific prote**ases**' because they contain a critical cysteine residue at the catalytic site and they cleave their protein substrates after aspartate residues. Many caspases have been identified and all are initially synthesized as the inactive precursors/zymogens called **procaspases**. The activation of **procaspase 8** is a critical event responsible for the serial activation of other caspases in the pathway. By convention, the cells relying on the caspase-dependent activation of apoptosis are called **type I cells**.

22

- ***Intrinsic apoptotic pathway*:** A hallmark of this pathway is the release of **cytochrome *c*** from the mitochondria into the cytosol. The protein cytochrome *c* is an important mobile component of the electron transport chain located in the inner mitochondrial membrane. Upon release, cytochrome *c* combines with **procaspase 9** molecules and other proteins to form a complex called **'apoptosome'** with subsequent activation of **caspase 9**. By convention, the cells requiring the mitochondria-dependent activation of caspases and apoptosis are called **type II cells**.
- ***Final common pathway*:** Ultimately both the extrinsic and intrinsic pathways, in type I or II cells, **converge** on certain shared series of biochemical events. This includes the activation of procaspases 3, 6 and 7, and irreversible damage to cellular proteins and DNA. This is aptly referred to as **death by a thousand tiny cuts**.

It is interesting to note that apoptosis is an energetically active, i.e. **ATP requiring** process. Further, **proapoptotic** (apoptosis favoring, e.g. p53 tumor suppressor protein) and **antiapoptotic** (apoptosis inhibiting, e.g. bcl-2 protein family) factors are in **balance** and each is genetically determined and regulated.

Biological Significance of Apoptosis

In the adult human body, early 100,000 cells are produced every second by mitosis and a similar number die by apoptosis. Taken together, apoptotic processes are of widespread biological significance, being involved in embryonic development, proliferation, differentiation, homeostasis, regulation of the immune system, and the removal of defective and harmful cells (Chemistry to Clinics 22.3).

Chemistry to Clinics 22.3: Clinical Significance of Apoptosis

1. Failure to correctly initiate apoptosis may result in cancer, autoimmune diseases and spread of infection.
2. Poorly-controlled or excessive apoptosis may lead to neurodegenerative disorders such as Alzheimer disease, Parkinson disease, Huntington disease and amyotrophic lateral sclerosis.
3. Gaining insight into the mechanisms and alterations by which components of the apoptotic machinery contribute to pathogenic processes, should allow the development of more effective, specific and better tolerated therapeutic approaches. It may include the targeted activation of proapoptotic tumor suppressors or the blockade of antiapoptotic genes in case of cancer. On the other hand, for the treatment of premature cell death seen in neurodegeneration, the inhibition of key proapoptotic molecules, such as caspases, might be promising.

For example

- During the **development of the brain and the reproductive organs**, nearly 50% of the cells that are initially formed die later by the time the systems attain maturity.
- Several millions of **T and B lymphocytes** are formed daily and nearly 95% die during genetic rearrangement and maturation.
- Cells **infected** by microbes are cleared by apoptosis (Fig. 22.6A).
- Autoreactive/self-reactive cells of the immune system are destroyed by apoptosis to **prevent autoimmune diseases** (Fig. 22.6B).
- Cells with **extensive DNA damage** that cannot be repaired are removed by apoptosis.

Genes that Regulate Apoptosis

Apoptosis, also called programmed cell death, occurs in many physiological and pathological conditions and is controlled by specific gene-regulated events. Cells undergoing apoptosis shrink, their chromatin condenses, DNA gets fragmented and membranes exhibit blebs.

Large families of genes that regulate apoptosis have been identified. These are designated by a series of words which have three letters beginning with b, e.g. bcl-2, bcl-x, bax, bad. Alterations in genes that regulate apoptosis may also result in neoplasia. Overexpression of bcl-2 protects lymphocytes from apoptosis and allows them to survive for longer period. This, in turn, causes steady accumulation of lymphocytes and results

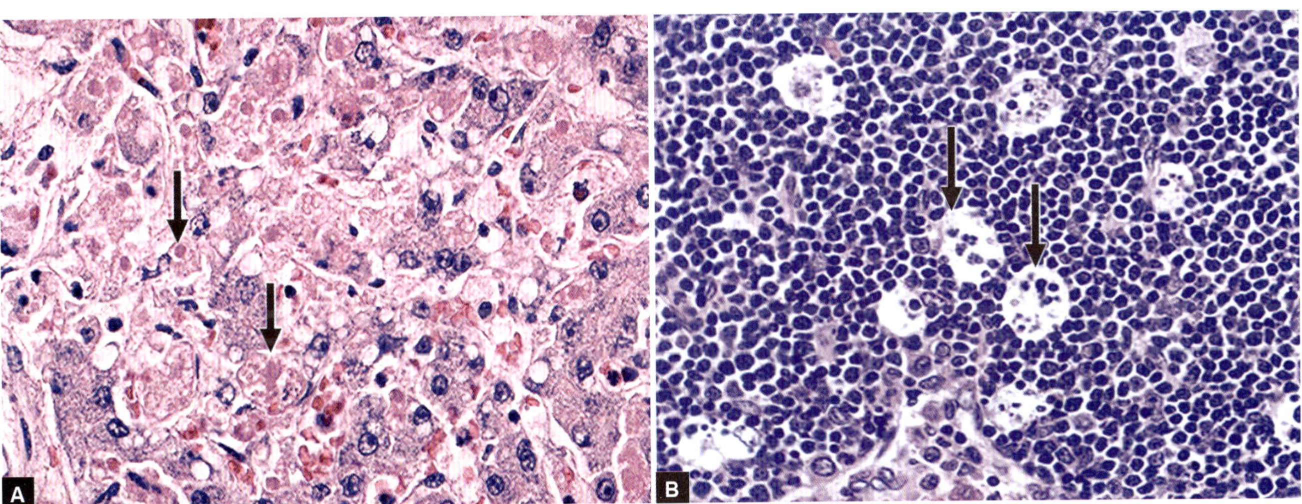

Fig. 22.6: (A) Apoptosis of liver cells (arrows) from injury by viral hepatitis. The cells are pink and without nuclei; (B) Apoptosis of lymphocytes in the fetal thymus. Individual cells fragment and are consumed by phagocytes to give the appearance of clear spaces filled with cellular debris (arrows)

in lymphadenopathy and bone marrow infiltration. On the other hand, bax opposes the action of bcl-2 and accelerates cell death. Hence, the relative levels of the two genes regulate cell proliferation.

BIOCHEMICAL CHANGES DURING TUMOR DEVELOPMENT

The biochemical profile of a malignant cell is different from that of the normal cell as it has a distinct type of metabolism (Table 22.7).

Once a cell becomes malignant, its composition and behavior does not remain static and there is always a tendency for the malignancy to increase.

Table 22.7: Biochemical comparison of a normal cell with a tumor cell

Parameter	Normal cell	Tumor cell
1. Ribonucleotide reductase activity	Normal	Enhanced
2. RNA and DNA synthesis	Normal	Enhanced
3. Pyrimidine catabolism	Normal	Suppressed
4. Rate of glycolysis	Normal	Enhanced
5. Isoenzyme profile	Normal	Altered
6. Synthesis of fetal proteins	No	Yes
7. Synthesis of specialized proteins	Yes	No
8. Inappropriate synthesis of growth factors/hormones	No	Yes

BIOCHEMICAL TUMOR MARKERS

A tumor marker is defined as a substance present in or produced by a tumor, or by the host cell in response to a tumor. Such a substance can be used to differentiate a tumor from the normal tissue or to determine the presence of a tumor based upon its measurement in the tissue, cells or body fluids. An **ideal** tumor marker is one which is both **specific** for a given type of cancer as well as **sensitive** enough to help in its early diagnosis.

Classification: Tumor markers can be classified into several groups such as enzymes and isoenzymes, hormones, oncofetal antigens, carbohydrate-epitopes or oncogene products (Table 22.8).

Applications

22

1. **Detection:** Screening in asymptomatic persons.
2. **Diagnosis:** Differentiate between benign and malignant conditions.

Table 22.8: Selected tumor markers with the type of cancer in which these are increased in serum

Tumor marker	Type of cancer
Enzymes	
Alkaline phosphatase	Bone, liver
Heat stable alkaline phosphatase	Uterus, ovary
Acid phosphatase	Prostate
Amylase	Pancreas
Hormones	
ADH	Adrenal cortex, pancreas, small cell lung cancer
Calcitonin	Medullary thyroid carcinoma
Growth hormone	Pituitary adenoma, renal and lung cancers
β-hCG	Testes, trophoblasts
Oncofetal antigens	
α-Fetoprotein (AFP)	Hepatocellular carcinoma
CEA	Colorectal, GIT, lungs, breast
Squamous cell antigen	Head and neck, cervix, lungs, skin
PSA	Prostate
Carbohydrate markers	
CA 125	Ovary, endometrium
CA 15-3	Breast, ovary
CA 19-9	Pancreas, GIT, liver
Proteins	
β_2-microglobulin	Multiple myeloma, B cell lymphoma
C-peptide	Insulinoma
Ferritin	Liver, lungs, breast, leukemias
Immunoglobulins	Multiple myeloma, lymphomas
Oncogenes	
K-ras mutation	Leukemias, lymphomas
c-myc translocation	B and T cell lymphomas, small cell lung cancer
bcl-2	Leukemias, lymphomas
c-erb B2 amplification	Breast, ovary, GIT
Mutations in tumor suppressor genes	
BRCA-1	Breast, melanoma
p53	Breast, colorectal, lungs, liver
Rb1	Retinoblastoma, osteosarcoma
DCC	Colorectal
Others	
Estrogen and progesterone receptors	Breast
Hydroxyproline (in urine)	Bone metastasis, multiple myeloma
Polyamines (in CSF)	Brain

3. **Monitoring/prognosis:** To assess the effect of treatment and predict the clinical outcome.
4. **Classification and staging:** To decide the type of treatment required.
5. **Localization:** Nuclear scanning of injected radioactive marker antibodies.
6. **Therapy:** Directed towards marker-containing cells.

BIOCHEMICAL BASIS OF CANCER THERAPY

As discussed above, the conversion of proto-oncogene to oncogene is caused due to translocation, rearrangement of chromosomes or mutation in gene, due to addition, deletion, duplication or viral infection. The DNA damage can be targeted by some of the drugs. In addition, different molecular biology techniques are also being developed to diagnose and treat cancer, including retroviral therapy, silencing of oncogenes and mutations in tumor suppressor genes. Amongst them, RNAi, zinc finger nucleases and CRISPR hold a brighter future towards creating a cancer free world.

L-Asparaginase

L-Asparaginase is an anticancer (antineoplastic or cytotoxic) chemotherapy drug that **stops the cancer cells from dividing and growing**. It is an **enzyme** that **hydrolyzes asparagines**, an amino acid necessary for the function of some neoplastic cells, such as lymphoblasts. In most human cells deficiency of L-asparagine can be compensated by alternative synthesis pathway through which L-asparagine is produced from aspartic acid and glutamine by asparagine synthethase. Depletion of L-asparagine from plasma by L-asparaginase results in inhibition of RNA and DNA synthesis with the subsequent blastic cell apoptosis. Since the cancer cells cannot make more asparagine, they die. Owing to the unique anticancer mechanism of action, L-asparaginase has been introduced to the multidrug chemotherapy in children and adults with acute lymphoblastic leukemia.

Alkylating Agents

Alkylating agents are a class of antineoplastic or anticancer drugs which act by inhibiting the transcription of DNA into RNA and thereby, stopping the protein synthesis. They do not alkylate DNA but cause covalent DNA adducts by substituting an alkyl group at the number 7 nitrogen atom of the purine ring of the DNA molecule. This, in turn, prevents the strands of the double helix DNA from linking, as they should. It causes breakage of the DNA strands and affects the ability of the cancer cell to multiply. Eventually, the cancer cell dies.

Alkylating agents were one of the first classes of drugs to be used against cancer. This, in turn, results in the formation of cross-links within the DNA chain and, thereby, causing cytotoxic, mutagenic and carcinogenic effects. This action occurs in all cells, but alkylating agents have their primary effect on rapidly dividing cells, which do not have time for DNA repair. Cancer cells are among the most affected because they are among the most rapidly dividing cells. The end result of the alkylation process results in the misreading of the DNA code and the inhibition of DNA, RNA and protein synthesis, and triggering of apoptosis in rapidly proliferating tumor cells. Different categories of alkylating agents include:

- The nitrogen mustards, e.g. mechlorethamine, cyclophosphamide, melphalan, bendamustine, etc.
- Ethylenamine and methylenamine derivatives like altretamine and thiotepa.
- Alkyl sulfonates such as busulfan.
- Nitrosoureas, e.g. carmustine, lomustine, streptozocin, etc. are a group of alkylating agents that can enter the brain because they are able to cross through the blood–brain barrier. These are useful in treating certain types of brain tumors.
- Triazenes like dacarbazine, procarbazine and temozolomide.
- The platinum-containing antineoplastic agents, which are referred to as platinum coordination complexes such as cisplatin, carboplatin, oxaliplatin, etc.

  Alkylating agents are the oldest type of chemotherapy and are used to treat many different types of cancer such as leukemia, lymphoma, Hodgkin's disease, multiple myeloma, and sarcoma, as well as breast, lung, and ovarian cancers.

Antimetabolites

Antimetabolites interfere with DNA and RNA by acting as a substitute for the normal building blocks of RNA and DNA. When this happens, the DNA cannot make copies of itself, and a cell cannot reproduce. They are commonly used to treat leukemias, cancers of the breast, ovary and the intestinal tract as well as other types of cancer. Commonly used antimetabolites include drugs like methotrexate, 5-fluorouracil (5-FU), etc.

- **Methotrexate** works by slowing, or stopping, the growth of the cancer cells and suppressing the immune system. It interferes with the growth of certain cells of the body, especially, the cells that reproduce quickly, like the cancer cells, bone marrow cells and the skin cells. It is used to treat certain types of cancer of the breast, skin, head and neck or lungs. Methotrexate is also in use to treat psoriasis and rheumatoid arthritis.

- **5-Fluorouracil** (5-FU) is an antimetabolite, an analog of pyrimidine (uracil), with the antineoplastic activity. Following its conversion to the active deoxynucleotide, 5-FU inhibits DNA synthesis, by inhibiting the conversion of deoxyuridylic acid (dUMP) to thymidylic acid (TMP) by the cellular enzyme thymidylate synthetase, and thus, reduces tumor growth.

Antitumor Antibiotics

Antitumor antibiotics are not like the antibiotics, which are used to treat infections, but they work by changing the DNA inside the cancer cells, to keep them from growing and multiplying, e.g. anthracyclines. These are antitumor antibiotics that interfere with enzymes involved in copying DNA, during the cell cycle. They bind with DNA, so it cannot make copies of itself, and a cell cannot reproduce. They are widely used for a variety of cancers.

Mitotic Inhibitors

Mitotic inhibitors are also called plant alkaloids. They are compounds derived from natural products, such as plants. They work by stopping cells from dividing to form new cells but can damage cells in all phases by keeping enzymes from making proteins needed for cell reproduction. Examples of mitotic inhibitors include the taxanes (which stabilize GDP bound tubulin in the microtubule, thereby inhibiting cell division, as depolymerization is prevented) and vinca alkaloids. They are used to treat many different types of cancer including breast, lung, myelomas, lymphomas and leukemias. These drugs may cause nerve damage, which can limit the amount that can be given.

Topoisomerase Inhibitors

These drugs are also called plant alkaloids. They interfere with enzymes called **topoisomerases**, which help separate the strands of DNA so they can be copied. Topoisomerase inhibitors are used to treat certain leukemias, as well as lung, ovarian, gastrointestinal, colorectal and pancreatic cancers.

Topoisomerase inhibitors are grouped according to which type of enzyme they affect:

- **Topoisomerase I inhibitors**, also called **camptothecins**, include irinotecan, irinotecan liposomal and topotecan.
- **Topoisomerase II inhibitors**, also called **epipodophyllotoxins**, include etoposide (VP-16), mitoxantrone (also acts as an *antitumor antibiotic*) and teniposide. Topoisomerase II inhibitors can increase the risk of a second cancer.

ROLE OF RNAi IN CANCER THERAPY

One of the methods used in cancer therapy is RNA interference (RNAi). RNAi refers to a member of noncoding RNAs (ncRNAs), which are not translated into proteins. RNAi is part of a small regulatory RNAs, including siRNAs (small interfering RNAs) and miRNAs (microRNAs). These small noncoding RNAs bind with other mRNAs and inhibit their translation into proteins. This result in the **loss of functions of genes** and prevent cancer from spreading. Knock downing of the gene products by RNAi exerts antiproliferative and proapoptotic effects.

There are different types of small synthetic RNAi such as siRNA, shRNA and bishRNA. The major advantage of RNAi in cancer therapy is targeting multiple genes of various cellular pathways involved in tumor progression. Such cancer therapy outweighs the others due to the silencing mechanism, and its specificity and the lack of side effects. Although, the RNAi method is fast, cheap and has a high efficiency, it has drawbacks that include incomplete knockdown and temporary prevention of gene function.

ROLE OF ONCOGENES IN CANCER TREATMENT

Several oncogenes have been targeted by various agents/drugs and gene therapies to inhibit, arrest, regulate or senescence their genes. For example, imatinib (ABL-kinase inhibitor) is being practiced to treat BCR-ABL. Gefitinib and erlotinib are used to target EGFR. VEGF oncogenes are targeted by bevacizumab or sorafenib. Sorafenib is also used to downregulate or inhibit B-Raf oncogene. These drugs are in use, sometimes in combination, to inhibit proliferation of oncogenes or downregulate signaling oncoproteins by gene replacements or knocking out oncogenes.

Genome Editing

In this technique, engineered nucleases which have specific domains, bind to the target site, followed by its cleavage. These nucleases have been shown to induce double-strand breaks (DSBs) in the target followed by the activation of DNA repair mechanisms. Two types of nucleases, which have been used, include programmable nucleases like zinc finger nucleases (ZFNs, also referred to as zinc finger proteins) and transcription-activator-like effector nucleases (TALENs).

- **Zinc finger nucleases:** Zinc finger nucleases (ZFNs) are the first nucleases to be used for gene editing. These are found as DNA-binding domains in eukaryotes. These are made up of 30 amino acids modules arranged in the form of an array of Cys2-His2- DNA-binding zinc fingers. These modules are used to a nuclease domain of FokI. The modules consist of 3–6 zinc fingers that can identify nucleotide triplets. The FokI nuclease functions only as dimers so a pair of zinc finger nucleases is needed to target any region in the genome. One ZFN will identify the sequence upstream of the genome region to be modified and other will identify downstream sequence. These arrays bind to the nearby DNA sequences that are in the opposite strands, to induce a double-stranded break in the specific region. The breaks are then repaired by different methods that can cause different changes in the specific region like point mutations or translocations. The ZFNs are being custom designed so that they can recognize all possible nucleotides and any specific region of DNA.
- **Transcription activator-like effector nucleases:** Transcription activator-like effector nucleases **(TALENs)** are similar to ZFNs, as they also need DNA-binding motifs and the same nuclease to edit the genome. The difference lies in the recognition of nucleotides as the TALENs domain identifies only one nucleotide instead of a triplet. Accordingly, the interactions between the TALEN domains and their target sites are stronger as compared to ZFNs.

  Using TALENs for cancer therapy have been shown to be very effective method. It needs two specifically engineered TALENs that can identify the sequences of DNA in the target gene on the opposite strands. It dimerizes the FokI nuclease cleavage domain in the TALENs, cleaving the sequence in the target gene. This causes double-stranded DNA breaks in the targeted gene. The lesion, due to the DNA break, is repaired by the end-joining DNA repair system. The target gene is altered due to the change in the reading frame. This gene editing technology can be used to treat the cancer cell lines efficiently, as it can target any gene in the genome.
- **CRISPR/Cas9 system:** CRISPR (Clustered Regularly Interspaced Short Palindromic Repeats) is a powerful tool for genome editing technology in cancer detection and treatment. The CRISPR system is much more efficient than ZFNs and TALENs and has many advantages. Firstly, the target design process is simpler for CRISPR as it depends upon the ribonucleotide complex formation, instead of DNA recognition. It can be designed easily and is much cheaper than designing nucleases, as this does not need different proteins for each target and eliminates laborious cloning steps. This can be used to target any specific sequence in the genome.

  CRISPR, primarily, constitutes two biological components, i.e. engineered sgRNA (single guide RNA) and Cas9. It requires noncoding tracrRNA, which triggers the processing of pre-crRNA via dsRNA-specific ribonuclease (RNase III), and Cas9 protein (only protein carrying out effective crRNA-mediated silencing of target). Different CRISPR–Cas systems have been, broadly, grouped into three types (I–III) depending upon diverse bacterial and archeal repeat sequences, genes, and their mode of action. SpCas9 (called *Streptococcus pyogenes* Cas9) is being in use currently for effective genome editing in eukaryotic organisms including humans.

CHEMOPREVENTION

As we know, cancer still imposes a global threat to public health. After decades of research on cancer biology and enormous efforts in developing anticancer therapies, we now understand that the majority of cancers can be prevented.

Chemoprevention is defined as the introduction of some of the **natural and/or synthetic substances in the diet, for preventing cancer**. Bioactive phytochemicals present in edible plants have been shown to reduce the risk of various types of cancer, particularly those of the lungs, stomach, colon, breast, prostate, etc. have been benefited by chemopreventive agents, sometimes called **nutraceuticals or nutriceuticals** (Table 22.9).

Recent trend is to **encourage enhanced consumption of fruits/vegetables**, which are natural sources of chemopreventive agents, at an early age.

Table 22.9: Chemopreventive nutraceuticals

- Vitamins A, C and E ('big three' antioxidants)
- Flavonoids
- Curcumin (major colored component of turmeric)
- Lunasin (a soy peptide)
- Poppy seeds
- Diallyl sulfide (in garlic and onion)
- Aqueous extracts of decaffeinated green or black tea

Antioxidant Vitamins

Antioxidant vitamins, e.g. vitamin A and carotenoids, vitamin E and vitamin C, have been shown to be the natural dietary inhibitors of carcinogenesis. They work by **various mechanisms**, i.e.:

- Inhibit the formation of free radicals as well as increasing their detoxification
- Stimulate immune system
- Inhibit nitrosamine formation
- Enhance cell-to-cell communication
- Metabolic detoxification of the carcinogen.

Ginsenosides

Ginsenosides are the saponins obtained from plant ginseng. Ginsenosides have been shown to elicit chemopreventive and chemotherapeutic effects in a wide range of animal models of experimental carcinogenesis. They have been reported to inhibit tumor angiogenesis, as well as the invasion and metastasis of various types of cancer cells. Ginsenosides compel tumor cells to commit suicide and arrest the proliferation of cancer cells. The major mechanisms of the anticarcinogenic effects of ginsenosides include:

i. The inhibition of oxidative damage and inflammation,
ii. The inhibition of tumor cell proliferation,
iii. The induction of cancer cell apoptosis,
iv. Antiangiogenic activity,
v. Inhibition of the invasion and metastasis of tumor cells, and
vi. The enhancement of the sensitivity of resistant cells to chemotherapeutic agents.

Some Important Questions

1. What is carcinogenesis? Describe in detail about chemical carcinogenesis.

2. What are oncogenes? How proto-oncogenes are activated?

3. What are cancer suppressor genes? Outline their protein products.

4. Differentiate between:

i. A benign tumor and a malignant tumor
ii. Direct reacting and indirect reacting carcinogens
iii. Initiator and promoter

5. Write notes on:

i. Metastasis
ii. Carcinogenesis
iii. Ames test
iv. Radiation carcinogenesis
v. Viral carcinogenesis
vi. Oncogenes
vii. Cell cycle
viii. Apoptosis
ix. DNA repair genes
x. Tumor markers
xi. Chemoprevention

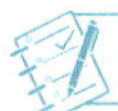

Multiple Choice Questions

1. High-fat low-fiber diet is associated with cancer of:

A. Oral cavity B. Esophagus
C. Stomach D. Colon

2. An increased risk of urinary bladder cancer is an occupational hazard in workers exposed to:

A. Azo dyes B. Aniline
C. Rubber D. All of the above

3. An increased risk of hepatocellular carcinoma may be due to exposure to:

A. Butter yellow
B. Saccharin
C. Aflatoxin B1
D. All of the above

4. Epstein-Barr virus (EBV) is associated with:

A. Nasopharyngeal carcinoma
B. Burkitt's lymphoma
C. B cell lymphoma
D. All of the above

5. The 'guardian of the genome' is:

A. pRb B. p53
C. c-erb B1 D. c-erb B2

6. The following is an antioncogene:

A. pRb B. hst-1
C. c-erb B1 D. c-erb B2

7. Hereditary nonpolyposis colon cancer (HNCC) is mainly attributed to a defect in genes regulating:

A. DNA repair
B. Apoptosis
C. Nuclear transcription
D. Cell cycle check points

8. Serum CEA is a marker for the following tumors *except*:

A. Colorectal B. Prostate
C. Lungs D. Breast

9. Serum AFP is a tumor marker for:

A. Ovary B. Testis
C. Liver D. Tongue

10. The following hormone may be ectopically produced in paraneoplastic syndrome:

A. PTHrP B. Calcitriol
C. Vasopressin D. All of the above

CHAPTER 23

Immunity

Competency Achievement: The student should be able to:

BI10.3 Describe the cellular and humoral components of the immune system and describe the types and structure of antibody

BI10.4 Describe and discuss innate and adaptive immune responses, self/nonself recognition and the central role of T-helper cells in immune responses

BI10.5 Describe antigens and concepts involved in vaccine development

The immune system is a host defense system comprising many biological structures and processes within an organism that protects it against disease. The main purpose of the immune system is to **identify self from nonself**, and defend the body from nonself proteins, such as viruses, bacteria, fungi, parasites and other pathogens. If the immune system is disrupted, it can lead to immunodeficiency and can attack itself, resulting in autoimmune disorders.

The immune system protects an organism from infection with various defenses of increasing specificity. Firstly, the **physical barriers** prevent pathogens, such as bacteria, viruses, etc. from entering the organism. If a pathogen breaches these barriers, the **innate immune response** provides an immediate but nonspecific response. If pathogens successfully evade the innate response, the innate response then activates **the adaptive immune response**. Both **innate** and **the adaptive immune responses** use **cell-mediated** as well as **humoral** components of the immune system.

COMPONENTS OF THE IMMUNE SYSTEM

The main lymphoid tissues of the immune system are the bone marrow and the thymus.

- **Bone marrow:** The bone marrow is extremely important to the immune system because all the body's blood cells (including T and B lymphocytes) originate in the bone marrow. **B lymphocytes** remain in the marrow to mature, while **T lymphocytes** travel to the thymus.
- **Thymus:** The thymus is a bilobed gland located above the heart, behind the sternum and between the lungs. The thymus is only active through puberty, and then it slowly shrinks and is replaced by fat and connective tissue. The thymus is responsible for producing the hormone **thymosin**, which, in turn, aids in the production of **T cells**. While in the thymus, T cells multiply, acquire different antigen receptors, and differentiate into helper T cells and cytotoxic T cells. Various proteins (e.g. CD4, CD8, etc.) are expressed on the T cell surface.

After the T and B lymphocytes have matured in the thymus and bone marrow, respectively, they travel to the lymph nodes and spleen, where they remain until the immune system is activated.

- **Lymph nodes:** Lymph nodes are located throughout the body.
- **The spleen:** The spleen is located in the upper left area of the abdomen, behind the stomach, and under the diaphragm. The main function of the spleen is to **filter the blood**. Healthy red blood cells easily pass through the spleen; however, damaged red blood cells are broken down by macrophages (large white blood cells specialized in engulfing and digesting cellular debris, pathogens and other foreign substances in the body) in the spleen. The spleen serves as a **storage unit for platelets** and **white blood cells**. The spleen aids the immune system by **identifying microorganisms that may cause infection**.

In addition to the lymph nodes and spleen, **mucosal-associated lymphoid tissues** (MALTs) and **gut-associated lymphoid tissues** (GALTs) play a vital role in the immune system, although they are considered to be part of the lymphatic system.

- **MALTs** are lymphoid tissues found in parts of the body where mucosa is present such as the **intestines, eyes, nose, skin** and **mouth**. They contain **lymphocytes** and **macrophages** that defend against pathogens attempting to enter from outside the body.
- **GALTs** are lymphoid tissues found in the **mucosa and submucosa** of the **gastrointestinal tract, tonsils, appendix** and **Peyer's patches in the small intestine.**

CELLS OF THE IMMUNE SYSTEM

Cells of the immune system include **phagocytes** and **lymphocytes**. Phagocytes internalize the pathogens and degrade them, while lymphocytes recognize the antigens on the pathogens.

Phagocytes

- Neutrophils and macrophages are the phagocytes that travel throughout the body in pursuit of invading pathogens. Phagocytes, such as polymorphonuclear neutrophils, bind to microorganisms, internalize and kill them (Chemistry to Clinics 23.1).

Chemistry to Clinics 23.1: Hypochlorous Acid

Activated neutrophils secrete hypochlorous acid (HOCl), which is more cytotoxic against microbes compared with H_2O_2. The body lacks direct enzymatic defenses against HOCl. Plasma albumin-SH groups and ascorbic acid protect against HOCl. Neutrophils contain 25 times more ascorbic acid than plasma, avoiding self-destruction.

  - **Neutrophils** are, normally, found in the bloodstream and are the most abundant type of phagocytes representing 50 to 60% of the total circulating leukocytes. During the acute phase of **inflammation**, particularly as a result of bacterial infection, neutrophils migrate towards the site of inflammation (in a process called chemotaxis) and are, usually, the first cells to arrive at the scene of infection.
  - **Macrophages** are the versatile cells that reside within the tissues, and produce a wide array of chemicals including enzymes, **complement proteins** and cytokines. They can also act as **scavengers** that rid the body of worn out cells and other debris, and as **antigen-presenting cells** that activate the adaptive immune response. **Pro-inflammatory** macrophages are called **M1 macrophages**, whereas the **noninflammatory** ones are designated **M2 macrophages**.
  - **Dendritic cells** are **phagocytes in tissues** that are in contact with the external environment. They are **located**, mainly **in the skin, nose, lungs, stomach** and **intestines**. Dendritic cells serve as a link between the bodily tissues and the innate and adaptive immune responses, as they present antigens to the T cells.

Phagocytosis: It is an important feature of the cellular innate immune response performed by the cells called phagocytes that engulf (or eat) pathogens (or particles). Phagocytes, generally, patrol the body, searching for pathogens, but can be called to specific locations by cytokines. Once a pathogen has been engulfed by a phagocyte, it becomes trapped in an intracellular vesicle, called a **phagosome**, which subsequently fuses with another vesicle, called **lysosome**. The pathogen is killed by the activity of the digestive enzymes, or following a respiratory burst that releases free radicals.

Leukocytes

- Leukocytes (white blood cells) act like independent, single-celled organisms and are the second arm of the innate immune system. The innate leukocytes include the phagocytes (macrophages, neutrophils and dendritic cells), innate lymphoid cells, mast cells, eosinophils, basophils and natural killer cells. They identify and eliminate pathogens either by attacking larger pathogen through contact or by engulfing and then killing microorganisms. Innate cells are also important mediators in lymphoid organ development and the activation of the adaptive immune response.
  - **Granulocytes:** Granulocytes are leukocytes that have granules in their cytoplasm. In this category are neutrophils, mast cells, basophils and eosinophils. **Mast cells** reside in connective tissues and mucous membranes, and regulate **inflammatory response**. They are most often **associated with allergy** and **anaphylaxis**. Basophils and eosinophils are related to neutrophils. They secrete chemical mediators that are involved in defending against parasites and play a role in allergic reactions, such as asthma.
  - **Lymphocytes:** Lymphocytes are the set of leukocytes which mediate adaptive immune response and, specifically, recognize individual pathogens. They fall into two categories, i.e. B lymphocytes and T lymphocytes.

B Lymphocytes

After formation and maturation in the **bone marrow** (hence, the name **B cell**), the **naive** ***B cells*** (**B lymphocytes**, or B cells, that have not been exposed to an antigen) move into the lymphatic system, to circulate throughout the body.

In the lymphatic system, naive B cells encounter an antigen, which starts the **maturation process for the B cells**. When naive B cells combat extracellular pathogens and their products, they release antibodies (the molecules which specifically recognize and bind to particular antigen) on their cell surface (i.e. ***membrane-bound antibodies***). These antibody molecules are large glycoproteins found in the blood and tissue fluids. B cells, thus, mediate **humoral immunity**.

After a naive B cell encounters an antigen, that fits or matches its membrane-bound antibody, it **quickly divides** in order to set off differentiation and become either a ***memory B cell*** or an ***effector B cell*** (also called a ***plasma cell***).

Memory B cells: Even when the infection has been overcome, some of the newly produced lymphocytes remain **available for restimulation** in case the antigen is encountered again, in future. These cells are called memory cells, since they retain the **immunological memory** of a particular antigen. The memory B cells express the same membrane-bound antibody as the original naive B cell, or the parent B cell.

Plasma B cells: Plasma B cells produce the same antibody as the parent B cell, but they are not membrane bound. Secreted antibodies work to identify free pathogens that are circulating throughout the body. These cells also express a specialized receptor, called **B cell receptors**, which assist with **antigen binding** as well as **internalization** and **processing of the antigen**.

B cell receptors also play an important role in **signaling pathways**. After the antigen is internalized and processed, the B cell can initiate signaling pathways, such as cytokine release, to communicate with other cells of the immune system.

T Lymphocytes

Once formed in the bone marrow, the T cells (*called T progenitor cells*) migrate to the thymus and become mature T cells (hence, these cells are called T cells or T lymphocytes). While in the thymus, the developing T cells start to express different types of receptors referred to as *T cell receptors* and other receptors called *CD4* and *CD8*.

All the T cells express T cell receptors, and either CD4 or CD8 but not both. Thus, some T cells express CD4 while the others express CD8 (Chemistry to Clinics 23.2).

Chemistry to Clinics 23.2: Cluster of Differentiation (CD)

These refer to specific cell surface proteins with diverse functions. Depending on the cell type, a CD may act as a receptor, ligand or adhesion molecule. The concept was applied for leukocytes (e.g. CD4+ are T helper cells, while CD8+ are cytotoxic T cells) but later expanded to include various other cell types (e.g. CD220 for insulin receptor). They are useful in immune-phenotyping, which identifies alterations in cell types in various disease conditions, e.g. depletion of CD4+ cells in HIV infection.

In order to mount an appropriate immune response, the T cell receptors recognize only those antigens that are bound to certain receptor molecules called ***major histocompatibility complex*** *(MHC)*. There are two types of MHC molecules, called MHC class I (MHCI) and MHC class II (MHCII). The MHC molecules are membrane-bound surface receptors on ***antigen-presenting cells***, like dendritic cells and macrophages.

CD4 and CD8 receptors play a role in T cell recognition and activation, by binding to either MHCI or MHCII.

After positive and negative selection, we are left with three types of mature T cells, with a variety of functions. These include:

- **Cytotoxic T cells:** They express CD8 and are responsible for the destruction of host cells, which have become infected by viruses or other intracellular pathogen.
- **Suppressor T cells:** They express CD4 and CD25. These cells help distinguish between self and nonself molecules, and by doing so, reduce the risk of autoimmune diseases. They also inhibit the production of cytotoxic T cells, when they are no longer needed. As suppressors of the immune system, they play an important role in maintaining homeostasis and, thus are also referred to as **T regulatory cells**.
- **Helper T cells:** Helper T cells (Th cells) express CD4 and help in the activation of B cells and other immune cells. They direct the immune response by secreting chemicals (the effector molecules), generally, referred to as **lymphokines**.

There are different types of helper T cells. These include:

- **T helper cells type 1 (Th1):** They interact with the mononuclear phagocytes and help them to destroy intracellular pathogens.

- **T helper cells type 2 (Th2):** This group of the helper T cells interacts with B cells and helps them to divide, differentiate and make antibodies.
- **T helper zero cells (Th0):** This group of T cells express cytokines from both the profiles.

  Differentiation of the CD4+ Th cells into Th1 and Th2 occurs only after they have been activated, during an immune response in the peripheral lymphoid system. Each type of the T cell produces a distinct set of effector molecules. For instance, Th1 cells release macrophage-activating effector molecules, such as interferon-γ and tumor necrosis factor-α, whereas Th2 cells produce B cell-activating effector molecules like interleukins 4, 5 and 15, among numerous other cytokines.

All types of the T cells recognize antigen when presented on the surface of the other cell by **major histocompatibility complex** (MHC) molecules.

MAJOR HISTOCOMPATIBILITY COMPLEX

All vertebrate cells express on their surfaces, a sample of peptides derived from the intracellular digestion of specific proteins in their cytosol. This expression, however, requires that the peptides should be bound to a specific class of integral membrane proteins/ antigens encoded by a set of genes referred to as the **major histocompatibility complex (MHC) genes**. Initially, MHC encoded antigens were detected on **leukocytes**; hence, they were also called **human leukocyte antigens (HLA)**.

HLA loci: Human beings carry six different **class I genes** (three from each parent) and six different **class II genes** that are present on the HLA loci, on chromosome 6. The three loci for class I genes are called HLA-A, HLA-B and HLA-C, while those for class II genes are called HLA-DP, HLA-DQ and HLA-DR. Because of **high polymorphism** between the HLA loci, it is very rare to find two persons (except monozygotic twins) with identical HLA. This is responsible for transplant rejection, unless the HLA genotypes of donor and recipient are closely matched. HLA is of physiological and clinical importance (Chemistry to Clinics 23.3).

MHC classes: The MHC gene encodes **three classes** of MHC proteins/antigens. These include class I proteins (presented to cytotoxic T cells), class II proteins (presented to helper T cells) and class III proteins or complement proteins (Table 23.1).

Chemistry to Clinics 23.3: Importance of HLA

- HLA plays a crucial role in **regulating the immune response** (Fig. 23.1).

  CD8 lymphocytes and their secretory proteins such as perforins and granzymes are responsible for direct killing of target cells recognized via MHCI. On the other hand, CD4 lymphocytes with the help of B cells combat the targets recognized via MHCII.
- Specific HLA types are associated with **disease susceptibility**, e.g. ankylosing spondylitis (HLA-B27), insulin-dependent diabetes mellitus (HLA-DR3/4), rheumatoid arthritis (HLA DR4), hemochromatosis (HLA-A3), myasthenia gravis (HLA-B8), etc.
- HLA **typing** is required before **organ transplantation**.

Table 23.1: Differences between class I and class II MHC

Class I MHC	Class II MHC
• Expressed on all cells	• Expressed on antigen-presenting cells (B cells, macrophages, dendritic cells)
• Present cytosolic proteins to cytotoxic T cells	• Present proteins internalized within endosomes to helper T cells
• Assisted by CD8 proteins	• Assisted by CD4 proteins
• Lead to direct killing of target cell	• Lead to enhancement of immune response

CELLULAR AND HUMORAL COMPONENTS OF THE IMMUNE SYSTEM

CELLULAR IMMUNE SYSTEM

Cellular or cell-mediated immune system refers to the immune system which is mediated by **T cells** (the **antigen-specific T cells**). Once the T cells encounter an antigen, they proliferate and differentiate into armed effector cells (**cytotoxic T cells**), which destroy the infected cells by **inducing apoptosis**. For this purpose, the antigen is presented to the surface of the antigen-presenting cells (**APCs**), along with the major histocompatibility complexes (**MHCs**). The major characteristic feature of the cellular immune system is that it **destroys the intracellular pathogens**.

HUMORAL IMMUNE SYSTEM

The humoral immune system refers to the immune system which is generated by the circulating **antibodies** that are produced and **secreted by plasma B cells**. For this purpose, **T helper cells stimulate plasma B cells** to produce antibodies. These antibodies generate

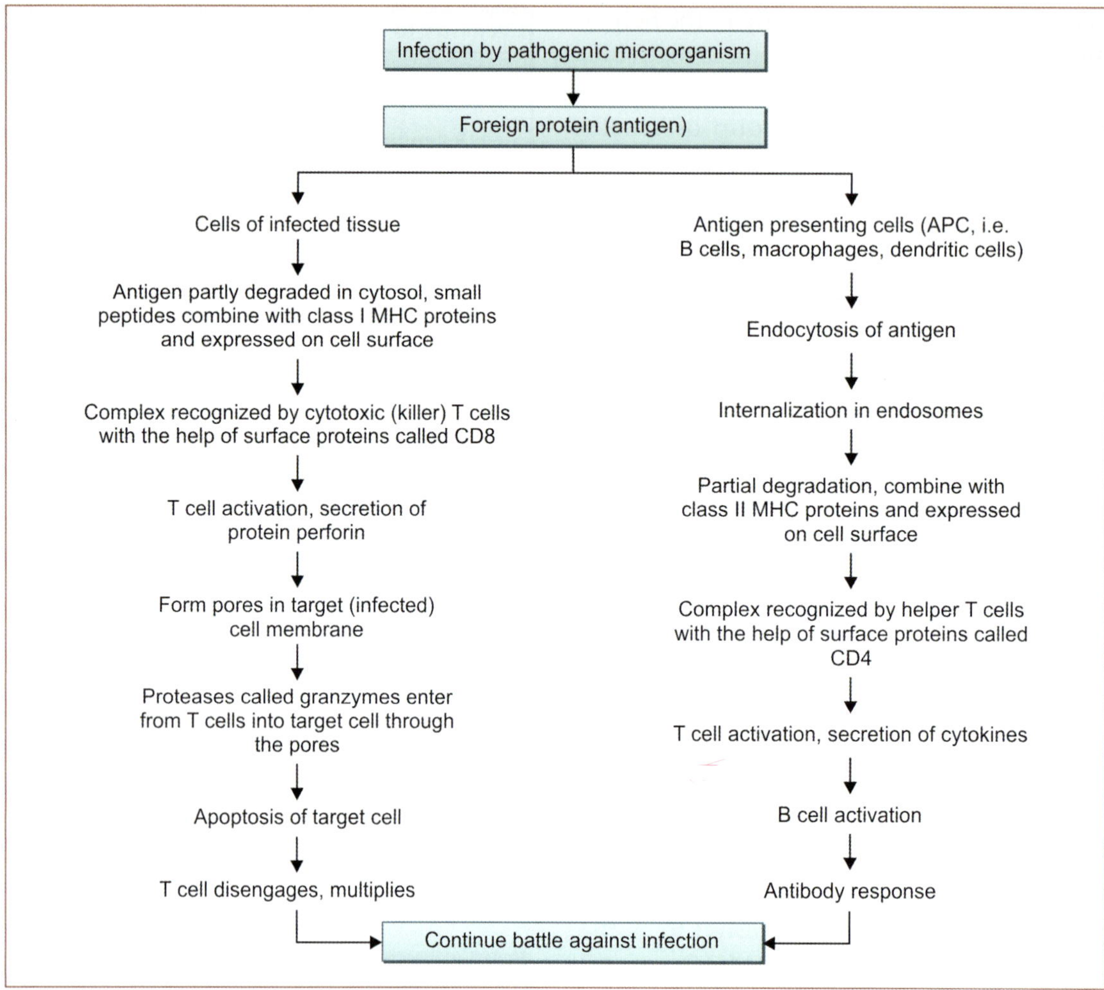

Fig. 23.1: Role of MHC in the regulation of immune response

specific immune response to a particular antigen (foreign material). The major characteristic feature of the humoral immune system is that it **destroys the extracellular pathogens**.

Difference between Cellular and Humoral Immune Systems

As discussed above, the cellular immune system is triggered by T cells, whereas the humoral immune system is triggered by B cells. The other difference between the two is that in the cellular immune system, T cells destroy infected cells by inducing apoptosis while the antigen-specific antibodies are produced in the humoral immune system (Table 23.2).

INFLAMMATION

23

Inflammation is a local response of a tissue to damage or infection. It is one of the first responses of the immune system to infection and has three principle components:

1. An increased blood supply to the area, bringing leukocytes and other serum components to the affected site.
2. An increase in capillary permeability, allowing exudation of serum proteins (antibody, complement, etc.) which are required to control infection.
3. An increase in leukocyte migration into the tissue.

Auxiliary cells including mast cells, basophils and platelets are important in initiation and development of acute inflammation. They act as a source of vasoactive mediators, such as histamine, which produce vasodilation, and increase vascular permeability. Mast cells are also the source of slow reacting inflammatory mediators including leukotrienes and prostaglandins, which contribute to a delayed component of acute inflammation. Clinically, an acute inflammation is characterized by the following classical signs:

Table 23.2: Difference between cellular and humoral immune systems

Humoral immune system	Cellular immune system
Humoral immune system refers to a component of the adaptive immune response, where B cells secrete antibodies, which circulate in the blood as a soluble protein	Cellular immune system refers to the other component of the adaptive immune response which is mediated by the activated antigen-specific T cells
It is mediated by T cells, B cells and macrophages	It is mediated by the helper T cells, cytotoxic T cells, natural killer cells and macrophages
Acts on extracellular microbes and their toxins	Acts on the intracellular microbes such as viruses, bacteria, parasites and tumor cells
B Cell receptors are involved	T Cell receptors are involved
Accessory surface molecules are Igα, Igβ, CD40, CD21 and Fc receptors	Accessory surface molecules are CD2, CD3, CD4, CD8, CD28 and integrins
Unprocessed antigens are recognized	Antigens are processed and presented by the MHC complexes
Plasma B cells secrete antibodies	T Cells secrete cytokines
Immune response is rapid	Immune response is a delayed type of hypersensitivity
Does not act on tumor cells and transplants	Acts on tumor cells and transplants

- **Redness:** Redness of the skin, due to locally increased blood circulation
- **Heat:** Either increase in local temperature, such as a warm feeling around a localized infection, or a systemic fever
- **Pain:** Local pain or painful joints
- **Swelling:** Swelling of the affected tissues, such as the joints affected by rheumatoid arthritis
- **Temporary loss of function**

Inflammation is produced by eicosanoids and cytokines, which are released by injured or infected cells. **Eicosanoids** include prostaglandins that produce fever and the dilation of blood vessels associated with inflammation, and leukotrienes that attract certain white blood cells (leukocytes). Common **cytokines** include interleukins that are responsible for communication between white blood cells, **chemokines** that promote chemotaxis and **interferons** that have anti-viral effects. **Growth factors** and **cytotoxic factors** may also be released. These cytokines and other chemicals recruit immune cells to the site of infection and promote healing of any damaged tissue following the removal of pathogens.

The process of acute inflammation is **initiated by** cells already present in all tissues, mainly, **macrophages**, **dendritic cells** and **mast cells**. These cells present receptors contained on the surface or within the cell, which recognize molecules that are broadly shared by pathogens but distinguishable from the host molecules.

Inflammation is stimulated by chemical factors released by injured cells and serves to establish a physical barrier against the spread of infection, and to promote healing of any damaged tissue following the clearance of pathogens. Chemical factors produced during inflammation such as histamine and leukotrienes, etc. sensitize pain receptors, cause local vasodilation of the blood vessels and attract phagocytes, especially, neutrophils. Neutrophils then trigger other parts of the immune system by releasing factors that summon additional leukocytes and lymphocytes. Cytokines produced by macrophages and other cells of the innate immune system mediate the inflammatory response.

TYPES AND STRUCTURE OF ANTIBODY

Antibodies are a diverse group of glycoproteins synthesized by the mature B lymphocytes called **plasma cells**. They are present either in the **free form** in plasma (constituting ≈20% of total plasma proteins, mainly the γ-globulins) and other biological fluids, or **bound** to the surface of B cells where they act as receptors for antigens. Since these are the globulins which bind to specific antigens, antibodies are also called immunoglobulins. The term **immunoglobulin**, thus, **is a structural concept** while **antibody is a functional one**.

STRUCTURE OF ANTIBODY

Salient features of the structure of an antibody molecule are summarized in Table 23.3.

Table 23.3: Salient features of the structure of an antibody molecule

1. An antibody has **four peptide chains**, which include **two H chains** and **two L chains.**
2. Each chain has **two regions** referred to as the **variable region** and the **constant region.**
3. Each variable region has **hypervariable sequences.**
4. An antibody has a **Y-shape** structure with **two arms** (called Fab fractions) and **a stem** (Fc fragment).
5. **Fab segments** are linked to **Fc segment** with **hinge region.**

1. An antibody has **four peptide chains**, which are bound to each other by the disulfide (–S–S–) linkages (Fig. 23.2).
   - Out of the four peptide chains (subunits), each antibody is comprised of **two** small peptide chains, called **L chains** (light chains), and **two** large peptide chains, referred to as **H chains** (heavy chains).
   - **L Chains:** There are **two types** of the L chains found in antibodies, which are designated as the **kappa chain (κ chain)** and the **lambda chain (λ chain)**. An antibody molecule has **two identical L chains**, i.e. it may have either two κ chains (as κ2) or two λ chains (as λ2) but never one κ chain and one λ chain (i.e. as κλ). These are referred to as **isotypes** and are present in all individuals. The κλ chains are more prevalent than the λ chains. Each L chain is about **≈25 kD** in size and has, nearly, **220 amino acids.**
   - **H Chains:** There are **five types** of the H chains found in antibodies. These are designated as **gamma (γ), alpha (α), mu (μ), delta (δ)** and **epsilon (ε)** chain. Each of these H chains is **specific to a class** of immunoglobulin (Ig). Accordingly, depending upon the presence of the H chain, immunoglobulins are classified into five groups and are designated as **IgG, IgA, IgM, IgD** and **IgE**. Each H chain is between **50–75 kD** in size and may have, nearly, **440–450 amino acids.**
   - The L chains and the H chains are **synthesized separately**, which are **subsequently assembled** to form a mature immunoglobulin molecule forming a tetramer, within the plasma cells. During assembly, each H chain is associated **with**

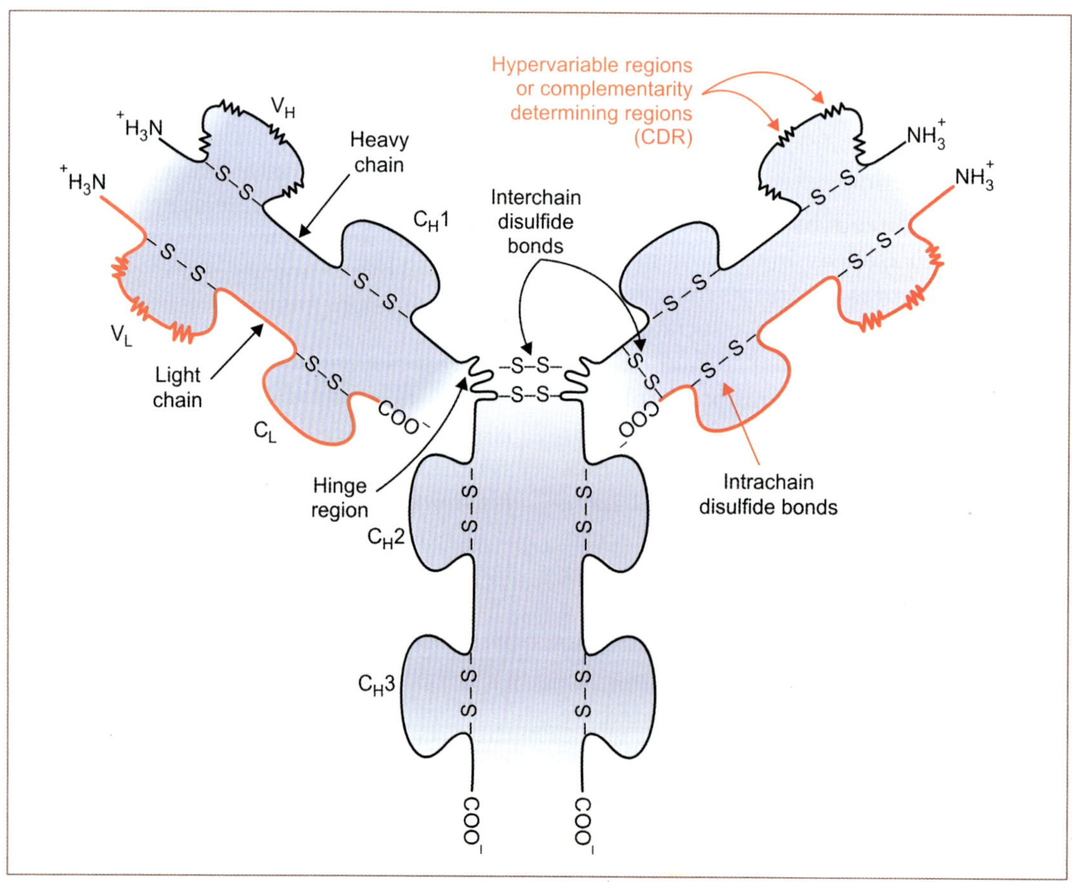

Fig. 23.2: Structure of an immunoglobulin

23

the L chain as well as to each other by the **–S–S– linkages**. An L chain is joined to an H chain in such a way that they run **parallel to each other**.

- In the structure of the antibody molecule, all the four chains are present in the **folded form** in **several discrete regions**, called **domains**. Each domain has, nearly, **110 amino acids**. An **L chain**, normally, has **two domains** while depending upon the class of the immunoglobulin, each of the **H chain** has **four** (or five) domains.

2. Each of these domains is referred to as the **variable region** and the **constant regions**.
   - Within each L and H chain of an immunoglobulin molecule, there are regions with **sequence homology**, referred to as the **constant regions**, as well as the **sequence variability**, called the **variable regions**.
   - **Variable regions:** Amino acid sequences in the N-terminal half of the L chains and one-quarter of the H chains are highly variable between different immunoglobulin molecules. Therefore, these N-terminal regions are called the variable regions (**V regions**). They are **heterogeneous** to the extent that no two V regions, from different humans, have identical amino acid sequences. V region determines **antigenic specificity** of the antibody. These regions, in the L chains and the H chains, are designated as V_L and V_H, respectively.
   - **Constant regions:** The remainder of the molecule, i.e. the C-terminal half of the L chain and the C-terminal three-quarter of the H chain, are **homologous** in sequence with the other L or H chains of the same class of immunoglobulin. These regions are called the constant regions (**C regions**). These regions in the L chains and the H chains are designated as the C_L and C_H, respectively. The constant region in the H chains is further subdivided into three homologous sequences of about 110 amino acids each. These are designated as C_H1, C_H2 and C_H3, respectively. These three segments of the C_H region are homologous to each other as well as to the C_L region. Each of these segments (sequence repeats) contains an intrachain disulfide bond. The μ and ε types of the H chains have four C_H regions, rather than three.
   - Thus, each **L chain** has **one variable region** and **one constant region**. These are referred to as V_L and C_L, respectively. On the other hand, each **H chain** has **one variable region** (V_H) but **three constant regions**, which are referred to as and C_H1, C_H2 and C_H3, respectively.
   - Whereas, the **variable region** is present **towards the N-terminal**, the **constant regions** are present **towards the C-terminal** of the protein chain.

Significance of the C_H region(s)

- C_H region determines the **antibody class** of an immunoglobulin, i.e. the differences in the sequence of the C_H region is responsible for characteristics of each class of immunoglobulin.
- It provides site for **binding of a complement protein**.
- It is also the site for the antibodies to **cross the placental membrane**.
- Depending upon the class of an immunoglobulin, variable amounts of **carbohydrates** (2–15%) are attached to C_H2 region.
- Amino acid sequences in the C_H regions, **in some cases**, also promote **polymerization** of the basic molecular structure (L2H2), which are covalently linked with each other with a peptide, referred to as the joining chain (**J chain**). Generally, immunoglobulins of the **IgA** class occur as **dimers** while **IgM** are found as **pentamers** (Fig. 23.3).

3. Antigenic specificity of an immunoglobulin molecule is responsible for recognition and binding of the antigen with the antibody. This ability of the antibody to recognize antigen resides in several short sequences that are located in **small loops** (short segments) within the V region. These sequences are referred to as **hypervariable regions** or **hypervariable sequences**.
   - Only **5–10 amino acids** in each hypervariable sequence contribute to the site where an antigen binds. This segment is referred to as antigen binding site (**ab site**). It is complementary to the topology of the antigen structure and, hence, it is called **complementarity-determining region** (CDR or complementarity determinant).
   - Three hypervariable sequences are, commonly, found in the V_L regions, while each of the V_H region, depending upon the type of antibody, has three or four hypervariable sequences.
4. An antibody has a **Y-shape** structure, i.e. it has **two arms**, referred to as the **Fab fragments**, and **a stem**, called **Fc fragment**.
   - When hydrolyzed by the enzyme papain, an immunoglobulin molecule, such as IgG, is cleaved into three fragments of nearly 50 kD each. Two of the identical fragments are obtained from the two arms. These are the sites, where antigen can bind. Hence, these **two fragments** are called **antigen binding fragments** (**Fab**). The third fragment, which is obtained from the **stem**, is called

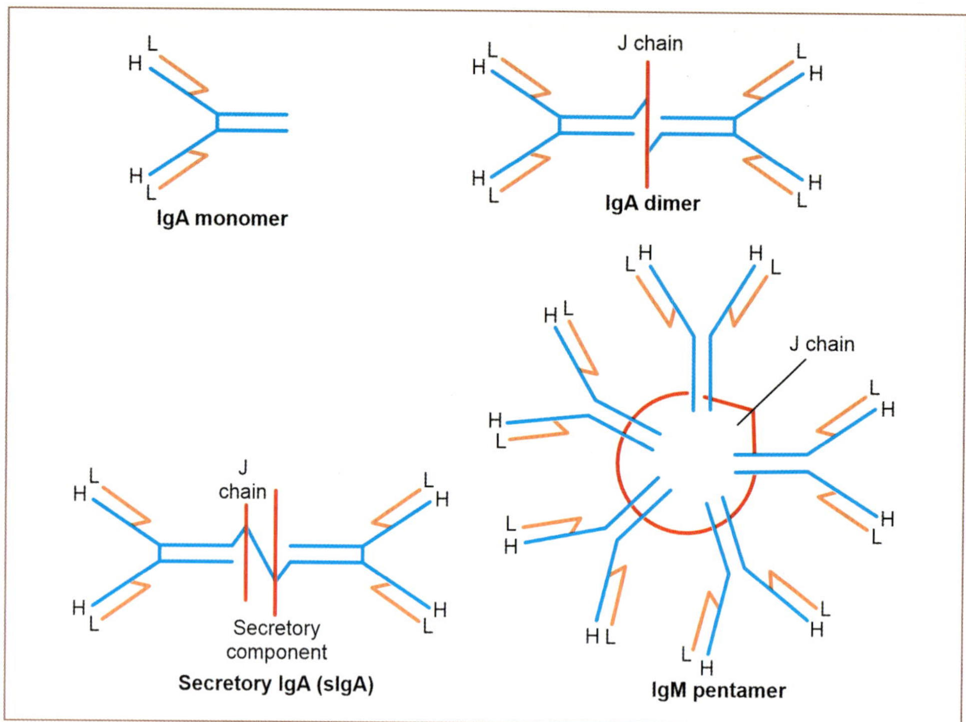

Fig. 23.3: Polymerization of immunoglobulin molecules

crystallizable fragment (**Fc**). It is called Fc due to the region that this fraction can be easily crystalized. On the other hand, when pepsin (a proteolytic enzyme) acts on an immunoglobulin molecule, it hydrolyzes the Fc fragment to its constituent amino acids, thereby leaving the 2 Fab fragments which remain connected with each other through the hinge region (Fig 23.4).

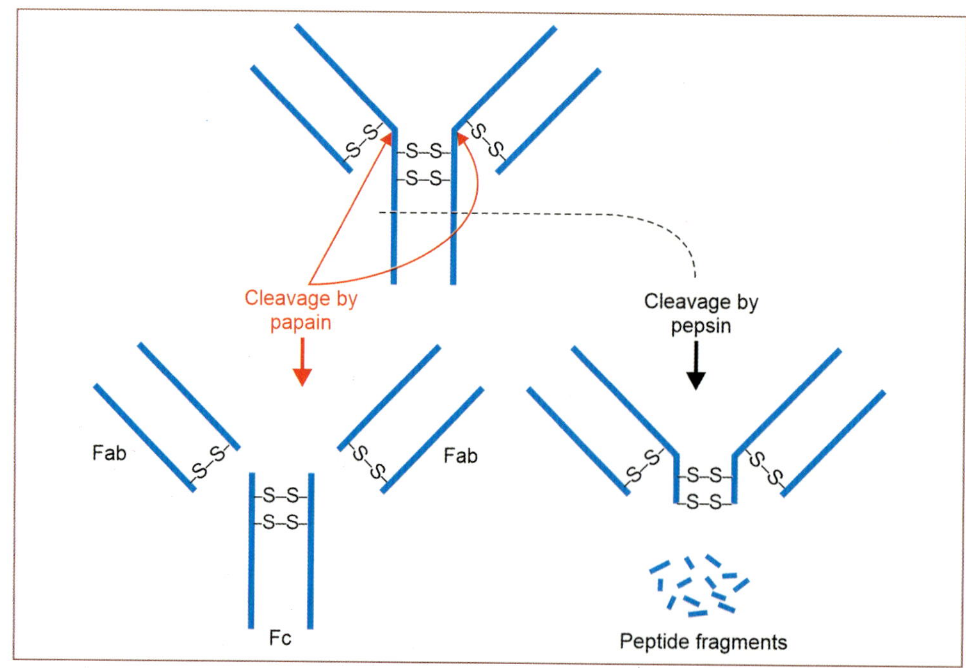

Fig. 23.4: Effects of papain and pepsin on an immunoglobulin molecule

- Each **Fab fragment** has entire L-chain and N-terminal-half of the H chain (i.e. $\mathbf{V_H}$ and $\mathbf{C_H1}$ **regions**).
- Since these **two Fab fragments** have the ability to **bind two antigens** independently, with the affinity similar to that of the intact antibody molecule, an immunoglobulin thus can bind two molecules of an antigen, simultaneously. Therefore, an **antibody is termed divalent**.
- The Fc fragment consists of the C-terminal half of the H chains (C_H2 and C_H3 regions) which are joined together by the disulfide bridges.

5. The two **Fab segments** are linked to the **Fc segment** with a flexible region, called **hinge region** (Fig 23.5).

The hinge region is present between C_H1 and C_H2 regions of the H chains. It confers **flexibility** to the antibody molecule and allows the two Fab fragments to move independently. This, in turn, helps them to bind two antigens simultaneously, that may be present at different distances, apart from each other. The hinge region contains one or more cysteine residues, which provide **interchain disulfide bridges**. It also controls interactions between different parts of the immunoglobulin molecule. Flexibility and proteolytic digestion by papain are facilitated by **proline** residues that are present in this part of the molecule.

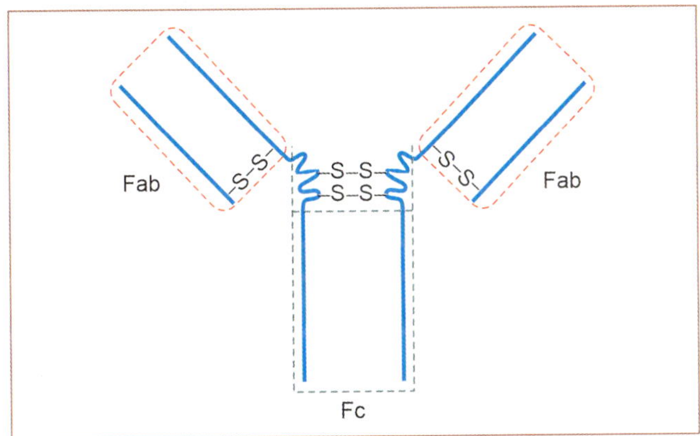

Fig. 23.5: Antigen binding (Fab) and crystallizable (Fc) fragments of immunoglobulin

TYPES OF ANTIBODIES

There are five types of antibodies (immunoglobulins), called IgG, IgA, IgM, IgD, and IgE. Each one it differs from others with respect to the type of its H chain. Various immunoglobulin classes have different physiological functions (Table 23.4).

Immunoglobulin G

Immunoglobulin G (IgG) is a major immunoglobulin produced by the plasma cells. It accounts for **70–75% of the total** immunoglobulins found in serum. IgG is the most important class of immunoglobulins that occurs in secondary immune response and is distributed evenly between the intravascular and the extravascular pools. Antibodies of the IgG class are **produced in response to most bacteria and viruses.** These antibodies **bind to macrophages and neutrophils,** and **promote phagocytosis.**

IgG has four subclasses, which are referred to as IgG_1, IgG_2, IgG_3, and IgG_4. Structurally, these **sub-**

Table 23.4: Types of immunoglobulins (Ig)

Ig class	Approximate molecular weight (kD)	H chain	Carbohydrate content (%)	Serum concentration (mg/dl)	Major physiological functions
IgG	146	γ	2–4	800–1500	• Placental transfer • Provides immunity to neonates
IgA	160–380	α	5–9	150–250	• Protects outer surfaces • sIgA is present in mucus secretions
IgM	970	μ	8–12	70–150	• First line of defense and is synthesized in neonates
IgD	160	δ	8–12	3–5	• Primary function unknown, acts as B cell receptor
IgE	190	ε	10–15	0.01–0.05	• Reaginic antibodies, implicated in allergic reactions • Release of histamine and other vasoactive amines

classes differ primarily, **in the hinge region**. It is the IgG_1 and IgG_3 both of which bind firmly, to Fc receptors of phagocytic cells and activate K cells (killer monocytes). The major effector mechanism of the human IgG_1 and IgG_3 subclasses is the activation of the classical pathway of a complement. In human beings, all the subclasses of IgG can cross placenta and confer high degree of passive immunity to the newborn.

Immunoglobulin A

Immunoglobulin A (IgA) accounts for about **15–20% of the total** serum immunoglobulins. In human beings, more than 80% of the IgA occurs as a monomer but in most other mammals, serum IgA is mainly dimeric.

IgA has two subclasses designated as IgA_1 and IgA_2. In human serum, IgA_1 is the predominant subclass. It accounts for 75–90% of total IgA in many secretions, such as in nasal secretion, tears, saliva, and milk. In the colon IgA_2 predominates.

Secretory IgA: Secretory IgA (sIgA) is the most important form of IgA. It is called secretory IgA since it is the predominant immunogloulin in seromucus secretions, such as saliva, colostrum, milk, and tracheobronchial and genitourinary secretions. It exists, mainly in the dimeric form, in association with another protein that is known as a secretory component. The sIgA is assembled during an active transport process, as the locally produced dimeric IgA passes across the mucosal epithelium. It is the sIgA, which is found in the bronchial, nasal, and intestinal mucous **secretions,** tear, milk, and colostrum. The sIgA provides initial defense against invading viral and bacterial pathogens, prior to their entry into the internal spaces. Its deficiency is the commonest disorder, which results in recurrent infections of the sinus and respiratory tract.

The sIgA may be of either of the two subclasses, i.e. it may be IgA_1 or IgA_2.

Immunoglobulin M

Immunoglobulin M (IgM) accounts for nearly **5–10% of the total** circulating immunoglobulins. An IgM molecule has abundance of oligosaccharide units, which are associated with the m chain. It also has an additional peptide chain, called joining chain (J chain), that assist in the process of polymerization, prior to its secretion, since most of the IgM in serum is **a pentamer**, consisting of five Y-shaped monomeric molecules which are **arranged around the J chain.**

23

IgM is the **first** immunoglobulin, which is synthesized by the cell, on introduction of an antigen into the host. IgM thus is called the **first line of defense**. It is the only immunoglobulin that **a neonate** normally synthesizes.

IgM is also the predominant antibody in primary immune response. It is largely confined to the intravascular pool and is frequently associated with the immune response to antigenically complex blood-borne infectious organisms. Once bound to its target, IgM is a potent activator of the classical pathway of a complement.

Immunoglobulin D

Immunoglobulin D (IgD) accounts for **less than 1% of the total** serum immunoglobulins. It is the major component of the surface membrane of many B cells and may play a role in antigen-triggered lymphocyte differentiation though its primary function is unknown.

Immunoglobulin E

Immunoglobulin E (IgE) is normally present in blood in **minute concentrations**. It is found on the surface membrane of basophils and mast cells, in all individuals. IgE also sensitizes cells on the mucosal surfaces, such as conjunctival, nasal, and bronchial mucosa and **protects** the host **against parasites**.

IgE is commonly associated with the **allergic diseases**, such as hay fever and asthma. When an antigen cross-links some of the attached IgE molecules, **mast cells** are stimulated to **release histamine** and other vasoactive amines, which, in turn, are responsible for vascular permeability and smooth muscle contraction.

Antibody Variants

- **Isotypes:** Isotypes are variants in molecules seen in all normal persons, e.g. classes and subclasses of immunoglobulins (IgG, IgM, IgA, etc.). Isotypic variation depends upon heavy chain make up such as IgG possesses the γ heavy chain isotype, IgM has μ, IgA has α, and so on.
- **Allotypes:** Allotypes represent slight differences in the amino acid sequences of heavy or light chains of different individuals (the differences are localized to the constant region of the heavy and light chains). The allotypes have been identified on the $\gamma1$, $\gamma2$, $\gamma3$, and $\alpha2$ heavy chains, and on the κ light chain. Knowledge of allotypes is important in antibody engineering and development of monoclonal antibodies to improve immunotherapy.
- **Idiotypes:** Idiotypes are the variations in the variable regions, particularly in the highly variable segments, of an antibody. These variations are individually

specific to each immunoglobulin molecule and determine the binding specificity of the antigen-recognition site.

POLYCLONAL ANTIBODIES

An antigen stimulates the production of antibodies by a mixture of B cells. These antibodies are called polyclonal antibodies since these are **directed against different epitopes** on the antigen and thus are not monospecific. Various immunoglobulins thus represent a **heterogeneous**, polyclonal mixture of antibodies. These are the products of **different clones of plasma cells**.

MONOCLONAL ANTIBODIES

Monospecificity: Benign or malignant proliferation of a **single clone** produces antibodies which are directed against the binding site for only **a particular epitope** of an antigen. These antibodies are called monoclonal antibodies, i.e. the antibodies of defined specificity, produced from an immortal clone of cells and are **homogeneous**.

Production: It is based on the **hybridoma technology** (Fig. 23.6).

- Immortal myeloma cells (B cells with the potential for unlimited replication but unable to produce antibodies) maintained in a tissue culture laboratory are **fused** with B cells isolated from the spleen of animal immunized with a particular antigen (against which monoclonal antibodies are desired to be produced).
- Normally, myeloma cells synthesize purines (required for DNA synthesis) by *de novo* pathway only since they lack the purine salvage pathway enzyme hypoxanthine guanine phosphoribosyl transferase (HGPRTase, hence these **myeloma cells are designated HGPRTase$^-$**).
- The fused hybridoma cells are grown in **'HAT'** (**h**ypoxanthine-**a**minopterin-**t**hymidine) medium. Aminopterin blocks the *de novo* pathway, therefore hybridoma cells are exclusively dependent on the salvage pathway for which HGPRTase gene is acquired from the splenocytes-derived HGPRTase$^+$ B cells. Hypoxanthine and thymidine are the substrates for DNA synthesis.

Applications: Because of their **specificity, monoclonal antibodies are used for various purposes**:

1. **To detect and quantify various proteins** by Western blot or immunohistochemistry.
2. **To determine the nature of the infectious agent**, e.g. types of bacteria.
3. **To subclassify** both **normal and tumor cells**, e.g. lymphocytes and leukemic cells.
4. **Used as immunotherapeutic agents** (Chemistry to Clinics 23.4).

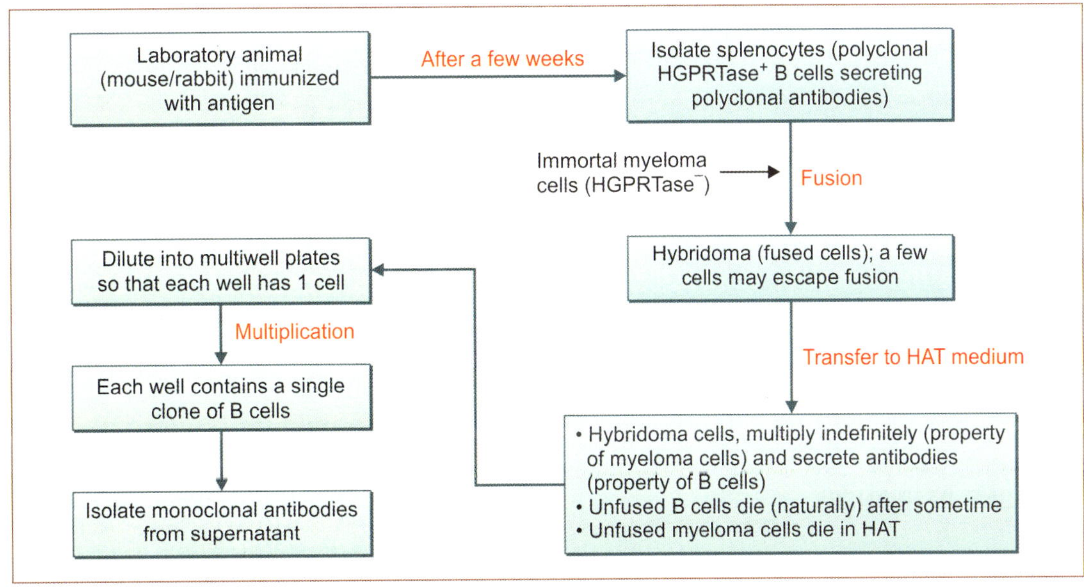

Fig. 23.6: Production of monoclonal antibodies by hybridoma technology

Chemistry to Clinics 23.4: Monoclonal antibodies as therapeutic agents

Monoclonal antibodies target specific epitopes implicated in disease processes and hence are employed as drugs. By convention, the suffix 'mab' (for '**m**onoclonal **a**nti**b**ody') is tagged with the drug. They are useful in the treatment of diverse clinical conditions:

1. Autoimmune diseases: Infliximab for Crohn's disease and rheumatoid arthritis.
2. Age-related macular degeneration: Ranibizumab.
3. Postmenopausal osteoporosis: Denosumab.
4. Allergic bronchial asthma: Omalizumab.
5. Renal transplant rejection: Muromomab.
6. Cancer: Trastuzumab (breast cancer), rituximab (lymphoma, leukemia).

The **advantages** of monoclonal antibodies over conventional drugs include:

1. Higher target specificity.
2. Lower systemic side effects.
3. Longer half-life.
4. Higher barrier for generic competition in the pharmaceutical industry.

MECHANISM OF ACTION OF ANTIBODIES

Antibodies destroy the pathogens in three ways:

- They bind to the specific molecules on the surface of the pathogen, thereby, **neutralizing the pathogen**. This, in turn, prevents entry of the pathogen to the cell.
- Thereafter, the antibody-bound pathogens are subjected to phagocytosis by macrophages and other cells, by the process called **opsonization**.
- The binding of antibodies to the pathogens also **activates the complement system**. During this process, the complement proteins bind to the antibody-bound pathogens and recruit the phagocytic cells.

INNATE AND ADAPTIVE IMMUNE RESPONSES

As discussed above, immune response refers to the ability of the body to defend itself against infection and disease, and comprises different organs and tissues, and cells that work together.

TYPES OF IMMUNE RESPONSES

Immune responses of the body to a foreign molecule can be classified in two ways based on the time and mode of development.

- **Based on the time of development,** the immune response can be classified as the **innate immune response** and the **adaptive** (also referred to as acquired) **immune response** (Table 23.5).

Table 23.5: Innate immunity versus acquired immunity

Innate immunity	Acquired/adaptive immunity
• By virtue of genetic make-up of an individual	• Acquired as the individual grows up
• No prior antigenic stimulus, i.e. immunization or contact with microorganisms is required	• Prior antigenic stimulus is required
• Present since birth, hence no lag phase	• Definite lag phase following antigenic challenge

- **Based on the mode of development,** the immune response can be classified as **active** and **passive** immune responses (Table 23.6).

Table 23.6: Active immunity versus passive immunity

Active immunity	Passive immunity
• **Produced** actively by the host's immune system	• **Received** passively by the host without participation of the immune system
• Requires antigenic challenge	• Introduction of ready-made antibodies
• Effective and durable	• Less effective and transient
• Lag phase is required to generate the immune response	• No lag phase
• Immunological memory present; subsequent challenge serves as booster	• No immunological memory is present; subsequent challenge is less effective
• Not applicable in immunocompromised host	• Applicable in immunocompromised host

Both the **active** and the **passive** immune responses may be either natural or artificial (Fig. 23.7).

The **natural immunity** may be either attained by exposure to the specific microorganisms or received by the fetus from the mother. On the other hand, **artificial immunity** refers to **vaccination/ immunization**, which employs live or killed microorganisms, their products, or the preformed antibodies.

23

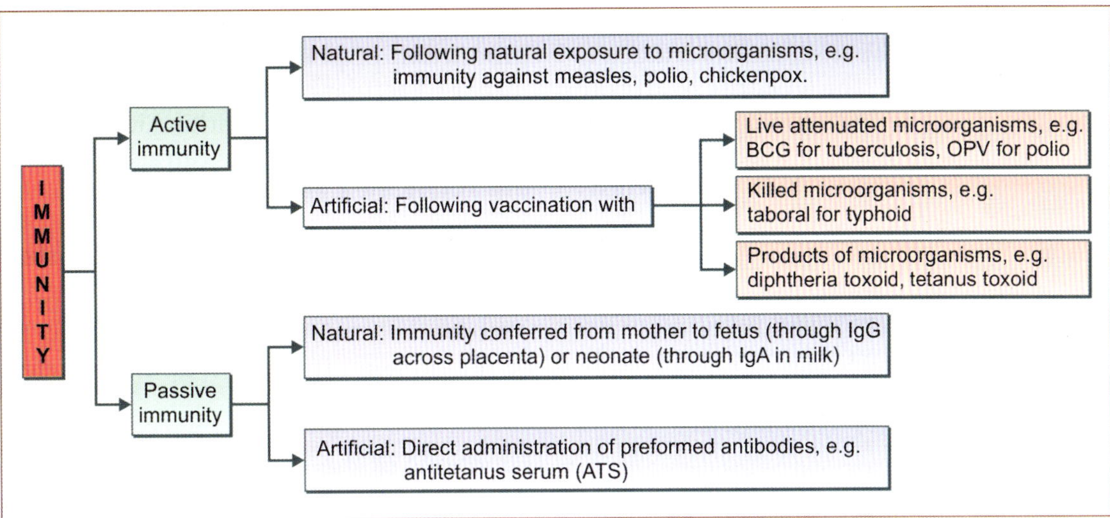

Fig. 23.7: Active and passive immunity

INNATE IMMUNE RESPONSE

Innate (or **nonspecific**) immune response is **immediate** and is referred to as the **first line of defense against pathogens**. It consists of physical, chemical and cellular defenses, the main purpose of which is to immediately prevent the spread and movement of the pathogens throughout the body.

Neutrophils are considered the first responders of the innate immune response, which include **natural killer cells** (NK cells). These lymphocytes that do not directly attack invading microbes, rather NK cells destroy compromised host cells, such as tumor cells or virus-infected cells, recognizing them by a condition known as **missing self** (the cells with the low levels of a cell-surface marker called MHC I). The MHC makeup on the surface of these cells is altered and the NK cells become activated through recognition of missing self. Thus, they do not require activation in order to kill cells that are missing self. Normal body cells are not recognized and attacked by NK cells because they express intact (self) MHC antigens.

The major components of the innate immune response include:

- **Recruitment of the immune cells to the site of infection**, through the production of chemical factors, including specialized chemical mediators, called **cytokines**.
- **Activation of the complement cascade**, to identify bacteria and activate cells, and promote clearance of the antibody complexes or the dead cells.
- **Identification and removal of the foreign substances**, which are present in the organs, tissues, blood and lymph, **by the specialized white blood cells.**
- **Activation of the adaptive immune system**, through the process referred to as **antigen presentation**.

ADAPTIVE IMMUNE RESPONSE

Adaptive immune response, also referred to as **acquired immunity**, is the **second line of defense** against pathogens. It is also called **specific immunity**, since it is specific to the presented pathogen. Although, the adaptive immune response is meant to attack the nonself pathogens but sometimes, can make errors and attack the self cells. When this happens, an autoimmune disease, such as rheumatoid arthritis, can develop.

Unlike the innate immune response which attacks based on the identification of the general threat, the adaptive immune response is **activated by exposure to pathogens** and uses an **immunological memory** to learn about the threat, and enhance the immune response, accordingly. The adaptive immune response is much **slower to respond** to threats and infections than the innate immune response, which is primed and ready to fight all times. However, the effect of the adaptive immune response is **long-lasting, highly specific** and is **sustained long-term by memory T cells.** The hallmark of the adaptive immune system is clonal expansion of the lymphocytes, i.e. the rapid increase of T and B lymphocytes from one, or a few, cell(s) to millions. Each clone that originates from the original T or B lymphocyte has the same antigen receptors as the original one, and fights the same pathogen.

Thus, adaptive immune response generates an **antigen-specific immune response**, i.e. the antigen is first recognized through the receptors of the lymphocytes and then the immune cell clones are produced, to attack that particular antigen. Thereafter, multiple defense mechanisms, such as **phagocytosis** and the **complement system**, are to recognize and neutralize the pathogen.

The adaptive immune response also creates **immunological memory**, i.e. after an initial response to the specific pathogen; it leads to an enhanced response to the subsequent encounters with that same pathogen. This process forms the **basis of vaccination**.

Cells of the Adaptive Immune Response

Cells of the adaptive immune response are also referred to as the **immune effector cells**, such as the **natural killer T lymphocytes** and **B lymphocytes**. They carry out an immune function in response to a stimulus, e.g. **activated T lymphocytes destroy pathogens**, via **cell-mediated response**. **Activated B cells secrete antibodies** that aid in mounting an immune response. Effector cells are also involved in the destruction of cancer.

On the other hand, the **noneffector cells** are the **antigen-presenting cells** (APCs), such as **dendritic cells, regulatory T cells, tumor-associated macrophages** and the **myeloid-derived suppressor cells**. These cannot cause tumor death, of their own, but prevent the immune action of the effector cells and allow tumors to grow.

COMPLEMENT SYSTEM

Complement system is a biochemical cascade that attacks the surfaces of foreign cells. It contains over 30 different proteins and is named for its ability to complement the killing of pathogens by antibodies. Complement is the major humoral component of the innate immune response.

In humans, this response is activated by complement binding to antibodies that have attached to these microbes or the binding of complement proteins to carbohydrates on the surfaces of microbes. This recognition signal triggers a rapid killing response. The speed of the response is a result of signal amplification that occurs after sequential proteolytic activation of complement molecules, which are also proteases. After complement proteins initially bind to the microbe, they activate their protease activity, which, in turn, activates other complement, proteases, and so on. This produces a catalytic cascade that amplifies the initial signal by controlled positive feedback. The cascade results in the production of peptides which attract immune cells, increase vascular permeability, and opsonize (coat) the surface of a pathogen, marking it for destruction. This deposition of complement can also kill cells directly by disrupting their plasma membrane.

Constituents of the Complement System

The complement system consists of approximately 30 protein molecules constituting nearly 10% of total serum proteins. It is one of the major defense systems of the body.

Functions of the Complement System

1. Control of inflammatory reactions and chemotaxis.
2. Clearance of immune complexes.
3. Cellular activation and antimicrobial defense.
4. Development of antibody responses.

Activation of the Complement System

Various components of the complement system interact with each other and with other elements of the immune system. Complement activation is a **cascade reaction** with each component sequentially acting on the other. Three principle pathways are involved in complement activation. These are:

- The **classical pathway** which is activated by antibody bound to antigen.
- The **lectin pathway** activated by carbohydrates.
- The **alternative pathway** activated in the presence of various microbial pathogens.

All the three pathways converge on the activation of the third component (C3, Chemistry to Clinics 23.5).

Chemistry to Clinics 23.5: Complement System and Disease

1. All three pathways of complement activation generate enzymes which cleave C3 into two fragments, i.e. C3a and C3b. Further, an important role of the complement system is to generate opsonins, proteins that stimulate phagocytosis by neutrophils and macrophages. A major opsonin is C3b. Patients with inherited deficiency of C3 are subjected to repeated bacterial infections.
2. Complement activation is a major effector in immunopathological diseases.

HYPERSENSITIVITY

The adaptive immune response provides specific protection against infection with bacteria, viruses, parasites or fungi. It provides rapid protection against a repeated challenge with the same or similar foreign organism or toxin. Some immune responses, however, give rise to an excessive or inappropriate reaction, referred to as hypersensitivity. It is an exaggerated form of an appropriate response and includes:

- **Type I or immediate hypersensitivity:** It is characterized by the production of **IgE** antibodies against foreign proteins that are commonly present in the environment, e.g. pollens, animal dander or dust mite. These antibodies bind specifically to high affinity receptors on mast cells and basophils which contain histamine. Conditions that are associated with type I hypersensitivity include hay fever, bronchial asthma, atopic dermatitis and anaphylaxis (Chemistry to Clinics 23.6).

Chemistry to Clinics 23.6: Anaphylaxis

It is an antigen-specific immune reaction mediated primarily by IgE. It results in vasodilation and constriction of smooth muscles including those of the bronchus and may result in death. Anaphylaxis occurs when a patient with immediate hypersensitivity is exposed to a relevant allergen in such a way that antigen enters the circulation rapidly. This can occur after a beesting, an injection of penicillin, eating an allergen or even following a therapeutic allergen injection for hyposensitization. It is an emergency and the treatment requires prompt administration of adrenaline.

- **Type II or antibody-mediated hypersensitivity:** These reactions are caused by **IgG or IgM** antibodies against cells surface or extracellular matrix antigens or to intracellular components. Antibodies trigger a cytotoxic reaction and damage cells/tissues by activating the complement system and by binding and activating effector cells carrying Fc receptors, e.g. autoimmune hemolytic anemia. Damage to tissue may be produced by antibodies to basement membrane, to intracellular adhesion molecules or to receptors, e.g. myasthenia gravis.
- **Type III or immune complex disease:** It occurs when excess **antigen–antibody complexes** are formed in the circulation that cannot be cleared by macrophages or other cells in the reticuloendothelial system. Accumulation of such complexes can trigger either a complement or a cell-mediated local reaction. Systemic lupus erythematosus (SLE) is a classical disease in which immune complexes are involved.
- **Type IV or cell-mediated reactions:** These are reactions in which **specific T cells** are the primary effector cells. Contact sensitivity (e.g. to nickel) and graft rejection are the examples of T cells causing unwanted responses.

SELF/NONSELF RECOGNITION

In immunology, **self molecules** are those **components of an organism's body** that can be distinguished from foreign substances by the immune system. Conversely, **nonself molecules** are those which are recognized as **foreign molecules**. One class of nonself molecules are the **anti**body **gen**erators, called **antigens** (the substances that bind to the specific immune receptors and elicit an immune response).

The self/nonself discrimination is at the very core of immunology. Both, **innate** and **adaptive immune responses** depend upon the ability of the immune system **to distinguish between the self and the nonself molecules**.

As mentioned above, the lymphocytes (or white blood cells) are the central players in the immune systems of all vertebrates. Each individual T lymphocyte expresses unique receptors for antigens (called T cell antigen receptor or TCR), as a result of unique rearrangements of the TCR gene elements within each T cell, as it develops. In order to mount an appropriate immune response, the T cell receptors recognize only those antigens that are bound to certain receptor molecules called ***major histocompatibility complex*** *(MHC)*. These MHC molecules are the membrane-bound surface receptors present on the ***antigen-presenting cells***, like dendritic cells and macrophages. The CD4 and CD8 receptors play a role in T cell recognition and activation, by binding to either MHC I or MHC II.

In order to make sure that T cells perform properly, once they have matured and released from the thymus, they undergo selection processes:

- **Positive selection:** This ensures MHC restriction by testing the ability of MHC I and MHC II to **distinguish between self** and **nonself proteins**. In order to pass the positive selection process, T cells must be capable of binding to only **self-MHC molecules**. If these cells bind **nonself MHC molecules**, they fail the positive selection process and **are eliminated by apoptosis**.
- **Negative selection:** Negative selection tests for self tolerance, for the binding capabilities of the CD4 and CD8 receptors, specifically. For example, if a T cell binds, via CD4 or CD8, to a self-MHC molecule that is not presenting an antigen or a self-MHC molecule that is presenting a self-antigen, it will fail negative selection and be eliminated by apoptosis.

  These two selection processes are put into place to protect our own cells and tissues against our own immune response.

The TCRs which bind, well enough, to the complex of an MHC glycoprotein with a particular antigenic peptide, trigger activation of T cells, enabling them to participate in immune defense. Moreover, the process of TCR gene rearrangement, which unfolds differently in each developing T cell, regularly produces TCRs that can recognize self-peptide/ MHC protein complexes with high affinity.

Thus, the immune system has the capacity to distinguish between **self** (body cells) and **nonself** (foreign materials) and reacts to the presence of a foreign material with an immune response that eliminates the intruding material from the body.

Disorders of the immune system can result in **autoimmune diseases, inflammatory diseases** and **cancer**. **Immunodeficiency** occurs when the immune system is less active than normal, resulting in recurring and life-threatening infections. It can either be the result of a **genetic disease**, such as severe combined immunodeficiency, **acquired conditions** such as HIV/ AIDS, or the **use of immunosuppressive medication**. In contrast, **autoimmunity** results from a hyperactive immune system attacking normal tissues as if they were foreign organisms. Common autoimmune diseases include rheumatoid arthritis, diabetes mellitus type 1 and systemic lupus erythematosus. **Cancer cells** can **undergo unchecked proliferation**, **producing self-antigens** that are **tolerated by the immune system**, rather than being targeted for destruction.

CENTRAL ROLE OF T-HELPER CELLS IN IMMUNE RESPONSES

The **T helper cells** (**Th cells**), also known as **CD4+ cells**, are a type of T cells that play an important role in the immune system, particularly, in the adaptive immune response. These cells help suppress or **regulate immune responses**. They also help the activity of other immune cells by releasing **cytokines**. They are also essential in **antibody-class switching**, **activation** and **growth of cytotoxic T cells** and in maximizing **bactericidal activity of phagocytes**, such as macrophages.

- Mature Th cells express surface protein CD4 and are referred to as **CD4+ T cells**. The CD4+ T cells are, generally, treated as having a pre-defined role in the immune system. For example, when an antigen presenting cell (APC) expresses an antigen on MHC class II, the CD4+ T cell help them through a combination of **cell-to-cell interactions** and **release of cytokines**.
- The CD154, also called **CD40 ligand** or **CD40L**, is a cell surface protein that mediates the Th cells function in a contact-dependent process. This protein is a member of the TNF superfamily of molecules and binds to CD40 on antigen presenting cells (APC), which leads to many effects depending on the target cell type.
- CD154 also acts as a costimulatory molecule and is, particularly, important on a subset of T cells, called T follicular helper cells (TFh cells). On the TFh cells, CD154 promotes B cell maturation and function, by engaging CD40 on the B cell surface and facilitate cell-to-cell communication.
- A defect in this gene has been shown to result in inability in immunoglobulin class switching and, in turn, associated with hyper IgM syndrome.
- Absence of CD154 also stops the formation of germinal centers and, therefore, prohibits antibody affinity maturation.
- The importance of Th cells can also be shown in HIV, the virus that, primarily, infects CD4+ T cells. In the advanced stages of the HIV infection, loss of function of the CD4+ T cells leads to symptomatic stage of infection, known as the acquired immunodeficiency syndrome (AIDS).
- There are also other disorders, such as lymphocytopenia, which result in the absence or dysfunction of the CD4+ T cells. These disorders produce symptoms, many of which are fatal.

ANTIGENS

Any molecule that triggers an immune response is called an **immunogen**. An immunogen may be an **antigen**, **hapten** or **allergen**.

ANTIGEN

An **antigen** is a molecule that can bind to its corresponding antibody. An antigen may be a protein, carbohydrate or nucleic acid and can be specifically recognized by the adaptive elements of the immune system, i.e. by B cells or T cells, or both. Thus, **all immunogens are antigens but all antigens may not be immunogenic**, e.g. hapten, antigen inducing immune tolerance, etc.

- Antigen molecules are recognized by receptors on lymphocytes. B lymphocytes usually recognize intact antigen molecules while T lymphocytes recognize antigen fragments on the surface of the cells.
- Each antibody binds to a restricted part of the antigen, called an **antigenic determinant** or **epitope**.

A particular antigen can have several different epitopes or repeated epitopes. Antibodies are specific for the epitopes rather than for the whole antigen molecule. In proteins, an antigenic determinant generally comprises only 6 or 7 amino acids.

An antigen is any substance that is capable of stimulating an immune response, specifically, activating lymphocytes to produce antibody, or to attack the antigen directly. Such a substance is also called **immunogen**.

In general, two main divisions of antigens are recognized, i.e. foreign antigens (or heteroantigens) and autoantigens (or self-antigens).

- **Foreign antigens** originate from outside the body, e.g. parts of, or substances, produced by viruses or microorganisms (such as bacteria and protozoa), as well as substances in snake venom, certain proteins in foods, and components of serum and red blood cells from other individuals.
- **Autoantigens**, on the other hand, originate within the body. Normally, the body is able to distinguish self from nonself, but in persons with autoimmune disorders, normal bodily substances provoke an immune response, leading to the generation of autoantibodies.

The antigen may **originate from within the body** (**self-antigen**) or **from the external environment** (**nonself**).

The immune system is supposed to identify and attack nonself invaders from the outside world or modified/harmful substances present in the body and usually does not react to self-antigens under normal homeostatic conditions due to negative selection of T cells in the thymus.

HAPTEN

Hapten is a small molecule which can act as an epitope but is **incapable by itself**, of eliciting an antibody response. It can induce synthesis of antibodies only when covalently attached to some large molecule. Though a hapten needs its attachment to a large molecule to elicit antibody production, it retains the ability to bind strongly to the antibody even after it has been detached from the carrier molecule.

ALLERGEN

An allergen is an antigen that gives rise to **immediate hypersensitivity**. It is an agent, e.g. pollen, dust or animal dander that causes IgE-mediated hypersensitivity reactions popularly called **'allergies'** (Chemistry to Clinics 23.7).

Chemistry to Clinics 23.7: Allergies

Th1/Th2 imbalance: A popular hypothesis, often referred to as the hygiene model, proposes that the children who are not exposed to enough antigens or innocuous microorganisms from soil or water early in their childhood, do not adequately develop their Th1 response. This leads to an imbalance toward Th2 responses. Even though this hypothesis is disputed as being grossly oversimplified, it is undisputed that the various manifestations of allergic inflammation are the result of wrongly activated Th2 cells.

Chemical mediators: The symptoms of bronchial asthma ultimately depend on the presence of Th2 cells, which secrete a characteristic cytokine repertoire on antigen challenge. One of the cytokines, interleukin-4, activates B cells to produce IgE antibodies, which bind to mast cells, eosinophils and other airway cells, via receptors that are specific for the Fc portions of the antibodies. On subsequent encounters with the antigen, IgE cross-linking, on the mast cells and the eosinophils, occurs. This leads to their activation, releasing histamine and leukotrienes, which in turn, cause bronchoconstriction and mucus hypersecretion. These and other inflammatory factors further recruit inflammatory cells, including additional Th2 cells, to the lung, resulting in a damaging immunological positive feedback cycle. Almost similar biochemical mechanisms operate in other allergies such as food allergies, skin allergies (e.g. urticaria), etc.

Management: Avoidance of allergens (if identified), type 1 antihistaminics, mast cell stabilizers, corticosteroids and desensitization.

CONCEPTS INVOLVED IN VACCINE DEVELOPMENT

A **vaccine** is a biological preparation that provides active acquired immunity to a particular infectious disease. **A vaccine** typically **contains an agent** that resembles **a disease-causing microorganism** and is often made from weakened or killed forms of the microbe, its toxins, or one of its surface proteins. The agent stimulates the body's immune system to recognize the agent as a threat, destroy it, and to further recognize and destroy any of the microorganisms associated with that agent that it may encounter in the future.

Vaccines are examples of antigens in an immunogenic form, which are intentionally administered to a recipient to induce the memory function of adaptive immune response toward the antigens of the pathogen invading that recipient.

Vaccine antigens include whole live pathogens (modified to reduce the virulence), individual pathogen components (e.g. protein or polysaccharides) and the genetic material of the pathogen (i.e. naked DNA/RNA) which can direct the production of the vaccine antigen in the recipient.

The immune system recognizes vaccine agents as foreign, destroys them and remembers them. When the virulent version of an agent is encountered, the body recognizes the protein coat on the virus, and thus is prepared to respond, by first neutralizing the target agent before it can enter cells, and secondly by recognizing and destroying infected cells before that agent can multiply to vast numbers.

Lack of response commonly results from genetics, immune status, age, health or nutritional status. It also might fail for genetic reasons if the host's immune system includes no strains of B cells that can generate antibodies suited to reacting effectively and binding to the antigens associated with the pathogen.

A number of innovative vaccines are also in development and in use

- **Dendritic cell vaccines** combine dendritic cells with antigens in order to present the antigens to the body's white blood cells, thus stimulating an immune reaction. These vaccines have shown some positive preliminary results for treating brain tumors and are also tested in malignant melanoma.
- **DNA vaccination:** An alternative, experimental approach to vaccination called **DNA vaccination**, created from an infectious agent's DNA, is under development. Some cells of the immune system that recognize the proteins expressed will mount an attack against these proteins and cells expressing them. Because these cells live for a very long time, if the pathogen that normally expresses these proteins is encountered at a later time, they will be attacked instantly by the immune system. One potential advantage of DNA vaccines is that they are very easy to produce and store.
- **Recombinant vector:** By combining the physiology of one microorganism and the DNA of another, immunity can be created against diseases that have complex infection processes.
- **RNA vaccine** is a novel type of vaccine which is composed of the nucleic acid RNA, packaged within a vector such as lipid nanoparticles. **A number of RNA vaccines are under development to combat the COVID-19 pandemic**.
- **T cell receptor peptide vaccines** are under development for several diseases using models of Valley Fever, stomatitis and atopic dermatitis. These peptides have been shown to modulate cytokine production and improve cell-mediated immunity.
- **The use of plasmids** has been validated in preclinical studies as a protective vaccine strategy for cancer and infectious diseases. The overall efficacy of plasmid DNA immunization depends on increasing the plasmid's immunogenicity while also correcting for factors involved in the specific activation of immune effector cells.

While most vaccines are created using inactivated or attenuated compounds from microorganisms, synthetic vaccines are composed mainly or wholly of synthetic peptides, carbohydrates, or antigens.

Generations of Vaccines

First generation vaccines are whole-organism vaccines—either live and weakened, or killed forms. Live, attenuated vaccines, such as smallpox and polio vaccines, are **able to induce killer T cell** (T_C or CTL) **responses, helper T cell (T_H) responses** and **antibody immunity**.

Second generation vaccines were developed to reduce the risks from live vaccines. These are subunit vaccines, **consisting of specific protein antigens** (such as tetanus or diphtheria toxoid) or **recombinant protein components** (such as the **hepatitis B surface antigen**). They can **generate T_H and antibody responses**, but not killer T cell responses.

DNA vaccines are examples of third generation vaccines. Clinical trials for DNA vaccines to prevent HIV are underway.

IMMUNODEFICIENCY

An immunodeficiency disorder may affect the cellular and/or the humoral immunity. A **primary immunodeficiency** results from an abnormality in the development of the immune mechanisms due to a specific genetic defect (involving lymphopoiesis, phagocytosis or complement) and is usually present **since birth** (Fig. 23.8).

On the other hand, a **secondary immunodeficiency** affects an already developed/mature immune system due to one or more **acquired cause(s)** (Table 23.7).

AUTOIMMUNE DISEASE

The immune system of the body is geared to detect an antigen that is foreign to the body, i.e. it distinguishes **self from the nonself** antigenic determinants so as to **avoid autoreactivity**. Due to various reasons, such as loss of self-tolerance, genetic mutation, interaction with drugs or certain types of infections, the immunological machinery of an individual sometimes starts forming **antibodies against one's own tissues or cells**. Such a disorder is referred to as an autoimmune disease.

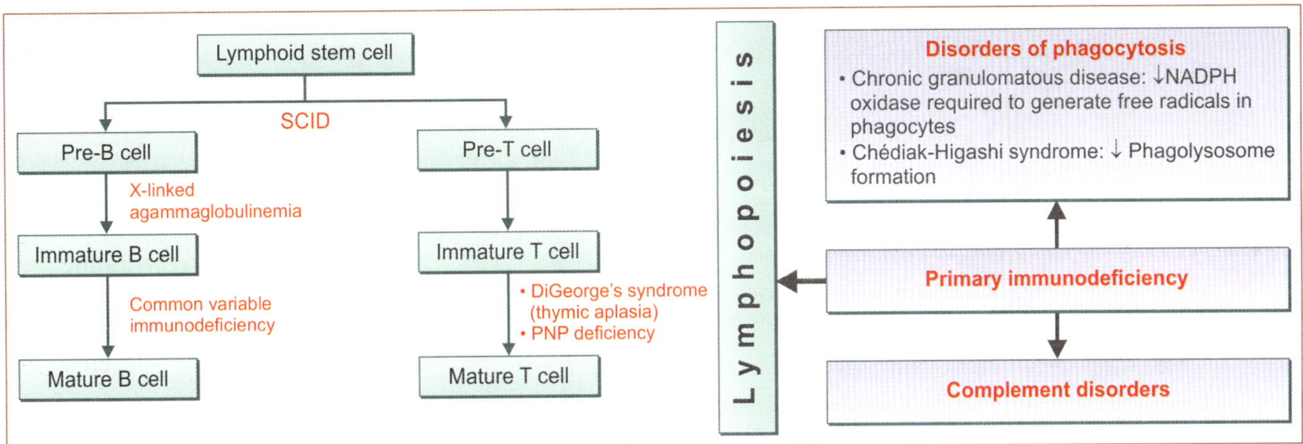

Fig. 23.8: Primary immunodeficiency. SCID (severe combined immunodeficiency due to adenosine deaminase deficiency involves both B and T lymphoid precursors) while PNP (purine nucleoside phosphorylase) deficiency involves immature T cells in the thymus

Table 23.7: Secondary immunodeficiency
• **Malnutrition:** ↓ Ig synthesis
• **Infection:** Tuberculosis, HIV
• **Renal disease:** Proteinuria
• **Malignancy:** ↓ Lymphocytes (leukemia), ↑abnormal Igs (multiple myeloma)
• **Anticancer drugs:** Bone marrow suppression
• **Prolonged corticosteroid therapy:** Immunosuppression
• **Loss of self-regulation and targeting self-antigens:** Autoimmunity

Autoimmune diseases range from **single organ (or cell) type disorder** which involve specific immune reaction directed against only a particular organ or cell type (such as Graves' disease or insulin dependent diabetes mellitus) to **multisystem disease** which are characterized by lesions in many organs and are associated with multiple autoantibodies (e.g. rheumatoid arthritis). Some of the autoimmune diseases are listed in Table 23.8.

ACQUIRED IMMUNODEFICIENCY SYNDROME (AIDS)

AIDS is a viral disease caused by human T cell lymphotropic virus, called human immunodeficiency virus (HIV), with severe depletion of **CD4+ T cells.**

HUMAN IMMUNODEFICIENCY VIRUS

Structural Organization of the Virus

The HIV is roughly spherical with a diameter of 120 nm (Fig. 23.9).

- It is composed of **two copies of single-stranded RNA** enclosed in a protein capsid made of **p24.**
- Each RNA strand is associated with the enzymes crucial to the life cycle of the virus such as **reverse**

Table 23.8: Some autoimmune diseases

Autoimmune disease	Target tissue	Effects
Graves' disease	Thyroid gland	↑ Thyroid hormone secretion
Insulin-dependent diabetes mellitus	Pancreatic β-cells	↓ Insulin secretion
Addison's disease	Adrenal cortex	↑ Na^+ excretion, K^+ retention
Myasthenia gravis	Acetylcholine receptor at neuromuscular junctional synapse	Progressive muscle weakness
Rheumatoid arthritis	Joint connective tissue	Inflammation of joints (arthritis)
Systemic lupus erythematosus	Tissue components, e.g. DNA, phospho-neurological lipids, etc.	Joint and muscle pain, anemia, disturbance, etc.
Pernicious anemia	Gastric parietal cells or intrinsic factor	Megaloblastic anemia

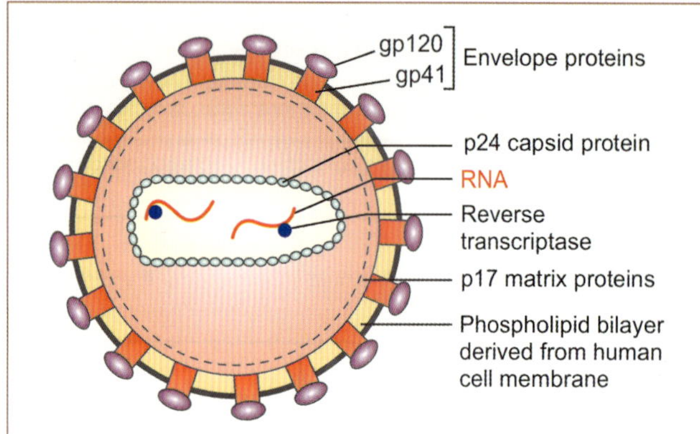

Fig. 23.9: Structural organization of human immunodeficiency virus (HIV)

transcriptase, integrase, ribonuclease and proteases.

- The capsid is again surrounded by a protein matrix made of **p17** that is enclosed in a phospholipid bilayer envelope derived from a human host cell membrane.
- Embedded in the viral envelope are Env proteins, each consisting of a cap made of three molecules of glycoprotein 120 (**gp120**) and a stem made up of three molecules of glycoprotein 41 (**gp41**).

Viral Tropism

The term viral tropism refers to which cell types the HIV infects. The virus can infect a variety of immune cells such as **CD4+ T lymphocytes, macrophages and microglial cells**.

- Viral entry into the target cells is mediated through the interaction of gp120 with its receptors, i.e. the $CD4^+$ molecules, besides some coreceptors.
- A commonly employed coreceptor is the β-chemokine receptor **CCR5** (CC chemokine receptor-5). The CC chemokine proteins have 2 adjacent cysteine residues near their amino terminus. Interestingly, people with a specific mutation known as **CCR5-Δ32, are resistant to HIV**.

Viral Replication

- Following the binding of gp120 with its receptors, the viral envelope **fuses** with the host cell membrane with the release of capsid, RNA and associated viral enzymes into the cytosol (Fig. 23.10).
  - The reverse transcriptase liberates the single-stranded RNA from the attached viral proteins and copies it into a **complementary DNA molecule**. The reverse transcription is **extremely error-prone** and the resulting mutations play an

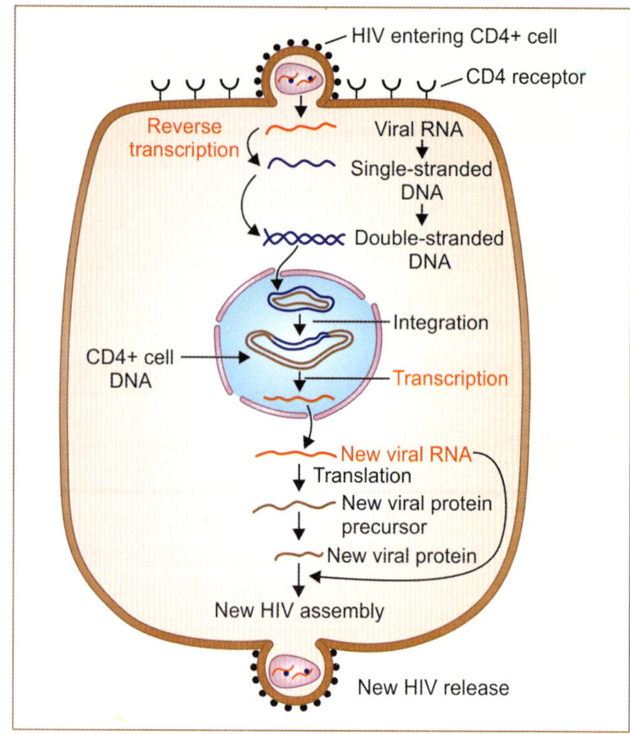

Fig. 23.10: HIV replication

important role in allowing the virus to **evade the immune system as well as in the development of drug resistance**.
  - The reverse transcriptase also has ribonuclease activity that degrades the viral RNA during the synthesis of cDNA.
  - Further, it possesses DNA-dependent DNA polymerase activity that copies the sense cDNA strand into an antisense DNA.
  - Together, the cDNA and its complement form a double-stranded viral DNA that is then transported to the host cell nucleus. All these events occur during the microtubule-based transport of the viral contents from the host cell membrane to the nucleus.
- The **incorporation of the viral DNA into the host cell genome** is carried out by the viral integrase.
  - This integrated viral DNA may lie **dormant**, explaining the **latent stage** of HIV infection.
  - On the other hand, during **active viral replication**, the integrated viral DNA is transcribed into mRNA which leaves the nucleus and is translated to form viral polyproteins, which are appropriately cleaved by the viral proteases into individual functional proteins, including the viral enzymes.
- Finally, the entire virus is **assembled and released**, ready to infect another cell.

Some Important Questions

1. What are immunoglobulins? Describe the structure of an immunoglobulin.

2. Classify immunoglobulins. Describe the functions of each class of immunoglobulin.

3. Describe:

i. The action of papain and pepsin on an immunoglobulin molecule
ii. Significance of the C_H regions in an immunoglobulin molecule
iii. Antibody diversity
iv. Class switching
v. Autoimmune diseases
vi. Immune response

4. Write notes on:

i. Immunity
ii. Antigen
iii. Hapten
iv. Complement system
v. Hypervariable sequences
vi. Hinge region
vii. Monoclonal antibodies
viii. AIDS
ix. Immunization
x. Isotypes
xi. MHC
xii. Cluster of differentiation

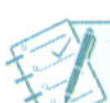

Multiple Choice Questions

1. Administration of antitetanus serum (ATS) is an example of:

A. Natural active immunity
B. Artificial active immunity
C. Natural passive immunity
D. Artificial passive immunity

2. The following is an antigen presenting cell (APC):

A. T cell and B cell B. Macrophage
C. Dendritic cell D. All of the above

3. The following is true for a hapten:

A. Small molecule capable of acting as an epitope
B. Elicits antibody response only when covalently linked to a carrier
C. Can bind to antibody even after being detached from the carrier
D. All of the above

4. The accumulation of immune complexes in SLE is an example of hypersensitivity reaction type:

A. I B. II
C. III D. IV

5. The complement system participates in the following *except*:

A. Regulation of chemotaxis
B. Clearance of immune complexes
C. Type I hypersensitivity
D. Antibody response

6. Complementarity determining regions (CDR) in an Ig molecule refer to:

A. Hypervariable sequences in the V-region
B. C_H region
C. J chain
D. C_L region

7. The highest serum concentration is of:

A. IgE B. IgD
C. IgA D. IgG

8. The variation in different Ig H and L chain classes and subclasses is called_______.

A. Isotype B. Idiotype
C. Allotype D. Any of the above

9. Monoclonal antibodies are used to:

A. Quantify proteins
B. Detect microorganisms
C. Classify normal and tumor cells
D. All of the above

10. The following is an autoimmune disease:

A. Folate deficiency anemia
B. Pernicious anemia
C. Iron deficiency anemia
D. Hemorrhagic anemia

Answer to MCQs

Chapter 1: Cell and Subcellular Components

1. A	2. C	3. C	4. C	5. C	6. B	7. D	8. A
9. A	10. A						

Chapter 2: Enzymes

1. A	2. D	3. B	4. D	5. B	6. D	7. C	8. B
9. C	10. C						

Chapter 3: Chemistry and Metabolism of Carbohydrates

1. D	2. A	3. D	4. A	5. D	6. C	7. C	8. A
9. C	10. C						

Chapter 4: Chemistry and Metabolism of Lipids

1. D	2. B	3. A	4. A	5. A	6. B	7. B	8. D
9. D	10. D						

Chapter 5: Chemistry and Metabolism of Proteins

1. A	2. D	3. D	4. A	5. C	6. B	7. D	8. B
9. C	10. C						

Chapter 6: Metabolism and Homeostasis

1. B	2. B	3. A	4. C	5. D

Chapter 7: Chemistry and Metabolism of Nucleotides

1. C	2. D	3. A	4. A	5. C	6. C	7. C	8. D
9. B	10. C						

Chapter 8: Vitamins

1. A	2. B	3. A	4. D	5. A	6. D	7. B	8. C
9. D	10. D						

Chapter 9: Biochemical Processes Involved in Generation of Energy in Cells

1. A	2. B	3. B	4. B	5. D	6. A	7. D	8. A
9. C	10. D						

Chapter 10: pH, Water, Electrolytes and Acid–Base Balance

1. B	2. C	3. A	4. A	5. B	6. A	7. D	8. A
9. B	10. A						

Chapter 11: Minerals

1. A	2. C	3. D	4. A	5. A	6. D	7. D	8. D
9. A	10. A						

Chapter 12: Metabolism of Hemoglobin

1. D 2. D 3. D 4. A 5. C

Chapter 13: Organ Function Tests

1. C 2. B 3. B 4. D 5. B 6. A 7. A 8. D
9. C 10. C

Chapter 14: Structure and Functions of Nucleic Acids

1. A 2. A 3. C 4. B 5. B 6. A 7. B 8. A
9. B 10. B

Chapter 15: Processes of Replication, Transcription and Translation

1. A 2. C 3. A 4. A 5. C 6. C 7. C 8. D
9. C 10. B

Chapter 16: Gene Mutations and Regulation of Gene Expression

1. D 2. C 3. B 4. D 5. D

Chapter 17: Applications of Molecular Technologies

1. C 2. D 3. B 4. D 5. C

Chapter 18: Xenobiotics

1. C 2. D 3. D 4. A 5. D

Chapter 19: Antioxidant Defense System and Oxidative Stress

1. D 2. D 3. B 4. C 5. D

Chapter 20: Nutrition

1. B 2. D 3. D 4. A 5. D

Chapter 21: Extracellular Matrix

1. D 2. A 3. C 4. D 5. D 6. C 7. A 8. B
9. D 10. A

Chapter 22: Oncogenesis

1. D 2. D 3. D 4. D 5. B 6. A 7. A 8. B
9. C 10. D

Chapter 23: Immunity

1. D 2. D 3. D 4. C 5. C 6. A 7. D 8. A
9. D 10. B

Index

L

M

N

O

P

R

S